HANDBOOK OF
(CENTRAL) AUDITORY PROCESSING DISORDER

Volume I
Auditory Neuroscience and Diagnosis

HANDBOOK OF (CENTRAL) AUDITORY PROCESSING DISORDER

Volume I
Auditory Neuroscience and Diagnosis

Edited by

Frank E. Musiek, Ph.D.
Gail D. Chermak, Ph.D.

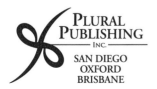

PLURAL
PUBLISHING
INC.
SAN DIEGO
OXFORD
BRISBANE

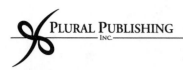

5521 Ruffin Road
San Diego, CA 92123

e-mail: info@pluralpublishing.com
Web site: http://www.pluralpublishing.com

49 Bath Street
Abingdon, Oxfordshire OX14 1EA
United Kingdom

ISBN-13: 978-1-59756-056-6
ISBN-10: 1-59756-056-1
Library of Congress Cataloging-in-Publication Data:

Handbook of (central) auditory processing disorder / [edited by] Frank
    E. Musiek, Gail D. Chermak.
        v. ; cm.
    Includes bibliographical references and index.
    Contents: v. 1. Auditory neuroscience and diagnosis – v. 2. Comprehensive
intervention.
    ISBN-13: 978-1-59756-056-6 (hardcover : v. 1)
    ISBN-10: 1-59756-056-1 (hardcover : v. 1)
    ISBN-13: 978-1-59756-057-3 (hardcover : v. 2)
    ISBN-10: 1-59756-057-X (hardcover : v. 2)
    1. Word deafness. 2. Hearing disorders. 3. Language acquisition.
4. Auditory perception.   I. Musiek, Frank E. II. Chermak, Gail D.
    [DNLM: 1. Language Development Disorders–diagnosis.
WL 340.2 H2353 2006]
RC394.W63H362 2006
617.8–dc22
                                                            2006021068

CONTENTS

FOREWORD

The concept of an auditory-specific perceptual disorder in children is more than 50 years old. It was first suggested by Helmer Myklebust, a psychologist originally interested in the evaluation of deaf children. At Northwestern University in the 1950s Myklebust set up a clinic to examine children suspected of hearing loss and to counsel their parents. As a graduate student in audiology at the time, I was privileged to participate in these pediatric evaluations and to learn, at first hand, the variety and breadth of auditory disorders. As child after child came through the clinic, Myklebust began to realize that some of the children with apparent hearing problems had normal audiograms. The symptoms described by parents and teachers could not be attributed to peripheral hearing sensitivity loss. They heard faint sounds normally in the controlled acoustic environment of the test booth, but in the real acoustic world, with its many sources of noise and competing speech, these children seemed unable to successfully suppress this background competition to selectively attend to a particular source. Myklebust supposed that such problems reflected an auditory-specific perceptual deficit, making it difficult to attend selectively.

In the more than five decades that have elapsed since those seminal observations, the reality of the problem has been verified many times over, but discovering the underlying mechanism of such auditory processing disorders remains an elusive goal. Into this void many ideas have flowed. Some have been helpful; others less so. Ideas founded on careful research based on a plausible conceptual framework have advanced our understanding of the phenomenon. Ideas of what someone thinks might be the problem, based on anecdotal evidence and exhaustive lists of symptoms, have not been as helpful and have often set us back.

The editors of this important volume, Drs. Frank Musiek and Gail Chermak, have pioneered the kinds of thoughtful studies basic to understanding, diagnosing, and treating auditory processing disorders. In this Handbook they have assembled a truly impressive group of national and international contributors to virtually every aspect of the problem. They bring us up to date on the latest findings from the standpoint of behavioral assessment, electrophysiologic measures, and the neurobiology of the disorder, all relevant to the identification and diagnosis of this troubling malady.

James Jerger, Ph.D.
Dallas, Texas

ABOUT THE EDITORS

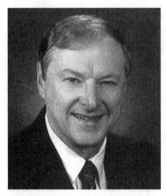

Frank E. Musiek, Ph.D.

Dr. Musiek is Professor and Director of Auditory Research in the Department of Communications Sciences and Professor of Otolaryngology, School of Medicine, University of Connecticut. He has published more than 160 articles and book chapters in the areas of auditory evoked potentials, central auditory disorders, auditory neuroanatomy, and auditory pathophysiology. He has developed the dichotic digits, frequency and duration patterns and gaps in noise (GIN) tests as well as the dichotic interaural intensity difference (DIID) auditory training procedure. He has also authored or edited six books and three monographs.

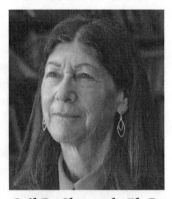

Gail D. Chermak, Ph.D.

Dr. Chermak is Professor and Chair of the Department of Speech and Hearing Sciences at Washington State University. She held the Washington State University College of Liberal Arts Edward R. Meyer Distinguished Professorship in 1999–2002 and received the College's Distinguished Faculty Award in 2002. She holds the Certificate of Clinical Competence in Audiology and is a Fellow of the American Academy of Audiology (AAA) and the American Speech-Language-Hearing Association (ASHA). Funded by the Kellogg Foundation, the World Institute on Disability, and the Fulbright American Republics Research Program, she has traveled extensively, consulting with public and private agencies in the area of rehabilitation service delivery. She has chaired and served on a number of national professional committees and task forces, including the ASHA Work Group on Central Auditory Processing Disorder (CAPD), which recently completed a technical report and position statement. Presently, she serves on the AAA's CAPD Task Force. She is an assistant editor for the *Journal of the American Academy of Audiology* and serves as editorial consultant for several other professional and scientific journals. She has published extensively and delivered numerous workshops, nationally and internationally, on differential diagnosis, assessment and rehabilitation of CAPD. Her coauthored articles and letters to the editor on CAPD and attention deficit hyperactivity disorder were named by her peers as among the best in diagnostic audiology in four of the last five consecutive years. Her 1997 book, *Central Auditory Processing Disorders: New Perspectives*, co-authored with Frank Musiek, has become a landmark volume in the field.

PREFACE

Central auditory processing disorder ([C]APD) is a deficit in neural processing of auditory stimuli that is not due to higher-order language, cognitive, or related factors, yet (C)APD may lead to or be associated with difficulties in higher-order language, learning, cognitive, and communication functions. The comorbidity of (C)APD with a range of language, learning, and communication disorders is the result of brain organization, about which we have learned much in recent years. The perspectives contained in this two-volume Handbook reflect major advances in auditory neuroscience and cognitive science, particularly over the last two decades since then President George H. Bush proclaimed the 1990s the "Decade of the Brain." Since that proclamation, we have witnessed great strides in basic and clinical research in neuroscience and cognitive science with considerable impact on the diagnosis and treatment of (C)APD. The multidisciplinary efforts of thousands of scientists and health care professionals have led to greater insights regarding the nature of (C)APD, brain organization and function, and directions for more efficient diagnosis (or diagnostic procedures) and efficacious interventions. With the recognition that neuroplastic changes in the brain underlie learning and rehabilitation, there is every reason to embrace an aggressive and optimistic approach to intervention knowing that behavioral interventions that appropriately stimulate plastic neural tissues should lead to positive change.

This Handbook provides comprehensive coverage of the field of (C)APD in children, adults, and older adults, involving the range of developmental (i.e., neurobiologic) and acquired (i.e., aging and neurologic diseases, disorders, and insults, including neurodegenerative diseases) origins. Volume I focuses on auditory neuroscience foundations, diagnostic principles and procedures, and multidisciplinary assessment. Volume II concentrates on rehabilitation and professional issues. The complexity and heterogeneity of (C)APD, combined with the heterogeneity of learning and related disorders, challenge scientists and clinicians as they attempt to understand and differentially diagnose individuals with listening deficits, language comprehension problems, attention deficits, learning disabilities and other related behavioral, emotional, and social difficulties. This Handbook offers up-to-date, comprehensive coverage of auditory neuroscience and clinical science needed to accurately diagnose, assess, and treat the auditory and related deficits of individuals with (C)APD.

This Handbook is intended to serve three primary audiences. First, the contributing authors have written a comprehensive set of manuals for clinicians, primarily audiologists, speech-language pathologists and psychologists, and for other related health care professionals as well. This Handbook also should serve as a reference source for a range of clinical scientists engaged in research related to audition and speech perception. Finally, but not any less a focus of our efforts, are graduate students, for whom we hope this Handbook can serve as a textbook(s) for use in the classroom and in support of their clinical experiences.

The approaches and recommendations offered in this Handbook are not intended to serve as a sole source of guidance for the differential diagnosis and intervention of individuals with (C)APD. Rather, the views and methods of the 33 contributing authors are designed to assist the clinician by providing a framework for decision-making and implementing diagnostic and treatment strategies. They are not intended to replace clinical judgment or to establish a protocol for all individuals with (C)APD. Individual differences and circumstances, including the presence of comorbid conditions, require flexibility and adaptation.

Notwithstanding considerable scientific, technologic, and clinical strides forward, we still have much more to learn. Continued research is needed to fully answer some of the longstanding questions, as well as the new questions that arise continually as new knowledge begets new questions. Collaboration between clinicians and scientists—combining the clinician's firsthand knowledge of clinical needs with the researcher's expertise in the scientific method—provides a powerful approach to asking the right questions and obtaining enduring answers. Indeed, the authors contributing to this Handbook reflect this very collaboration between scientists and clinicians. Only through continued collaboration can we generate truly creative and innovative approaches to questions and problems, and accelerate the pace of discovery. In so doing, we will continue to advance our understanding of the central auditory nervous system and its intersections with cognitive and language domains that lead to the complex and heterogeneous clinical profiles of (C)APD. It is imperative that we take advantage of the momentum that has taken us to our current level of understanding and clinical practice, as described in this Handbook.

In closing, we hope that the knowledge shared in this Handbook leads to improved health and well-being of individuals with (C)APD, their families, and their communities.

Frank E. Musiek
Gail D. Chermak

CONTRIBUTORS

Jill Anderson, Au.D.
Research Assistant/Ph.D. Candidate
Department of Communication
    Sciences and Disorders
University of Cincinnati
Cincinnati, Ohio
Chapter 9

Douglas D. Backous, M.D., FACS
Director, Otology, Neurotology and
    Skull Base Surgery
Director, The Listen for Life Center at
    Virginia Mason Medical Center
Seattle, Washington
Chapter 18

Doris-Eva Bamiou, M.D., MSC, MPhil
Consultant in Audiological Medicine
    and Hon Senior Lecturer
Neuro-otology Department National
    Hospital for Neurology and
    Neurosurgery
Institute of Child Health (University
    College London)
Chapter 11

Karen Banai, Ph.D.
Department of Communication
    Sciences
Northwestern University
Evanston, Illinois IL
Chapter 4

Jane A. Baran, Ph.D.
Professor
Department of Communication Disorders
University of Massachusetts Amherst
Amherst, Massachusetts
Chapter 7

Teri James Bellis, Ph.D.
Associate Professor and Chair
Department of Communication
    Disorders

The University of South Dakota
Vermillion, South Dakota
Chapters 5 and 13

Gail D. Chermak, Ph.D.
Professor and Chair
Department of Speech and Hearing
    Sciences
Washington State University
Pullman, Washington
Chapters 1, 15, and 19

Rebekah E. Clemen
Research Assistant
Seattle Pacific University
Seattle, Washington
Chapter 18

Susan E. Fulton, M.A.
Ph.D. Candidate
Department of Communication
    Sciences & Disorders
University of South Florida
Tampa, Florida
Chapter 2

James W. Hall III, Ph.D.
Clinical Professor and Chief of
    Audiology
Department of Communicative
    Disorders
University of Florida
Gainsville, Florida
Chapter 12

Annette Hurley, Ph.D.
Assistant Professor
Department of Communicative
    Disorders
Louisiana State University Health
    Sciences Center
New Orleans, Louisiana
Chapter 14

Raymond M. Hurley, Ph.D.
Associate Professor
Department of Communication
    Sciences and Disorders
University of South Florida
Tampa, Florida
Chapters 2 and 14

Kristin N. Johnston, Au.D.
Audiologist
Department of Communicative Disorders
University of Florida
Gainsville, Florida
Chapter 12

Robert W. Keith, Ph.D.
Professor
Director of Medical Education
Department of Otolaryngology-Head
    and Neck Surgery
University of Cincinnati Medical Center
Cincinnati, Ohio
Chapter 9

Nina Kraus, Ph.D.
Hugh Knowles Professor
Department of Communication Sciences
Neurobiology and Physiology
Otolaryngology
Northwestern University
Evanston, Illinois
Chapter 4

Sridhar Krishnamurti, Ph.D.
Associate Professor
Department of Communication Disorders
Auburn University
Auburn, Alabama
Chapter 8

Art Maerlender, Ph.D.
Assistant Professor and Director
Clinical School Services and Learning
    Disorders Program
Department of Psychiatry
Dartmouth Medical School
Lebanon, New Hampshire
Chapter 17

Frank E. Musiek, Ph.D.
Professor and Director of Auditory
    Research
Department of Communication Sciences
Professor of Otolaryngology
School of Medicine
University of Connecticut
Storrs, Connecticut
Chapters 1 and 19

Dennis P. Phillips, Ph.D.
Killam Professor in Psychology
Department of Psychology
Dalhousie University
Halifax, Nova Scotia
Chapter 3

Gail J. Richard, Ph.D., CCC-SLP
Professor and Chair
Department of Communication
    Disorders and Sciences
Eastern Illinois University
Charleston, Illinois
Chapter 16

Ronald L. Schow, Ph.D.
Professor
Department of Communication
    Sciences and Disorders, and
    Education of the Deaf
Idaho State University
Pocatello, Idaho
Chapter 6

J. Anthony Seikel
Professor, Communication Sciences &
    Disorders, and Education of the Deaf
Idaho State University
Pocatello, Idaho
Chapter 6

Jennifer Brooke Shinn, Ph.D.
Assistant Professor and Director of
    Audiology
Chandler Medical Center
University of Kentucky
Lexington, Kentucky
Chapter 10

To my wonderful family, Erik, Amy, Justin, and Sheila

FM

To my parents, Zee and Martin, and
my children, Alina and Isaac

GC

SECTION I

Auditory Neuroscience

CHAPTER 1

AUDITORY NEUROSCIENCE AND (CENTRAL) AUDITORY PROCESSING DISORDER

An Overview

FRANK E. MUSIEK AND GAIL D. CHERMAK

The initial section of the first volume of this two-volume Handbook is devoted to selected aspects of auditory neuroscience as its relates to the diagnosis of central auditory processing disorder ([C]APD). This emphasis on science is consistent with the view of the Handbook editors and contributors that those who are involved in the diagnosis (as well as the intervention) of (C)APD must be well grounded in auditory neuroscience.

Knowledge of auditory neuroscience is, at times, difficult to attain. By its nature, science is complex and not always easily accessible. In addition, it is often not high on the "to do" list of busy clinicians juggling what may seem at times like an endless array of competing priorities and demands. Nonetheless, clinicians must find the time necessary to examine the science that underlies their clinical prac-

tices, in particular the science underlying central auditory test construction and interpretation before administering a central auditory processing test battery in the clinical setting.

By devoting several chapters of this Handbook to auditory neuroscience, we hope to provide clinicians, students, and researchers ready access to this crucial information. By placing the science chapters before the chapters focused on clinical practice, it is our intention that they will be read first.

Our focus on science also is intended to communicate the important role of the scientific "attitude" and the scientific method of inquiry for the clinical process. The scientific "attitude" is one that appreciates the scientific method, which is objective, open, and data-based. The scientific attitude begets an approach to knowledge acquisition that is broad and inclusive, recognizing that knowledge pertinent to one's particular area of interest can originate from many different disciplines and methodologies.

Scientific thinking begins with curiosity that leads to identifying a problem, generating a hypothesis to solve the problem, testing the hypothesis, and ultimately applying the solution to benefit people. These same attitudinal and thought processes and methodologies are as critical to clinical practice as they are to science. Science cannot be separated from clinical services and visa versa —advances in one leads to commensurate progress in the other domain. Conversely, lagging developments in one delays progress in the other. Clinicians tell scientists what is important to examine. Scientists deploy strong research designs to obtain enduring answers to clinicians' questions. Working together, knowledge summates and clinical services improve.

Overview of the Science Section

The science section begins with Ray Hurley's chapter on psychoacoustic considerations and implications for diagnosis of (C)APD. Dr. Hurley's longstanding interest in speech perception and (C)APD makes him an ideal author to explore these relationships. Dr. Hurley brings considerable research and clinical experience to his chapter. He guides the reader through the number of psychoacoustic principles that are key to developing and using behavioral, central auditory processing tests.

In explaining the neurobiology of the central auditory nervous system (CANS), Dennis Phillips demonstrates his unmatched ability as an auditory neuroscientist to bridge the gap between science and clinic. Dr. Phillips' interests in the auditory system are broad and far-ranging, both from the standpoint of the nature of the processing executed by the system (i.e., spatial, spectral, temporal) and from the standpoint of the perspective and level of analysis with which it is studied (e.g., psychophysical, neurophysiologic). In his chapter, he covers the basic neuroscience of the ascending auditory system, with some emphasis on how the brain establishes a sensory representation of the stimulus. He applies his experience in auditory neurophysiology and psychophysics to provide an informed view of auditory temporal processing and auditory system plasticity, and closes his chapter with a critical analysis of the neurophysiologic relationship between central auditory processing and language.

Next, Nina Kraus, who has been on the forefront of central auditory processing for a number of years, examines neurobiologic processes underlying the perception of speech and learning-associated brain plasticity. Her distinguished research career has been motivated by her keen interest in the linkages between neural encoding of sound in the CANS, the resultant perception of those sounds, and the subsequent incorporation of sound or speech perception into higher-level language skills (e.g. spoken language processing, reading, spelling). Germane to this chapter is her line of research demonstrating a fundamental, biological basis for speech-sound perception deficits in some school-age children with learning disabilities and (C)APD. Although

Dr. Kraus also has provided the field important research in regard to the cortical processing of sound using middle-latency and mismatched negativity evoked potentials, her chapter reflects some of her latest research regarding neural encoding of speech in the auditory brainstem with implications for the diagnosis of (C)APD, and for auditory training remediation strategies.

Auditory Neuroscience: Implications for (C)APD

To acknowledge and also encourage advances in neuroscience, the decade from 1990 to the year 2000 was designated as the Decade of the Brain. Many technologic breakthroughs have influenced our ability to study the brain and many of the developments in neuroscience carry implications crucial to our understanding of, and clinical advances in, (C)APD.

There have been numerous linkages between advances in auditory neuroscience and (C)APD. One of the classic links between auditory neuroscience and (C)APD was seen in the development of auditory pattern perception tests. The early animal studies performed by Neff, Butler, and Diamond demonstrated that ablation of the auditory cortex in cats resulted in their inability to correctly recognize patterns of sound (Neff, 1961). Even with training, these animals could not reach the levels of performance documented before surgical ablation. These findings were utilized by Pinheiro and Ptacek (1971) in the development of the frequency (pitch) pattern test for humans. Clinical research studies in humans

essentially yielded the same results that the Neff, Butler, and Diamond studies had produced with animals (Musiek & Pinheiro, 1987). Hence, the development of an efficient and popular (C)APD test that has been used for many years was directly linked to early neuroscience research.

Dichotic testing is another example of the linkage between auditory neuroscience and clinical practice. Dichotic testing, which has long been used to assess the CANS, reveals deficits in the ear contralateral to the compromised hemisphere (Figure 1–1). Doreen Kimura's original research identified the basis for interpreting dichotic laterality effects

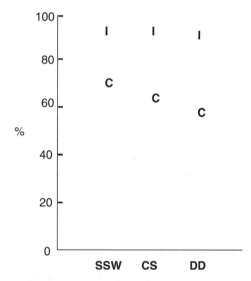

Figure 1–1. The performance (in percent correct) on three dichotic listening tests (CS = competing sentences, SSW = staggered spondaic words, DD = dichotic digits) for patients with confirmed cortical lesions primarily involving auditory regions in one hemisphere. Note there is significantly better performance for the ear ipsilateral (I) to the lesion than for the ear contralateral to the lesion (C).

(Kimura, 1961). In her original study, Kimura (1961) recruited individuals with well-defined lesions limited to the temporal lobe in one hemisphere. She clearly demonstrated that temporal lobe damage affected dichotic listening performance—primarily in the ear contralateral to the lesioned hemisphere. She explained this finding on the basis of physiologically stronger contralateral neural pathways that contain more fibers than the ipsilateral pathways. When the contralateral route was compromised due to the left temporal lobe lesion, the remaining intact pathways (i.e., both ipsilateral pathways and the contralateral pathway routed to the opposite side) were dominant, resulting in a right ear deficit on the dichotic listening task in patients with left hemisphere lesions. Kimura (1961) also showed that left hemisphere damage exerted a greater effect on dichotic listening for speech than did right hemisphere lesions. Many years later, functional magnetic resonance imaging (fMRI) data obtained by Hugdahl et al. (1998) supported Kimura's original observations and theoretical explanation regarding the suppression of the ipsilateral neural tracks and dominance of the contralateral neural tracks during dichotic listening. The fMRI data also indicated more activity in the posterior left temporal plane than in the right plane for dichotic speech stimuli. Both the Kimura and the Hugdahl et al. studies have provided scientific grounding for the clinical use of dichotic listening tests.

The auditory brainstem response (ABR) demonstrates yet another linkage between science and clinic. The ABR has long been used as an audiologic test for brainstem dysfunction. It is well known that certain patterns of ABR results are reliably associated with central auditory dysfunction of the brainstem. That is, when the later waves (III, IV, V) of the ABR are compromised with the earlier waves unaffected, there is a high probability of CANS involvement at the level of the brainstem (see Figure 1-2). The basis for these patterns and their interpretation derive from basic studies on generator sites and lesion effects on animals (Moller, 2000; Wada and Starr 1983a, 1983b). This basic research has enabled clinicians using ABR to differentiate peripheral from central auditory involvement.

The recent development of the Gaps-in-Noise (GIN) test demonstrates the continuing linkage between science and practice (Musiek et al., 2005). Although data on the psychoacoustic underpinnings of many gap detection procedures have been available for many years (Plomp, 1964), the real source of information needed to develop a clinical gap detection procedure comes from animal data that showed major effects of auditory cortex ablations Syka et al. (2002). Similar results were obtained from humans with cortical lesions and animals with cortical ablations. This is yet another case where the animal data were predictive of clinical findings with humans.

The clarification that auditory neuroscience provides relative to pathophysiology is another example of the link between basic science and clinic. For example, research demonstrating the effects of auditory cortex ablations on auditory detection in primates has informed our understanding of the underlying pathophysiology of CANS dysfunction. Although it has been well documented over the years that central lesions do not influence pure tone detection thresholds, Heffner and Heffner (1986) presented contrary findings that certainly were thought provoking. These researchers demonstrated

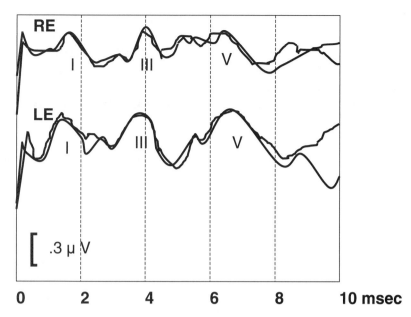

Figure 1–2. An ABR of a patient with a midline brainstem lesion of the caudal pons. Note the increased III-V latencies bilaterally, but most obvious on the left side, consistent with a brainstem lesion.

poorer pure tone detection thresholds after auditory cortex ablations in the ear contralateral to the lesion, although the animals did recover their hearing sensitivity in time. The clinical implication is an important one in that it poses the possibility that in severe cortical damage (other than central deafness) there may be an effect on pure tone detectability, which may be recovered over time.

Also revealing the role of auditory neuroscience in clarifying the pathophysiology of auditory dysfunction is the work by Masterton and colleagues (1992) who, by sectioning ipsilateral versus contralateral lateral lemnisci (LL), demonstrated that the contralateral LL serves a more significant role for detection and frequency discrimination than does the ipsilateral LL. This contralateral dominance is consistent with longstanding anatomic data indicating more con-

tralateral than ipsilateral fibers in the LL and underlies clinical data which show contralateral deficits on behavioral central auditory tests for lesions in the more rostral pons (Musiek et. al., 1988).

Implications of Clinical Findings for Auditory Neuroscience

Although there are many more examples demonstrating the impact of auditory neuroscience in clinical practice, we move on to provide examples of the reverse effect whereby clinical findings impact auditory neuroscience. One recent example of the impact of clinical findings with human subjects for auditory neuroscience concerns the function of the insula.

For years the function of the insula has been uncertain. A few studies suggested that the insula might be involved in audition; however, these studies were mostly ignored (see Bamiou et al., 2003). A rather dramatic clinical report was published in 1995 that did much to change the thinking about the functional role of the insula (Habib et al., 1995). Habib et al. studied an individual who incurred a stroke involving the insula on the right side and then a few days later a stroke involving the insula on the left side. Interestingly, after the second stroke the patient demonstrated central deafness, despite the fact that Heschl's gyrus was unaffected and intact on both sides. Clearly, this clinical report has had a resonating impact on auditory neuroscience related to function of the insula.

Another example of human behavioral findings influencing science involves the corpus callosum. Although animal research had demonstrated electrophysiologically the importance of the corpus callosum (Berlucchi, 1972), findings with human subjects ultimately clarified the underlying science. Although Berlucchi's data demonstrated the influence of myelin on interhemispheric transfer times, it was not until humans with "split brains" were studied that the importance of the corpus callosum was realized. The original studies demonstrated that split-brain patients showed essentially no responses to left ear stimuli, but only in a dichotic listening mode using speech stimuli. If speech stimuli were presented monaurally no deficits were noted (Musiek et al., 1984). The dichotic listening findings demonstrated the role of the corpus callosum in the transfer of information from one hemisphere to the other. In conjunction with other test battery findings, interhemispheric transfer deficits related to damage of the callosum are now rather routinely inferred from left ear deficits on clinical dichotic listening tests.

Clinical Decision Analysis

Clinical decision analysis (CDA) provides the clinician with a quantitative and systematic approach to evaluate the performance of diagnostic tests (see Turner, Robinette, & Bauch, 1999 for review). CDA focuses on a test's sensitivity (i.e., ability of a test to identify correctly those individuals who have the dysfunction), specificity (i.e., ability of a test to identify correctly those individuals who do not have the dysfunction), and efficiency (i.e., a test's combined sensitivity and specificity). Although specificity typically decreases as sensitivity increases, tests can be constructed that offer high sensitivity with an acceptable degree of specificity needed for clinical use. The alteration of pass/fail criteria can influence the sensitivity and specificity of a test. This changing of criteria can help the clinician achieve the desired outcome for the test by manipulating the sensitivity and specificity. If one measures test sensitivity and specificity for a progression of criteria, a receiver operating characteristic (ROC) curve can be constructed to visualize the variation of sensitivity (i.e., hit rate or true positive rate) versus false alarm rate (i.e., false positive rate) for different pass/fail criteria. (See Chapters 6 and 7 for discussion of CDA and sensitivity and specificity.)

Also related to a test's clinical utility are the concepts of validity and reliability. Reliability (i.e., consistency or stability of a measure) is essential to validity; however, reliability does not ensure validity. Validity, and in particular construct validity, which is probably the most important form of validity, refers to the fundamental question: *what* does the test measure?. In the case of central auditory testing, the clinician must employ tests and procedures that not only provide a *consistent* measure of function, but also provide a *true, legitimate* measure of CANS integrity. Ascertaining that a test is valid (e.g., through comparison of its content to the domain being measured, correlation (or factor analysis) with other supposedly valid tests of that domain, amassing convergent, divergent, and other evidence that the presumed construct is what is being measured) does not mean that the test is sensitive (or specific). CDA is necessary to quantify a test's sensitivity and specificity. The audiologist's central auditory test battery must consist of valid (and therefore reliable) measures of CANS function. Such tests and procedures will not be useful clinically, however, unless they are also highly sensitive to CANS dysfunction and at the same time capable of excluding as normal those individuals who do not present CANS dysfunction. Such measures present the test efficiency needed to accurately diagnose (C)APD.

Neuroanatomy of the Human Brain Revisited

Both the scientist and the clinician interested in (C)APD are highly dependent on the anatomic correlates of their laboratory or clinical test findings, respectively. In fact, interest in anatomic correlates has fueled advances in functional imaging, which has in turn heightened interest in the anatomy of the human brain. As the anatomy of the human brain has re-entered the spotlight, the limitations of anatomic methods have come under scrutiny. It appears that the anatomic knowledge needed to establish important correlations may fall a bit short. Much of this knowledge shortcoming is the result of the fact that much of the information on human neuroanatomy is based on animal models, which in actuality are quite different from humans—especially at the cortical level (see Musiek & Baran, 2007; Wise, 2003).

Interesting questions have evolved about the human brain—especially in regard to auditory regions (Leonard, Puranik, Kildau, & Lombardino, 1998). It has been shown that the primary auditory region in humans, Heschl's gyrus, can be two or three gyri (Musiek & Reeves 1990). Also, at times it is very difficult to know where Heschl's gyrus ends and the planum temporale begins because of the morphology of the tissue in that area of the brain (Rubens, 1977). Perhaps the biggest question mark about human brain anatomy centers on the morphology of the Sylvian fissure. The Sylvian fissure, which is a guide to most of the auditory regions of the cortex, courses along the superior fringe of the superior temporal gyrus. The difficulty lies in the fact that the Sylvian fissure is highly variable in its morphology. At times it courses straight back, but at times the posterior one-quarter may also turn up (termed an ascending ramus) or down (descending ramus). This can change the precise position of associated structures, including the planum temporale, supramarginal gyrus and angular gyrus (see Rubens, 1977, Musiek and Baran, 2007 for review. These morphologic alterations have implications for establishing anatomic correlates to test findings, evoked potentials, and yes, even functional imaging. Clearly, the anatomic variability of the human brain must be studied further so that clinicians and scientists have a solid dependable reference to support a better working knowledge for clinical practice.

Communication Between Clinician and Scientist

The many examples of linkage between auditory neuroscience and clinic underscore the importance of this relationship to advances in the field of (C)APD. There is no denying these links exist and that the linkages are strengthened through the hard work of clinicians and scientists. It would also be fair to say that communication among clinicians, clinical investigators, and basic scientists often is lacking. Given the importance of this communication, we propose several means to improve the communication process.

As discussed in other chapters in this Handbook, attitude plays a key role in communication. Auditory neuroscientists must take an interest in clinical problems and clinicians must be aware of the issues confronting the basic researcher. Effort must be expended so that colleagues active in each arena are aware of each other's progress. (See Chapter 19.)

Probably one of the biggest hurdles to communication is understanding each other's "language." For example, the acronym CAP is interpreted by physiologists as *compound action potential*; however, to most clinicians, CAP is likely to mean central auditory processing! Familiarizing oneself with terminology is a first step toward improving communication. One way to become familiar with terminology and to achieve the larger goal of communication would be served by cli-

nicians and scientists attending sessions in the other's area at major conferences. Also, clinicians and scientists should at least browse some of the key journals in each other's areas on a more regular basis, focusing on those reports carrying implications for one's clinical practice or research. For example, journals such as *Hearing Research*, *Journal of the Acoustical Society of America*, *Journal of Neuroscience*, and the *Journal of the Association for Research in Otolayrngology* are science journals that frequently contain articles pertinent to clinicians. Likewise, auditory neuroscientists should become familiar with the *Journal of the American Academy of Audiology*, *International Journal of Audiology*, and the *American Journal of Audiology*, which are primarily clinically oriented journals. A journal such as *Ear and Hearing* publishes both basic research and clinical reports and should serve as informative "crossover" reading.

Perhaps one of the most useful approaches to foster communication between the clinician and scientist is to spend time in each other's lab or clinical setting, observing each other's daily routine. This is an invaluable experience that can establish rapport and provide knowledge and insights that benefit the scientist's research and the clinician's patients. This in turn can lead to shared information sessions and even collaborative projects that bridge clinical and research interests.

Summary

In this introductory chapter, we emphasized the important role of the scientific "attitude" and the scientific method of inquiry for the clinical process. Following a brief overview of the auditory neuroscience chapters in this volume, we provided examples of the impact of advances in auditory neuroscience for (C)APD diagnostic approaches and the reciprocal role of clinical studies in fueling basic science. The chapter concludes with several suggestions to improve interdisciplinary communication and augment the mutually beneficial relationship between scientists and clinicians.

References

Bamiou, D., Musiek, F., & Luxon, L. (2003). The insula (Island of Reil) and its role in auditory processing: Literature review. *Brain Research Reviews, 42,* 143-154.

Berlucchi, G. (1972). Anatomical and physiological aspects of visual functions of corpus callosum. *Brain Research, 37,* 371-392.

Habib, M., Daquin, G., Milandre, L., Royere, M., Ray, M., Lanteri, A., Salamon, G., & Khalil, R. (1995). Mutism and auditory agnosia due to bilateral insular damage—role of the insula in human communication. *Neuropsychologia, 3,* 327-339.

Heffner, H., & Heffner, R. (1986). Effect of unilateral and bilateral auditory cortex lesions on the discrimination of vocalizations by Japanese macaques. *Journal of Neurophysiology, 56,* 683-701.

Hugdahl, K., Heiervang, E., Nordby, H., Smievoll, A. I., Steinmetz, H., Stevenson, J., & Lund, A. (1998). Central auditory processing, MRI morphometry and brain laterality: Applications to dyslexia. *Scandinavian Audiology Supplement, 49,* 26-34.

Kimura D. (1961). Some effects of temporal lobe damage on auditory perception. *Canadian Journal of Psychology, 15,* 157-165.

Leonard, C., Puranik, C., Kildau, J., & Lombardino, L. (1998). Normal variation in the frequency and location of human auditory cortex landmarks. Heschl's gyrus: Where is it? *Cerebral Cortex, 8,* 397-406.

Masterton, R. B., Granger, E. M., & Glendenning, K. K. (1992). Psychoacoustical contribution of each lateral lemniscus. *Hearing Research, 63,* 57-70.

Moller, A. R. (2000). *Hearing: Its physiology and pathophysiology.* New York: Academic Press.

Musiek, F. E., & Baran, J. A. (2007). *The auditory system: Anatomy, physiology and clinical correlates.* Boston: Allyn & Bacon.

Musiek, F. E., Gollegly, K. M., Kibbe, K. S., & Verkest, S. B. (1988). Current concepts on the use of ABR and auditory psychophysical tests in the evaluation of brainstem lesions. *American Journal of Otology, 9,* 25-33.

Musiek, F. E., Kibbe, K., & Baran, J. (1984). Neuroaudiological results from split-brain patients. *Seminars in Hearing, 5*(3), 219-229.

Musiek, F. E., & Pinheiro, M. (1987). Frequency patterns in cochlear, brainstem, and cerebral lesions. *Audiology, 26,* 79-88.

Musiek, F. E., & Reeves, A. G. (1990). Asymmetries of the auditory areas of the cerebrum. *Journal of the American Academy of Audiology, 1,* 240-245.

Musiek, F. E., Shinn, J. B., Jirsa, R., Bamiou, D. E., Baran, J. A., & Zaidan, E. (2005) The GIN© (Gaps-in-Noise) Test performance in subjects with confirmed central auditory nervous system involvement. *Ear and Hearing, 26,* 608-618.

Neff, W. (1961). Neural mechanisms of auditory discrimination. In W. Rosenblith (Ed.), *Sensory communication* (pp. 259-278). New York: Wiley & Sons.

Pinheiro, M. L., & Ptacek, P. H. (1971). Reversals in the perception of noise and tone patterns. *Journal of the Acoustical Society of America, 49,* 1178-1782.

Plomp, R. (1964). Rate of decay of auditory sensation. *Journal of the Acoustical Society of America, 36,* 277-382.

Rubens, A. B. (1977). Anatomical asymmetries of human cerebral cortex. In S. Harnad, R. Doty, L. Goldstein, J. Jaynes, & G. Krauthamer (Eds.), *Lateralization in the nervous system*. New York: Academic Press.

Syka, J., Rybalko, N., Mazelova, J., & Druga, R. (2002). Gap detection in the rat before and after auditory cortex ablation. *Hearing Research, 172,* 151–159.

Turner, R., Robinette, M., Bauch, C. (1999). Clinical decisions. In F. E. Musiek & W. Rintelmann (Eds.), *Contemporary perspectives in hearing assessment* (pp. 437–464). Boston: Allyn & Bacon.

Wada, S. I., & Starr, A. (1983a). Generation of auditory brain stem responses (ABRs). II. Effects of surgical section of the trapezoid body on the ABR in guinea pigs and cat. *Electroencephalography and Clinical Neurophysiology, 56*(4), 340–351.

Wada, S. I., & Starr, A. (1983b). Generation of auditory brain stem responses (ABRs). III. Effects of lesions of the superior olive, lateral lemniscus and inferior colliculus on the ABR in guinea pig. *Electroencephalography and Clinical Neurophysiology, 56*(4), 352–366.

Wise, R. J. (2003). Language systems in normal and aphasic human subjects: Functional imaging studies and inferences from animal studies. *British Medical Bulletin, 65,* 95–119.

CHAPTER 2

PSYCHOACOUSTIC CONSIDERATIONS AND IMPLICATIONS FOR THE DIAGNOSIS OF (C)APD

RAYMOND M. HURLEY AND SUSAN E. FULTON

The purpose of this chapter is threefold: (1) to review selected aspects of traditional and contemporary psychoacoustics; (2) to focus on psychoacoustic phenomena that may have a direct bearing on a (central) auditory processing disorder ([C]APD) evaluation; and (3) to convince the reader that the study of psychoacoustics within the context of (C)APD is needed. Beginning with the third purpose, we note that the rationale that Zeng and colleagues (Zeng, Oba, Garde, Sininger, & Starr, 2001) provided for the psychoacoustic study of auditory neuropathy can apply equally well to the study of (C)APD. First, the basic auditory function of a listener with (C)APD needs to be described if we are ever to discover the reason for the common observation that an individual with (C)APD hears, but does not understand. Second, we need to

develop behavioral tests that can provide a more accurate differential diagnosis and identify underlying physiologic processes related to (C)APD. Third, the psychoacoustic study of (C)APD may provide insight into the development of (re)habilitation programs for the successful treatment of the listener with (C)APD. For a more conventional review/update on psychoacoustics, the reader is referred to selected textbooks (Gelfand, 2004; Moore, 1997; 1998; Yost, Popper & Fay, 1993) and textbook chapters (Humes, 1994; Kidd, 2002; Yost, 2000).

Psychoacoustics is the branch of psychophysics that is concerned with the relationship between a stimulus and the perception of that stimulus by the listener's sensory system. Psychoacoustics deals with how changes in the physical parameters of sound affect the psychological detection of that change and attempts to infer from a listener's responses what the stimulus has evoked in the auditory system. Naturally, each response from the listener consists of two aspects: (1) a change in the listener's sensory perception (sensitivity) and (2) the listener's response criteria (i.e., biases) that contribute to the response. Psychacoustic methodology is driven by attempts to control or at least minimize the effect of the listener's response bias on the actual response.

Classical Psychoacoustic Methods

The three classical psychoacoustic methods are: (1) method of limits, (2) method of adjustment, and (3) method of constant stimuli. Each method has positive and negative aspects, and each is used for absolute and difference threshold measures. Audiologists are familiar with the Békésy tracking method, which is an adaptation of both the method of limits and the method of adjustment.

Method of Limits

The method of limits is in part the foundation on which the well-known modified Hughson-Westlake procedure (Carhart & Jerger, 1959) is based. All the acoustic stimuli are under the control of the examiner who presents to the listener (subject) a series of acoustic stimuli that change in a predetermined step. The listener either responds indicating perception of the stimulus change or fails to respond signifying that the stimulus

change was not perceived. The procedure to estimate absolute threshold may be used in an ascending series with the starting signal being at a level predetermined to be below the listener's threshold. Or conversely, a descending series may be used beginning at a signal level predetermined to be above the listener's threshold. Conventionally, alternating descending and ascending series are utilized with a predetermined number of trials used in each series (run). The listener's response is recorded for each trial and the response reversal point is determined for each series (see Figure 2–1). The mean of the response reversal points defines the 50% threshold.

In the measurement of differential threshold, the method of limits test paradigm utilizes the presentation of two stimuli for each trial with the level of the first stimulus fixed and the level of the second stimulus varied in a predetermined step size. The subject's task is to determine if the second stimulus is greater than, less than, or the same as the first stimulus. The results of a differential threshold measure using the method of limits results in a range of values in which the second stimulus is: (1) greater that the first stimulus, (2) less that the first stimulus, or (3) equal to the first stimulus. The difference between the 50% point of the values between greater than and equal to and the 50% point between equal to and less than is referred to as the "interval of uncertainty" and is used in determining the just noticeable difference (jnd).[1] If the pluses and minuses in Figure 2–1 are substituted with the words "greater," "lesser," or "equal," then the figure would illustrate a differential sensitivity measure using the method of limits.

---

[1]The jnd is considered to be one-half the interval of uncertainty (Gelfand, 2004).

dB	Run	1	2	3	4	5	6	7
	Direction	Descend	Ascend	Descend	Ascend	Descend	Ascend	Descend
20		Yes						
18								
16		Yes	·					
14				Yes				
12		Yes	Yes	Yes		Yes		Yes
10			No	Yes	Yes	Yes	Yes	Yes
8		Yes	No	Yes	No	No	No	No
6			No	No	No		No	
4		No	No		No			
2			No					
	Threshold	6 dB	11 dB	7 dB	9 dB	9 dB	9 dB	9 dB

Figure 2–1. Illustration of the method of limits that result in an average threshold of 9 dB with the first descending trial not included in the average. Each (yes) indicates that the listener responded to the stimulus and each (no) indicates that the listener did not respond to the stimulus.

The method of limits suffers from two types of bias. First, because the stimulus presentation is under the control of the examiner, tester bias can come into play as it can in pure tone audiometry. Second, the listener's bias for anticipating the stimulus level at which the response reversal will occur in either the ascending or descending stimulus series can affect the results. In an attempt to control for these bias effects, an equal number of ascending and descending trials is often utilized or, alternatively, a random ascending-descending presentation schedule is used. In addition to the above biases, the method of limits' accuracy is affected by the step size used in the trial series. Too large a step size results in an imprecise estimate of threshold and too small a step size results in an ineffective use of test time. Step size selection by the experimenter is a balance between selecting a step size that is large enough to quickly arrive at threshold and small enough to offer the precision necessary for an accurate measure of threshold. Lastly, the method of limits does not allow a distinction in the listener's response between a true sensory change perceived by the listener and a change in the listener's response criterion (bias).

Method of Adjustment

The psychophysical method of adjustment differs from the method of limits in that the listener, not the examiner, controls the stimulus, although the examiner sets the initial level of the stimulus and the subject adjusts the stimulus according to the test instructions. The subject's adjustment of the stimulus variable is continuous via an unmarked dial and is not stepped as in the method of limits. Typically, the examiner has a control dial that is used to set the initial level of the stimulus which is unknown to the listener. This initial level is either below or above some preselected starting point, which is varied by the examiner. Obviously, if the initial level is above the listener's threshold, the trial will be a descending one with the listener decreasing the level of the stimulus until it is below threshold; conversely, if the starting level is below the listener's threshold, the trial will be an ascending one with the listener increasing the level of the stimulus until it is above threshold. Like the method of limits, the method of adjustment is applicable to both absolute and differential threshold measures.

Although the method of adjustment removes examiner bias, it is not without other problems. As the stimulus is for the most part under the control of the listener, the test paradigm can be affected by an undetected change in the listener's response criterion during a trial. Listeners have a tendency to undershoot or overshoot their threshold level by excessively decreasing or increasing the stimulus level. To control or at least minimize this exaggerated threshold effect, testers have used alternating ascending and descending trials. Furthermore, like the method of limits, the method of adjustment does not allow a distinction in the listener's response between a true sensory change perceived by the listener and a change in the listener's response criterion.

Method of Constant Stimuli

The method of constant stimuli differs from the method of limits and the method of adjustment by using a random stimulus presentation mode from a pretest selection of at least 10 stimulus levels (Humes, 1994), thus not utilizing an ascending and descending test paradigm. Typically, a minimum of 10 presentations per stimulus level is used in the test paradigm (Humes, 1994). In an absolute threshold measure, the examiner will preselect the stimulus levels and the step size, and randomize the presentation sequence. In addition to measuring absolute threshold, the method of constant stimuli can be used to measure differential threshold using a two-stimuli paradigm requiring the subject to make a judgment about the second stimulus in reference to the first stimulus. Again, the examiner will preselect the stimulus values for the two stimuli, the step size, and the presentation order. An advantage of the method of constant stimuli is that the examiner can get an estimation of a listener's guessing behavior by inserting blank or "catch" trials in the predetermined test schedule. The listener is to indicate "yes" or "no" through either a verbal or manual response for each stimulus presentation during the response interval, which is usually designated by two visual markers viewed by the subject. From the listener's responses, the percentage of correct responses are computed for each stimulus level and displayed in an S-shaped psychometric function (Figure 2–2). From the psychometric function, the 50% point or a more stringent criterion, for example, the 75% point, can define the threshold. The weakness of the method of constant stimuli is the test time required to obtain sufficient data points to construct the psychometric function.

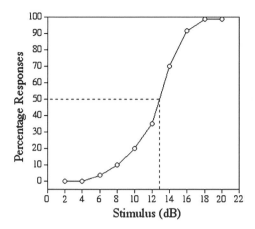

Figure 2–2. Illustration of a psychometric function depicting a 50% threshold of 13 dB.

Selective Adaptive Methods

Adaptive methods have increased the efficiency of absolute and differential threshold measures by utilizing test paradigms that converge on the threshold value by quickly eliminating values that are distant from the threshold value. In adaptive methods, the level of any given stimulus is determined by the listener's response to the previous stimulus. Adaptive test strategies often initially use a large step size that is reduced as the stimulus value gets closer to threshold.

Staircase Method

The staircase method (Levitt, 1971, 1978) is similar to the method of limits in that the stimulus value is decreased until the listener gives a negative response and then is increased until the listener gives a positive response. The difference

between the method of limits and the staircase method is that the testing sequence does not stop when the listener's response changes in the staircase method. Similar to the method of limits, a specific step size is utilized in the staircase method. A test sequence (run) is begun using a large step size in decreasing value until the listener gives a negative response. The test run reverses direction using a smaller step size that is generally one-half of the original one (Figure 2–3). The direction of the runs continues to be reversed at each change in the listener's response from positive to negative and negative to positive until six to eight reversals have occurred; the first reversal is not included. The 50% threshold point is determined by taking the average of the positive and negative reversal values, excluding the first reversal value. The staircase method is very efficient as it converges on the 50% point quickly, if the step size is neither too small nor too large. Too small a step size would result in unnecessary runs whereas too large a step size would result in a less than precise 50% threshold point.

Point Estimation by Sequential Testing (PEST)

Adaptations of the staircase method are the point estimation by sequential testing (PEST) method (Taylor & Creelman, 1967) and the transformed up-down procedure (Gelfand, 2004; Levitt, 1971, 1978). The PEST procedure utilizes a set of testing rules to either halve the stimulus level or double the stimulus level depending on the listener's response behavior. Although the staircase method can only measure the 50% threshold point, the PEST procedure can obtain any

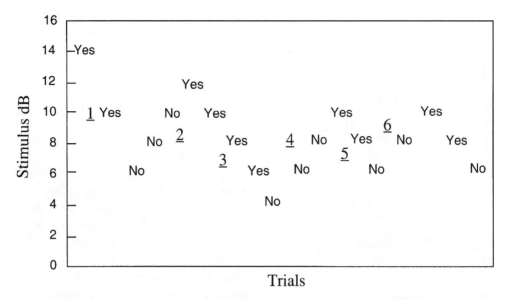

Figure 2–3. Illustration of the adaptive staircase method with each (*yes*) signifying a positive response and each (*no*) signifying a negative response. The first descending trial is not included in the average.

preselected point on the psychometric function. Similarly, a transformed up-down procedure can be used to estimate a point on the psychometric function that is above the 50% point; the 71% (70.7%) point is commonly used. The more stringent 71% criterion is obtained by altering the up-down rules such that an increase in stimulus value requires a different response criterion than a decrease in stimulus value. For example, an increase in stimulus value would require a negative response or a positive response followed by a negative response, whereas a decrease in stimulus value would require two positive responses. Like the traditional staircase method, neither the PEST nor the transformed up-down procedure accounts for the listener's guessing behavior or a change in the listener's response criterion.

Alternative Forced-Choice Methods

A "yes-no" response mode similar to the method of constant stimuli lends itself to evaluation using an interval forced-choice paradigm. A response interval is established during which the listener must respond "yes" or "no" to each presentation: a one-alternative (interval) forced-choice. More often than not, however, a multiple alternative (interval) forced-choice paradigm is utilized such as a two-alternative forced-choice procedure during which the listener must indicate in which of two intervals the stimulus is present. The multiple alternative (interval) forced-choice paradigm can be extended to three or four response intervals and can be paired with an adaptive procedure. In this combined paradigm, the stimulus value is adjusted according to a predetermined rule such as a 2-down 1-up criterion during which the stimulus value is reduced only after the listener has two successive correct responses. The stimulus value is increased after one error response that would result in the 71% point on the psychometric function. Other adaptive rules will estimate different points on the psychometric function. For example, a 3-down 1-up, and 4 down 1-up rules will estimate the 79% and 84% correct points on the psychometric function, respectively (Levitt, 1971).

Theory of Signal Detection

As mentioned in the previous sections, the "classical" and adaptive psychophysical methods do not separate a change in sensitivity from a change in the listener's response criterion (bias). On the other hand, the theory of signal detection (TSD) (Green & Swets, 1974; MacMillan & Creelman, 1991) does provide a procedure that separates a change in the listener's sensitivity from a change in the listener's response criterion (bias). Similar to the method of constant stimuli, the TSD procedure can utilize "catch" trials to estimate a listener's guessing behavior. For example, in a 100-trial run, a single stimulus value is presented during 50 trials and the rest of the trials contain no stimulus (i.e., catch trials). This test paradigm will result in four possible outcomes : (1) the signal is present and the subject says "yes"; (2) the signal is not present and the subjects says "no"; (3) the signal is present and the subject says "no"; and (4) the signal is not present and the subjects says "yes." These four

possible outcomes can be expressed in a 2 × 2 matrix. Figure 2–4 displays these four outcomes using the TSD nomenclature of hit rate, correct rejection rate, miss rate, and false alarm rate. Similar tables would subsequently be constructed for each stimulus value. From these matrices, a receiver operator characteristic (ROC) curve is constructed (see Figure 2–5) which plots the hit rate on the vertical axis (ordinate) against the false alarm on the horizontal axis (abscissa). The diagonal line in Figure 2–5 represents chance performance. Curves 1 and 2 depicted in Figure 2–5 represent the listener's sensitivity to two different stimulus values, whereas points A B, C and D, E, F represent the listener's response criterion to the two different stimulus values. In short, curves 1 and 2 depict different sensitivity to the stimulus value whereas points A B, C and D, E, F depict changes in the listener's response bias. If points A, B, C are at the same location as points D, E, F on their respective ROC curves, the listener's response bias

		Response	
		Yes	No
Stimulus	Present	Hit	Miss
	Absent	False Alarm	Correct Rejection

Figure 2–4. Illustration of the 2 × 2 matrix that would summarize the four possible stimulus-response outcomes for a series of test trials at the same stimulus value.

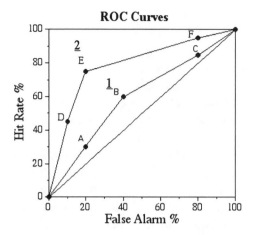

Figure 2–5. Illustration of ROC curves with the diagonal line representing a d' value of zero and curves 1 and 2 differ in sensitivity whereas points A, B, and C, and D, E, and F reflect different response criteria.

would be considered the same for the two ROC curves. A true change in the listener's sensitivity is reflected in an increase/decrease in the hit rate and no change in the false alarm rate. Conversely, a change in the listener's response bias results in proportional changes in both the hit and false alarm rates.

The listener's response bias can, however, be manipulated by the examiner through instructions given to the listener. For example, the listener can be encouraged to guess, which would result in an increase in the hit rate; however, because the listener's response bias is being manipulated, there would be a proportional increase in the false alarm rate. Or the listener could be instructed that guessing was frowned on, which would decrease the false alarm rate, but would increase the miss rate by changing the listener's response bias. The listener's response bias can also be manipulated by pairing a reward or, conversely, a

penalty to each response, such as a financial reward for each hit and a financial fine for each false alarm.

The index of sensitivity in TSD is the d' value which is the amount of separation between the distributions for the stimulus and nonstimulus (catch trials) conditions (i.e., separation between the hit rate and correct rejection rate). d' is a measure of the overlap of the hit rate and false alarm rate probability distribution curves, which in theory are normally distributed and have equal variance. As the overlap of the hit rate and false alarm rate probability distribution curves decreases, the d' value becomes larger signifying an increase in sensitivity. The most expedient way to determine d', assuming that the hit and false alarm rates are known, is to use available tables (Swets, 1964). Pictorially, the ROC curve that has the greatest displacement from the diagonal ($d' = 0.0$) toward the upper left corner where the hit rate is high and the false alarm rate is low, shows greater sensitivity to a stimulus value and produces the largest d' value (see Figure 2-5).

Clinical Decision Analysis

An outgrowth of TSD is clinical decision analysis (CDA) which has been used in the past to determine the efficacy of (C)APD tests (Hurley & Musiek, 1997; Singer, Hurley, & Preece 1998). In the CDA model, hit rate is the percentage of subjects correctly identified by a test score; the false alarm rate is the percentage of subjects incorrectly identified as positive by a test score; the miss rate is the percentage of subjects incorrectly identified as negative by a test score; the correct rejection rate is the percentage of subjects correctly identified as negative by a test score; and d' or A' is a measure of the overall performance of various test scores (Hyde, Davidson, & Alberti, 1991; Turner, Robinette, & Bauch, 1999). Although d' is dependent on the form of the hit rate and false alarm rate probability distribution cures, A' is not, as it is a nonparametric measure with values ranging from 0.50 for a test of no diagnostic value to 1.00 for the perfect diagnostic test. The formula to compute A' may be found in Turner et al. (1999). As audiology tests are known to have hit rates and false alarm rates that are not normally distributed or of equal variance (Turner et al., 1999; Turner & Nielsen, 1984), the nonparametric A' value is used in CDA as an indication of overall performance. For a comprehensive discussion of d' and A' see Turner and Nielsen (1984) and for an expanded treatment of CDA, the reader is referred to Hyde et al. (1991) and Turner et al. (1999). (See Chapter 7 for application of the CDA in the central auditory test battery.)

Differential Sensitivity: Frequency and Intensity

Many studies have sought to quantify the number of hertz (Hz) or decibels (dB) that is needed for the listener to detect the respective change in frequency or intensity. In short, the investigations have asked the questions, how large a Hz or dB difference must there be between two tones before the listener can detect a change? These measures of differential sensitivity are referred to as just-noticeable-difference (jnd) or difference limen (DL), and can be characterized as an absolute quantity or a relative quantity,

that is a ratio. The ratio, which is often referred to as the Weber fraction, is computed by dividing the absolute DL (Δ) value by the base value, that is, Df/f and DI/I for frequency (f) and intensity (I), respectively. For example, if the base value was 1000 Hz and the DL (Δ) was 10 Hz, the Δf/f ratio would be 0.01.

One might ask, why should differential sensitivity be studied within the context of (C)APD? Kidd (2002) identified three strong reasons for investigating DLs (jnds) for frequency and intensity which can be readily applied to the investigation of (C)APD. First, DLs will provide insight into how effectively a listener's auditory system codes the acoustic parameters of frequency and intensity. (See this chapter's section on differential sensitivity for frequency.) Second, DLs can be used to either develop models of hearing or to test normal/abnormal models of auditory function through such techniques as computer simulation. And third, a listener's DLs can be compared to normative standard values providing further insight into an impaired listener's auditory dysfunction(s). These three reasons are certainly sufficient to justify studying DLs in individuals suspected of having (C)APD (see Zeng et al., 2001).

Differential Sensitivity for Frequency

Historically, two paradigms have been used to measure differential sensitivity for frequency (Δf). The first paradigm is a frequency modulation (FM) technique where tones are modulated at a low rate of 2 to 4 Hz with the listener's task being to detect the change in modulation rate. The second paradigm has used a successive steady tone technique where the pulsed tones differ in frequency by a small amount and the listener's task is to indicate if the first or second tone is higher in frequency. The minimal amount of frequency change that a listener can detect between the successive tones is the DL value.

The seminal study by Shower and Biddulph (1931) was the first to successfully delineate the ear's differential sensitivity (DL) for frequency. By using the FM technique, they overcame the technologic limitation of that era which was the production of transient clicks that resulted from turning a pure tone signal on and off. Subsequent investigations (Harris, 1952; Moore, 1973; Wier, Jesteadt, & Green, 1977) using the successive pulsed tone technique were not in agreement with the Shower and Biddulph (1931) study. The main reason for the difference between the data of Shower and Biddulph (1931) and the more recent investigation of Weir et al. (1977) is attributed to the different test paradigms with the FM technique producing a stimulus with a more complex acoustic spectrum resulting in a different form of phase locking for neural coding than the successive pulsed tone technique (Gelfand, 2004; Moore, 1997). In addition to the measurement paradigm, the parameters of sensation level (SL) and tone duration will affect the absolute DL value (Moore, 1973; Weir et al., 1977).

The most recent investigations (Moore, 1973; Weir et al., 1977) have shown smaller DL values at low and mid-frequencies (<2000 Hz) and larger DL values at higher frequencies (>2000 Hz) (see Figure 2–6). The Weir et al. (1977) data at 40 dB SL, shows the DL value at 200 to 800 Hz to be approximately 1.0 to 1.5 dB and at 1000 to 2000 Hz to be approximately 2 to 3 dB. As illustrated in

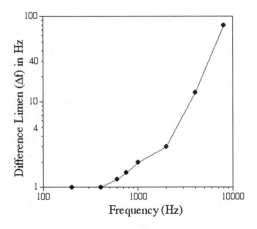

Figure 2–6. Illustration of frequency difference limen (Δf) at a sensation level of 40 dB from the work of Wier et al. (1977).

Figure 2-6, above 1000 Hz, the DL value increases to 16 to 18 dB in the region of 4000 Hz and rapidly increases above 4000 Hz to 67 to 70 dB in the region of 8000 Hz. These data are interpreted to be consistent with the VIIIth nerve's phase locking characteristics for frequency, which decreases at about 1000 to 2000 Hz and is absent above 4000 to 5000 Hz (Moore, 1997) with place information being responsible for frequency perception above 5000 Hz. Naturally, both place and phase locking mechanisms do not operate exclusive of one another with the place mechanism being in operation over the range of human hearing with phase locking resulting in better frequency discrimination up to 4000 to 5000 Hz (Moore, 1993).

Differential Sensitivity for Intensity

Historically the main methods to measure differential sensitivity for intensity (ΔI) have been modulation detection, increment detection, and intensity discrimination between successive pure tones (Moore, 1997). Using an adaptive two-alternative forced-choice technique (2AFC), the modulation detection paradigm would present an unmodulated interval and amplitude modulated (AM) interval to the listener whose task would be to indicate which interval contained the AM signal. The increment detection (continuous pedestal) paradigm using 2AFC would have a continuous tone occurring during both intervals, with one interval containing an increment superimposed on the continuous tone, much like the classic Short Increment Sensitivity Index (SISI) test (Jerger, Shedd, & Harford, 1959). The listener's task is to indicate which interval contains the increment. For the intensity discrimination between successive pure tones paradigm, the listener is presented two successive tones/pulses (gated pedestal) with one tone being more intense than the other tone and with each tone assigned to a separate interval. Again, the listener's task is to identify the interval that contains the more intense tone.

In the seminal study on differential sensitivity for intensity, Riesz (1928), like Shower and Biddulph, overcame the transient click problem of that era, which resulted from turning pure tones off and on by using amplitude modulated (AM) tones where two pure tones that differed slightly in frequency were presented simultaneously. For example, if a 1000-Hz and a 1003-Hz tone were presented simultaneously, the resulting tone would modulate (beat) at a rate equal to the frequency difference of the two stimuli, which in this case would be 3 Hz, which Riesz determined to be the optimum modulation rate to study DLs for intensity. Reisz's listeners adjusted the intensity

of the AM tone until they could detect the beats for a broad range of frequencies (35–10,000 Hz) presented at an equally broad range of SLs (0–100 dB). Weber's law predicts that the differential sensitivity fraction/ratio ($\Delta I/I$) will be constant irrespective of stimulus level or frequency. Riesz (1928), however, demonstrated that the $\Delta I/I$ had an intensity effect particularly at low SLs where the fraction was reduced as intensity increased. At moderate and high SLs, Riesz's data came close to approximating the prediction of Weber's law; the approximation is referred to as the "near miss" to Weber's law. Subsequent investigations (Florentine, Buus, & Mason, 1987; Jesteadt, Wier, & Green, 1977; Moore & Raab, 1974; Viemeister & Bacon, 1988) have likewise supported the "near miss" to Weber's law for the SL parameter.

In addition to an intensity effect for $\Delta I/I$, Riesz's (1928) data reflected a frequency effect; the $\Delta I/I$ was inversely related to frequency up to 1000 Hz (i.e., $\Delta I/I$ was reduced as frequency increased). Above 1000 Hz, Riesz's data were consistent with the prediction of Weber's law. Subsequent investigations (Jesteadt et al., 1977; Schacknow & Raab, 1973), however, did not support Riesz's findings. Specifically, Jesteadt et al. (1977) did not report a frequency effect, showing instead that $\Delta I/I$ was constant across frequencies at any given SL. Another investigation (Florentine et al., 1987) did find, in general, a frequency effect although there was not a strong frequency effect at analogous frequencies tested by Jesteadt et al. (1977). A compilation of results (Gelfand, 2004) suggests that Weber's law is consistent for a range of SLs, 10 to 40 dB (Rabinowitz, Lim, Braida, & Durlach, 1976) or 20 to

50 dB (Viemeister & Bacon, 1988), but shows an SL effect above and below these ranges. In short, DLs for intensity become smaller as the SL increases for mid-frequency stimuli (Gelfand, 2004).

Differing intensity DL results among investigations could be attributed to the test paradigm differences. Recall that Riesz (1928) used the AM methods, whereas Jesteadt et al. (1977) used the increment detection (continuous pedestal) method, and others (Florentine et al., 1987; Viemeister & Bacon, 1988) utilized the intensity discrimination between successive tones (gated pedestal) method. Turner, Zwislocki, and Filion (1989) compared the increment detection and successive tone methods and reported smaller intensity DLs for the increment detection method.

Profile Analysis

As reflected above, the traditional method for studying intensity discrimination used individual single frequencies, that is, noncomplex stimuli. Profile analysis (Green, 1988) is a contemporary paradigm which utilizes a multifrequency complex to study intensity discrimination. Typically, the stimulus is comprised of a 21-frequency complex, encompassing a range of frequencies such as, 300 to 3000 Hz or 200 to 5000 Hz, in which all the components are equally, logarithmically spaced along the frequency range and are of equal amplitude. In the typical two-alternative forced choice paradigm, the listener is presented with a standard (reference) stimulus of a 21-frequency complex in one interval and, in the other interval, a background stimulus made-up of a 20-frequency complex with a single frequency being greater in intensity than the other component frequencies (see

Figure 2–7). Naturally, the listener's task is to identify the interval that contains the signal/target frequency contained within the multifrequency background complex. The frequency of the target signal frequency is varied on each trial. To ensure that the listener is discriminating spectral shape rather than the overall spectrum level of the two stimuli, a roving-standard procedure is used whereby the intensity of the standard (reference) stimulus and target signal are randomly varied for each presentation.

The intensity discrimination threshold derived from a profile analysis task appears to be better than comparable DLs for single frequency paradigms. The profile analysis thresholds, however, are, affected by the frequency location of the increment component signal within the multifrequency background complex. When the frequency of the signal increment component is in the middle of the multifrequency complex (500–2000 Hz), the thresholds are smaller than when the increment frequency is closer to each end of the frequency range. The profile analysis thresholds are better when the range of frequencies that comprise the background stimuli widens and the number of frequency components within the range increases (Green, 1993). Conversely, the profile analysis threshold becomes poorer when components that are near in frequency to the target frequency are added (Green, 1993).

Loudness

Although the physical measure of sound is the decibel scale, the subjective measure (psychological attribute) of sound is loudness. Even though there are similar-

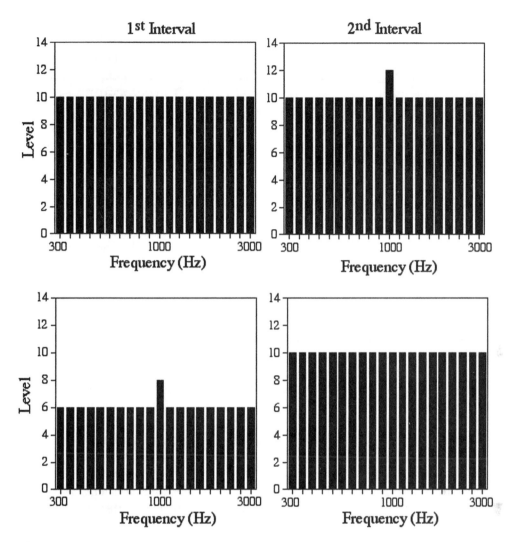

Figure 2–7. Illustration of profile analysis using a two-interval forced choice procedure with roving levels. The listener is to indicate which interval contains the signal level that differs from the background frequencies.

ities between the two measurements, such that loudness increases when intensity increases, they do not increase at the same rate, as illustrated by loudness contour curves, which are the common way to equate intensity and loudness. These contour curves plot the intensity of different frequencies as they are compared to the loudness of a 1000-Hz reference tone so as to be perceived as equal in loudness to the reference tone.

Fletcher and Munson (1933) established loudness contour curves by asking listeners to match the loudness of tones of varying frequency to the loudness of a 1000-Hz reference tone set at varying sound pressure levels (SPLs). Figure 2–8 displays an example of loudness contour

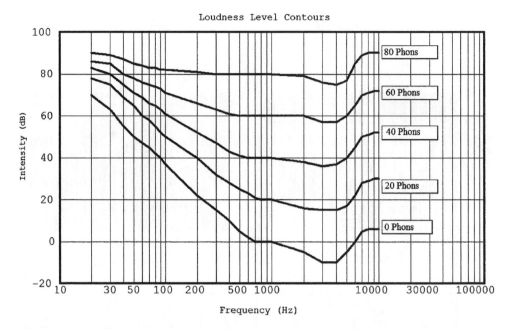

Figure 2–8. Illustration of equal loudness contours based on the data of Fletcher and Munson (1933). Frequencies are depicted along the x-axis and the perceived loudness intensity is along the y-axis. (Redrawn with permission from Harvey Fletcher, *The Journal of the Acoustical Society of America*, 5, 82. Copyright 1933, Acoustical Society of America.)

curves. Examination of these loudness contour curves shows that the sensation of loudness grows faster in the low frequencies than it does in the high frequencies. Notice how the rate of loudness grows steeper for low frequencies as the intensity of the reference decreases. Stated differently, more energy is required to reach the same loudness level as frequency decreases. The rate of loudness growth remains relatively flat across the mid-frequencies; however, an increase in the growth of loudness is noted in the extreme high frequencies. Note that the loudness contour curve at 0 phons equals the minimum audible field (MAF) threshold curve.

The phon is the unit of loudness level most commonly used and is referenced to a 1000-Hz tone at 40-dB SPL. As illus-trated in Figure 2–8, a tone with a loud-ness of 40 phons would match the loud-ness of a 40-dB SPL tone at 1000 Hz and a tone with a loudness of 20 phons would match the loudness of a 20-dB SPL tone at 1000 Hz. Thus, all the tones (fre-quencies) on a particular phon curve (equal loudness contour) are considered to be equal in loudness to the reference SPL level at 1000 Hz for that particular loudness contour.

Another way to depict loudness is the sone scale which provides a comparison in loudness between two stimuli (see Figure 2–9). Like the phon scale, the sone scale uses a 1000 Hz tone at 40-dB SPL as the reference. Thus, one sone equals the loudness level of 40 phons; two sones are twice the loudness of one sone; and three sones are three times the

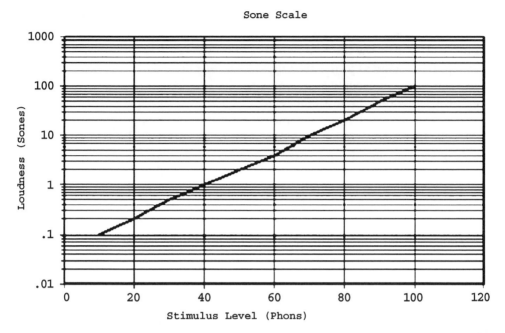

Figure 2–9. Illustration of sone scale with loudness in sones depicted as a function of stimulus level in phons such that 40-dB SPL or 40 phons equals one sone. A 10-dB increase in level (to 50-dB SPL) is equal to a doubling in loudness (2 sones). Another 10-dB increase in level (to 60 dB) is equal to another doubling in loudness (4 sones).

loudness of one sone. When loudness is expressed in sones, frequency is not relevant because the reference is the phon, which represents the same loudness level across frequencies.

Factors Affecting Loudness Perception

Duration affects loudness perception: the perceived loudness of a stimulus changes as the duration of the tone increases. Similar to absolute threshold and acoustic reflex threshold, loudness perception is affected by temporal integration (i.e., summation). (See Temporal Effects below.) Specifically, using a loudness balance paradigm with a long (500–1000 msec) reference tone and test

tones that vary (10–640 msec) in duration, Richards (1977) demonstrated that loudness perception increases up to approximately 80 msec. A small amount of additional loudness integration does occur beyond the 80-msec "critical duration." The 80-msec "critical duration" value has, however, been somewhat variable among studies (Gelfand, 2004). Sensation level (SL) for the loudness matching paradigm has been shown to affect temporal integration for loudness, with SLs between 20 and 50 dB demonstrating the maximum temporal integration.

Another loudness duration effect is loudness adaptation, which is the perceived decrease in the loudness of a long, steady tone that is fixed in intensity (Gelfand, 2004). For example, a reference tone is presented and a test tone is matched in loudness to that reference. The reference tone is presented for a few minutes followed by the test tone, which is matched in loudness to the reference tone. The next consecutive loudness match will show that the test tone-reference tone loudness match was at a lower dB level than the original loudness match, thus reflecting a loudness adaptation effect. Hellman, Mikiewicz, and Scharf (1997) found that loudness adaptation increased as the stimulus frequency increases and the SL decreases. Furthermore, maximum loudness adaptation occurs within 3 minutes of the stimulus onset.

Like duration, bandwidth affects loudness perception. If the loudness of two tones is compared, they will be perceived as the same loudness as long as they remain within the same critical bandwidth. Once they become more than a critical bandwidth apart, a noticeable increase in loudness will occur (Gelfand, 2004). Suppose a listener is presented with two pairs (sets) of tones that are close in frequency, all at the same intensity level. One set of tones is designated as the reference tones and the other set as the test tones. The listener's task is to compare the loudness of the test tones to the reference tones. The distance between the pair of comparison tones is gradually increased. The listener will perceive the two sets of tones as equal in loudness as long as they are a critical bandwidth apart. Once the distance between the test tones exceeds the critical bandwidth, while the reference tones remain constant, a significant increase in loudness perception will occur as the listener compares the test tone complex to the reference tone complex. Furthermore, a loudness summation effect has been reported to occur when more tones differing in critical bandwidth are added to the test tone complex (Florentine, Buus, & Bonding, 1978; Gelfand, 2004).

Pitch

The psychological attribute of frequency is pitch. High-frequency tones stimulating the basal end of the cochlea are perceived as high pitched, and low-frequency tones stimulating the apical end of the cochlea are perceived as low pitched. The basic unit of pitch is the mel, which is referenced to a 1000 Hz tone presented at 40 dB SPL and considered to be 1000 mels in value (Stevens & Volkmann, 1940; Stevens, Volkmann, & Newman, 1937). Thus, a 1000-Hz tone at 40-dB SPL has a loudness level of 40 phons or one sone, and a pitch level of 1000 mels. A comparison frequency that is considered to be double the pitch of 1000 mels would have a pitch of 2000 mels (see Figure 2–10).

As with loudness and intensity, pitch and frequency do not increase at the same rate: pitch perception increases at a slower rate than frequency. For example, a 3000-Hz tone will have a pitch of 2000 mels. Thus, the mel scale is a condensed/compressed scale when compared to the physical parameter of frequency, although there is a close relationship between any given pitch on the mel scale and the corresponding point of maximum displacement on the basilar membrane (Humes, 1994). To appreciate further the compressed relationship between frequency and the mel scale, the 0 to 20,000 Hz range of human hearing is compressed into 3500 mels, as shown in Figure 2–10.

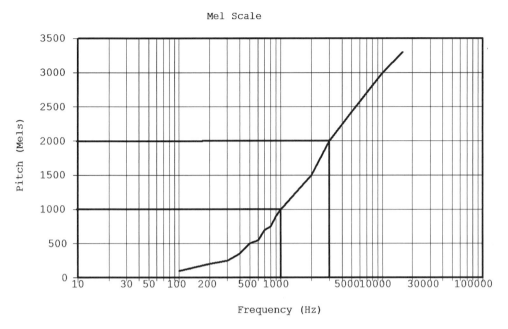

Figure 2–10. Illustration of a mel scale. In the low frequencies, pitch and frequency grow at a similar rate; however, as frequency is increased, pitch grows at a slower rate. A tripling of frequency from 1000 to 3000 Hz only doubles the pitch from 1000 to 2000 mels. (Redrawn from the *Journal of Psychology* with permission of the University of Illinois Press.)

Pitch Theories

There are two theories of pitch perception, the place theory and the temporal theory. The place theory assumes that the perceived pitch of a stimulus corresponds to the point of maximum displacement along the basilar membrane. The temporal theory implies that the perceived pitch of a stimulus is related to the temporal pattern of neuron firing (phase locking) produced by the frequency of the stimulus. The tonotopic organization of the cochlea and the close correspondence between pitch and basilar membrane displacement obviously play roles in our perception of pitch, and support the place theory of pitch perception. The temporal theory of pitch perception is supported by the "missing

fundamental" phenomenon, which is also known as "periodicity pitch," "residue pitch," or "virtual pitch" (Gelfand, 2004). Illustrating the missing fundamental phenomenon, listeners match the pitch of the complex tone to the fundamental frequency even when the complex tone is comprised only of the harmonics of the fundamental frequency, but devoid of the fundamental frequency itself. For example, a complex tone made up of a series of pure tones such as 400, 600, and 800 Hz will be perceived by the listener to have a pitch equal to 200 Hz, which is the fundamental frequency of this series of pure tones. Although no energy is present at 200 Hz, the listener will perceive the pitch of the complex stimulus as 200 Hz. Another way to demonstrate the missing fundamental phenomenon would be to present a high-frequency carrier tone that is pulsed at a slow rate. In this demonstration, the listener will choose a tone with the frequency matching the period of the pulse rate (Thurlow & Small, 1955). For example, if a 4000 Hz tone is interrupted every 2.5 msec, the listener will match the pitch of that tone to a frequency of 400 Hz as 25 msec is the period of a 400 Hz tone. Because the addition of appropriate ipsilateral masking to a multi-frequency complex tone will not mask the pitch of the fundamental frequency, a place theory cannot explain the missing fundamental phenomenon. Thus, what role do the two theories play in pitch perception? A temporal mechanism, namely, VIIIth nerve phase locking, appears to be responsible for low-frequency pitch perception and a place mechanism, tonotopic organization of the cochlea, is responsible for high-frequency pitch perception, with both mechanisms operating for mid-frequencies (Humes, 1994; Moore, 1997).

Nonsimultaneous or Temporal Masking

Nonsimultaneous masking refers to a change in detection threshold produced by a test paradigm where the masker and the test signal (probe) do not overlap in time. This psychoacoustic test paradigm is referred to as temporal masking and takes one of two forms, backward or forward. Backward masking refers to a test sequence where the test signal (probe) precedes the masker (i.e., the masking effect occurs backward in time). Forward masking refers to a test sequence where the masker precedes the test signal (see Figure 2–11). In both backward and forward masking paradigms, there is a time separation/delay between the probe and masker. In backward masking the probe is terminated before the onset of the masker. In forward masking, the masker is terminated before the onset of the probe. Forward masking appears to have been more thoroughly investigated

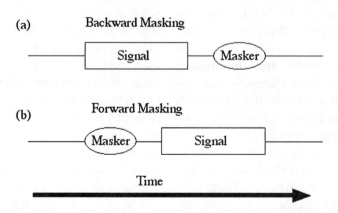

Figure 2–11. Illustration of (a) backward masking where the masker trails the signal and (b) forward masking where the masker leads the signal.

than backward masking, possibly because the backward masking effect is dependent on the amount of pretest practice the listeners have received (Moore, 1997), as well as attention to task plus the cognitive abilities of the listener (Kidd, 2002; Wright, 1998). Furthermore, minimal to no backward masking effect has been reported in listeners who have received considerable pretest instruction (Oxenham & Moore, 1994).

In comparing the reported backward and forward masking data, Gelfand (2004) offered several observations. First, backward masking provides more masking of the probe tone than does forward masking. Second, ipsilateral masking (probe and masker in the same ear) provides more masking than contralateral masking (probe and masker in opposite ears). Third, shorter delays between the probe and the masker result in greater masking effects. Fourth, the closer the probe and masker are in frequency, the greater the masking effect. In addition, the combination of backward and forward masking in a test paradigm provides a greater masking effect than the simple sum of the backward and forward masking obtained separately (Bilger, 1959; Elliott, 1969).

There is a precipitous reduction in the backward masking effect as the gap between the probe and the masker increases from 0 to 15 msec. Although the backward masking effect can still be seen when the gap is as great as 100 msec (Elliott, 1967), there is very little further reduction in the backward masking effect as the gap between the probe and the masker is extended from 15 to 100 msec. Similarly, there is a reduction in the forward masking effect, although less precipitous, as the gap between the masker and probe increases from 0 to 25 msec,

with a minimal forward masking effect occurring between 25 and 100 msec. In addition to the delay/gap parameter, temporal masking effects are influenced by the duration and intensity of the masker. Specifically, the forward masking effect increases for increments in masker duration up to approximately 20 msec (Moore, 1997), although some studies (Kidd & Feth, 1982; Zwicker, 1984) have reported an effect for masker duration of up to 200 msec. Similar masker duration effects have not been reported for backward masking (Moore, 1997). Increments in the intensity of the masker do not result in equivalent increments in the forward masking effect; roughly, a 10 dB increment in the masker will result in only a 3 dB increment in the masker effect (Gelfand, 2004; Moore, 1997). Comparable intensity effects for backward masking do not appear to have been thoroughly investigated.

Although the exact physiology underlying nonsimultaneous temporal masking is not well understood, it is hypothesized that temporal masking effects may have both peripheral and central components (Duifhuis, 1973; Gelfand, 2004; Moore, 1997). Specifically, the precipitous reduction in temporal masking as the gap between the probe and the masker increases from 0 to 15 to 25 msec has been viewed by some (Gelfand, 2004; Moore, 1997) to represent the peripheral component of temporal masking. Forward masking is thought to be primarily peripheral due to the continued response of the basilar membrane overlapping the response of the probe after the termination of the masker (Gelfand, 2004; Moore; 1997). Also underlying forward masking is the similarity between forward masking characteristics and the short-term adaptation/fatigue characteristics of the VIIIth nerve. Stated differently, the VIIIth nerve's responsiveness to the signal is reduced because of the short-term adaptation/fatigue produced by the masker (Kidd, 2002; Gelfand, 2004). Arguing against a dominant peripheral source for forward masking are the data from cochlear implant listeners (Chatterjee, 1999; Shannon, 1990) that approximates that of non-cochlear-implant listeners (Kidd, 2002). In other words, listeners devoid of the cochlea-VIIIth nerve connection produce forward masking patterns akin to listeners with a normal cochlea-VIIIth nerve connection. These data directly question whether the periphery is the predominate source of forward masking. Although it is hypothesized that backward masking, the least understood of the two temporal masking types, is predominately a centrally dominated phenomenon (Gelfand, 2004; Kidd, 2002), the hypothesis appears to be based more on speculation than research reports. The speculation may be derived from the previously mentioned observations (Kidd, 2002; Wright, 1998) that backward masking is significantly affected by attention factors and cognitive abilities.

Temporal Effects

Temporal Integration

A signal parameter that affects hearing sensitivity for tones is signal duration. Tones with durations of 200 to 300 msec will produce the lowest absolute thresholds. As the duration of a tone is increased from 30 msec to 300 msec, the absolute threshold will improve by 10 dB (i.e., a tenfold change in duration results in

a 10 dB increment in sensitivity). Conversely, a tenfold decrease in duration (from 300 msec to 30 msec) results in a 10 dB reduction in sensitivity. Tonal durations greater than 300 msec do not result in an improvement in absolute threshold. This duration effect is referred to as temporal integration/summation suggesting that the ear integrates the total stimulus energy over time, which can be described by a constant (i.e., threshold × pulse duration = constant). An alternative to the classic temporal integration model is the multiple look model, which states that the auditory system does not perform an integration function, but that the absolute threshold improves because longer stimulus duration provides more opportunity for the auditory system to sample the stimulus (Viemeister & Wakefield, 1991).

Temporal Resolution

The auditory system is required to discriminate small timing differences when processing speech. These differences can be changes over time in the envelope of the signal or changes in the amplitude modulation (AM) of the signal. The process of detecting these quick timing changes is referred to as temporal resolution and can be interrupted by hearing impairment, aging, maturational delay, and possibly (C)APD.

Gap Detection

A common method used to assess temporal resolution is to establish a gap detection threshold (GDT). The GDT is the smallest amount of silence between two signals (a sinusoid, broadband noise, or narrowband noise) that a listener can detect. Alternatively, the GDT paradigm may utilize two or more signal pairs with one signal burst containing the silent gap. In the previous paradigm, the listener's task is to indicate whether they hear two successive stimuli or one signal. In the latter paradigm, the listener's task is to indicate which of the stimulus pairs contain the gap. Another paradigm offered by a new gap detection test (Musiek, et al, 2005) utilizes a series of broadband noise segments that contain 0 to 3 gaps per segment with the gaps varying in duration. In any particular noise segment, the location and duration of the individual gaps is randomized (see Figure 2–12B).

In the simplistic GDT paradigm illustrated in Figure 2–12A, a narrowband noise signal is broken down into an initial segment followed by a silent gap followed by a final segment. The initial and final narrowband signals are referred to as markers. The length of the gap or time interval between the markers is then adjusted until the listener's GDT (the level just above where the listener cannot hear the gap) is established. At gap intervals below the GDT, the listener will perceive a constant narrow band of noise even though a silent gap is present.

When the same signal (narrow band of noise) is used as the initial marker (before the gap) as well as the final

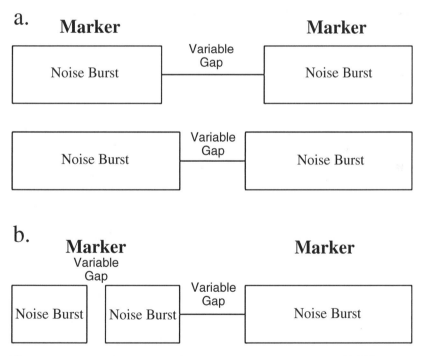

Figure 2–12. Illustration of gap detection threshold (GDT) paradigms. (a) The size of the gap between the two bands of noise (markers) is varied with the smallest gap that a listener can detect being the GDT. (b) The size of the gap between the two bands of noise (markers) is varied as is the size of the gap contained within a marker (Musiek et al., 2005).

marker (after the gap), the test is considered to be a within-channel GDT paradigm. According to the hypothesis that gap processing occurs centrally, the same perceptual channel is used to process the signal when it is presented in a within-channel paradigm. A within-channel GDT paradigm would be a monotic or diotic presentation of the marker-gap-marker test sequence with markers that are within a half octave of each other (Formby & Forrest, 1991). For example, the test sequence would begin with an initial 1000 Hz narrow band of noise followed by a gap followed by a final 1000 Hz narrow band of noise. An across-channel GDT paradigm could involve a dichotic presentation of the marker-gap-marker sequence with similar frequency markers, or a diotic/monaural presentation, but with dissimilar frequency markers (more than a half octave apart). For the across-channel paradigm, the test sequence would start with a 1000 Hz narrowband of noise followed by a gap, and then terminate with a 2000 Hz narrowband of noise. Generally, the within channel paradigm produces smaller GDTs, on the order of 2 to 24 msec, than the across channel paradigm, which are on the order of 14 to 50 msec (Formby, Gerber, Sherlock, & Magder, 1998; Grose, Hall, Buss, & Hatch, 2001; Lister, Koehnke, & Besing, 2000, 2002). According to the GDT central hypothesis, this type of test sequence is referred to as across channel because two processing channels are being utilized to accommodate the different inputs (Phillips, Taylor, Hall, Carr, & Mossip, 1997). One processing channel is used for the first marker and a second processing channel is used for the second marker. Because the GDT is similar when the test paradigm is presented dichoti-

cally or monaurally with dissimilar frequency markers, it has been suggested that the channels may be centrally located within the auditory system. (Formby, Gerber, Sherlock, & Magder, 1998; Phillips & Hall, 2000). In addition, the across-channel paradigm is thought to access higher order cortical auditory function than the within-channel paradigm, thus possibly tapping cortical mechanisms that are involved in speech perception (Formby et al., 1998; Phillips et al., 1997).

Hearing Loss and Aging Effects on GDT

GDTs have been found to be similar for listeners with hearing loss and listeners with normal hearing (Lister et al., 2000). This finding lends support to the theory that the perceptual channels for processing gap detection are centrally located because damage to the peripheral system (hearing loss) does not appear to affect the GDT. Conversely, there are studies that show either a larger GDT when a sensorineural hearing loss (SNHL) is present (DeFilippo & Snell, 1986; Florentine & Buus, 1984; Grose, Eddins, & Hall, 1989) or no difference in GDTs between normal and SNHL listeners. (Gordon-Salant & Fitzgibbons, 1999; Hall, Grose, & Buss, 1998; Moore, Peters, & Glasberg, 1992).

Strouse, Ashmead, Ohde, and Grantham (1998) found that there are age-related differences in temporal processing. Older listeners, without SNHL, were found to have higher GDTs which would appear to be an indication of an aging effect in the central auditory system. In a similar investigation, Snell and Frisina (2000) utilized GDTs as one method to measure age-related differences in temporal processing. They found that during adulthood changes in auditory processing take place as reflected in larger GDTs for the older group of subjects without SNHL. These results suggest that in the absence of peripheral hearing loss, aging of the auditory system affects temporal processing, which in turn affects speech perceptional abilities.

In summary, it is known that SNHL, aging, and maturation can affect the ability to discriminate fine temporal differences in a signal, which can affect performance on a GDT task. As the ability to detect fine differences in a signal is important when processing a speech signal, poor performance on a GDT task suggests an inability to hear the subtle acoustic changes in a speech signal that may result in speech perception difficulties. This would be especially true in the presence of background noise, where the fluctuations in the noise can obscure the fluctuations in the speech signal.

Temporal Modulation Transfer Function (TMTF)

Another way to study temporal resolution is to determine the temporal modulation transfer function (TMTF), which associates the depth of amplitude modulation (AM) to the modulation frequency. Specifically, a broadband noise of constant spectrum level is sinusoidally amplitude-modulated (see Figure 2–13). In a typical, two-alternative, forced choice paradigm, the listener is presented with a standard (reference) stimulus of a nonmodulated broadband noise in one interval and in the other interval, the sinusoidal amplitude-modulated (SAM) broadband noise that is the test stimulus. The listener's task is to identify the modulated signal. The modulation rate of the signal is varied and the listener's threshold for detection of the modulated signal is determined.

Modulated Signals

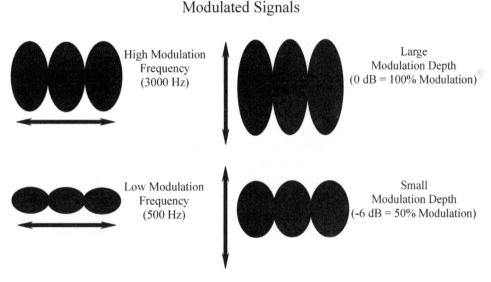

Figure 2–13. Illustrations of temporal modulated transfer function (TMTF) stimuli. The illustration on the left shows two stimuli of differing modulated frequency with the one on the top having a higher modulation rate than the illustration on the bottom. The illustration on the right demonstrates modulation depth with the one on the top having a larger modulation depth than the illustration on the bottom.

The faster the SAM rate, the closer in time the modulations occur, thus measuring temporal resolution. The TMTFs are measured according to the modulation depth, which is the depth (height) of the amplitude modulation (see Figure 2–13), with the TMTF being the point at which the listener can detect the smallest amplitude change in the modulated signal as compared to the nonmodulated signal. The TMTF can be depicted as a percent of modulation depth or expressed in decibels. Measured in this way, 0 dB would equal 100% modulation. As the modulation percentage decreases (i.e., smaller depth of modulation), the dB level becomes more negative (see Figure 2–13). For example, 50% modulation is equal to –6 dB and 25% modulation is equal to –12 dB (Gelfand, 2004). The human auditory system is most sensitive to modulation frequencies in the 2 to 50 Hz range and precipitously declines above 100 Hz (Bacon & Viemeister, 1985).

Masking Level Difference (MLD)

The masking level difference (MLD) is a psychoacoustic phenomenon in which detection or recognition of a monaurally or binaurally presented signal is improved in the presence of a binaurally competing noise. This improvement results from the auditory system's use of subtle binaural phase and amplitude level differences between simultaneously presented signals or masking noises. In two seminal articles, Hirsh (1948) and Licklider (1948) showed that the normal auditory system takes advantage of subtle, interaural time differences in the detection and/or recognition of binaurally presented acoustic stimuli producing a release from masking. This release from masking phenomenon is referred to as the MLD value.

The MLD represents an advantage in detection or recognition of the binaurally phase-altered condition in reference to the non-phase-altered condition (monaural or binaural reference). Specifically, the signal or noise in one ear is adjusted in phase from 0 to 180° relative to the signal or noise in the other ear, while the other signal or noise remains in phase interaurally. This results not only in a separation of starting phase between the two ears, but also an increase in perceptual loudness level due to the addition of waveform amplitudes that overlap (coincide) during the binaural correlation process.

Listeners with normal auditory brainstem function demonstrate a release from masking under MLD conditions, whereas listeners with certain types of auditory pathology do not demonstrate a comparable masking release. The relevant literature indicates that the MLD mechanism is located centrally, but its function can be affected by the status of the peripheral auditory system. For example, investigators have demonstrated that individuals with longstanding unilateral conductive hearing loss have reduced MLD performance, with MLD recovery occurring after the resolution of the conductive hearing loss (Hall & Grose, 1993; Wilmington, Gray, & Jahrsdoerfer, 1994). Cullen and Thompson (1974) reported equivalent MLD values for a group of normal hearing subjects and four clinical subjects who had undergone temporal lobe resections, suggesting that a bilaterally intact auditory reception cortex is not necessary for a release from masking to occur. Cullen and Thompson concluded that the MLD phenomenon is the result of two ear interaction at a subthalamic level. Subsequent studies (Lynn, Gilroy, Taylor, & Leisea, 1981; Olsen & Noffsinger, 1976; Olsen, Noffsinger, & Carhart, 1976; Quaranta & Cervellera, 1977) have shown that clinical subjects with brainstem lesions do not produce the characteristic release from masking that is reflected in the MLD measure, whereas lesions of the subcortex and cortex do not affect the MLD values. Thus, the expectation is that the results of the auditory brainstem response (ABR) and the MLD should coincide (Hannley, Jerger, & Rivera, 1983) because the MLD and some waves of the ABR are generated within the same or adjacent anatomic structures. Subsequent reports, however, do not confirm this expectation (Hurley, Hurley, & Berlin, 2002; Levine et al., 1994). A possible reason for this discrepancy is that the MLD may be dependent on phase locking by individual neurons to *some portion* of the stimulus, whereas the ABR is dependent not only on phase locking but also having all the neurons phase locking to the *same phase* of the stimulus (i.e., group synchrony) (Levine et al., 1994). Collectively, these and other results suggest that cross-correlation processes at the mid-brainstem level are responsible for the MLD.

Basic Characteristics of MLD

The MLD is generally computed in two ways: (1) the percentage improvement in the detection or recognition of an auditory signal in reference to the non-phase-altered condition or (2) the decibel (dB) improvement in the detection of an auditory signal in reference to a non-phase-altered condition. Conventional MLD nomenclature uses (S) as the signal

designation, (N) as the noise designation, (m) as the monaural designation, (o) as the binaural homophasic designation, and (π) as the binaural antiphasic designation (see Figure 2-14). The most common MLD conditions are: (1) SoNo, in which both the signal and the noise are in phase interaurally; (2) SπNo, in which the signal is 180° out of phase interaurally and the noise is in phase interaurally; and (3) SoNπ, in which the noise is 180° out of phase interaurally while the signal is in phase interaurally. In the monaural MLD paradigm, the largest MLD value is obtained for the SmNo (6-9 dB) condition followed by the SmNπ condition (3-6 dB), both referenced to SmNm. For the binaural paradigm, the largest MLD value occurs at SπNo (13-15 dB) followed by SoNπ (10-13 dB) (Gelfant, 2004; Hurley et al., 2002; Jefferss, 1972; Olsen, Noffsinger, & Carhart, 1976). One of the major variables that affect the magnitude of the MLD is the stimulus test frequency.

Several studies (Flanagan & Watson, 1966; Hirsh, 1948; Hirsh & Burgeat, 1958) have shown that the largest MLD values occur at 300 Hz decreasing above and below this frequency. The MLD values are minimal above 1500 Hz because of the auditory system's inability to transmit high frequencies effectively. Release from masking seen for stimuli which contain frequencies above 1500 Hz most likely is accounted for by interaural differences in level. Thus, the MLD is primarily a low-frequency phenomenon.

Another important parameter is the bandwidth of the binaurally competing noise. The magnitude of the MLD value appears to approach an asymptote when the noise reaches a 40 to 50 dB spectrum level (Dolan, 1968; Townsend, 1969). MLDs at low noise intensities, albeit

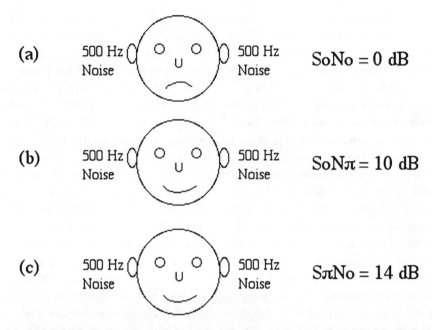

(a) 500 Hz Noise ... 500 Hz Noise $SoNo = 0 \ dB$

(b) 500 Hz Noise ... 500 Hz Noise $SoN\pi = 10 \ dB$

(c) 500 Hz Noise ... 500 Hz Noise $S\pi No = 14 \ dB$

Figure 2–14. Illustration of masking level difference (MLD) for three typical conditions with the signal being a 500-Hz pure tone and the masker being a narrow band of noise center at 500 Hz. The values for the SoNp and SpNo conditions are mean values taken from the data of Hurley et al. (2002).

reduced, may be the result of internal noise interacting with low intensity external noise producing an effective masker (Soderquist & Lindsey, 1979). This internal noise is the low-frequency jitter produced by the auditory system. A narrowband noise yields much larger MLDs for $S\pi No$ condition than a wideband noise as long as the narrowband is not smaller than the critical band of the test signal it masks. Narrower bandwidths of noise, however, do not change the detection or recognition performance for the SoNo condition (Jefferss, 1972). Variables that do not appear to significantly affect the magnitude of the MLD are age, gender, or central auditory dysfunction above the brainstem.

Theories of MLD Function

There are two theoretical models of MLD function, the lateralization-vector (L-V) theory (Jeffress, 1972) and equalization and cancellation (EC) theory (Durlach, 1972). Simplistically presented, the L-V theory states that a central process, primarily correlation processes within the central nervous system, is responsible for the MLD phenomenon. The L-V theory is based on two mechanisms that need to work sequentially: (1) a peripheral mechanism to preserve and transmit the signal and (2) a central mechanism to compare temporal information from both ears The central mechanism converts differences in time of arrival to differences in place by neural summation and reads the arriving impulses from the two ears, and then neurally delays the impulses from the ear that leads in time. This model hypothesizes that the MLD advantage in detection is provided by a lateral shift in the auditory image to one ear produced by differences in both time and level. In short, the L-V model is based on the premise the phase difference between the ears results in time of arrival differences at the central processor, which results in the release from masking effect.

The equalization and cancellation (EC) model is a nonphysiologic, electrical analogue model. The EC model postulates that the stimuli to the two ears are normally adjusted to approximate equality (equalization) and then, when the signal is altered 180° in phase interaurally, the waveform in one ear is subtracted from the waveform in the other ear resulting in a cancellation effect. The result of this subtraction is the perception of the signal alone. A pivotal component in this model is the EC factor which is the ratio between the binaural input relative to one of the monaural inputs. Thus, the EC factors describe the change in the signal-to-noise ratios, and, therefore, the change in the masked threshold produced by the binaural processing. In the EC model, processing of binaural stimuli takes place in three basic components: (1) two band pass filters representing the two ears; (2) an EC mechanism that receives the binaurally processed signal; (3) and a decision device that receives either the monaural signals directly from the band-pass filters or the binaural signal from the EC mechanism. Ideally, the EC mechanism improves the signal-to-noise ratio by transforming the total signal received at one input relative to the total signal received at the other input in such a way that the masking components become exactly the same in both channels (the E process), and then subtracting the signal in one channel from that in the other (the C process). If these operations are perfectly performed, the masking signal is completely eliminated.

Binaural Hearing

The old adage that two ears are better than one is certainly true as in more sensitive binaural DLs for both frequency and intensity relative to monaural DLs. Likewise, the binaural absolute threshold for pure tones and spondaic words is approximately 2 to 3 dB better than a monaural threshold due to binaural summation (Gelfand, 2001). In addition, binaural summation results in binaurally presented sound being perceived at twice the loudness level as monaurally presented sound (Marks, 1978; see Figure 2–15). Furthermore, binaural speech intelligibility is, on average, better than monaural speech intelligibility particularly in the presence of background noise (Moore, 1998). In short, binaural listening provides advantages in hearing sensitivity, loudness perception, general speech perception, and speech perception in adverse listening conditions.

Binaural Fusion and Binaural Beats

Two interesting binaural phenomena observed under headphones and involving the central auditory system are binaural fusion and binaural beats. Binaural fusion

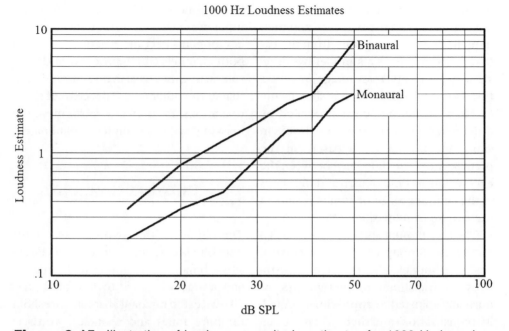

Figure 2–15. Illustration of loudness magnitude estimates for 1000 Hz based on data from Marks (1978). The lower line on the graph shows average loudness magnitude estimates for monaural listening, while the upper line on the graph shows loudness magnitude estimates for binaural listening. (Redrawn with permission from L. E. Marks, *Journal of the Acoustical Society of America, 64,* 107–113. Copyright 1978, Acoustical Society of America.)

is the sensation of hearing a fused auditory signal at midline. For example, if two recordings of word lists are created by using a high-pass filter and a low-pass filter and the modified lists are presented dichotically, the listener's word identification performance for the modified word lists will be similar to identification of the original (i.e., unfiltered) word list (Bornstein, Wilson, & Combron, 1994). The human auditory system combines the high pass information in one ear and the low pass information in the other ear to derive a *fused* word. In this scenario, the stimuli are the same words with different filtering characteristics. If completely different stimuli are presented to each ear, there will be no fusion in the midline as signals must be similar for the

fusion effect to occur (Cherry & Sayers, 1957). The fusion phenomenon is frequency sensitive in that, if different high-frequency tones are presented to the ears of a listener, the listener will report hearing separate tones; however, if a low-frequency tone is superimposed over both high-frequency tones, the listener will report hearing a fused auditory signal (Leaky, Sayers, & Cherry, 1958). The probable site of a "fusion mechanism" (Cherry & Sayers, 1957) is within the central auditory system where a cross-correlation analysis takes place.

Another interesting phenomenon, which occurs with binaural fusion, is binaural beats. Beats occur when two stimuli, close in frequency, are presented simultaneously to one ear resulting in a waxing and waning perception (Gelfand, 2004). Beats will also occur when tones close in frequency are presented dichotically to each ear. For example, if a 600-Hz tone is presented to the right ear and a 603-Hz tone is presented to the left ear, the listener will perceive a 600-Hz tone at midline that waxes and wanes in loudness at a rate of three per second. The binaural beat phenomenon will occur for two frequencies that are 2 to 10 Hz apart, and may be perceived until the frequency separation is approximately 20 Hz apart. After this point, the stimuli are perceived as two separate tones lateralized to each individual ear. The binaural beat phenomenon is optimal for frequencies between 300 and 600 Hz (Licklider, Webster, & Hedlun, 1950). Like, binaural fusion, the binaural beat phenomenon involves processing within the central auditory system with the superior olive complex being implicated as the control center (Wernick & Starr, 1966).

Directional Hearing

One of the advantages of being a two-eared listener is the ability to locate a sound source in the everyday listening environment. Localization ability is based on two parameters of a signal that become modified through travel from a sound source to each ear. The two parameters are time of arrival differences and intensity differences between the ears. If the signal is presented to the right side of the head, it has to travel farther to reach the left ear, compared to the right ear, resulting in an interaural time difference (ITD) and an interaural intensity difference (IID). Neither of these interaural differences is consciously perceived by the listener who hears a fused single sound.

ITD varies as a function of the azimuth (angle) relative to the head position (see Figure 2–16). ITDs increase from zero when the sound source is either directly in front of the listener or directly behind the listener (0° or 180° azimuth), to a maximum when the sound source is to either side (90° azimuth) of the listener (Feddersen, Sandel, Teas, & Jeffress, 1957). The ITD and IID effects are frequency specific. The wavelengths of low-frequency tones are long enough to bend around the head creating an ITD between the ears which provides a localization clue. For high-frequency tones, the IID serves as the localization cue because the wavelength of high-frequency tones is too short to bend around the head; therefore, a "head shadow" effect occurs resulting in an IID between ears (see Figure 2–17). The IID is negligible at low frequencies, but can be as large as 20 dB at high frequencies (Fedderson et al., 1957). In addition to ITD and IID, spectral changes in the stimulus brought about by the folds of the pinna coupled with reflections from the head and torso provide localization cues. These pinna-induced spectral changes assist the listener in locating an elevated sound source, front/back discrimination, and monaural localization (Middlebrooks, 1992). Listeners' localization abilities are most accurate below 1000 Hz and above 4000 Hz, whereas most listener localization errors occur between 2000 and 4000 Hz. Lastly, localization is better for complex stimuli than for pure tones (Stevens & Newman, 1936).

Directional hearing also involves the ability to identify small changes in position of the sound source, that is, the minimum audible angle. Listeners are able to identify the smallest change in location of a sound source when the frequency is below 1500 Hz and above 2000 Hz

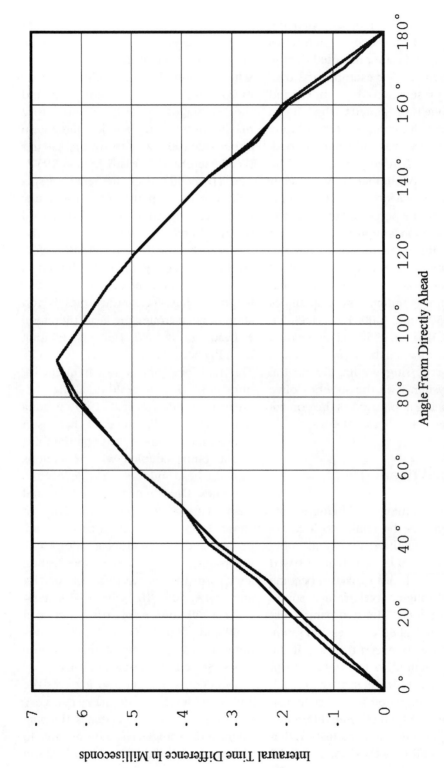

Figure 2–16. Illustration of interaural time differences (ITD) as a function of azumith from the head (Fedderson et al., 1957). Note that there is no ITD between ears when the signal is directly in front (0° azimuth) or behind (180° azumith) the listener. The largest ITD occurs when the signal is presented directly to the opposite ear (90° azumith). (Redrawn with permission from W. E. Feddersen, *The Journal of the Acoustical Society of America, 29,* 988. Copyright 1957, Acoustical Society of America.)

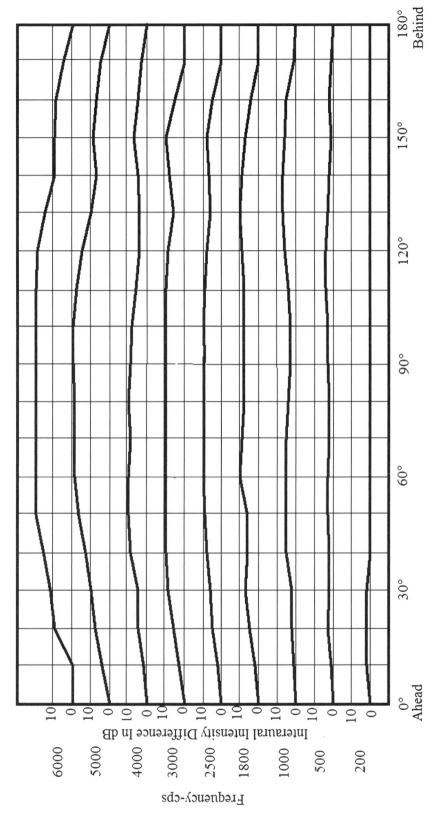

Figure 2–17. Illustration of interaural intensity differences (IID) as measured by frequency (Fedderson et al., 1957). IID is negligible between ears at 200 Hz. As the frequency becomes higher, the amount of IID between ears becomes larger, increasing to approximately 20 dB at 6000 Hz. (Redrawn with permission from W. E. Feddersen, *The Journal of the Acoustical Society of America, 29,* 988. Copyright 1957, Acoustical Society of America.)

(Mills, 1958, 1972). Between 1500 Hz and 2000 Hz, listeners demonstrate the poorest ability to discriminate a change in the sound source location. Listeners are able to discriminate 1° to 2° changes in azimuth when a sound source is located at a 0° azimuth or directly in front of them because small changes in location result in large ITDs (Mills, 1958). The poorest discrimination of azimuth degree change in the minimal audible angle occurs when the sound source is located to either side (90° and 270° azimuth) of the listener because the IID remains the same despite large changes in sound source location (Gelfand, 2004). This lateral head area is designated the "cone of confusion" reflecting the poor discrimination of the minimal audible angle changes (Gelfand, 2004). Despite the fact that there is a large area in which listeners have difficulty discriminating fine changes in the direction of a sound source, listeners are able to compensate with head movement which constantly changes the direction of the "cone of confusion," thus minimizing its effect (Moore, 1998).

Lateralization

A psychoacoustic phenomenon related to localization is lateralization. The major difference between localization and lateralization paradigms is that the former uses a sound field to deliver test stimuli while the latter utilizes earphones to deliver the test stimuli. Binaural presentations of stimuli that are equal in frequency and intensity, and have no significant interaural temporal differences, will result in a fused perception with the listener hearing only one sound in the midline. A change in interaural intensity will

result in the well-known Stenger effect, with the listener perceiving one sound that is lateralized to the ear receiving the greater intensity. Binaural presentation of two stimuli equal in intensity, but differing in frequency will result in the listener perceiving two stimuli. In the lateralization paradigm, the use of earphones allows one to vary independently the IID and ITD; however, in a localization paradigm, IID and ITD cannot be separated due to sound field presentation.

A common paradigm to study IID and ITD utilizes a two-alternative forced-choice design with successive presentations of binaural stimuli that have an interaural difference (i.e., IID or ITD). One stimulus will be the same at each ear whereas the other stimulus will have an IID or ITD. The listener indicates if the second stimulus was different from the first stimulus or if the second stimulus changed location relative to the first stimulus. Using the first paradigm, Yost (1974) studied phase discrimination (ITD) by presenting a reference stimulus that had an interaural phase difference (θ) creating lateralization to one side of the head followed by presentation of a test stimulus that had varying amounts of phase differences ($\Delta\theta$) larger than the reference stimulus ($\theta + \Delta\theta$). Yost's findings are illustrated in Figure 2–18A. Note that interaural phase discrimination was the best at 0° and 360°, which corresponds to zero phase differences between the ears. The poorest interaural phase discriminations were seen at 180°, where the test signals lateralized to one side. Phase difference ($\Delta\theta$) discrimination was essentially the same for frequencies up to 900 Hz, but much poorer at 2000 Hz. These findings suggest that interaural phase appears to be an important cue for low-frequency lateralization, but not for

(a)

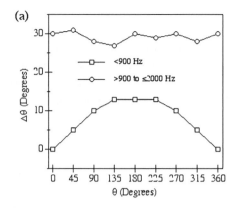

(b)

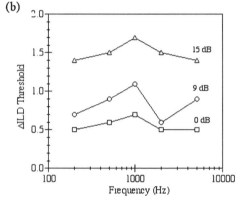

Figure 2–18. (a) The amount of interaural phase change (Δθ) needed to discriminate a lateralization change from a reference (θ). (Adapted and redrawn with permission from William A. Yost, *The Journal of the Acoustical Society of America*, *83*, 1846. Copyright 1988, Acoustical Society of America.) (b) Interaural intensity difference (IID) thresholds as a function of frequency from 200–5000 Hz. (Redrawn with permission from William A. Yost, *The Journal of the Acoustical Society of America*, *55*, 1299. Copyright 1974, Acoustical Society of America.)

higher frequency lateralization, a finding consistent with the role of timing cues for localization.

Figure 2–18B depicts IID discrimination as a function of frequency from 200 to 5000 Hz. IID is rather constant across frequency for a particular lateralization site, with a slight increase at 1000 Hz. The 0, 9, and 15 dB designations in Figure 2–18B are the IID values used to produce lateralization sites at the midline, halfway between the midline and the left ear, and the left ear, respectively. Clearly, the midline lateralization site produced the best IID discrimination, with the poorest IID discrimination occurring at the left ear lateralization site. Although lateralization research suggests that ITD is the main clue for low frequencies, interaural time also seems to provide the binaural system cues for complex high-frequency sounds that may be modulated by a low-frequency component (Yost, 2000). For example, consider three stimuli, a 250 Hz tone, a 3000 Hz tone, and a 3500 Hz tone that are amplitude modulated (AM) by a 250 Hz tone. Listeners will be able to detect an ITD for the 250 Hz tone, but not for the 3000 Hz tone. On the other hand, listeners will detect an ITD for the 3500 Hz tone that is AM by a 250 Hz tone (Gelfand, 2004). In summary, lateralization research indicates that IID is the cue for high frequencies, and ITD is the cue for low frequencies and for complex stimuli that consist of a high-frequency carrier that undergoes low-frequency repetition.

With the advent of virtual reality technology, a sound field environment can be simulated accurately by using each listener's head-related transfer function (HRTF) for each ear to create stimuli containing the necessary perceptual cues that can be well controlled through earphone presentation. Due to individual differences in skull, torso, and pinna, the HRTF must be determined for each listener so that the amplitude and phase spectra contain the cues unique to the listener for an earphone virtual reality test paradigm to be accurate. A number of investigations comparing individualized versus nonindividualized HRTFs to assess simulated localization performance demonstrated poorer performance when listeners used other than their own HRTF in the virtual reality experiment (Middlebrooks, 1999; Møller, Sorensen, Jensen, & Hammershoi, 1996; Wenzel, Arruda, Kistler, & Wightman, 1993). At least one study comparing sound field localization and earphone simulated localization reported correlation coefficients of 0.97 to 0.98 between the actual sound location and the subject's sound field judgments and correlations of 0.83 to 0.96 between the actual sound location and the subject's simulated virtual reality earphone judgments (Wightman, et al., 1987). See Chapter 11 for additional discussion of binaural listening and clinical measurement of binaural fusion, localization, lateralization, and other measures of binaural interaction.

Summary

The goals of this chapter were to provide a brief review of classic and contemporary psychoacoustic methods and phenomena, indirectly highlight aspects of psychoacoustics that might apply to (C)APD diagnosis, and leave the reader wondering why basic psychoacoustic profiles of listeners with (C)APD have yet to be created. High precision in measuring human test performance is one of the basic foundations of "evidence-based audiology" (Bess, 1995; Cox, 2005). In order to exact this precision, however, each examiner must understand that any given behavioral response to an auditory test stimulus could be a true indication of the listener's perception, a guess on the part of the listener, or a change in the listener's response criterion (bias) (see Silman, Silverman, & Emmer, 2000). Coupling sound measurement methods with psychoacoustic profiling should lead to a better understanding of the perceptual deficit(s) that listeners with (C)APD experience and better define the heterogeneous profiles seen in (C)APD. Technologic advances such as virtual source auditory testing (Besing & Koehnke, 1995; Koehnke & Besing, 1996) need to be paired with psychoacoustics to study (C)APD. Lastly, before psychoacoustic profiling can be used to guide customized treatment for (C)APD, additional psychoacoustic data from listeners with confirmed (C)APD are needed.

References

Bacon, S. P., & Viemeister, N. F. (1985). Temporal modulation transfer functions in normal-hearing and hearing-impaired subjects. *Audiology, 24,* 117–134.

Besing, J., & Koehnke, J. (1995). A test of virtual auditory localization. *Ear and Hearing, 16,* 220–229.

Bess, F. H. (1995). Evidence-based audiology. *American Journal of Audiology, 4,* 5.

Bilger, R. C. (1959). Additivity of different types of masking. *Journal of the Acoustical Society of America, 31,* 1107–1109.

Bornstein, S. P., Willson, R. H., & Combron, N. K. (1994). Low-and-high-pass filtered Northwestern University Auditory Test No. 6 for monaural and binaural evaluation. *Journal of the American Academy of Audiology, 5,* 259–264.

Budd, T. W., Hall, D. A., Gonclaves, M. S., Akeroyd, M. A., Foster, J. R., Palmer, A. R., Head, K., & Summerfield, A. Q. (2003). Binaural specialization in human auditory cortex: An fMRI investigation of interaural correlation sensitivity. *NeuroImage, 20,* 1783-1794.

Carhart, R., & Jerger, J. (1959). Preferred method for clinical determination of pure-tone thresholds. *Journal of Speech and Hearing Disorders, 16,* 340-345.

Chatterjee, M. (1999). Temporal mechanisms underlying recovery from forward masking in multielectrode-implant listeners. *Journal of the Acoustical Society of America. 105,* 1853-1863.

Cherry, E. C., & Sayers, B. McA. (1957). "Human cross correlator" A technique for measuring certain parameters of speech perception. *Journal of the Acoustical Society of America, 28,* 889-896.

Cox, R. (2005). Evidence-based practice in provision of amplification. *Journal of the American Academy of Audiology, 16,* 419-438.

Cullen, J. K., & Thompson, C. L. (1974). Masking release for speech in subjects with temporal lobe resections. *Archives of Otolaryngology, 100,* 113-116.

DeFilippo, C. L., & Snell, K. B. (1986). Detection of a temporal gap in low-frequency narrow-band signals by normal-hearing and hearing-impaired listeners. *Journal of the Acoustical Society of America, 80,* 1354-1358.

Dolan, T. R. (1968). Effects of masker spectrum level on masking level differences at low signal frequencies. *Journal of the Acoustical Society of America, 44,* 1507-1512.

Duifhuis, H. (1973). Consequences of peripheral frequency selectivity for nonsimultaneous masking. *Journal of the Acoustical Society of America, 54,* 1471-1188.

Durlach, N. I. (1972). Equalization and cancellation theory. In J. V. Tobias (Ed.), *Foundations of modern auditory theory* (Vol, 2, pp. 369-462). New York: Academic Press.

Elliott, L. L. (1967). Development of auditory narrow-band frequency contours. *Journal of the Acoustical Society of America, 42,* 143-153.

Elliott, L. L. (1969). Masking of tones before, during, and after brief silent periods in noise. *Journal of the Acoustical Society of America, 45,* 1277-1279.

Feddersen, W. E., Sandel, T. T., Teas, D. C. & Jeffress, L. A. (1957). Localization of high frequency tones. *Journal of the Acoustical Society of America, 29,* 988-991.

Flanagan, J. L., & Watson, B. J. (1966). Binaural unmasking of complex signals. *Journal of the Acoustical Society America, 40,* 456-468.

Fletcher, H., & Munson, W. A. (1933). Loudness, its definition, measurement, and calculation. *Journal of the Acoustical Society of America, 5,* 82-105.

Florentine, M., & Buus, S. (1984). Temporal gap detection in sensorineural and simulated hearing impairments. *Journal of Speech and Hearing Research, 27,* 449-455.

Florentine, M., Buus, S., & Bonding, P. (1978). Loudness of complex sounds as a function of the standard stimulus and the number of components. *Journal of the Acoustical Society of America, 64,* 1036-1040.

Florentine, M., Buus, S., & Mason, C. R. (1987). Level discrimination as a function of level for tones from 0.25 to 16 kHz. *Journal of the Acoustical Society of America, 81,* 1528-1541.

Formby, C., & Forrest, T. G. (1991). Detection of silent temporal gaps in sinusoidal markers. *Journal of the Acoustical Society of America, 89,* 830-837.

Formby, C., Gerber, M., Sherlock, L., & Magder. L. (1998). Evidence for an across-frequency, between-channel process in asymptotic monaural temporal gap detection. *Journal of the Acoustical Society of America, 103,* 3554-3560.

Gelfand, S. A. (2001). *Essentials of audiology,* New York: Thieme Medical Publishers.

Gelfand, S. A. (2004). *Hearing: An Introduction to psychological and physiological acoustics* (4th ed., pp. 243-431), New York: Marcel Dekker.

Gordon-Salant, S., & Fitzgibbons, P. (1999). Profile of auditory temporal processing in older listeners. *Journal of Speech Language and Hearing Research, 42,* 300–311.

Grantham, D. W. (1984). Interaural intensity discrimination: Insensitivity at 1000 Hz. *Journal of the Acoustical Society of America, 75,* 1190–1194.

Green, D. M. (1988). *Profile analysis: Auditory intensity discrimination.* New York: Oxford University Press.

Green, D. M. (1993). Auditory intensity discrimination. In W. A. Yost, A. N. Popper, & R. R. Fay (Eds)., *Human psychophysics* (pp. 13–55). New York: Springer-Verlag.

Green, D. M., & Swets, J. A. (1974). *Signal detection theory and psychoacoustics.* New York: Kreiger.

Grose, J. H., Eddins D. A., & Hall, J. W. (1989). Gap detection as a function of stimulus bandwidth with fixed high-frequency cutoff in normal-hearing and hearing-impaired listeners. *Journal of the Acoustical Society of America, 86,* 1747–1755.

Gross, J. H., Hall, J. W., Buss, E., & Hatch, D. (2001). Gap detection for similar and dissimilar gap markers. *Journal of the Acoustical Society of America, 109,* 1158–1595.

Hall, J. W., & Grose, J. H. (1993). Short-term and long-term effects on the masking level difference following middle ear surgery. *Journal of the American Academy of Audiology, 4,* 307–312.

Hall, J., Grose, J., & Buss, E. (1998). Temporal analysis and stimulus fluctuation in listeners with normal and impaired hearing. *Journal of Speech Language and Hearing Research, 41,* 340–354.

Hannley, M., Jerger, J. F., & Rivera, V. M. (1983). Relationship among auditory brain stem responses, masking level differences and the acoustic reflex in multiple sclerosis. *Audiology, 22,* 20–33.

Harris, J. D. (1952). Pitch discrimination. *Journal of the Acoustical Society of America, 24,* 750–255.

Hellman R., Mikiewicz, A., & Scharf, B. (1997). Loudness adaptation and excitation patterns: Effects of frequency and level. *Jour-*

nal of the Acoustical Society of America, 101,* 2176–2185.

Hirsh, I. J. (1948). The influence of interaural phase on summation and inhibition. *Journal of the Acoustical Society America, 20,* 536–544.

Hirsh, I. J., & Burgeat, M. (1958).Binaural effects in remote masking. *Journal of the Acoustical Society America, 30,* 827–832.

Humes, L. E. (1994). Psychacoustic considerations in clinical audiology. In J. Katz (Ed.), *Handbook of clinical audiology* (4th ed., pp. 56–72). Baltimore: Williams and Wilkins.

Hurley, R. M., Hurley, A., & Berlin, C. I. (2002). The effect of midline petrous apex lesions on tests of afferent and efferent auditory function. *Ear and Hearing,. 23,* 224–234.

Hurley, R. M., & Musiek, F. M. (1997). Effectiveness of three central auditory processing (CAP) tests in identifying cerebral lesions. *Journal of the American Academy of Audiology, 8,* 257–262.

Hyde, M. L., Davidson, M. J., & Alberti, P. W. (1991). Auditory test strategy. In Jacobson, J. T. & Northern, J. L. (Eds.), *Diagnostic audiology* (pp. 295–322). Austin, TX: Pro-Ed.

Jeffress, L. A. (1972). Binaural signal detection vector theory. In J. V. Tobias (Ed.), *Foundations of modern auditory theory* (Vol. 2, pp. 351–368). New York: Academic Press.

Jerger, J., Shedd, J. L., & Harford, E. (1959). On the detection of extremely small changes in sound intensity. *Archives of Otolaryngology, 69,* 200–211.

Jesteadt, W., Wier, C. C., & Green, D. M. (1977). Intensity discrimination as a function of frequency and sensation level. *Journal of the Acoustical Society of America, 61,* 169–177.

Kidd, G. (2002). Psychoacoustics. In J. Katz (Ed.), *Handbook of clinical audiology* (5th ed., pp. 33–49). Philadelphia: Lippincott Williams and Wilkins.

Kidd, G., & Feth, L. L. (1982). Effects of masker duration in pure-tone forward masking. *Journal of the Acoustical Society of America, 72,* 1384–1386.

Koehnke, J., & Besing, J. M. (1996). A procedure for testing speech intelligibility in a virtual listening environment. *Ear and Hearing, 17*, 211-217.

Leaky, D. M., Sayers, B., & Cherry, E. C. (1958). Binaural fusion of low and high frequency sounds. *Journal of the Acoustical Society of America, 30*, 222-223.

Levine, R. A., Gardner, J. C., Fullerton, B. C., Stufflebeam, S. M., Carlisle, E. W., Furst, M., & Rosen, B. R. (1994). Multiple sclerosis lesions of the auditory pons are not silent. *Brain, 117*, 1127-1141.

Levitt, H. (1971). Transformed up-down methods in psychoacoustics. *Journal of the Acoustical Society of America, 49*, 467-477.

Levitt, H. (1978). Adaptive testing in audiology. *Scandanavian Audiology, 6*(Suppl.), 241-291.

Licklider, J. C. R. (1948). The influence of interaural phase relations upon masking of speech by white noise. *Journal of the Acoustical Society America, 20*, 150-159.

Licklider, J. C. R., Webster, J. C., & Hedlun, J. M. (1950). On the frequency limits of binaural beats. *Journal of the Acoustical Society of America, 22*, 468-473.

Lister, J. J., Besing, J. M., & Koehnke, J. D. (2002). Effects of age and frequency disparity on gap duration discrimination. *Journal of the Acoustical Society of America, 11*, 2793-2800.

Lister, J. J., Koehnke, J. D., & Besing, J. M. (2000). Binaural gap duration discrimination in listeners with impaired hearing and normal hearing. *Ear and Hearing, 21*, 141-150.

Lynn, G. E., Gilroy, J., Taylor, P. C., & Leisea, R. P. (1981). Binaural masking level difference in neurological disorders. *Archives of Otolaryngology, 107*, 357-362.

MacMillian, N. A., & Creelman, C. D. (1991). *Detection theory: A user's guide.* Cambridge, MA: Cambridge University Press.

Marks, L. E. (1978). Binaural summation of loudness of pure tones. *Journal of the Acoustical Society of America, 64*, 107-113.

Middlebrooks, J. C. (1992). Narrow-band sound localization related to external ear acoustics. *Journal of the Acoustical Society of America, 92*, 2607-2624.

Middlebrooks, J. C. (1999). Virtual localization improved by scaling nonindividualized external-ear transfer functions in frequency. *Journal of the Acoustical Society of America, 106*, 1493-1510.

Mills, A. W. (1958). On the minimal audible angle. *Journal of the Acoustical Society of America, 30*, 237-246.

Mills, A. W. (1972). Auditory localization. In J. V. Tobias (Ed.), *Foundations of modern auditory theory* (Vol. 2, pp. 301-348). New York: Academic Press.

Møller, H., Sorensen, M. F., Jensen, C. B., & Hammershoi, D. (1996). Binaural technique: Do we need individual recordings? *Journal of Audio Engineering Society, 44*, 451-469.

Moore. B. J. C. (1973). Frequency difference limen for short duration tones. *Journal of the Acoustical Society of America, 54*, 610-619.

Moore. B. J. C. (1993). Frequency analysis and pitch perception. In W. A. Yost, A. N. Popper, & R. R. Fay (Eds.), *Human psychophysics* (pp. 56-115), New York: Springer-Verlag.

Moore, B. C. J. (1998). *Cochlear hearing loss.* London, UK: Whurr Publishers Ltd.

Moore, B. C. J. (1997). *An introduction to the psychology of hearing.* London, UK: Academic Press.

Moore, B. C. J., Peters, R. W., & Glasberg, B. R. (1992). Detection of temporal gaps in sinusoids by elderly subjects with and without hearing loss. *Journal of the Acoustical Society of America, 92*, 1923-1932.

Moore, B. C. J., & Raab, D. H. (1974). Pure-tone intensity discrimination: Some experiments relating to the "near miss" to Weber's law. *Journal of the Acoustical Society of America, 55*, 1049-1054.

Musiek, F. E., Shinn, J. B., Jirsa, R., Bamiou, D-E., Baran, J. A., & Zaidan, E. (2005). GIN (gap-in-noise) test performance in subjects with confirmed central auditory nervous system involvement. *Ear and Hearing, 26,* 608–618.

Olsen, W. O., & Noffsinger, D. (1976). Masking level differences for cochlear and brainstem lesions. *Annals of Otology, Rhinology and Laryngology, 85,* 820–825.

Olsen, W. O., Noffsinger, D., & Carhart, R. (1976). Masking level differences encountered in clinical populations. *Audiology, 15,* 287–301.

Oxenham, A. J., & Moore, B. C. J. (1994). Modeling the additivity of nonsimultaneous masking. *Hearing Research, 80,* 105–118.

Phillips, D. E., & Hall, S. E. (2000). Independence of frequency channels in auditory temporal gap detection. *Journal of the Acoustical Society of America, 108,* 2957–2963.

Phillips, D. P., Taylor, T. L., Hall, S. E., Carr, M. M., & Mossop, J. E. (1997) Detection of silent intervals between noises activating difference perceptual channels: Some properties of "central" auditory gap detection. *Journal of the Acoustical Society of America, 101,* 3694–3705.

Quaranto, A., & Cervellera, G. (1977). Masking level differences in central nervous system disease. *Archives of Otolaryngology, 103,* 482–484.

Rabinowitz, W. M., Lim, L. S., Braida, L. D., & Durlach, N. I. (1976). Intensity perception: VI, summary of recent data on deviations from Weber's law for 1000 Hz tone pulses. *Journal of the Acoustical Society of America, 59,* 1506–1509.

Riesz, R. R. (1928). Differential intensity sensitivity of the ear for pure tones. *Physiological Review, 31,* 867–875.

Richards, A. M. (1977). Loudness perception for short-duration tones in masking noise. *Journal of Speech and Hearing Research, 20,* 684–693.

Schacknow, R. N., & Raab, D. H. (1973). Intensity discrimination of tone bursts and the form of the Weber function. *Perception and Psychophysics, 14,* 449–450.

Shannon, R. V. (1990). Forward masking in patients with cochlear implants. *Journal of the Acoustical Society of America, 88,* 741–744.

Shower, E. G., & Biddulph, R. (1931). Differential pitch sensitivity of the ear. *Journal of the Acoustical Society of America, 2,* 275–287.

Silman, S., Silverman, C. A., & Emmer, M. B. (2000). Central auditory processing disorders and reduced motivation: three case studies. *Journal of the American Academy of Audiology, 11,* 57–63.

Singer, J., Hurley, R. M., & Preece, J. (1998). Effectiveness of central auditory processing (CAP) tests with children. *American Journal of Audiology, 7,* 7384.

Snell, K. B. & Frisina, D. R. (2000). Relationships among age-related differences in gap detection and word recognition. *Journal of the Acoustical Society of America, 107,* 1615–1626.

Soderquist, D. R., & Lindsey, J. W. (1970). Masking level differences as a function of noise spectrum level, frequency and signal duration. *Journal of Auditory Research, 10,* 276–282.

Stevens, S. S., & Newman, E. B. (1936). The localization of actual sources of sound. *American Journal of Psychology, 48,* 297–306.

Stevens, S. S., & Volkmann, J. (1940). The relation of pitch to frequency: A revised scale. *American Journal of Psychology, 53,* 329–353.

Stevens, S. S., Volkmann, J., & Newman, E. B. (1937). A scale for the measurement of the psychological magnitude pitch. *Journal of the Acoustical Society of America, 8,* 185–190.

Strouse, A., Ashmead, D. H., Ohde, R. N., & Grantham, D. W. (1998). Temporal processing in the aging auditory system. *Journal of the Acoustical Society of America, 104,* 2385–2399.

Swets, J. A. (1964). *Signal detection and recognition by human observers.* New York: John Wiley and Sons.

Taylor, M. M., & Creelman, C. D. (1967). PEST: Efficient estimate on probability function. *Journal of the Acoustical Society of America, 41*, 782-787.

Townsend, T. H. (1969). *Binaural unmasking as a function of earphone and masker level,* unpublished doctoral dissertation, Purdue University, Lafayette, IN.

Thurlow, W. R., & Small, A. M. (1955). Pitch perception of certain periodic auditory stimuli. *Journal of the Acoustical Society of America, 27*, 132-137.

Turner, C. W., Zwisocki, J. J., & Filion, P. R. (1989). Intensity discrimination determined with two paradigms in normal and hearing-impaired subjects. *Journal of the Acoustical Society of America, 86*, 109-115.

Turner, R. G., & Nielsen, D. W. (1984). Application of clinical decision analysis to audiological tests. *Ear and Hearing, 5*, 125-133.

Turner, R. G., Robinette, M. S., & Bauch, C. D. (1999). Clinical decisions. In F. E. Musiek & W. F. Rintelmann (Eds.), *Contemporary perspectives in hearing assessment* (pp. 437-464). Needham Heights, MA: Allyn and Bacon.

Viemeister, N. F., & Bacon, S. P. (1988). Intensity discrimination, and magnitude estimation for 1-kHz tones. *Journal of the Acoustical Society of America, 84*, 172-178.

Viemeister, N. F., & Wakefild, S. P. (1991). Temporal integration and multiple looks. *Journal of the Acoustical Society of America. 90*, 858-865.

Wenzel, E. M., Arruda, M., Kistler, D. J., & Wightman, F. L. (1993). Localization using non-individualized head-related transfer functions. *Journal of the Acoustical Society of America, 94*, 111-123.

Wernick, J. S., & Starr, A. (1966). Electrophysiological correlates of binaural beats in superior olivary complex of cat. *Journal of the Acoustical Society of America, 40*, 1276.

Wier, C. C., Jesteadt, W., & Green, D. M. (1977). Frequency discrimination as a function of frequency and sensation level. *Journal of the Acoustical Society of America, 61*, 178-184.

Wightman, F. L., Kistler, D. J., & Perkins, M. E. (1987). A new approach to the study of human sound localization. In W. Yost & G. Gourevitch (Eds.). *Directional hearing.* New York: Springer-Verlag.

Wilmington, D., Gray, L., & Jahrsdoerfer, R. (1994). Binaural processing after corrected congential unilateral conductive hearing loss. *Hearing Research, 74*, 99-114.

Wright, B. A. (1998). Specific language impairment: abnormal auditory masking and the potential for its remediation through training. In A. R. Palmer, A. Reese, A. Q. Summerfield, & R. Mededis (Eds.), *Psychological and physiological advances in hearing* (pp. 604-610) London: Whurr Publishing.

Yost W. A. (1974). Discriminations of interaural phase differences. *Journal of the Acoustical Society of America, 55*, 1299-1303.

Yost, W. A. (2000). *Fundamentals of hearing: an introduction.* (4th ed., pp. 149-225). San Diego, CA: Academic Press.

Yost, W. A., & Dye, R. H. (1988). Discrimination of interaural differences of level as a function of frequency. *Journal of the Acoustical Society of America, 83*, 1846-1851.

Yost, W. A., Popper, A. N., & Fay, R. R. (1993). *Human psychophysics.* New York: Springer-Verlag.

Zeng, F-G, Oba, S., Garde, S., Sininger, Y., & Starr, A. (2001). Psychoacoustics and speech perception in auditory neuropathy. In Y. Sininger & A. Starr (Eds.), *Auditory neuropathy* (pp. 141-161). San Diego, CA: Singular.

Zwicker, E. (1984). Dependence of post-masking duration and its relation temporal effects in loudness. *Journal of the Acoustical Society of America, 75*, 219-223.

CHAPTER 3

AN INTRODUCTION TO CENTRAL AUDITORY NEUROSCIENCE

DENNIS P. PHILLIPS

Introduction

All the conscious and unconscious operations executed on any auditory sensation we have probably involve activity in the central auditory nervous system (CANS). The list of those operations—which might include generation of the perceptual event, resolving it in spectrum and time and space, differentiating it from other auditory sensations, recognition and identification of the event, and so on—can appear daunting in itself. So too can the plethora of empirical articles on the central auditory underpinnings of those functions, and the theoretical frameworks in which those articles are cast. Nevertheless, if we are ever to have a penetrating comprehension of central auditory processing, some attempt must

be made to examine the relation between the subjective experience of hearing and the neural machinery that mediates it— and both of those in the context of a firm understanding of the stimulus. Fortunately, we are becoming increasingly aware that the anatomy and physiology of the central auditory system follows specifiable principles or rules, as does human auditory perception. In at least some instances, it has become possible to show that there is an orderly mapping of auditory function visualized in the neurophysiology with that seen psychophysically.

This chapter provides an overview of central auditory neuroscience, from auditory nerve to auditory cortex, and points to some psychophysical corollaries of central auditory function as they emerge. The chapter was composed with two goals in mind. One is to provide the reader with a brief, stand-alone summary of auditory neuroscience and its perceptual correlates, and enough referencing, to provide the reader with a qualitative comprehension of principles of auditory neuroscience, and a means of tracking it further. The second goal is to provide a foundation for the rest of this book. Ultimately, a knowledge of central auditory neuroscience must embrace normal function, dysfunction, development, and aging. To that end, principles of central auditory neuroscience need to be described in a way that enables comprehension of the level of the system, and the fashion in which pathologic and developmental processes operate to exert the effects that they do.

These are tall orders, and the best that a single chapter can do is provide an outline. Many of the references cited are review articles or recent empirical ones that address important conceptual issues. What follows begins with an account of the auditory nerve, because it is the physiology and connectivity of the auditory nerve that sets some of the resolution and organization of information available to the brain. We then work our way through the cochlear nuclei, the superior olivary complex, the auditory midbrain, and then the thalamus and cortex. At each of those stations, we explore identifiable neural circuits and their functions. Having laid out the afferent auditory system in this serial, anatomic way, we then take a functional approach, first, by devoting some time to neuroplasticity, and second, by exploring temporal aspects of central auditory processing. Both of these are topics of intense current investigation in their own right, and both have been implicated in the genesis of central auditory processing disorders ([C]APD) or their remediation.

The Auditory Nerve

The afferent auditory nerve is made up of spiral ganglion neurons whose dendrites contact the inner hair cells of the cochlea, and whose axons depart the cochlea through the internal auditory meatus, ultimately to contact cells of the cochlear nuclei. The cochlea can be construed as a linear array of filters, with those for high frequencies arising in the basal turn and those for low frequencies being located in the apical turns. This tonotopic organization is a consequence of the strictly mechanical properties of the basilar membrane, in particular, its stiffness and width gradients from base to apex. The selectivity and sensitivity of the mechanical tuning at any given point is shaped by the passive mechanics of the basilar membrane at that site and by the active contribution of the outer hair cells (OHCs; Dallos, 1992). The latter serve both to increase the sensitivity of the response and to enhance the frequency tuning (Ruggero & Rich, 1991). A rough metaphor might be that the outer hair cells serve as lock-in amplifiers, with the OHC shortening and lengthening responses linked to upward and downward motions of the basilar membrane, respectively. It is in this way that the outer hair cells' contractile response adds to the passive mechanical response. The magnitude of the OHC mechanical response depends on the size of the OHC electrical one, which in turn depends on the magnitude of the basilar membrane's mechanical response at that site. The OHC contribution is decidedly nonlinear. It is greatest for frequencies at or near the one to which that site is most sensitive.

Each spiral ganglion cell receives its input from a single inner hair cell; there are no (neural) longitudinal interactions between cochlear nerve cells (Spoendlin, 1967), which consequently function independently, each driven entirely by its single input. In this sense, cochlear nerve cells "inherit" their properties from a unitary source. Their frequency tuning is slave to that of the inner hair cell they innervate, and therefore to that of the basilar membrane at that site (Narayan, Temchin, Recio, & Ruggero, 1998; Sellick, Patuzzi, & Johnstone, 1982). Each nerve cell is thus characterized by a characteristic frequency (CF) to which it is most sensitive and narrowly tuned. The auditory nerve, then, can be thought of as an array of fibers across which are mapped the frequency filters of the cochlea: which frequencies are present in the stimulus will be expressed in which neurons of the array are activated. It is, of course, the independence of these frequency channels that permits frequency-specific hearing losses after local cochlear damage. Because cochlear pathology typically affects outer hair cells (and so the fine frequency tuning of the transduction process), the consequence of OHC damage is not merely a loss of sensitivity to sound, but also an impaired ability of the cochlea to execute a spectral decomposition of the sound: there is a "blurred" mapping of the sound energy through the impaired sector of the cochlea onto the auditory nerve array.

The spike discharge patterns of cochlear neurons are determined in large part by the physiology of the hair cell–afferent fiber synapse (Ruggero, 1992). For low-frequency stimuli, spike discharges in cochlear neurons are phase-locked to upward motions of the basilar membrane. This is because it is upward motions of the membrane that depolarize the inner hair cell and thus

elicit neurotransmitter release; downward motions of the basilar membrane hyperpolarize the hair cell and thus prevent neurotansmitter release. Phase-locking is strongest at very low frequencies, but is statistically detectable in responses to frequencies as high as 2.5 to 3 kHz or so. Accordingly, in addition to the tonotopic ("place") code above, a second representation of sound frequency resides in the timing of action potentials in the nerve cell array activated by the sound: the intervals between spikes are informative about periodicities in the stimulus. Precisely how pitch (the subjective correlate of stimulus frequency) is recovered from interspike intervals by the brain is unclear, but there is little doubt that sounds that produce pitch percepts also evoke responses whose interspike intervals are directly related to the temporal stucture of the stimulus and thus also to the pitch (Cariani & Delgutte, 1996). This is true even of sounds that contain no energy, or no special concentration of energy, at the pitch frequency; this is made possible, of course, by the fact that the time waveform of the stimulus has a periodicity at the pitch frequency. Thus, we have two neural substrates for pitch. A spectral representation resides in the identities of the cochlear neurons activated by the sound, and in the firing rates across the activated neural array. A temporal code resides in the temporal distribution of spikes within and across cochlear output channels activated by the stimulus. For relatively low frequencies (e.g., in the musical range), both codes are available concurrently, and it is an intriguing question as to how the two representations contribute to the pitch percept (see Cariani & Delgutte, 1996; Oxenham, Bernstein, & Penagos, 2004).

At higher frequencies, the biophysical coupling of basilar membrane motion and inner hair cell neurotransmitter release is not synchronized on such a fine-grained moment-by-moment basis, and the result is a steady depolarization of the hair cell for as long as the stimulus is present. It follows that for as long as the stimulus is present, there is continuous release of neurotransmitter by the hair cell, and thus a continuous train of action potentials generated in the auditory nerve fiber. In practice, tone- or noise-burst stimuli evoke a highly time-locked onset response, which then adapts to a steady firing rate (Ruggero, 1992). The firing rate itself is determined by the relation between the spectral content of the stimulus and the nerve cell's frequency-intensity response ranges. Most cochlear nerve cells have monotonic spike rate-intensity functions, although they vary in the extent to which firing rates saturate at high stimulus levels. In general then, one can conceptualize the activity of each cochlear nerve cell as indicating the presence, amplitude, and timing of stimulus energy within its narrow frequency passband.

Cochlear Nucleus

The cochlear nucleus has three broad nuclei: a ventral division (VCN), which is divisible into anteroventral (AVCN) and posteroventral (PVCN) nuclei, and a dorsal nucleus (DCN). Each axon of the auditory nerve bifurcates as it enters the cochlear nucleus, with one branch innervating AVCN, and the second branch innervating PVCN en route to DCN (Rhode, 1991). This constitutes an early expression of parallel processing, that is,

a divergent projection upon multiple target nuclei, which are then able to execute separate operations on the same input simultaneously. In each of these nuclei, the entering auditory nerve axons terminate in an orderly tonotopic fashion, so that a sheet of neurons comes to be innervated by each cochlear site in each of the three divisions of the nucleus. Thus, the AVCN, PVCN, and DCN contain relatively complete representations of the cochlear partition, and stimulus processing continues to be executed on a frequency-by-frequency basis.

Functional specialization within the cochlear nucleus has been studied extensively (see Rhode, 1991 and Rhode & Greenberg, 1992 for review). One striking specialization occurs in the AVCN. So-called "spherical bushy cells" of the AVCN are cells with relatively poorly developed dendritic trees and cell membranes that have a low input resistance. In the low-frequency region of the AVCN, individual bushy cells are innervated directly by small numbers of auditory nerve axons via elaborate synapses termed "endbulbs of Held." The presynaptic terminal is large and wraps partially around the postsynaptic cell body. There are numerous synaptic contacts made via this specialization, with the result that the low input resistance of the postsynaptic cell is met by a large synaptic current. In turn, this means that the postsynaptic cell's behavior becomes dominated by a very small number of auditory nerve inputs (as few as 1–4; Rhode, 1991). In particular, the timing of postsynaptic spikes tends faithfully to reflect that of the auditory nerve input ("spike-in/spike-out" transmission). Low-frequency cochlear output is often phase-locked, and this synaptic specialization preserves the temporal organization of the input, and therefore information about the phase of the stimulus at the eardrum. In turn, the cells of the medial superior olive (MSO) derive their inputs bilaterally from spherical bushy cells of the VCN (Cant, 1991), and are thus able to compare the timing of phase-locked spikes arriving from the two VCNs. This comparison is informative about the relative phases of the stimuli at the two ears, which is important in sound localization (see below). A second group of AVCN cells, the "globular bushy cells" also receive inputs from the auditory nerve via endbulb contacts; the globular bushy cells have large axons (and therefore high axonal conduction velocities) and project upon nuclei of the trapezoid body.

A quite different specialization is seen in some cells of the PVCN. "Octopus cells" (multipolar neurons) have large, relatively unbranched dendrites that appear to be oriented somewhat across the tonotopic array of input fibers, with the result that they receive input from relatively broad cochlear segments. Physiologic studies show these neurons to have broader frequency tuning curves than other cells of the VCN, which is consistent with the anatomic organization of their inputs. The discharge patterns evoked by tone-burst stimuli in these neurons are often dominated by a very precisely timed onset transient; the jitter in (standard deviation of) first spike latency can be as low as a few tens of microseconds, which is again consistent with a highly convergent input (Rhode, 1991) because variability in first spike timing declines with increases in the number of inputs. The phase-locking of spikes by some of these neurons is among the most temporally precise of any cells in the central auditory system, including the auditory nerve. The axonal outputs of these cells are directed toward the periolivary nuclei and the contralateral ventral nucleus of the lateral lemniscus (Schwartz, 1992).

The output neurons of the DCN are fusiform cells. They receive input from the auditory nerve and from local inhibitory circuitry. They direct their outputs to the contralateral auditory midbrain, especially the inferior colliculus. DCN cells are excited by a narrow range of tone frequency-intensity conjunctions ("response area"), but they also are inhibited by tones falling in domains that flank the excitatory one. It is possible to categorize DCN cells according to the organization of these inhibitory response areas (Young & Brownell, 1976), and subsequent studies have offered evidence on which morphologic cell types are characterized by various patterns of inhibitory inputs, and on the organization of the connectivity between the cell types (Rhode & Greenberg, 1992). For the present purposes, at least two new physiologic response properties emerge from this circuitry. One is that, because the inhibitory response areas flank the excitatory one at the cell's CF, the cell can develop a marked sensitivity to stimulus bandwidth. It is thus not simply the presence of stimulus energy within the excitatory response area, but also the distribution of energy across the excitatory and inhibitory response area(s), that determines discharge rates in these cells. A second feature to emerge from the inhibitory circuitry in at least some DCN cells is the presence of an inhibitory input at CF. Often the excitatory input at CF is the more sensitive, but the presence of both means that these cells have a nonmonotonic spike rate–intensity function for CF (and nearby) tones.

Neurons with nonmonotonic rate responses to tone pulses or other signals are increasingly common at more rostral sites in the auditory pathway, and the apparent "tuning" to stimulus level has been incorporated into accounts of the central representation of sound intensity. The responses of central neurons also become increasingly dominated by sound onsets (Phillips, Hall, & Boehnke, 2002). Because responses to variations in stimulus level are typically studied without also covarying stimulus rise-time, it is important to determine independently whether the responses to differences in sound level are actually driven by the plateau level of the sound or by the dynamics of sound pressure change at sound onset (Heil, 1997). In practice, it is often the latter (Heil, 1997; Phillips, Hall, Guo, & Burkhard, 2001). For sustained responses, this issue may be moot because the sustained response enables a separation of the "code" for ongoing stimulus level from the response to the onset transient. Nevertheless, the striking dominance of onset responses seen rostrally, and the rethinking of exactly which stimulus parameter is encoded in the rate-response function, raises new questions about the contribution of forebrain and hindbrain mechanisms to the mediation of perceived loudness.

Superior Olivary Complex

The superior olivary complex (SOC) is a bilateral structure that contains a number of separable cell groups distinguished by their cytoarchitecture, connectivity, and function. For the purposes of the present chapter, two cell groups are important: the medial (MSO) and lateral (LSO) superior olivary nuclei. Their particular significance derives from the fact that these nuclei are crucially involved in the neural encoding of the binaural cues for the spatial location of sounds. Both nuclei are tonotopically organized, and neurons of both nuclei ultimately derive their inputs from both ears. These two features of their inputs confer on the SOC the ability to execute interaural stimulus comparisons, and to do so on a frequency-by-frequency basis. The frequency specificity of the interaural disparity coding is important. Interaural time (ITD) and level (ILD) differences are the principal binaural cues used in sound localization. They derive from the travel time of sound around the head and the acoustic shadow cast by head and pinnae, respectively. The magnitudes of the cues vary with the size of the receiver's head, the azimuth of the sound source, and the spectral composition of the sound itself. For spectrally rich sources, each frequency component generates its own ITD and ILD, and the distribution of these provides a wealth of information about source azimuth— but this wealth is usable only if the nervous system encodes the interaural disparities at each frequency independently. It is because the nervous system does indeed encode interaural disparities in a frequency-specific way that localization performance is so much more acute for broad-band sources than for very narrow-band ones.

The MSO receives direct projections from the AVCN bilaterally (Cant, 1991). Interestingly, it is often the case that the particular AVCN cells that contribute to this innervation are the same ones that receive endbulb innervation from the auditory nerve (Oertel, Wu, & Hirsch, 1988) and which thus carry very faithful information about the phase of the stimulus at the ears. In turn, MSO cells are able to execute a temporal coincidence detection on the spike trains arriving from the two cochlear nuclei and, through that mechanism, encode the relative phases of sounds at the two ears. That is, the phase-locked spike trains evoked in the cochlear nerve are conferred upon the bushy cell axons, and the recipient MSO cells can compare the timing of spikes from the two sides. What results is a neural sensitivity to interaural phase expressed as a cyclical relation of MSO cell spike count to interaural phase, with the period of the cycle being equal to the period of the sound at the two ears (Yin & Chan, 1990).

In principle, coincidence detection could be mediated using exclusively excitatory mechanisms. In practice, however, it seems likely that the neural encoding of ITDs also relies on glycine-mediated inhibition (Brand, Behrend, Marquardt, McAlpine, & Grothe, 2002). If one imagines the afferent spike trains from either AVCN as constituting phase-locked half-periods of excitation, then the inhibition expresses itself as half-periods inserted between the excitatory ones. The "insertion" is probably achieved through inhibitory neurons satellite to the MSO, activated in parallel by the AVCN input. Variations in ITD will now cause shifts in the relative timing of excitation/inhibition from one side and excitation/inhibition from the other side, and will do so on a cycle-by-cycle basis. The result is that the modulation of spike rate evoked by variations in ITD is deeper than could be achieved by excitatory mechanisms alone. The greater the modulation of spike rate

by the stimulus manipulation, the more salient is the neural signal.

In practice, the neural path length from the contralateral ear is usually the longer, so that in order for the spikes from the two AVCNs to arrive synchronously at the MSO, the phase of the stimulus at the contralateral ear must precede that at the ipsilateral ear; that is, the interaural stimulus timing difference offsets the neural travel time difference from the two ears. This has the consequence that the relation of spike rate to ITD is not only cyclical; spike rates are greatest for ITDs favoring the contralateral ear, minimal for ITDs favoring the ipsilateral ear, and the functions are disposed such that their steepest slopes are associated with very small ITDs (McAlpine, Jiang, & Palmer, 2001). It seems to be the case that the ITDs associated with peak responses are systematically longer for cells with lower CFs (which, of course, have longer periods). The result is that the steep portion of the spike count versus ITD function is usually associated with very small ITDs (McAlpine et al., 2001) and therefore with azimuths near the midsagittal plane. This point is illustrated in Figure 3-1, which shows idealized spike count versus ITD functions for cells of relatively low, medium, and high CFs. Note that spike count is a cyclical function of ITD for each of the neurons, and that, because peak spike rates are associated with longer ITDs in the lower-CF cells, the steep portion of the function is associated with relatively small ITDs. The absolute range of ITDs that an individual will encounter depends on head size, source location, and source frequency, but small ITDs are the ones most likely to occur naturally (shaded area in Figure 3-1). Now, it is the steep part of the function

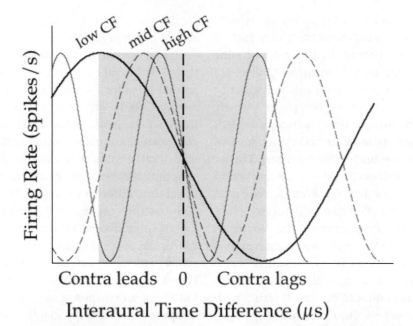

Figure 3–1. Idealized spike rate-versus-ITD functions for neurons of relatively low, medium, and high CF. Shaded area indicates the range of ITDs associated with near-midline azimuths. Each of the three neurons shows a cyclical relation of spike count to ITD, which is expected of a coincidence-detector mechanism working on two phase-locked inputs. Note that for each neuron, spike rates are high for ITDs that favor the contralateral ear. This reflects the fact that the neural path length is longer from the contralateral ear than the path length from the ipsilateral ear. Importantly, irrespective of CF, the steep part of the function is always centered at small ITDs.

in which neural firing rate most unambiguously specifies ITD and, through the azimuth-ITD relation, source location. This may be one reason why free-field sound localization acuity is greater for sources near the midline (Middlebrooks & Green, 1991; Phillips & Brugge, 1985).

ITD coding is usually studied at the neuron's CF, but the phenomena seen in responses to CF tones often extend to responses to off-CF frequencies. One fascinating concept to emerge from studies of ITD coding at different frequencies within a neuron's effective range is that

of "characteristic delay" (see Yin & Kuwada, 1983, for studies of this at the level of the inferior colliculus). For many cells, the ITD functions obtained with different frequencies coincide at a single ITD. When the coincidence is at a peak in the delay functions, then the coincidence usually is at an ITD favoring the contralateral ear; when the characteristic delay occurs at the trough in the delay functions, the characteristic ITD commonly favors the ipsilateral ear. The net result of this is that the ITDs evoking the most vigorous responses, and often also the most highly differentiated responses, are associated with contralateral azimuths. The axonal outputs of the MSO project most heavily on the ipsilateral dorsal nucleus of the lateral lemniscus (DNLL) and central nucleus of the inferior colliculus (ICC), so the contralateral bias in the representation of spatial information developed in the MSO is conferred upon higher centers.

Neurons of the LSO receive an excitatory input from the VCN of the same side. From the contralateral side, the VCN projects upon the medial nucleus of the trapezoid body (MNTB) adjacent to the LSO. This connection is excitatory. In turn, the MNTB projects upon the LSO, and this connection is inhibitory. The excitation exerted on both the LSO and MNTB by projections from the cochlear nucleus is mediated by an excitatory amino acid neurotransmitter, and the inhibition exerted on the LSO by the MNTB is mediated by glycine (Wu & Kelly, 1992). Both the inputs to LSO cells are intensity-dependent, with the strength of the excitatory and inhibitory drives being monotonically related to peripheral stimulus level. This means that the spike output of LSO cells is a sensitive function of the relative levels of the stimuli at the two ears, that is, a sensitive function of ILD. The inputs and the outputs of the LSO are responses sustained for the stimulus duration. Studied with transient stimuli, however, LSO cells (and therefore their inputs) display a familiar latency-intensity relation, with first-spike latencies inversely related to stimulus level. Because the responses to transients (e.g., clicks) are also transient, LSO cells are susceptible to a time-intensity trading, such that the effects of an ILD favoring one ear can be offset by an ITD favoring the opposite ear.

The general form of ILD sensitivity in the LSO is a sigmoidal relation of spike count to ILD, with high spike rates associated with ILDs favoring the ipsilateral ear, and the steep portion of the spike count function associated with ILDs near zero. Studied with virtual space technology, many LSO cells have spatial receptive fields occupying the ipsilateral acoustic hemifield, and medial borders near the midline (Tollin & Yin, 2002). The axonal outputs of the LSO are directed most heavily to the contralateral DNLL and ICC. These connections are excitatory, and because they are crossed, they have the consequence of conferring on those centers a contralateral bias in the representation of ILDs, paralleling the one offered by the MSO for ITDs.

Figure 3–2 shows idealized spike count versus ILD functions as might be obtained from neurons rostral to the LSO; it illustrates their general form after the decussation. Spike rates are high when the ILD significantly favors the contralateral ear, and near zero for ILDs favoring the ipsilateral ear. The steep portions of the functions are associated with small ILDs. The absolute values of naturally occurring ILDs vary with head size, sound source frequency, and source azimuth, but it is always true that the slope of the function relating ILD size to source azimuth is steepest for near-midline azimuths (Irvine, 1987). This means that the neural code (spike rate) for the stimulus information (ILD size) is most unambiguous for cue values that themselves most precisely specify source azimuth (Phillips & Brugge, 1985). If psychophysical acuity for sound localization reflects stimulus precision "mapped through" the neural code, then it is no surprise that behavioral acuity for source location is greatest at the midline.

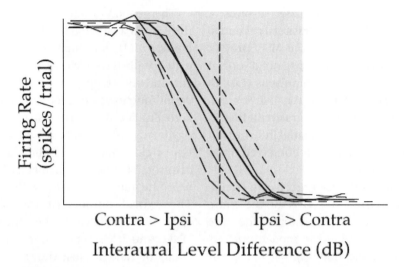

Figure 3–2. Idealized spike rate-versus-ILD functions. Note that spike rates are high, and relatively undifferentiated, for ILDs significantly favoring the contralateral ear, and that they are low, and undifferentiated, for ILDs significantly favoring the ipsilateral ear. This means that spike rate is the most unambiguous indicator of ILD (and therefore of source azimuth) for small ILDs (shaded area). Shaded area also indicates the range of ILDs associated with near-midline azimuths.

Some cells of the MSO, the LSO, and some of the surrounding cell groups of the olivary complex are those whose axons form the last leg of the descending, efferent auditory system (Warr, 1992; see also Spoendlin, 1967), that is, they are olivocochlear neurons. The olivocochlear neurons are typically divided into lateral and medial systems. The lateral one consists mostly of fine axons from cells in or near the LSO; these ultimately project toward the inner hair cells of the ipsilateral ear, where they terminate on the afferent nerve endings serving the inner hair cells. The medial pathway arises from larger cells outside the MSOs. Their large, myelinated axons generally cross the midline to innervate the contralateral ear. These fibers innervate the base of the outer hair cells

directly. The olivocochlear system, perhaps especially that serving the outer hair cells, may ultimately be shown to have effects on cochlear sensitivity. Let us consider one with a clear psychophysical expression. Focused auditory attention can operate selectively within the frequency domain (Scharf, Quigley, Aoki, Peachey, & Reeves, 1987). It can manifest, for example, as better detection thresholds for tone pips of an attended frequency than for tone pips of nonattended frequencies. There is a clear "tuning" of the phenomenon, which is perhaps what we would expect of a system working in a frequency-specific fashion. Recent evidence from neurologic case studies, specifically in patients who have had their olivocochlear axons cut, indicates that activity of the olivocochlear pathways may serve to dampen sensitivity in nonattended frequency channels, thus giving a sensitivity advantage to the attended channel (Scharf, Magnan, Collet, Ulmer, & Chays, 1994). Note that, in this case, olivocochlear activity does not "add" in some way to sensitivity in the attended channel, but rather, it dampens sensitivity in the nonattended ones.

Inferior Colliculus

The central nucleus of the inferior colliculus (ICC) is a mandatory synaptic station for auditory sensory information ascending beyond the auditory midbrain. It is a laminated, tonotopically organized structure, surrounded by pericentral (ICP) and external nuclei (ICX). ICP and ICX also receive auditory input, but their functions are less well known, save for the fact that ICX is multimodal and is likely involved in the neural circuitry mediating head and pinna movements. The ICC receives significant projections from the LSO bilaterally, from the ipsilateral MSO, and from the DNLL bilaterally. The projections onto the ICC are highly differentiated, not only in the sense that they respect the tonotopy developed more caudally, but in the sense that there are regional differences in anatomic convergence patterns within the ICC. In turn, this means that there are regional differences in neuronal physiology as well. Thus, one caudal, predominantly high-frequency region of the ICC receives inputs jointly from the contralateral LSO and the contralateral DCN, and neurons in that region of the ICC thus "inherit" the properties of those afferent sources (e.g., sensitivity to interaural level differences, and a nonmono-

tonic spike rate-versus-intensity profile; Oliver, Beckius, Bishop, & Kuwada 1997; Semple & Aitkin, 1981).

As mentioned above, the crossed projection from the LSO is excitatory; the projection from the ipsilateral LSO is, however, inhibitory and probably mediated by glycine (Glendenning, Baker, Hutson, & Masterton, 1992). Note that this arrangement preserves the contralaterality of spatial representation in the LSOs' projections onto the ICC. The DNLL projections onto the ICC appear to follow a similar functional pattern. In this case, it is the crossed projection that is inhibitory, likely mediated by gamma-aminobutyric acid (GABA: Shneiderman, Oliver, & Henkel, 1988). If we recall that the MSO and LSO inputs to the DNLL confer a distinctly contralateral bias in the spatial representation there, then the fact that the crossed DNLL projection to the ICC is inhibitory would again function to preserve the contralaterality of spatial representation in the recipient ICC.

The further question is whether this inhibitory circuitry in some way does more than simply "preserve" the contralaterality of spatial representation in the ICC. Does it enhance spatial coding? There is evidence that interfering with DNLL function unilaterally interferes with the neural coding of interaural level (Li & Kelly, 1992a) and time differences (Kidd & Kelly, 1996) in the contralateral ICC; the spike rate-versus-interaural disparity functions less precisely indicate the disparity size or sign in the presence of DNLL inactivation. What is less clear is whether the spike rate-versus-disparity functions in the ICC of intact animals are any "sharper" or more precise than those seen in the nuclei providing their input. That is, does the inhibitory circuitry improve the precision of the code above that seen in the SOC, or does it maintain the precision of SOC coding in the face of converging inputs from additional sources that would otherwise degrade the code in the ICC? We do not yet have good answers to these questions.

A second way of thinking about this general issue is to ask whether spatial coding in the ICC has acquired some qualitatively new feature (i.e., one not seen more caudally), rather than having sharpened a pre-existing neural code. In this regard, Spitzer and Semple (1993, 1998) studied the responses of brainstem auditory neurons to dynamic interaural phase differences, that is, stimuli which provide information about source *movement* rather than sound source *location*. They showed that the response rate of ICC neurons evoked by a given interaural phase disparity depended on the immediately preceding stimulus-response history; in contrast, MSO response rates more closely reflected the instantaneous interaural delay, irrespective of the stimulus history. These findings suggest that there is an emergence of sensitivity to dynamic stimulus features at the level of the ICC; it remains to be determined exactly what circuitry is responsible for this emergence.

Medial Geniculate Body and Auditory Cortex

The medial geniculate body contains a parvocellular ventral nucleus (MGv) in which neurons are arranged in sheetlike layers, each deriving its input from a single cochlear place, and arranged tonotopically. The MGv is surrounded by a number of other nuclei, the most notable of which are the magnocellular, medial division (MGm) and the dorsal division (MGd). There is some evidence of a parallelism in the pathways linking the midbrain and thalamus such that ICC preferentially projects upon MGv through the brachium of the inferior colliculus, whereas the nuclei surrounding the ICC project upon the nuclei abutting the MGv (Calford & Aitkin, 1983; Winer, 1992). This parallel organization involving the parvocellular and magnocellular divisions of the medial geniculate body should not be confused with the "magno" and "parvo" streams of processing in primate vision. In the primate visual system, the magno and parvo streams arise in the retina, extend into the lateral geniculate body, and then to the striate cortex and beyond (Livingstone & Hubel, 1988); they are largely independent pathways, each sampling the sensory epithelium, but with different stimulus feature selectivities (color versus luminance, sensitivity to motion or not, contrast sensitivity, different periodic temporal responses), by neurons with different receptive field sizes and adaptive properties (transient and sustained). In the auditory system, there is little evidence for magnocellular and parvocellular "streams" of processing in this sense of the term. And although there are certainly auditory system neurons whose responses are dominated by "transient" or "sustained" discharge patterns (Phillips et al., 2002), these neurons are not organized into streams in the way that they may be in vision. Accordingly, allusions to magnocellular and parvocellular "streams" of processing in audition (e.g., Stein, 2001) or to "transient subsystems" (Galaburda, Menard, & Rosen, 1994) are to be interpreted skeptically.

Neurons in MGv are narrowly tuned to tone frequency, have short response latencies, and show the familiar patterns of binaural input and interaction (Clarey, Barone & Imig, 1992). Cells of the MGm and MGd tend more often to be broadly tuned to frequency, and those of the MGd particularly often have longer latencies and show irregular, habituating responses to acoustic stimulation. Some of them are multimodal.

The auditory cortex is a broad area of the temporal cortex that is responsive to acoustic stimulation. It is divisible into a number of separable "fields" or territories, based on cytoarchitecture, and/or the presence or absence of a tonotopic map, and/or patterns of connectivity with the thalamus and other cortical fields. Some of the fields are tonotopically organized, and these typically receive thalamic input from MGv, with the densest such projection serving the primary auditory cortex (AI; Winer, 1992). The nontonotopic fields receive thalamic afferents more heavily loaded in favor of the MGm and MGd. The MGm projection is perhaps particularly interesting, because it targets almost all the cortical auditory fields, and in this way reflects its own input, which is very convergent even at the level of individual neurons. In cats, the primary field is surrounded by other tonotopic fields, which typically take their names from their spatial position in relation to AI (e.g., anterior field, posterior field) and the probably nontonotopic field AII, which appears to contain broadly tuned neurons (Reale & Imig, 1980). In primates, AI abuts a near-mirror image rostral field, and these are flanked by so-called "lateral belt" fields, at least some of which are also tonotopic (Merzenich & Brugge, 1973).

The thalamocortical connections in the auditory system are largely reciprocal (Winer, 1992). There are dense and quite orderly projections from deep layer V and layer VI back to the thalamus and to the inferior colliculus. These projections form "loops" between the midbrain, thalamus, and cortex, and these loops may be a medium through which the cortex is able to "select" or modulate the relative strengths of inputs across the tonotopic (or other) representational dimension (Suga, Yan, & Zhang, 1997; Yan & Suga, 1996; Zhang, Suga, & Yan 1997; see also below). The cortex is also the origin of a longer descending, efferent auditory pathway which ultimately reaches the cochlea (Warr, 1992).

In the tonotopic fields, and we shall deal mostly with AI because it is the most well-studied, the tonotopic organization is expressed in the form of roughly parallel, striplike assemblies of neurons, each deriving its input from a particular cochlear site, and thus a convergent input from the sheet of MGv neurons representing the same cochlear place. These "iso-CF" strips of cells span most of the cortical layers, and the strips themselves are spatially arrayed according to CF, forming the familiar tonotopic "map." Borders between adjacent tonotopic fields are typically marked by a reversal in the tonotopic sequence of neural CFs so that the tonotopic maps of adjacent fields are somewhat mirror images of each other.

Within AI's tonotopic map, there are patches of tissue distinguished by their cells' other neurophysiologic properties. The majority of cortical auditory neurons are binaurally influenced (Semple & Kitzes, 1993), and there are local territories or patches of cortical tissue dominated by cells expressing one or other form of binaural interaction (Imig & Adrian, 1977). Some patches of tissue contain cells with predominantly "suppressive" binaural interactions (typically, though not always, reflecting an excitatory input from the contralateral ear and an inhibitory one from the ipsilateral ear). Others contain cells with predominantly "summative" binaural interactions (often reflecting a net excitatory input from each ear). At least some of these patches are elongated and are oriented orthogonal to the iso-CF lines of the tonotopic map. It is likely that cells with suppressive binaural interactions are the neurons which have free-field spatial receptive fields occupying the contralateral acoustic hemifield, with the azimuthal location of the receptive field's medial border being determined by the relative sensitivities and strengths of the contralateral excitatory and ipsilateral inhibitory inputs (Middlebrooks & Pettigrew, 1981; Rajan, Aitkin, Irvine, & McKay, 1990; Samson, Clarey, Barone, & Imig, 1993). The neurons with summative binaural interactions are likely the same neurons that have spatial receptive fields centered on the midline, or which are omnidirectional.

The corticocortical connectivities of "suppressive" and "summative" binaural patches may differ (see Hackett & Phillips, 2006 for review). Cells with suppressive binaural interactions have connections which tend to be restricted to cortical targets in the same cerebral hemisphere (Imig & Reale, 1981), whereas cells with summative interactions tend to have stronger callosal connectivity (Imig & Brugge, 1978). There is good reason to link "suppressive" binaural interactions with free-field spatial selectivity for the contralateral auditory hemifield, and "summative" binaural interactions with free-field spatial selectivity for midline locations or with omnidirectionality (Clarey, Barone, & Imig, 1992; Hackett

& Phillips, 2006). Taken together, these data suggest that the spatial information carried by intrahemispheric connectivity is dominated by the contralateral auditory hemifield, whereas the spatial information carried interhemispherically is not. In this regard, unilateral lesions of the auditory cortex in animals produces sound localization deficits that are restricted to sources in the contralateral auditory hemifield, and there is an auditory "neglect" syndrome in man characterized by inattentiveness to (or "extinction" for) sources contralateral to parietal cortical damage (Phillips, 2001).

In man, there are further psychophysical expressions of this hemifield-specific organization. There is growing evidence that spatial processing in man is mediated by two perceptual channels, each with hemifield azimuthal tuning (left or right), and medial borders that overlap at the midline (Boehnke & Phillips, 1999; Phillips & Hall, 2005; see also Stecker, Harrington, & Middlebrooks, 2005 for a neurophysiologic counterpart in animals). Spatial processing of sources near the midline likely depends on the outputs of both perceptual channels, whereas spatial processing of sources deep in one or other auditory hemifield likely is dominated by one or other perceptual channel. This organization of processing may contribute to the perception of speech in noisy free-field environments. If a listener's task is to repeat speech presented concurrently with a noise masker, then the perceptual benefit of a 90-degree separation of speech and noise is close to 1.3 dB when the speech and noise are located in the same acoustic hemifield, and closer to 8.6 dB when the speech and noise are on opposite sides of the midline (Phillips, Vigneault-MacLean,

Hall, & Boehnke, 2003). It is thus not the absolute separation of speech and noise alone which offers the perceptual advantage, but rather the extent to which the speech and noise fall into separate spatial channels and are thus available for selective scrutiny. This phenomenon may well extend to include other forms of spatial competition, for example, cocktail party paradigms. The extent to which the phenomenon reflects specifically binaural processing, or the signal to noise advantage for the speech at the ear nearer the speech (after Hirsh, 1950), is unclear. (This is not a small point. It is true that most auditory cortical neurons are binaurally influenced, and that interaural cues contribute to the azimuthal location of receptive field medial borders. However, the pinnae can become highly directional receivers for high-frequency sources, and this spatial selectivity is superimposed on neural spatial selectivity that would otherwise arise from binaural processing of ILDs due to head shadows alone. The pinna directionality could potentially saturate the ILD coding system for favored frequencies so that although neurons in the cortex may be binaurally influenced, their responses may become dominated by events at one—the contralateral—ear. This effect would presumably be most marked for high frequencies and for sources located in the acoustical axis of the pinna.)

A second "patchy" organization of the primary auditory cortex is based on the frequency-level "response areas" or response ranges of the neurons therein. Neurons with strongly nonmonotonic spike count-versus-level functions tend to be located toward the middle of the iso-CF strips (Phillips, Orman, Musicant, & Wilson, 1985; Phillips, Semple, Calford,

& Kitzes, 1994) in patches that do not respect the boundaries of the "binaural" ones. Recall that these are neurons with strong inhibitory response domains that flank the excitatory one at CF, and they often display exceptionally narrow frequency tuning. The differential location of these neurons toward the center of AI likely underlies the narrow bandwidth tuning and poorer responses to wideband sounds seen in neural activity in the same region (e.g., Schreiner & Mendelson, 1990).

The patchy distribution of neurons according to their neurophysiologies leads us to important inferences for how we construe stimulus "representation" in the auditory cortex. Tonotopic maps are *not* representations of stimulus frequency. If it were that simple, then the pattern of excitation across the cortical mantle would be predictable from knowledge of the stimulus frequency alone, and it is not (Phillips et al., 1994). Tonotopic maps simply describe the spatial arrangement of neurons according to their CFs. The cortical *representation* of a stimulus resides in the distribution of responses in space (and time) across the cortex. Even for a stimulus as simple as a tone pulse of a specified frequency, the pattern of excitation evoked depends on the ear stimulated and the plateau level of the tone, and it takes the form of discontinuous patches of activation distributed along the relevant iso-CF strip (for low-level tones) and sometimes quite far from it (in the case of high-amplitude tones). Sometimes, the middle parts of an iso-CF strip can be devoid of activity in the presence of high-amplitude tones at that CF—because those territories are occupied by cells with nonmonotonic rate-responses (Phillips et al., 1994). The fact that stimulus representation may not be in the form of neat, linear maps is in many ways functionally irrelevant. What matters is that the putative neurophysiologic representation of a stimulus parameter is as differentiated as is the perceptual dimension it supports (see also Middlebrooks, Xu, Eddins, & Green, 1998; Stecker et al., 2005). That is, there usually must be an orderly one-to-one relation between brain state and subjective experience.

Cortical Coding of the Temporal Structures of Sounds

The fashion in which the cortex is able to encode the temporal properties of auditory stimuli is a key topic. Studied with transient stimuli, temporal jitter in single neuron mean first-spike latencies (i.e., the precision with which the cortex is able to "time-stamp" a stimulus event) can be significantly less than a millisecond (Phillips & Hall, 1990). This is more than sufficient to encode the timing of the phonetically important events in speech, and is comparable to that seen in the cochlear nerve. (The spectral content of the acoustic event is represented by the pattern of activity across the tonotopic array; see above, and Wang, Merzenich, Beitel, & Schreiner, 1995; Phillips et al., 1994). By contrast, the ability of cortical cells to establish a temporal code for periodic events is much poorer than that seen in the cochlear nerve; cortical neurons can entrain to periodicities up to only a few tens of hertz (Eggermont, 1991, 1994). This would be insufficient to encode glottal pulse rates on a temporal basis, and is over an order of magnitude poorer than the upper limit of temporal coding of stimulus periodicities by the cochlear nerve. The poverty of cortical responses to periodic stimuli—in the face of the temporal precision of responses to transients—may reflect a synaptic depression driven by the periodicity (Eggermont, 2002). It is perhaps because of the dominance and temporal precision of transient responses in the cortex that auditory cortical lesions have different effects on the perception of speech sounds at the level of pitch and phonetics (see below).

Temporal issues are important to understanding cortical function for a second reason. The responses of cortical cells to successive stimuli are not independent, especially if the stimulus events are in close temporal proximity. Thus, the response to a specified frequency modulation (FM) depends very much on whether it occurs as an isolated event (e.g., an FM tone pulse) or as a modulation of a continuous carrier (Phillips, 1988; see also Malone & Semple, 2002 for evidence of stimulus context effects on the coding of trapezoidal ITD changes). Likewise, the response to one binaural tone can be significantly altered by the presence of a preceding "conditioning" tone (Reale & Brugge, 2000; Zhang, Nakamoto & Kitzes, 2005; see also Brosch & Schreiner, 2000). This may be one of the reasons why laterality percepts for tone pulses of a given frequency are so markedly influenced by stimulus history at that frequency (Phillips & Hall, 2005). The mechanisms mediating these kinds of sequential interactions are still being worked out, but likely include short-term adaptive tracking of effective stimulus level (Malone & Semple, 2002; Phillips, 1985, 1988; Phillips et al., 2002) and inhibition (Calford & Semple, 1995; Eggermont, 1991). The general point is that cortical neural responses are sensitive to the recent stimulus history.

A further issue, raised at the outset of this chapter, concerns the neural coding of the pitch of complex sounds, particularly those stimuli with no energy (or no special concentration of energy) at the pitch frequency. We have already remarked that stimuli arousing nonspectral pitch percepts must rely on a temporal coding process, and there is direct evidence that lower auditory neurons display interspike intervals related to the period of the perceived pitch frequencies of such sounds (see Cariani & Delgutte, 1996). Direct recordings from the primary auditory cortex of primates have failed to find evidence of neurons responsive to pitch frequency; rather, the responses are dominated by the relation between the spectral content of the sound and the neuron's frequency response area (Fishman, Reser, Arezzo, & Steinschneider, 1998; Schwarz & Tomlinson, 1990). However, at least some neurons in a border region between the primary field (AI) and rostral and lateral belt fields in the primate may be sensitive to nonspectral pitch, and display tuning to pitch frequency (Bendor & Wang, 2005). How it is that the temporal code expressed in the auditory hindbrain is converted to a spike-rate code in pitch-tuned cortical neurons is unclear, but the location of the relevant cortical neurons near the border of the low-frequency part of AI is compatible with human brain-imaging data suggesting the existence of a peri-AI cortical region activated by temporal pitch stimuli in a perhaps homologous region (Patterson, Uppencamp, Johnsrude, & Griffiths, 2002).

Finally, the issue of temporal gap detection warrants some mention. Temporal gap detection is a behavioral measure of auditory temporal acuity. Historically, the method has provided a measure of the shortest detectable period of silence ("gap detection threshold") inserted roughly at the temporal midpoint of an otherwise homogeneous, ongoing stream of sound. Depending on the spectral content of the stimulus in which the gap is inserted, gap thresholds may be as low as 1 to 2 ms. Gap thresholds are lowest for wide-band sounds (Eddins, Hall, & Grose, 1992), probably because information about the presence of the gap is being carried by more than one channel of cochlear output. This means that a central perceptual processor can recover the temporal event by integrating information being transmitted roughly synchronously by separate, independent frequency channels. Studied with narrow-band noises, and noise band pairs containing synchronous gaps, human gap thresholds are better for noise band pairs than for single noise bands, but are independent of noise band spectral separation (Hall, Grose, & Saju, 1996). This finding is consistent with the notion that the perceptual recovery of the gap is facilitated by the synchronous transmission of the event in multiple frequency channels.

Gap detection took on new interest when it became clear that acuity for gaps bounded by different markers is poorer (sometimes by an order of magnitude or more) than is acuity for gaps bounded by identical sounds (Formby, Gerber, Sherlock, & Magder, 1998; Grose, Hall & Buss, 1999; Phillips, Taylor, Hall, Carr, & Mossop, 1997). In practice, detection of gaps in the historical "within-channel" design of stimulus likely reflects the detection of a discontinuity in the time course of activity aroused by the stimulus in the relevant perceptual channel (see Figure 3–3, upper); it may reduce to the detection of the onset of the sound marking the end of the silent period (Florentine, Buus, & Geng, 1999; Oxenham, 1997; Phillips et al., 1997, 2002). By contrast, detection of the silent period in the "between-channel" paradigm may require some kind of relative timing process to be executed on the offset of activity in the perceptual channel serving the leading marker and the onset of activity in the channel serving the trailing marker (Figure 3–3, lower: Phillips et al., 1997; Phillips & Hall, 2000, 2002). Particular interest in the nature and properties of

mechanisms mediating between-channel gap detection derives from the fact that gap thresholds for between-channel stimuli that model the structure of stop-consonant vowel syllables tend to average 20 to 40 ms (Phillips & Hall, 1997; Phillips & Smith, 2004). This is the range of values taken by many voice onset time phonetic boundaries, and so between-channel gap detection acuity may be a natural psychophysical parameter exploited by the speech system in the generation of voice onset time phonetic boundaries (after Kuhl & Miller, 1978; Phillips & Smith, 2004).

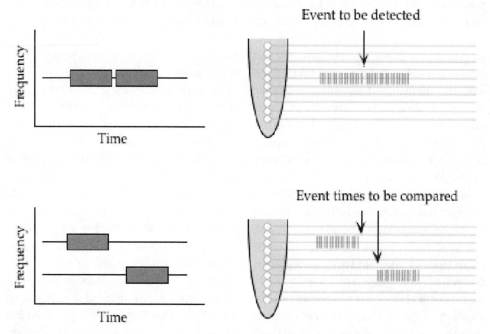

Figure 3–3. Schematic depiction of within-channel (*upper*) and between-channel (*lower*) temporal gap detection stimuli, and the perceptual operations required to perform the tasks. Left side shows the time course of the stimuli, center shows a schematic layout of the cochlea, and right side depicts the time course of activity in the neural-perceptual channels activated by the stimuli. In within-channel gap detection, the perceptual operation is the detection of a discontinuity in the activity of the channel excited by the stimulus. In the between-channel case, detection of the silent period requires a relative timing of the offset of the leading marker and the onset of the trailing marker.

Especially in anesthetized animals, cortical neural responses tend to be dominated by brief responses time-locked to discrete stimulus events, notably stimulus onsets or amplitude increments (Phillips et al., 2002). Studied with wideband noise stimuli in within-channel paradigms, cortical neural responses to gap detection stimuli take the form of an onset response to the beginning of the leading marker, and another onset response time-locked to the beginning of the trailing marker (Eggermont, 1995, 1999). Neurophysiologic "gap threshold" is thus the shortest-duration gap for which there is a detectable onset response to the trailing marker. When the gap occurs "late" in the noise signal (e.g., 500 ms after the onset of the leading marker), these neurophysiologic thresholds can be as short as about 5 ms (Eggermont, 1995), and most fall in the range below 15 ms (Eggermont, 1999). If the temporal gap follows a very short leading marker (e.g., 5 ms), then neurophysiologic gap thresholds are longer, averaging around 40 ms, and with a wide range (>10 to <60 msec: Eggermont, 1999). There is psychophysical evidence of a similar pattern of dependence of within-channel gap threshold on the temporal position of the silent period in some, though not all, human listeners (cf. Phillips et al., 1997, 1998; Snell & Hu, 1999). That is, gap thresholds are sometimes best (lowest) for silent periods not in close temporal proximity to the onset of leading marker or the offset of the trailing one (i.e., when the leading or the trailing marker is very short: Snell & Hu, 1999). Interestingly, it may be that the most highly practiced listeners show the smallest effects of leading marker duration. This raises the possibility that skilled listeners are more able to rely on the activity of the subset of the neurons displaying the "best" acuity, and that one form of perceptual learning is the process of learning how to do this.

The cortical coding of between-channel gap detection stimuli has not been studied directly. Eggermont (2000) has modeled cortical responses to between-channel gap stimuli, based on (a), direct measurement of the onset and postonset inhibitory responses driven by wideband stimuli, and (b) the assumptions that information from different frequency-specific channels converges on broadly tuned cortical cells and that it is the activity of these cells which are the neurophysiologic correlates of psychophysical performance. Certainly, the modeling effort provided a strikingly accurate neurophysiologic prediction of perceptual between-channel gap detection performance (Eggermont, 2000). It is, however, an open question as to whether one needs to explain the psychophysical performance on the basis of individual neurons receiving input from both frequency (or other) channels. Perhaps all that is required are temporally segregated responses to leading marker offset and trailing marker onset, without any special requirement that those responses come from the same neurons.

Plasticity in the Central Auditory System

"Plasticity" is an umbrella term. For the present purposes, it encompasses any change in the organization of the auditory system and the behavior which the system mediates. Some of these changes are genetically programmed to proceed independently of acoustic experience (e.g., the embryologic development of the auditory system); some may be activity-dependent and/or experience-dependent (e.g., perceptual learning) and/or dependent on "critical periods." The paragraphs that follow describe examples of different levels of plasticity.

Neonatal cochlear ablations can cause quite dramatic rewiring in the auditory brainstem. Recall that in the normal animal, the VCN projects upon the MSO bilaterally. MSO neurons have oriented dendrites, with a lateral arm receiving input from the VCN of the same side, and the medial arm receiving input from the contralateral VCN (Cant, 1991). Following a neonatal unilateral cochlear lesion, ectopic projections arise from the VCN serving the intact ear: this VCN can come to innervate both the medial and lateral dendrites of cells in both MSOs (Kitzes, Kageyama, Semple, & Kil, 1995; Russell & Moore, 1995). It is also possible for the VCN serving the intact ear to come to innervate the ipsilateral MNTB, as opposed to the contralateral one. In gerbils, at least, this reorganization of connectivity occurs before the onset of hearing and may be restricted to that period; it is therefore unlikely to depend on auditory experience (Russell & Moore, 1995). There is significant shuffling of afferent connectivity to the ICC following unilateral cochlear lesions in neonates, and the reorganized connections support vigorous responses to stimulation at the intact ear, indicating that those connections are functional (Kitzes et al., 1995). In cats that receive unilateral neonatal cochlear ablations cells of the auditory cortex ipsilateral to the intact ear are more likely to receive (especially excitatory) input from that ear than do cells in normal animals (Reale, Brugge, & Chan, 1987).

In adult rats, one can experimentally lesion the superior olivary complex. After recovery from the surgery, such animals can exhibit remarkably normal binaural input patterns among neurons in both the ICC (Sally & Kelly, 1992) and auditory cortex (Kelly & Sally, 1993). The sensitivity of ICC cells to interaural level differences is also remarkably normal in appearance in these animals (Li & Kelly, 1992b). It is not currently known if these neurons show normal sensitivity to interaural temporal parameters. The presence of any binaural input itself suggests either that substantial rewiring has taken place following the lesion, or that there are other pre-existing media of binaural convergence, knowledge of which has perhaps been overshadowed by interest in the olivary nuclei. Certainly, there are many decussations of the auditory pathways (Hutson, Glendenning, & Masterton, 1991), and many or all of these are potentially capable of mediating binaural convergence. They include the corpus callosum (Kitzes & Doherty, 1994). This line of work, then, also serves to remind us that binaural interaction is a "layered" process, occurring not just once at the olivary nuclei and then being transmitted upstream without modification; rather, it may occur repeatedly through the convergent connectivity of the afferent auditory system. (See also the description, above, of the role of the DNLL in binaural interactions.)

There has been considerable effort afforded to exploring the consequences of partial cochlear lesions in adult animals. This issue is of interest clinically because experimental cochlear ablations in animals might simulate naturally occurring peripheral hearing loss in man. There have been compelling demonstrations that the tonotopic map in the auditory cortex is affected by frequency-restricted cochlear lesions in adult animals (Rajan, Irvine, Wise, & Heil, 1993; Robertson & Irvine, 1989; Schwaber, Garraghty, & Kaas, 1993). The reorganization takes the form of a loss of representation of the lesioned cochlear sector, and an expansion of the representation of the "perilesional," adjacent cochlear sites. The reorganization is not instantaneous. Studied in acutely lesioned animals, shortly following the ablation, neurons in the affected cortical places show somewhat broad, insensitive tuning to tonal stimulation (Robertson & Irvine, 1989). Studied in chronic animals 2 to 11 months after the lesion, however, neurons in those cortical regions come to acquire more normal sensitivities, frequency tuning, and response latencies for stimuli of the "new" CFs (Rajan et al., 1993). Note that, in normal animals, the vast majority of cortical cells are binaurally influenced, and the CFs of inputs from the two ears are closely matched in individual neurons; the tonotopic maps obtained for the two ears are therefore highly similar. In the cortex of animals with a unilateral, partial cochlear lesion, the tonotopic maps for the two ears are out of register in the reorganized sector. This mismatch may be a central neural correlate of binaural diplacusis because the activity of neurons in the reorganized sector is ambiguous with respect to indicating the presence of a frequency of the normal CF at the intact ear, or a frequency of the remapped CF at the damaged ear.

It is of interest to ask whether the expanded cortical representation of the perilesional cochlear places supports superior frequency discrimination at frequencies represented by those perilesional cochlear sites. We can make the assumption that frequency-restricted hearing loss in man causes the same representational changes in the cortex as are seen in animals; that assumption made, frequency discrimination at the "edge" frequencies appears to be no better than at frequencies served by the healthy cochlear sectors (Irvine, Rajan, & McDermott, 2000). It is possible that human frequency discrimination is already as good as the neural machinery can support, so that the provision of further cortical representational space still leaves the neural machinery at a ceiling level of performance.

A further form of plasticity is that associated with auditory learning. In the auditory forebrain, neurons which are narrowly tuned to frequency or amplitude, for example, those which might be found in primary auditory cortex, will undergo shifts in their CFs and even their optimal stimulus levels in response to behavioral training (Edeline, Pham, & Weinberger, 1993; Weinberger, 1997; Weinberger, Javid, & Lepan, 1993). Most of these changes appear to be shifts in selectivity within the limits of the "untrained" frequency-intensity response range. Figure 3–4 presents an idealized case. In the untrained animal, the spike count versus frequency function of a neuron shows some selectivity, and one can identify a "best" frequency to which the cell is most responsive. If the animal is then behaviorally conditioned so that an off-best-frequency stimulus takes on particular behavioral significance, then the best frequency shifts to match that of the relevant frequency. Almost all the published cases (at least, of which this author is aware) are of instances in which the shift in preferred frequency remains within the limits of the effective frequency range in the untrained animal.

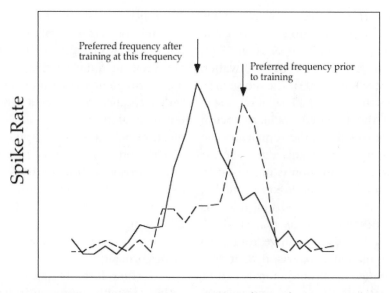

Figure 3–4. Idealized spike rate-versus-frequency functions of a single cortical neuron before and after behavioral conditioning at a single frequency within the effective response range. Note that both before and after conditioning, the neuron has a preferred frequency within its effective response range, but that the frequency preference within that range is malleable.

There is good evidence that even the excitatory frequency-intensity receptive field centered at CF itself is the envelope of convergent inputs (Phillips & Hall, 1992), so these behavioral conditioning-induced shifts might reflect a selection process exerted on the relative contributions of those inputs (after Suga et al., 1997; Zhang et al., 1997). At least some of this plasticity may be enabled by cholinergic input from the nucleus basalis of the basal forebrain because explicit pairing of electrical microstimulation of the nucleus basalis with acoustic tonal stimulation can cause these kinds of response selectivity changes, even without behavioral training (Weinberger, 1997). In the same vein, exogenous acetylcholine paired with tonal stimulation also can produce stimulus-specific shifts in recep-

tive field organization (Metherate & Weinberger, 1990).

Another expression of learning-induced plasticity has been revealed in some neurons of the secondary auditory cortical fields (Diamond & Weinberger, 1986). Neurons in these fields often have broad-frequency tuning or undifferentiated, disorderly responses across the frequency domain. This broad tuning necessarily indicates a highly convergent afferent input. When a frequency within the response range is explicitly paired with a conditioning stimulus (forepaw shock), then a striking selectivity for the frequency of the behaviorally-relevant stimulus can develop. It is reversed by extinction procedures. Once again, the neurons behave as if the behavioral conditioning process exercises some kind of selection process on the effective afferent input array.

Studies of learning-induced plasticity thus offer two means by which the representation of a stimulus in the cortex might be modified. Within a tonotopic field, there may be modest shifts in the stimulus selectivity of individual neurons whose frequency response ranges are close to the stimulus frequency of interest, so that the profile of activity aroused across the tonotopic field by a particular stimulus becomes selectively stabilized or enhanced. Within a nontonotopic field containing very broadly tuned elements, behavioral conditioning can impose a selectivity on a previously undifferentiated pattern of responsiveness. Both of these expressions of plasticity may contribute to the formation of long-term "templates" for the recognition or discrimination of acoustic signals, including speech ones (after Blumstein & Stevens, 1980; Stevens, 1980). Thus, if speech perception is conceptualized as an on-line, somewhat context-dependent, matching of the acoustic signal with internal representations of phonetic spectral templates, then these learning-induced plasticities may be some of the factors that mediate template formation.

A further question concerns the effects of learning-induced plasticity on the internal organization of tonotopic (or other) cortical maps. Recanzone et al. (1993) trained primates in a frequency discrimination task, and studied cortical neural physiology before and after successful training. They found expanded tonotopic representations of the test frequencies, although no significant changes in selectivity of frequency tuning, or changes in response latencies, of neurons in the reorganized area. A more recent study in cats (Brown, Irvine, & Park, 2004) showed no such change in tonotopy in animals successfully trained in a frequency discrimination task. That is, they showed changes in behavioral performance in the absence of overt changes in the neurophysiology of the primary auditory cortex. There is, of course, no special reason why the neurophysiologic changes that mediate the behavioral ones need to be located in the primary auditory field. Nevertheless, these findings raise important questions about exactly what form will be taken by the plastic changes associated with auditory perceptual learning, and at what loci they will be found. We do not yet have complete answers to these questions.

Finally, there is the question of whether one should necessarily expect to see expansion of activated cortical territories in situations of successful learning. The development of proficiency at a given skill, especially one that requires the coordinated activity of many brain regions, may reflect an increase in neural processing efficiency. This could be expressed in an increased automaticity of processing and less cortical tissue devoted to the task, rather than more. Indeed, human brain imaging has provided an empirical precedent for this kind of hypothesis in the domain of language learning (Zhang, Kuhl, Imada, Kotani, & Tohkura, 2005). An unqualified adherence to a "bigger is better" view of brain function may therefore be unwise.

Temporal Processing and Developmental Language Disorders

Like "plasticity," "temporal processing" and variants of it like "rapid auditory temporal processing," are umbrella terms. Rosen (1992) performed a valuable service in using the speech stimulus as a reminder of the various temporal grains of the stimulus and the information they carry. Thus, voice pitch information resides largely in glottal pulse rates; periodicities of this sort can be discriminated with close to tens of microsecond resolution. Segmental (phonetic) information has a coarser grain (milliseconds to tens of milliseconds), and suprasegmental information (e.g., intonation contours) is expressed over even longer time scales. Stimulus dimensions with different temporal grains and time structures (e.g., transient vs. periodic) are likely encoded using different neural strategies, rendering them differentially susceptible to pathology (Phillips, 1995; Phillips & Hall, 1990). Thus, some neurologic patients can show a deficit in the discrimination of phonetic information while having little trouble discriminating voice gender; others are unable to interpret prosody but retain the ability to extract the phonetic identity of a speech stimulus.

Sounds are, by their very nature, physical events distributed in time, and so there is a sense in which it is almost inevitable that a neural "sound" processing deficit is also a "temporal" processing deficit. Because the time structures of sounds come in so many forms, and because the processing of successive acoustic events is not independent for any of a number of reasons (temporal integration window width, masking time courses, adaptation, etc.), it is not particularly helpful to describe an impaired listener as having an impairment of temporal processing. Moreover, as Klein and Farmer (1995; see also Klein, 2002) point out, we need to distinguish the "processing of time" (that is, the establishing of a veridical neural-perceptual representation of the time structure of the stimulus) from the "time of processing" (i.e.,

the duration required to execute the relevant neural processes that lead to the perception of a specified acoustic event). This distinction is rarely made, and while the two processing deficits may often go hand-in-hand, in principle they need not do so. This point may be particularly relevant in studies of children, in whom the developmental improvement in perceptual performance across age may reflect changes in the "efficiency" of auditory processing in the presence of a steady adultlike temporal resolution (cf. Hill, Hartley, Glasberg, Moore, & Moore, 2004; Stuart, 2005; Stuart et al, 2006; Stuart & Phillips, 1996).

One "rapid auditory temporal processing" deficit that has received much attention is that seen in some children with developmental language disorders. Let us use it as a medium for illustrating analytic approaches to understanding the nature of temporal processing problems. Tallal & Piercy (1973a, 1973b) showed that children with what was then called "developmental aphasia" had difficulty repeating the sequence of two brief, nonverbal sounds if the sounds were in close temporal proximity. Discrimination of the two sounds also was impaired under the same temporal constraints. Tallal and Piercy noted that if the two sounds were significantly lengthened or presented at wide intersound intervals, then repetition of the sequence, and discrimination of the elements in it, improved, often to normal. Thus, it was the conjunction of sound brevity and rapid temporal succession that was the source of the problem, and not either one of those parameters alone. The same authors went on to demonstrate that sequencing and discrimination impairments extended to stop-consonant perception, but not to the perception of steady vowels; this pointed to the possibility that the rapid sequence of events at stop consonant onset (onset burst, aspiration, formant transitions and their temporal relations) in some way exceeded the processing capacity of affected individuals. Interestingly, using synthetic speech sounds, they showed that vowel-vowel syllables in which the duration of the first vowel approximated that of a stop-consonant, were subject to the same processing difficulty as were consonant-vowel syllables. By extending ("stretching") the consonant onset (formant transitions, in their study) in time, and thus providing more "time" for processing successive elements in the stream of sound, the sequencing and discrimination problems were overcome (Tallal & Piercy, 1974, 1975).

It thus seems that it was specifically not the "transitional nature" of consonant onsets that was the source of the perceptual difficulty, but the brevity of that event when it was immediately followed by another event (the vowel). Certainly the evidence presented was consistent with this view, although it would have been informative to know whether affected children had difficulty discriminating the properties of isolated frequency-sweep stimuli. In any case, it is perhaps unlikely that the perceptual system tracks the successive periods in the formant transition waveform in an individuated way that results in a conscious percept of the glide direction in a speech sound; rather, the percept tends to be of a single event that has a particular quality which we label as "b," for example. This is somewhat akin to perceiving the location of a low-frequency sound source on the basis of ITDs: there is no sense in which we "hear" successive, individuated periods of the sound at each ear and their temporal relations. Rather we perceive a single event which has the quality of being "over there."

With the deficit specified in the way that Tallal and Piercy had, subsequent references to the problematic stimuli for language learning-impaired children being the "rapid formant transitions" are imprecise: do we mean that the rate of change of frequency, on a period-by-period analysis, is too fast for the system to process? Or that the formant transition event is brief and in such close temporal proximity to other sounds that there is some interference with it being processed properly? These two questions speak to very different mechanisms, so the language with which we describe temporal processing and its disorders needs to be very precise.

Ambiguity in the use of terms arises again in the "magnocellular" theory of developmental language disorders. As mentioned earlier, the retinogeniculocortical visual pathway has at least two streams (magnocellular and parvocellular) distinguished by cell soma size and a number of physiologic properties (Livingstone & Hubel, 1988). A "magnocellular theory of dyslexia" emerged from the fact that there is some evidence for a deficit selectively in the magnocellular processing stream of the visual system in dyslexics (Livingstone et al., 1991), that is, in the processing system most responsive to high-stimulus temporal frequencies ("processing of time"), with the greater axonal conduction velocities ("time of processing"), and whose neurons have responses dominated by a transient component. The hypothesis has been extended to audition (Galaburda et al., 1994; Stein, 2001) because of the finding of a modest decrement in cell size in the medial geniculate body; it has done so, however, without any cautionary preamble that the auditory system does not have magnocellular and parvocellular streams of processing (or "transient subsystems") in the same sense that vision does. The magnocellular hypothesis has since evolved into a theory about large neurons and rapid processing, rather than about specifically sensory processing *per se* (Stein, 2001). The intended connotations of the term "magnocellular hypothesis" have thus undergone significant change over time.

There has been recent attention on the ability of the auditory systems of language learning-impaired individuals to support the normal encoding of stimulus periodicities, especially periodic amplitude or frequency modulations of tonal or other carriers. Reasons for interest in this issue stem from the facts that (a) the magnocellular hypothesis emphasizes "fast" stimuli, and (b) the rate of change of stimulus events in spoken language is in the order of 2 to 50 Hz (e.g., Rosen, 1992), a distribution of temporal frequencies that is easily within range of the normal auditory system to encode. Note, however, that in the stream of sound that constitutes speech, it may be true that changes in envelope amplitude occur as fast as every 2 to 50 ms; but the events so spaced are spectrally different from each other (e.g., consonantal burst, onset of voicing), so there is no special burden on individual neurons to respond to all of them. This is a very different situation to that in studies of temporal frequency coding, in which the stimulus is strictly periodic (i.e., a repetition of the same waveform) and the same neurons likely contribute to the temporal response (see also Phillips, 1988). This means that studies of responses to periodic stimulus changes do not necessarily inform us about the mechanisms that encode aperiodic or discrete stimulus changes.

Stefanatos, Green, and Ratliff (1989) were among the first to provide electrophysiologic evidence that the brains of developmental dysphasics were apparently less sensitive to periodic frequency modulations than those of controls. This general point has been confirmed by others: There seems to be consistent evidence that the brains of dyslexics are poorer than those of controls at supporting electrophysiologic responses to periodic frequency (FM) or amplitude modulations (McAnally & Stein, 1996; Menell, McAnally, & Stein, 1999), and that dyslexics appear to be perceptually less sensitive to such modulations (Menell et al., 1999; Talcott et al., 1999; Witton et al., 1998). Interestingly, the behavioral deficits seem to be most marked at low-modulation frequencies (e.g., Witton et al., 1998). Moreover, sensitivity to such modulations appears to be highly correlated with word and nonword reading performance (McAnally & Stein, 1996; Menell et al., 1999; Talcott et al., 1999; Witton et al., 1998). The relationship between sensitivity to low-frequency periodic FMs and reading performance extends to normal (i.e., unselected) children (Talcott et al., 2000; Witton et al., 1998).

These are fascinating findings in their own rights, and we have no particular wish to dispute them (but see Bishop, Carlyon, Deeks, & Bishop, 1999 and Van der Lely, Rosen, & McClelland, 1998 for evidence of developmental language deficits in the absence of concurrent—though not necessarily a history of earlier and predisposing—auditory temporal processing ones). However, in the context of the present discussion of the magnocellular hypothesis and rapid auditory temporal processing, two points warrant attention. First, periodic frequency modulations are not the same thing as the more discrete or singular frequency modulations that compose formant transitions in speech, so the relevance of any deficit in periodicity processing to phonology and speech perception is not immediately clear. In this regard, periodic amplitude or frequency modulations are by definition not examples of "transients," despite assumptions or inferences to the contrary (e.g., Stein, 2001; Stein & Talcott, 1999; Stein & Walsh, 1997), so there is little sense in which sensitivity to such periodicities informs us about "transient" stimulus processing. Indeed, neurophysiologic studies of single-cell coding of transient and periodic FMs indicate that the coding principles may be quite different (Phillips, 1988). This is an important point because if the hypothesis is that the reading or language deficit is attributable to a "transient system" defect, then the probes of that system actually have to challenge transient coding efficiency; it is not at all clear that periodicity coding does this. It is possible that the magnocellular auditory subsystem hypothesis has confused "transient" in the sense of being concerned with the neural coding of transient stimulus features, with "transient" in the sense of not responding in a sustained fashion.

Second, the impaired FM sensitivity was restricted to low FM frequencies of a tonal carrier (e.g., 2 Hz and 40 Hz, but not 240 Hz: Witton et al., 1998). Witton et al (1998) point out that in the case of (only) the highest (240 Hz) FM rate, the distribution of energy in the stimulus exceeds a critical band, so that the discrimination of a tone with an FM from one without the FM could be based on spectral cues rather than on any tracking of the temporal variations in the stimulus. However, for the two low FM rates, a "rapid temporal processing defect" might be expected to affect responses to the higher of the two FM rates differentially. For example, if the defect in the system was in the form of a temporal jitter in the neural code (after Miranda & Pichora-Fuller, 2002), then a constant level of temporal jitter would be larger in relation to the period of the high-frequency FM, and so would be expected to affect performance at that FM rate differentially. In practice, however, the magnitude of the difference between dyslexics' and normal listeners' FM detection thresholds was either comparable at the two low FM rates, or was larger at the lowest rate (Witton et al., 1998). This may be somewhat awkward to explain for the magnocellular theory or for a rapid auditory temporal processing account of developmental language disorders.

Summary

Our goal in this chapter has been to provide a description of central auditory neuroscience sufficiently broad that the reader has a basis to pursue further study of the topic in its own right, and to provide a foundation for later chapters in this volume. As we worked our way through the ascending auditory sensory pathway, we saw some instances in which there are comprehensible links between the physical properties of a stimulus dimension, the neural representation of the stimulus dimension, the psychophysical correlates of that dimension, and the behavioral effects of damage to structures housing the neural representation. We have seen this in the domains of spatial hearing, and sound-time structure. We then explored the notion of neuroplasticity, and found that term to be an umbrella one—it encompasses a form of plasticity driven by dramatic events during a critical period early in development, and also the plasticity which constitutes everyday perceptual learning in adulthood. In the domain of auditory temporal processing and its involvement with developmental language-learning impairment, we saw another umbrella term. What, exactly, is "rapid auditory temporal processing"? Is it a reference to the efficiency or speed with which perceptual operations are performed, or a reference to the time structure of the stimulus to be encoded? If the latter, do we mean "rapid" in the sense of high-frequency periodicities, or perhaps spectrally different transient events in close temporal proximity? There is good reason to believe that the mechanisms required for the perceptual timing of events in the same or different spectral (or binaural) channels are very different (Eggermont, 2000; Phillips et al., 1997), differentially relevant to speech processing (e.g., Phillips & Smith, 2004), and differentially susceptible to the effects of aging (Lister, Besing, & Koehnke, 2002; Lister, Koehnke, & Besing, 2000). Whenever a term has more than one meaning, it is crucial that the intended meaning be specified precisely. If there is a single general lesson to be learned from this chapter, it is that the most comprehensive understanding of auditory processing is going to depend on detailed, comprehensive knowledge of the stimulus, the neural representation of the stimulus, and the psychological dimensions of the percept aroused by the stimulus.

Acknowledgments. The preparation of this chapter, and some of the work cited herein, was supported by grants from the Natural Sciences and Engineering Research Council of Canada, the Canadian Language and Literacy Research Network, and the Killam Trust, to the author. Special thanks are due to Susan E. Hall for being an active collaborator in some of the work described in this chapter, for preparing the illustrations, and for her editorial commentaries. Thanks also to Dr Ray Klein, Dr Susan Boehnke, and Susan Hall for countless discussions on what constitutes temporal processing.

References

Bendor, D., & Wang, X. (2005). The neuronal representation of pitch in primate auditory cortex. *Nature, 436*, 1161–1165.

Bishop, D. V. M., Carlyon, R. P., Deeks, J. M., & Bishop, S. J. (1999). Auditory temporal processing impairment: Neither necessary nor sufficient for causing language impairment in children. *Journal of Speech Language and Hearing Research, 42*, 1295–1310.

Blumstein, S. E., & Stevens, K. N. (1980). Perceptual invariance and onset spectra for stop consonants in different vowel environments. *Journal of the Acoustical Society of America, 67*, 648–662.

Boehnke, S. E., & Phillips, D. P. (1999). Azimuthal tuning of human perceptual channels for sound location. *Journal of the Acoustical Society of America, 106*, 1948–1955.

Brand, A., Behrend, O., Marquardt, T., McAlpine, D., & Grothe, B. (2002). Precise inhibition is essential for microsecond interaural time difference coding. *Nature, 417*, 543–547.

Brosch, M., & Schreiner, C. E. (2000). Sequence sensitivity of neurons in cat primary auditory cortex. *Cerebral Cortex, 10*, 1155–1167.

Brown, M., Irvine, D. R. F., & Park, V. N. (2004). Perceptual learning on an auditory frequency discrimination task by cats: Association with changes in primary auditory cortex. *Cerebral Cortex, 14*, 952–965.

Calford, M. B., & Aitkin, L. M. (1983). Ascending projections to the medial geniculate body of the cat: Evidence for multiple, parallel pathways through the thalamus. *Journal of Neuroscience, 3,* 2365-2380.

Calford, M. B., & Semple, M. N. (1995). Monaural inhibition in cat auditory cortex. *Journal of Neurophysiology, 73,* 1876-1891.

Cant, N. B. (1991). Projections to the lateral and medial superior olivary nuclei from the spherical and globular bushy cells of the anteroventral cochlear nucleus. In R. A. Altschuler, R. P Bobbin,. B. M.Clopton, & D. W. Hoffman, (Eds.), *Neurobiology of hearing. The central auditory system* (pp. 99-119). New York: Raven Press.

Cariani, P., & Delgutte, B. (1996). Neural correlates of the pitch of complex tones. I. Pitch and pitch salience. *Journal of Neurophysiology, 76,* 1698-1716.

Clarey, J. C., Barone, P., & Imig, T. J. (1992). Physiology of thalamus and cortex. In A. N. Popper, & R. R. Fay (Eds.), *The mammalian auditory pathway: Neurophysiology* (pp. 232-334). New York: Springer-Verlag.

Dallos, P. (1992). The active cochlea. *Journal of Neuroscience, 12,* 4575-4585.

Diamond, D. M., & Weinberger, N. M. (1986). Classical conditioning rapidly induces specific changes in frequency receptive fields of single neurons in secondary and ventral ectosylvian auditory cortical fields. *Brain Research, 372,* 357-360.

Eddins, D. A., Hall, J. W., & Grose, J. H. (1992). The detection of temporal gaps as a function of frequency region and absolute noise bandwidth. *Journal of the Acoustical Society of America, 91,* 1069-1077.

Edeline, J-M., Pham, P., & Weinberger, N. M. (1993). Rapid development of learning-induced receptive field plasticity in the auditory cortex. *Behavioral Neuroscience, 107,* 539-551.

Eggermont, J. J. (1991). Rate and synchronization measures of periodicity coding in cat primary auditory cortex. *Hearing Research, 56,* 153-167.

Eggermont, J. J. (1994). Temporal modulation transfer functions for AM and FM stimuli in cat auditory cortex. Effects of carrier type, modulating waveform and intensity. *Hearing Research, 74,* 51-66.

Eggermont, J. J. (1995). Neural correlates of gap detection and auditory fusion in cat auditory cortex. *NeuroReport, 6,* 1645-1648.

Eggermont, J. J. (1999). Neural correlates of gap detection in three auditory cortical fields. *Journal of Neurophysiology, 81,* 2570-2581.

Eggermont, J. J. (2000). Neural responses in primary auditory cortex mimic psychophysical, across-frequency-channel, gap-detection thresholds. *Journal of Neurophysiology, 84,* 1453-1463.

Eggermont, J. J. (2002). Temporal modulation transfer functions in cat primary auditory cortex: Separating stimulus effects from neural mechanisms. *Journal of Neurophysiology, 87,* 305-321.

Fishman, Y. I., Reser, D. H., Arezzo, J. C., & Steinschneider, M. (1998). Pitch vs. spectral encoding of harmonic tone complexes in primary auditory cortex of the awake monkey. *Brain Research, 786,* 18-30.

Florentine, M., Buus, S., & Geng, W. (1999). Psychometric functions for gap detection in a yes-no procedure. *Journal of the Acoustical Society of America, 106,* 3512-3520.

Formby, C., Gerber, M.J., Sherlock, L. P., & Magder, L. S. (1998). Evidence for an across-frequency, between-channel process in asymtotic monaural temporal gap detection. *Journal of the Acoustical Society of America, 103,* 3554-3560.

Galaburda, A. M., Menard, M. T., & Rosen, G. D. (1994). Evidence for aberrant auditory anatomy in developmental dyslexia. *Proceedings of the National Academy of Sciences, USA, 91,* 8010-8013.

Glendenning, K. K., Baker, B. N., Hutson, K. A., & Masterton, R. B. (1992). Acoustic chiasm V: Inhibition and excitation in the ipsilateral and contralateral projections of LSO. *Journal of Comparative Neurology, 319,* 100-122.

Grose, J. H., Hall, J. W., & Buss, E. (1999). Modulation gap detection: Effects of modulation rate, carrier separation, and mode of presentation. *Journal of the Acoustical Society of America, 106*, 946-953.

Hackett, T. A., & Phillips, D. P. (2006). The auditory forebrain callosal and non-callosal neural systems. In J. A. Winer & C. E. Schreiner (Eds.), *The auditory cortex.* New York: Springer-Verlag.

Hall, J. W., Grose, J. H., & Saju, J. (1996). Gap detection for pairs of noise bands: Effects of stimulus level and frequency separation. *Journal of the Acoustical Society of America, 99*, 1091-1095.

Heil, P. (1997). Auditory onset responses revisited. II. Response strength. *Journal of Neurophysiology, 77*, 2642-2660.

Hill, P. R., Hartley, D. E. H., Glasberg, B.R., Moore, B.C.J., & Moore, D. R. (2004). Auditory processing efficiency and temporal resolution in children and adults. *Journal of Speech, Language, and Hearing Research, 47*, 1022-1029.

Hirsh, I. J. (1950). The relation between localization and intelligibility. *Journal of the Acoustical Society of America, 22*, 196-200.

Hutson, K. A., Glendenning, K. K., & Masterton, R. B. (1991). Acoustic chiasm IV: Eight midbrain decussations of the auditory system in the cat. *Journal of Comparative Neurology, 312*, 105-131.

Imig, T. J., & Adrian, H. O. (1977). Binaural columns in the primary auditory field (AI) of cat auditory cortex. *Brain Research, 138*, 241-257.

Imig, T. J., & Brugge, J. F. (1978). Sources and terminations of callosal axons related to binaural and frequency maps in primary auditory cortex of the cat. *Journal of Comparative Neurology, 182*, 637-660.

Imig, T. J., & Reale, R. A. (1981). Ipsilateral corticocortical projections related to binaural columns in cat primary auditory cortex. *Journal of Comparative Neurology, 203*, 1-14.

Irvine, D. R. F. (1987). Interaural intensity differences in the cat: Changes in sound pressure level at the two ears associated with azimuthal displacements in the frontal horizontal plane. *Hearing Research, 26*, 267-286.

Irvine, D. R. F., Rajan, R., & McDermott, H. J. (2000). Injury-induced reorganization in adult auditory cortex and its perceptual consequences. *Hearing Research, 147*, 188-199.

Kelly, J. B., & Sally, S. L. (1993). Effects of superior olivary complex lesions on binaural responses in rat auditory cortex. *Brain Research, 695*, 237-250.

Kidd, S. A., & Kelly, J. B. (1996). Contribution of the dorsal nucleus of the lateral lemniscus to binaural responses in the inferior colliculus of the rat: Interaural time delays. *Journal of Neuroscience, 16*, 7390-7397.

Kitzes, L. M., & Doherty, D. (1994). Influence of callosal activity on units in the auditory cortex of ferret (*Mustela putorius*). *Journal of Neurophysiology, 71*, 1740-1751.

Kitzes, L. M., Kageyama, G. H., Semple, M. N., & Kil, J. (1995). Development of ectopic projections from the ventral cochlear nucleus to the superior olivary complex induced by neonatal ablation of the contralateral cochlea. *Journal of Comparative Neurology, 353*, 341-363.

Kitzes, L. M., & Semple, M. N. (1985). Single-unit responses in the inferior colliculus: Effects of neonatal cochlear ablation. *Journal of Neurophysiology, 53*, 1483-1500.

Klein, R M. (2002). Observations on the temporal correlates of reading failure. *Reading and Writing: An Interdisciplinary Journal, 15*, 207-232.

Klein, R. M., & Farmer, M. E. (1995). Dyslexia and a temporal processing deficit: A reply to the commentaries. *Psychometric Bulletin and Review, 2*, 515-526.

Kuhl, P. K., & Miller, J. D. (1978). Speech perception by the chinchilla: Identification functions for synthetic VOT stimuli. *Journal of the Acoustical Society of America, 63*, 905-917.

Li, L., & Kelly, J. B. (1992a). Inhibitory influence of the dorsal nucleus of the lateral lemniscus on binaural responses in the rat's inferior colliculus. *Journal of Neuroscience, 12*, 4530-4539.

Li, L., & Kelly, J. B. (1992b). Binaural responses in rat inferior colliculus following kainic acid lesions of the superior olive: Interaural intensity difference functions. *Hearing Research*, *61*, 73-85.

Lister, J., Besing, J., & Koenhke, J. (2002). Effects of age and frequency disparity on gap discrimination. *Journal of the Acoustical Society of America*, *111*, 2793-2800.

Lister, J. J., Koehnke, J. D., & Besing, J. M. (2000). Binaural gap duration discrimination in listeners with impaired hearing and normal hearing. *Ear and Hearing*, *21*, 141-150.

Livingstone, M., & Hubel, D. (1988). Segregation of form, color, movement, and depth: Anatomy, physiology, and perception. *Science*, *240*, 740-749.

Livingstone, M. S., Rosen, G. D., Drislane, F. W., & Galaburda, A. M. (1991). Physiological and anatomical evidence for a magnocellular defect in developmental dyslexia. *Proceedings of the National Academy of Sciences, USA*, *88*, 7943-7947.

Malone, B. J., & Semple, M. N. (2002). Context-dependent adaptive coding of interaural phase disparity in the auditory cortex of awake macaques. *Journal of Neuroscience*, *22*, 4625-4638.

McAlpine, D., Jiang, D., & Palmer, A. R. (2001). A neural code for low-frequency sound localization in mammals. *Nature Neuroscience*, *4*, 396-401.

McAnally, K. I., & Stein, J. F. (1996). Auditory temporal coding in dyslexia. *Proceedings of the Royal Society of London Series B*, *263*, 961-965.

Menell, P., McAnally, K. I., & Stein, J. F. (1999). Psychophysical sensitivity and physiological response to amplitude modulation in adult dyslexic listeners. *Journal of Speech, Language and Hearing Research*, *42*, 797-803.

Merzenich, M. M., & Brugge, J. F. (1973). Representation of the cochlear partition on the superior temporal plane of the macaque monkey. *Brain Research*, *50*, 275-296.

Metherate, R., & Weinberger, N. M. (1990). Cholinergic modulation of responses to single tones produces tone-specific receptive field alterations in cat auditory cortex. *Synapse*, *6*, 133-145.

Middlebrooks, J. C., & Green, D. M. (1991). Sound localization by human listeners. *Annual Review of Psychology*, *42*, 135-159.

Middlebrooks, J. C., & Pettigrew, J. D. (1981). Functional classes of neurons in primary auditory cortex of the cat distinguished by sensitivity to sound location. *Journal of Neuroscience*, *1*, 107-120.

Middlebrooks, J. C., Xu, L., Eddins, A. C., & Green, D. M. (1998). Codes for sound-source location in nontonotopic auditory cortex. *Journal of Neurophysiology*, *80*, 863-881.

Miranda, T. T., & Pichora-Fuller, M. K. (2002). Temporally jittered speech produces performance intensity, phonetically balanced rollover in young normal-hearing listeners. *Journal of the American Academy of Audiology*, *13*, 50-58.

Narayan, S. S., Temchin, A. N., Recio, A., & Ruggero, M. A. (1998). Frequency tuning of basilar membrane and auditory nerve fibers in the same cochleae. *Science*, *282*, 1882-1884.

Oertel, D., Wu, S. H., & Hirsch, J. A. (1988). Electrical characteristics of cells and neuronal circuitry in the cochlear nuclei studied with intracellular recordings from brain slices. In G. M Edelman, W. E. Gall, & W. M. Cowan (Eds.), *Auditory function* (pp. 313-336). New York: Wiley.

Oliver, D. L., Beckius, G. E., Bishop, D. C., & Kuwada, S. (1997). Simultaneous anterograde labeling of axonal layers from lateral superior olive and dorsal cochlear nucleus in the inferior colliculus of cat. *Journal of Comparative Neurology*, *382*, 215-229.

Oxenham, A. J. (1997). Increment and decrement detection in sinusoids as a measure of temporal resolution. *Journal of the Acoustical Society of America*, *102*, 1779-1790.

Oxenham, A. J., Bernstein, J. G. W., & Penagos, H. (2004). Correct tonotopic representation is necessary for complex pitch perception. *Proceedings of the National Academy of Sciences, USA*, *101*, 1421-1425.

Patterson, R. D., Uppencamp, S., Johnsrude, I. S., & Griffiths, T. D. (2002). The processing of temporal pitch and melody information in auditory cortex. *Neuron, 36,* 767–776.

Phillips, D. P. (1985). Temporal response features of cat auditory cortex neurons contributing to sensitivity to tones delivered in the presence of continuous noise. *Hearing Research,* 19, 253–268.

Phillips, D. P. (1988). The neural coding of simple and complex sounds in the auditory cortex. In J. S. Lund (Ed.), *Sensory processing in the mammalian brain. Neural substrates and experimental strategies* (pp. 172–203). New York: Oxford University Press.

Phillips, D. P. (1995). Central auditory processing: A view from auditory neuroscience. *American Journal of Otology, 16,* 338–352.

Phillips, D. P. (2001). Introduction to the central auditory nervous system. In A. F. Jahn & J. Santos-Sacchi (Eds.), *Physiology of the ear* (2nd ed., pp. 613–638). San Diego, CA: Singular Publishing Group.

Phillips, D. P., & Brugge, J. F. (1985). Progress in neurophysiology of sound localization. *Annual Review of Psychology, 36,* 245–274.

Phillips, D. P., & Hall, S. E. (1990). Response timing constraints on the cortical representation of sound time structure. *Journal of the Acoustical Society of America,* 88, 1403–1411.

Phillips, D. P., & Hall, S. E. (1992). Multiplicity of inputs in the afferent path to cat auditory cortex neurons revealed by tone-on-tone masking. *Cerebral Cortex, 2,* 425–433.

Phillips, D. P., & Hall, S. E. (2000). Independence of frequency channels in auditory temporal gap detection. *Journal of the Acoustical Society of America, 108,* 2957–2963.

Phillips, D. P., & Hall, S. E. (2002). Auditory temporal gap detection for noise markers with partially overlapping and non-overlapping spectra. *Hearing Research, 174,* 133–141.

Phillips, D. P., & Hall, S. E. (2005). Psychophysical evidence for adaptation of central auditory processors for interaural differences in time and level. *Hearing Research, 202,* 188–199.

Phillips, D. P., Hall, S. E., & Boehnke, S. E. (2002). Central auditory onset responses, and temporal asymmetries in auditory perception. *Hearing Research, 167,* 192–205.

Phillips, D. P., Hall, S. E., Guo, Y-Q., & Burkard, R. (2001). Sensitivity of unanesthetized chinchilla auditory system to noise burst onset, and the effects of carboplatin. *Hearing Research, 155,* 133–142.

Phillips, D. P., Hall, S. E., Harrington, I. A., & Taylor, T. L. (1998). "Central" auditory gap detection: A spatial case. *Journal of the Acoustical Society of America, 103,* 2064–2068.

Phillips, D. P., & Irvine, D. R. F. (1981). Responses of single neurons in physiologically defined area AI of cat cerebral cortex: Sensitivity to interaural intensity differences. *Hearing Research, 4,* 299–307.

Phillips, D. P., Orman, S. S., Musicant, A. D., & Wilson, G. F. (1985). Neurons in the cat's primary auditory cortex distinguished by their responses to tones and wide-spectrum noise. *Hearing Research, 18,* 73–86.

Phillips, D. P., Semple, M. N., Calford, M. B., & Kitzes, L. M. (1994). Level dependent representation of stimulus frequency in the cat's primary auditory cortex. *Experimental Brain Research, 102,* 210–226.

Phillips, D. P., & Smith, J. C. (2004). Correlations among within- and between-channel auditory temporal gap detection thresholds in normal listeners. *Perception, 33,* 371–378.

Phillips, D. P., Taylor, T. L., Hall, S. E., Carr, M. M., & Mossop, J. E. (1997). Detection of silent intervals between noises activating different perceptual channels: Some properties of "central" auditory gap detection. *Journal of the Acoustical Society of America, 101,* 3694–3705.

Phillips, D. P., Vigneault-MacLean, B., Hall, S. E., & Boehnke, S. E. (2003). Acoustic hemifields in the spatial release from masking of speech by noise. *Journal of the American Academy of Audiology, 14,* 518–524.

Rajan, R., Aitkin, L. M., Irvine, D. R. F., & McKay, J. (1990). Azimuthal sensitivity of neurons in primary auditory cortex of cats. I. Types of sensitivity and the effects of variations in stimulus parameters. *Journal of Neurophysiology, 64*, 872-887.

Rajan, R., Irvine, D. R. F., Wise, L. Z., & Heil, P. (1993). Effect of unilateral partial cochlear lesions in adult cats on the representation of lesioned and unlesioned cochleas in primary auditory cortex. *Journal of Comparative Neurology, 338*, 17-49.

Reale, R. A., & Brugge, J. F. (2000). Directional sensitivity of neurons in the primary auditory (AI) cortex of the cat to successive sounds ordered in space and time. *Journal of Neurophysiology, 84*, 435-450.

Reale, R. A., Brugge, J. F., & Chan, J. C. K. (1987). Maps of auditory cortex in cats reared after unilateral cochlear ablation in the neonatal period. *Developmental Brain Research, 34*, 281-290.

Reale, R. A., & Imig, T. J. (1980). Tonotopic organization in cat auditory cortex. *Journal of Comparative Neurology, 192*, 265-291.

Recanzone, G. H., Schreiner, C. E., & Merzenich, M. M. (1993). Plasticity in the frequency representation of primary auditory cortex following discrimination training in adult owl monkeys. *Journal of Neuroscience, 13*, 87-103.

Rhode, W. S. (1991). Physiological-morphological properties of the cochlear nucleus. In R. A Altschuler,. R. P. Bobbin, B. M. Clopton, & D. W. Hoffman (Eds.), *Neurobiology of hearing. The central auditory system* (pp. 47-77). New York. Raven Press.

Rhode, W. S., & Greenberg, S. (1992). Physiology of the cochlear nuclei. In A. N. Popper, & R. R. Fay (Eds.), *The mammalian auditory pathway: Neurophysiology* (pp. 94-152). New York: Springer.

Robertson, D., & Irvine, D. R. F. (1989). Plasticity of frequency organization in auditory cortex of guinea pigs with partial unilateral deafness. *Journal of Comparative Neurology, 282*, 456-471.

Rosen, S. (1992). Temporal information in speech: Acoustic, auditory and linguistic aspects. *Philosophical Transactions of the Royal Society of London Series B, 336*, 367-373.

Ruggero, M. (1992). Physiology and coding of sound in the auditory nerve. In A. N Popper, & R. R. Fay (Eds.), *The mammalian auditory pathway: Neurophysiology* (pp. 34-93). New York: Springer.

Ruggero, M., & Rich, N. C. (1991). Furosemide alters organ of Corti mechanics: Evidence for feedback of outer hair cells upon the basilar membrane. *Journal of Neuroscience, 11*, 1057-1067.

Russell, F. A., & Moore, D. R. (1995). Afferent reorganization within the superior olivary complex of the gerbil: Development and induction by neonatal, unilateral cochlear removal. *Journal of Comparative Neurology, 352*, 607-625.

Sally, S. L., & Kelly, J. B. (1992). Effects of superior olivary complex lesions on binaural responses in rat inferior colliculus. *Brain Research, 572*, 5-18.

Samson, F. K., Clarey, J. C., Barone, P., & Imig, T. J. (1993). Effects of ear plugging on single-unit azimuth sensitivity in cat primary auditory cortex. I. Evidence for monaural direction cues. *Journal of Neurophysiology, 70*, 492-511.

Scharf, B., Magnan, J., Collet, L., Ulmer, E., & Chays, A. (1994). On the role of the olivocochlear bundle in hearing: A case study. *Hearing Research, 75*, 11-26.

Scharf, B., Quigley, S., Aoki, C., Peachey, N., & Reeves, A. (1987). Focussed auditory attention and frequency selectivity. *Perception and Psychophysics, 42*, 215-223.

Schreiner, C. E., & Mendelson, J. R. (1990). Functional topography of cat primary auditory cortex: Distribution of integrated excitation. *Journal of Neurophysiology, 64*, 1442-1459.

Schwaber, M. K., Garraghty, P. E., & Kaas, J. H. (1993). Neuroplasticity of the adult primary auditory cortex following cochlear hearing loss. *American Journal of Otology, 14*, 252-258.

Schwartz, I. R. (1992). The superior olivary complex and the lateral lemniscal nuclei. In D. B. Webster, A. N. Popper, & R. R. Fay (Eds.), *The mammalian auditory pathway: Neuroanatomy* (pp. 117-167). New York: Springer-Verlag.

Schwarz, D. W. F., & Tomlinson, R. W. W. (1990). Spectral response patterns of auditory cortex neurons to harmonic complex tones in alert monkey (*Macaca mulatta*). *Journal of Neurophysiology, 64*, 282-298.

Sellick, P. M., Patuzzi, R., & Johnstone, B. M. (1982). Measurement of basilar membrane motion in the guinea pig using the Mössbauer technique. *Journal of the Acoustical Society of America, 72.* 131-141.

Semple, M. N., & Aitkin, L. M. (1981). Integration and segregation of input to the cat inferior colliculus. In J. Syka, & L. M. Aitkin (Eds.), *Neuronal mechanisms of hearing* (pp. 155-161). New York: Plenum Press.

Semple, M. N., & Kitzes, L. M. (1993). Binaural processing of sound pressure level in cat primary auditory cortex: Evidence for a representation based on absolute levels rather than interaural level differences. *Journal of Neurophysiology, 69*, 449-461.

Shneiderman, A., Oliver, D. L., & Henkel, C. (1988). Connections of the dorsal nucleus of the lateral lemniscus: An inhibitory parallel pathway in the ascending auditory system? *Journal of Comparative Neurology, 276*, 188-208.

Snell, K. B., & Hu, H-L. (1999). The effect of temporal placement on gap detectability. *Journal of the Acoustical Society of America, 106*, 3571-3577.

Spitzer, M. W., & Semple, M. N. (1993). Responses of inferior colliculus neurons to time-varying interaural phase disparity: Effects of shifting the locus of virtual motion. *Journal of Neurophysiology, 69*, 1245-1263.

Spitzer, M. W., & Semple, M. N. (1998). Transformation of binaural response properties in the ascending auditory pathway: Influence of time-varying interaural phase disparity. *Journal of Neurophysiology, 80*, 3062-3076.

Spoendlin, H. H. (1967). Innervation patterns in the organ of Corti in the cat. *Acta Otolaryngologica, 67*, 239-254.

Stecker, G. C., Harrington, I. A., & Middlebrooks, J. C. (2005). Location coding by opponent neural populations in the audi-

tory cortex. *Public Library of Science, 3*, 520-528.

Stefanatos, G. A., Green, G. G. R., & Ratliff, G. G. (1989). Neurophysiological evidence of auditory channel anomalies in developmental dysphasia. *Archives of Neurology, 46*, 871-875.

Stein, J. (2001). The magnocellular theory of developmental dyslexia. *Dyslexia, 7*, 12-36.

Stein, J., & Talcott, J. (1999). Impaired neuronal timing in developmental dyslexia—the magnocellular hypothesis. *Dyslexia, 5*, 59-77.

Stein, J., & Walsh, V. (1997). To see but not to read. The magnocellular theory of dyslexia. *Trends in Neuroscience, 20*, 147-152.

Stevens, K. N. (1980). Acoustic correlates of some phonetic categories. *Journal of the Acoustical Society of America, 68*, 836-842.

Stuart, A. (2005). Development of auditory temporal resolution in school-aged children revealed by word recognition in continuous and interrupted noise. *Ear and Hearing, 26*, 78-88.

Stuart, A., Givens, G. D., Walker, L. J., & Elangovan, S. (2006). Auditory temporal resolution in normal-hearing preschool children revealed by word recognition in continuous and interrupted noise. *Journal of the Acoustical Society of America, 119*, 1946-1949.

Stuart, A. M., & Phillips, D. P. (1996). Word recognition in continuous and interrupted broadband noise by young normal-hearing, older normal hearing, and presbyacusic listeners. *Ear and Hearing, 17*, 78-489.

Suga, N., Yan, J., & Zhang, Y. (1997). Cortical maps for hearing and egocentric selection for self-organization. *Trends in Cognitive Sciences, 1*, 13-20.

Talcott, J. B., Witton, C., McClean, M., Hansen, P. C., Rees, A., Green, G. G. R., & Stein, J. F. (1999). Can sensitivity to auditory frequency modulation predict children's phonological and reading skills? *NeuroReport, 10*, 2045-2050.

Talcott, J. B., Witton, C., McLean, M. F., Hansen, P. C., Rees, A., Green, G. G. R., & Stein, J. F. (2000). Dynamic sensory sensitivity and children's word decoding skills. *Proceedings of the National Academy of Sciences, USA, 97*, 2952-2957.

Tallal, P., & Piercy, M. (1973a). Defects of non-verbal auditory perception in children with developmental aphasia. *Nature, 241*, 468-469.

Tallal, P., & Piercy, M. (1973b). Developmental aphasia: impaired rate of non-verbal processing as a function of sensory modality. *Neuropsychologia, 11*, 389-398.

Tallal, P., & Piercy, M. (1974). Developmental aphasia: Rate of auditory processing and selective impairment of consonant perception. *Neuropsychologia, 12*, 83-93.

Tallal, P., & Piercy, M. (1975). Developmental aphasia: the perception of brief vowels and extended stop consonants. *Neuropsychologia, 13*, 69-74.

Tollin, D. J., & Yin, T. C. T. (2002). The coding of spatial location by single units in the lateral superior olive of the cat. I. Spatial receptive fields in azimuth. *Journal of Neuroscience, 22*, 1454-1467.

Van der Lely, H. K. J., Rosen, S., & McClelland, A. (1998). Evidence for a grammar-specific deficit in children. *Current Biology, 8*, 1253-1258.

Wang, X., Merzenich, M. M., Beitel, R, & Schreiner, C. E. (1995). Representation of a species-specific vocalization in the auditory cortex of the common marmoset: Temporal and spectral characteristics. *Journal of Neurophysiology, 74*, 2685-2706.

Warr, W. B. (1992). Organization of olivo-cochlear efferent systems in mammals. In D. B. Webster, A. N. Popper, & R. R. Fay (Eds.), *The mammalian auditory pathway: Neuroanatomy* (pp. 410-448). New York: Springer-Verlag.

Weinberger, N. M. (1997). Learning-induced receptive field plasticity in the primary auditory cortex. *Seminars in Neuroscience, 9*, 59-67.

Weinberger, N. M., Javid, R., & Lepan, B. (1993). Long-term retention of learning-induced receptive field plasticity in the auditory cortex. *Proceedings of the National Academy of Sciences, USA, 90*, 2394-2398.

Winer, J. A. (1992). The functional architecture of the medial geniculate body and the primary auditory cortex. In D. B. Webster, A. N. Popper, & R. R. Fay (Eds.), *The mammalian auditory pathway: Neuroanatomy* (pp. 222-409). New York: Springer-Verlag.

Witton, C., Talcott, J. B., Hansen, P. C., Richardson, A. J., Griffiths, T. D., Rees, A., Stein, J. F., & Green, G. G. R. (1998). Sensitivity to dynamic auditory and visual stimuli predicts nonword reading ability in both dyslexic and normal readers. *Current Biology, 8*, 791-797.

Wu, S. H., & Kelly, J. B. (1992). Synaptic pharmacology of the superior olivary complex studied in mouse brain slice. *Journal of Neuroscience, 12*, 3084-3097.

Yan, J., & Suga, N. (1996). Corticofugal modulation of time-domain processing of biosonar information in bats. *Science, 273*, 1100-1103.

Yin, T. C. T., & Chan, J. C. K. (1990). Interaural time sensitivity in medial superior olive of cat. *Journal of Neurophysiology, 64*, 465-488.

Yin, T. C. T., & Kuwada, S. (1983). Binaural interactions in low-frequency neurons in inferior colliculus of the cat. III. Effects of changing frequency. *Journal of Neurophysiology, 50*, 1020-1042.

Young, E. D., & Brownell, W. E. (1976). Responses to tones and noise of single cells in dorsal cochlear nucleus of unanesthetized cats. *Journal of Neurophysiology, 39*, 282-300.

Zhang, J., Nakamoto, J. T., & Kitzes, L. M. (2005). Modulation of level response areas and stimulus selectivity of neurons in cat primary auditory cortex. *Journal of Neurophysiology, 94*, 2263-2274.

Zhang, Y., Kuhl, P. K., Imada, T., Kotani, M., & Tohkura, Y. (2005). Effects of language experience: Neural commitment to language-specific auditory patterns. *NeuroImage, 26*, 703-720.

Zhang, Y., Suga, N., & Yan, J. (1997). Corticofugal modulation of frequency processing in bat auditory system. *Nature, 387*, 900-903.

CHAPTER 4

NEUROBIOLOGY OF (CENTRAL) AUDITORY PROCESSING DISORDER AND LANGUAGE-BASED LEARNING DISABILITY

KAREN BANAI AND NINA KRAUS

(Central) auditory processing disorder (abbreviated here APD) is defined as a deficit in the processing of auditory information, despite normal hearing thresholds, that primarily involves the auditory modality (ASHA, 2005; Jerger & Musiek, 2000). This umbrella definition encompasses a wide variety of perceptual and cognitive manifestations. APD thus cannot be reduced to a single anatomic site or impaired process in the auditory system. The question of whether such a nonspecific definition can really benefit research, diagnosis, and treatment notwithstanding, in this chapter we focus on the physiologic processes thought to underlie the perception of auditory aspects that fall within the realm of APD. We review evidence for specific physiologic processes and anatomic sites contributing to normal and abnormal auditory processing. In particular we review studies of the physiology and anatomy of: (1) auditory temporal processing, (2) auditory perception in noise, (3) representation and discrimination of acoustic features and (4) binaural processing. We also present evidence for (5) training-related neural plasticity of these processes where such evidence exists, focusing on training studies aimed at populations with symptoms of APD. The physiologic processes reviewed here with their accompanying perceptual correlates are summarized in Table 4–1. To our knowledge, physiologic and anatomic studies of APD diagnosed populations have been rare. On the other hand, many studies have focused on auditory processing in populations diagnosed with language-based learning disabilities (e.g., specific language impairment [SLI] and

Table 4–1. Auditory Processing Deficits: Perception and Neurophysiology

Perceptual Difficulty	Proposed Neurophysiologic Correlates
Temporal Processing	
Temporal resolution	Delayed onset of auditory brainstem response (ABR) to speech
Temporal order judgment[1]	Abnormal cortical representation of sound under temporal stress
Backward masking detection	Delayed ABR wave V in masked conditions
Modulation detection	Reduced amplitude modulation following response (AMFR)
Auditory Perception in Noise	
Processing of speech in noise[1]	Abnormal suppression of otoacoustic emissions (OAE), speech-evoked ABR; cortical representation of speech in noise,[2] frequency following response (FFR) magnitude.[2]
Representation and Discrimination of Acoustic Features (Speech and Nonspeech)	
Discrimination of acoustic features[1]	Abnormal cortical representation of sound; immature cortical responses;[2] abnormal mismatched negativity response (MMN).[2]
Speech perception[1]	Delayed speech-evoked ABR onset; reduced magnitude of the FFR in F1 frequency range; abnormal cortical lateralization and N1 responses.
Speech discrimination[1]	Abnormal MMN[2] and P3 (not reviewed here)
Binaural Processing	
Sound localization, dichotic listening[1]	Abnormal binaural interaction components (BIC)
Training-Related Plasticity	
[1]Improve with training and [2]Exhibit training-related plasticity in the LLD population	

dyslexia) in which symptoms of APD are often present. Throughout the chapter we will use the general term LLD (language-based learning disorder) to refer to this population. The principles we present here derive, therefore, from our understanding of the normal auditory system as applied to a wide array of studies in clinical populations intersecting with APD.

Temporal Processing

Temporal processing in the auditory system is defined, broadly, as the ability of the auditory system to represent and process changes in the acoustic signal that occur over time (e.g., the temporal envelope of the signal), and to its ability to process brief transient acoustic events (e.g., sound onset and consonants). Adequate auditory perception requires good temporal resolution on the time scale of microseconds for the processing of binaural cues, milliseconds for processing of temporal synchrony, tens of milliseconds for the processing of speech transients and voicing information, and hundreds of milliseconds to seconds for the processing of prosodic and suprasegmental cues. In addition, in order to make sense of our environment, the intact auditory system needs to be sensitive to the order in which acoustic events occur (e.g., "on" vs. "no") and be able to transition between those time scales and integrate information from all the time scales to create a unitary auditory percept. Indeed, evidence suggests that encoding of temporal information into a coherent form begins as early as the cochlear nucleus and continues up to the auditory cortex (Frisina, 2001; Griffiths, Uppenkamp, Johnsrude, Josephs, & Patterson, 2001).

The measurement of auditory evoked potentials provides a window into temporal processing, providing information about neural timing with fractions of a millisecond precision. Available recording techniques enable the study of timing along the ascending auditory pathway from the XIIIth nerve to the auditory cortex and indeed most of our information on temporal processing in humans comes from such studies. Additional information, in particular regarding cortical temporal processing comes from studies of patients with cortical lesions. However, it should be noted that due to the complex pattern of connectivity in the auditory pathway (e.g., massive feedback connections), and the relative nature of perception (i.e. its dependence on context) it is hard to attribute a specific perceptual deficit to a specific anatomic location along the pathway without additional information (Eggermont & Ponton, 2002; Phillips, 1995).

Temporal Resolution

Of particular interest here is the brainstem's response to sound. Transient acoustic events evoke a pattern of voltage changes in the auditory brainstem. The resulting waveform provides information about brainstem nuclei along the ascending auditory pathway (see Hood, 1998; Jacobsen, 1985 for reviews). Converging evidence suggests that learning-impaired populations show normal click-evoked auditory brainstem responses (ABR) (Grontved, Walter, & Gronborg, 1988a, 1988b; Jerger, Martin, & Jerger, 1987; Lauter & Wood, 1993; Mason & Mellor, 1984; McAnally & Stein, 1997; Purdy, Kelly, & Davies, 2002), yet about a third of all individuals diagnosed with language-based learning problems manifest reduced temporal synchrony at the level of the upper brainstem (i.e., lateral lemniscus, inferior colliculus) in response to speech sounds (Banai, Nicol, Zecker, & Kraus, 2005; Cunningham, Nicol, Zecker, Bradlow, & Kraus, 2001; King, Warrier, Hayes, & Kraus, 2002; Wible, Nicol, & Kraus, 2004) and backward masked signals (Marler & Champlin, 2005).

The speech-evoked ABR may be conceptualized as the neural code of a speech syllable (reviewed in Johnson, Nicol, & Kraus, 2005). To a consonant-vowel syllable, the onset response (waves V, A) represents the burst onset of a voiced consonant, whereas later portions likely represent the offset of the onset burst or the onset of voicing (wave C) and the offset of the stimulus (wave O). The harmonic portion of the speech stimulus gives rise to the frequency-following response (FFR, waves D, E, and F) (Galbraith, Arbagey, Branski, Comerci, & Rector, 1995; Krishnan, 2002). The FFR is characterized as a series of transient neural events phase locked to the periodic information within the stimulus (Marsh & Worden, 1968; Sohmer & Pratt, 1977). Disruption of either the onset or the FFR is likely to result in impaired representation of important segmental and suprasegmental information, respectively, within the speech sound thus degrading the input into higher levels of the auditory system (Kraus & Nicol, 2005). A characteristic brainstem response to the speech syllable /da/ is shown in Figure 4–1. Like the familiar click-evoked ABR, speech-evoked ABRs can be obtained from an individual subject with relative ease, making it an objective biological marker of auditory processing (Johnson et al., 2005; Russo, Nicol, Musacchia, & Kraus, 2004).

Using this measure in large groups of normal learning children and children

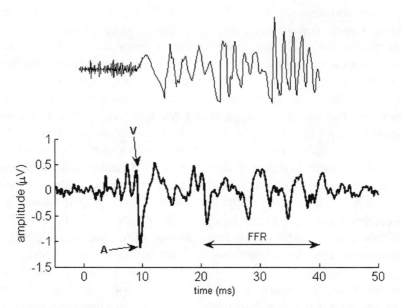

Figure 4–1. *Top:* Stimulus waveform (amplitude vs. time) of the speech syllable /da/. The first 10 ms correspond to the consonant portion whereas the larger amplitude portion from 10 to 40 ms corresponds to the vowel portion of the syllable. *Bottom:* the corresponding brainstem evoked response (speech-ABR) recorded from a typically developing 9-year-old child. Waves V and A marked on the response waveform correspond to the brainstem's response to the initial portion of the syllable, whereas the FFR corresponds to the vowel.

diagnosed with LLD has shown that children with LLD present abnormalities of both the onset response and the magnitude of the FFR. King et al. (2002) demonstrated that wave A of the onset response was at least 1 SD delayed in 20 of the 54 listeners with LLD they studied, and that these listeners also had delayed waves C and F. Wible et al. (2004) further studied the differences in brainstem encoding of speech between normal learning and children with LLD. They concluded that children with LLD had markedly shallower slopes of the transition between onset waves V and A, suggesting a more sluggish response in these children. They also showed that the amplitude of the FFR was significantly reduced among LLD children in the frequency region corresponding to the first formant (F1) of the /da/ stimulus used. Similarly, Cunningham et al. (2001) demonstrated that the magnitude of the FFR in response to a stimulus presented in background noise was reduced in a group of LLD children in the F1 frequency range. The magnitude of the response in the fundamental frequency (F0) range on the other hand was found to be normal in both quiet (Wible et al., 2004) and noise (Cunningham et al., 2001). Recently, Banai et al. (2005) estimated, in the largest sample yet studied with speech-ABR, that 30% of children with LLD show onset responses that are abnormal at the 2 SD level when a unifying onset score was created based on the latencies of onset waves V and A, as well as the duration and slope of the transition between them.

A similar phenomenon was recently shown with more simple stimuli. Marler and Champlin (2005) studied ABR elicited by tone bursts in a group of children with LLD (specifically diagnosed with

SLI). They reported that even though wave V latencies did not differ between children with normal learning and children with LLD when tone bursts were presented alone, wave V of the LLD group was significantly delayed when the same tone was presented immediately followed by a noise burst (backward masking condition). It may be that a similar mechanism underlies abnormal onset responses to speech sounds (which are potentially masked by the steady state portion of the stimulus) and masked nonspeech sounds. Supporting this notion, children with LLD and elevated backward masking detection thresholds also have abnormal brainstem encoding of speech sounds (Johnson, Nicol, Zecker, Wright,& Kraus, 2004).

Neurons in the auditory system, including the auditory brainstem, show a high degree of sensitivity to oxygen shortage during development. A recent study of rats who suffered from experimentally induced anoxia at birth showed that one consequence of this oxygen shortage was a degraded click-ABR (Strata et al., 2005). It may be that a similar process contributes to abnormal ABRs measured to complex sounds in children with LLD. Although click ABR in these children are typically within clinical norms, they tend to be delayed (Song et al., 2006). It is therefore possible that scalp-measured ABR in humans are not sensitive enough to document this minute effect and that deficits are therefore observed only in response to more complex stimuli.

Taken together with the perceptual deficits present among individuals with LLD, this combined body of research suggests that processing of rapidly changing spectrally complex information at the level of the brainstem is one

likely source of APD. It is anticipated that the brainstem response to speech sounds will be incorporated into the clinical evaluation of APD (e.g., see BioMAP™ —Biological Marker of Auditory Processing, Bio-logic Systems Corp, Mundelein, IL). Furthermore, as explained in detail in the relevant sections below, brainstem timing was found to correlate with the robustness of the cortical response in noise (Wible, Nicol, & Kraus, 2005), and the majority of individuals with abnormal cortical detection of rare acoustic events also have delayed speech-evoked ABRs (Banai et al., 2005). Thus, deficient brainstem timing may affect the cortical response to sound.

The timing of the N1 evoked response is sometimes considered an index of temporal processing at the cortical level. However, as it is optimally evoked with a stimulation rate slower than 2 Hz (Hall, 1992), and as the response is probably less affected by the physical characteristics of the stimulus, but rather by its functional significance (Kraus & McGee, 1992), it may be more useful to consider it as representing the initial cortical processing of the auditory signal. Its manifestations in individuals with LLD are discussed further under Representation of Acoustic Features.

Encoding of Stimulus Temporal Envelope

Another measure of auditory encoding of stimulus structure can be obtained by recording the amplitude modulation following response (AMFR). This response encodes the frequency of the fluctuations in the amplitude envelope of an amplitude-modulated (AM) sound. The magnitude of this response has been found to be reduced in individuals with dyslexia, meaning they need deeper (larger) signal modulation to detect its presence compared to controls. This physiologic finding corresponds with behavioral findings of higher AM detection thresholds (McAnally & Stein, 1997; Menell, McAnally, & Stein, 1999), and suggests that auditory encoding of signal modulation difficulties may lead to perceptual difficulties in following such temporal modulations in speech. For a discussion of the role of temporal information in speech see Rosen (1992). The AMFR has multiple thalamic and cortical generators (Herdman et al., 2002; Kuwada, Batra, & Maher, 1986), with subcortical generators probably contributing to the processing of fast modulations (>80 Hz) and cortical ones to the processing of slower (<40 Hz) rates. However, behavioral evidence suggests that individuals with dyslexia have similar deficits across all modulation rates (Lorenzi, Dumont, & Fullgrabe, 2000; Menell et al., 1999), and the magnitudes of their AMFR were similarly reduced across the range from 10 to 320 Hz rates (Menell et al., 1999).

Temporal Order/Sequencing of Rapid Acoustic Events

Perceptual organization of sound, such as determining temporal order, is typically thought of as a function of the auditory cortex (see Näätänen, Tervaniemi, Sussman, Paavilainen, & Winkler, 2001 for review). Nagarajan et al. (1999) presented poor readers with pairs of brief tones, asking them to determine the order in which the tones were presented (high-low; low-high; high-high; low-low, a task originally used by Tallal with a language-impaired population) and recorded their evoked magnetic responses to the tone pairs. Poor readers had a normal response to the first tone, but had a significantly reduced response to the second one when interstimulus interval (ISI) within the pair was short (100 or 200 ms), but not when it was longer (i.e., 500 ms). These neurophysiologic findings were consistent with better behavioral performance in the long ISI condition. These data suggest that, although the basic cortical response in poor readers may be intact, representation of successive signals is impaired. Bishop and McArthur (2004) reported similar results in the population diagnosed with SLI. They reported enhanced correlations between the cortical response to a single tone and the response to tone pairs in individuals with SLI, indicating a less reliable processing of tone sequences. Bishop and McArthur suggested that these findings reflect immature auditory processing among some individuals with SLI. Similarly, Temple et al. (2000) using nonverbal analogues of a formant transition found a disruption of the neural response to the transient stimulus in subjects with dyslexia. They showed that an area in the left prefrontal cortex that became activated among normal readers in response to a rapidly transient stimulus, but not in response to a slower transition, did not show this increased activation in dyslexics in response to rapidly changing stimuli. Moreover, Poldrack et al. (2001) reported that an area within the left inferior frontal cortex (pars triangularis), that is specifically involved in phonological processing, also showed changes in activation that were related to the degree of compression of a speech signal (i.e., temporal processing). These findings suggest that areas that are not typically considered auditory areas have

an important role in auditory processing. Yet, because these areas are not sensitive to specific acoustic characteristics, some other functional property must be shared between "simple auditory" and phonological processing.

To summarize, populations diagnosed with LLD such as dyslexia and SLI are characterized by abnormalities in several different aspects of temporal processing as measured by imaging and electrophysiologic techniques. Importantly, these populations also manifest difficulties in the perception of temporal information. Some individuals with LLD have difficulties in tasks requiring temporal order judgments (Cacace, McFarland, Ouimet, Schrieber, & Marro, 2000; Farmer & Klein, 1995; Heath, Hogben, & Clark, 1999; Nagarajan et al., 1999; Tallal, 1980; Tallal & Piercy, 1973), *detection of amplitude and frequency modulations in sound* (Lorenzi et al., 2000; Menell et al., 1999; Rocheron, Lorenzi, Fullgrabe, & Dumont, 2002; Talcott et al., 2003; Witton, Stein, Stoodley, Rosner, & Talcott, 2002) *and detection of backward masked tones* (Griffiths, Hill, Bailey, & Snowling, 2003; Marler, Champlin, & Gillam, 2002; Wright et al., 1997). *Overall, it is estimated that 30 to 50% of individuals diagnosed with dyslexia also manifest an auditory perceptual deficit characteristic of APD* (Amitay, Ahissar, & Nelken, 2002; King, Lombardino, Crandell, & Leonard, 2003; Ramus, 2003). It has been suggested, most notably by Tallal and her colleagues, that such a pattern of deficits should lead to difficulties in the representation and discrimination of consonants characterized by brief formant transitions and consequently to difficulties in phonological processing and reading which are the hallmarks of dyslexia (Tallal, 1980; Tallal, Miller, & Fitch, 1993). Subsequent studies have indeed shown that many individuals with language-based learning problems, have poorer phonemic discrimination in addition to their reading and phonological deficits suggesting a possible link between temporal processing and literacy (Adlard & Hazan, 1998; Breier, Fletcher, Denton, & Gray, 2004; Breier et al., 2001; Cornelissen, Hansen, Bradley, & Stein, 1996; Joanisse, Manis, Keating, & Seidenberg, 2000; Reed, 1989; Rosen & Manganari, 2001; Ziegler, Pech-Georgel, George, Alario, & Lorenzi, 2005). Poor discrimination is not, however, restricted only to rapidly changing consonants, but found also for vowels (e.g. Putter-Katz et al., 2005; Rosen & Manganari, 2001). Also, it should be noted that speech perception deficits are probably mostly characteristic of children with a history of SLI (Joanisse et al., 2000).

Neurophysiology of Perception in Noise

A hallmark of APD is unusual difficulties in speech understanding in noisy environments (Chermak, Hall, & Musiek, 1999; Chermak, Tucker, & Seikel, 2002). Individuals with LLD show abnormal physiologic responses to sound at the cortical level when it occurs in background noise. Cunningham et al. (2001) investigated cortical and brainstem responses in normal learning children and children with LLD in response to speech stimuli in quiet and in noise. Physiologic responses at both the cortical and brainstem level did not differ between groups in ideal listening conditions (i.e., quiet). On the other hand, both cortical and brainstem responses of children with LLD were significantly reduced when

the same /da/ stimulus was presented in noise. This pattern of neurophysiologic findings matched the observed pattern of perceptual deficits whereby children with LLD had normal discrimination thresholds in quiet, but significantly elevated thresholds in noise. Both perception and cortical responses significantly improved, however, when the stimuli were presented in a cue-enhanced "clear speech" mode. At the brainstem level, cue enhancement improved the timing of the onset response, but had no effect on response magnitude. Wible, Nicol and Kraus (2002) showed that repeated presentations of a stimulus in noise resulted in less reliable P1/N1/P2/N2 cortical responses (i.e., lower correlations between responses to repeated stimuli) in a subset of children with LLD, but not in normal learning children, suggesting that the LLD system is more sensitive to the stresses of a noisy listening situation. Warrier, Johnson, Hayes, Nicol and Kraus (2004) found that the correlation between cortical responses in quiet and noise (i.e., the degree of response degradation by noise), which serves to test the reliability of the cortical response in noise, also was severely reduced in about 20% of LD participants tested. Further studies showed a strong correlation between the brainstem onset response and the degree of degradation of cortical correlation in noise (Wible et al., 2005) and that only the subset of children with LLD with abnormal brainstem timing are likely to show severely abnormal cortical responses in noise (King et al., 2002). Furthermore, only in this group did listening training (i.e., Earobics) result in significant enhancement of the reliability of cortical function in noise (Hayes, Warrier, Nicol, Zecker, & Kraus, 2003; King et al., 2002). This abnormal physiology coincides with poor perception of speech in noise (Cunningham et al., 2001). Furthermore, while children with LLD with both normal and abnormal brainstem timing alike also show poor discrimination of speech in quiet listening conditions, only among those children with LLD with abnormal brainstem timing did speech discrimination improve following listening training (King et al., 2002). *Taken together, these findings imply that among children with LLD, physiologic processing of speech in noise is abnormal at both the brainstem and cortical levels, and that encoding of speech in noise can be improved with either training or the use of cue enhanced stimuli.*

Taking a somewhat different approach, based on evidence linking the medial olivocochlear bundle (MOCB) of the lower brainstem to hearing in noise, Muchnik et al. (2004) objectively tested the function of the MOCB system in children diagnosed with APD using otoacoustic emissions (OAE) with and without acoustic stimulation of the contralateral ear. In the normal population, contalateral stimulation suppresses the OAE (e.g. Collet et al., 1990), probably reflecting the inhibitory control of the MOCB on the outer hair cells. Muchnik et al. (2004) reported that the suppression effect was significantly reduced in the APD group compared to normal controls, characterizing 11 of 15 children in the APD group. Furthermore, 80% of the children with APD in this study exhibited severely impaired speech perception in noise. These findings provide evidence for abnormal function of the descending auditory pathway in APD, and taken together with the cortical and higher brainstem findings summarized above, likely suggest an important top-down effect in APD.

Representation and Discrimination of Acoustic Features

Information about representation of sound at the level of the auditory cortex can be obtained by recording the obligatory cortical response to sound (P1/N1/P2/N2), whereas information on deficits in acoustic discrimination is most commonly obtained from the mismatch negativity response (MMN) (Näätänen, 1992). The MMN is generated in response to a change in a repetitive sequence of stimuli, that is, when rare acoustic stimuli are presented amidst common (standard) stimuli in an oddball paradigm. Under such presentation conditions, the brain generates a negative potential in response to the rare element, even when the difference between the standard and rare stimuli is barely perceptible. The MMN probably has several generators including the thalamocortical pathway, the auditory cortex, and frontal brain regions (Kraus et al., 1994; Rinne, Alho, Ilmoniemi, Virtanen, & Näätänen, 2000; Sams, Kaukoranta, Hamalainen, & Näätänen, 1991).

Representation of Acoustic Features

The ability of the cortex to adequately represent the acoustic stimulus is critical to our ability to further process the stimulus in functionally significant ways (e.g., discriminate, categorize, identify). In the dyslexic population, several studies have shown abnormal N1 responses to nonspeech and speech sounds (i.e., pseudowords and vowels) (Helenius, Salmelin, Richardson, Leinonen, & Lyytinen, 2002);

nonspeech sounds with temporal or spectral deviance, and syllables differing in voice onset time (VOT) or second formant (Moisescu-Yiflach & Pratt, 2005); 2000-Hz tone bursts (Pinkerton, Watson, & McClelland, 1989); and consonants and vowels (Putter-Katz et al., 2005). Fewer left-lateralized responses also have been reported (Heim, Eulitz, & Elbert, 2003), as well as abnormal cerebral asymmetry to speech sounds (Duara et al., 1991; Gross-Glenn et al., 1991; Leonard et al., 2001). Furthermore, it has been suggested that the generating sources of these potentials within the auditory system may vary between typically developing children and children with dyslexia (Heim et al., 2003; Heim et al., 2000). At birth, N1 responses to consonant-vowel syllables (/ga/, /ba/, /da/) of children with familial risk for dyslexia and SLI are different from those of not-at-risk newborns (Guttorm et al., 2001). Furthermore, N1 responses to syllables at birth are predictive of later development of language and literacy skills (Espy, Molfese, Molfese, & Modglin, 2004; Molfese, 2000). Later components of the auditory evoked response to speech-sounds at birth also have been linked to risk for dyslexia and to language and memory development (Guttorm et al., 2005; Guttorm et al., 2001; Molfese & Molfese, 1985, 1997); however, those components may not represent uniquely auditory processing and, therefore are not discussed further here.

Other studies failed to documents differences in the basic auditory cortical representation between typically developing individuals and individuals with LLD. Thus, in optimal listening conditions, the cortical representation of basic acoustic features (N1/P2/N2) in many individuals with learning problems may be intact, even though it is typically degraded in nonideal situations such as those involving noisy environment or rapid stimulus rate (Cunningham, Nicol, Zecker, & Kraus, 2000; Nagarajan et al., 1999; Wible et al., 2002).

In the SLI population, evidence suggests that the obligatory cortical response may be abnormal, at least in some diagnosed individuals. Neville, Coffey, Holcomb, and Tallal (1993) reported that N1 amplitudes to a pure tone were reduced and N1 latencies delayed only among language-impaired children with abnormal auditory temporal processing and poor reading. McArthur and Bishop (2004) reported that individuals with SLI had age-inappropriate N1/P2/N2 responses to tonal stimuli. In a subsequent study, a subgroup of individuals with SLI had abnormal N1-P2 responses to both nonverbal tonally complex stimuli and to vowels (McArthur & Bishop, 2005). Taken together, these findings suggest that at least among some individuals with SLI the language deficit may be related to a more general auditory processing disorder.

To summarize, in subgroups of individuals with LLD the basic cortical representation of sound, manifested in the N1/P2 evoked response may be abnormal in response to both speech and nonspeech sounds.

Fine-Grained Auditory Discrimination

One hallmark of adequate perception is our ability to discriminate fine acoustic differences between similar stimuli. Such fine grained auditory discrimination of both speech and nonspeech elements is known to be impaired among many individuals with LLD (Adlard & Hazan, 1998; Ahissar, Protopapas, Reid, & Merzenich,

2000; Amitay et al., 2002; Banai & Ahissar, 2004; Ben-Yehudah, Banai, & Ahissar, 2004; Cacace et al., 2000; De Weirdt, 1988; Fischer & Hartnegg, 2004; France et al., 2002; McAnally & Stein, 1996; Mengler, Hogben, Michie, & Bishop, 2005; Walker, Shinn, Cranford, Givens, & Holbert, 2002). Physiologically, the MMN has been used to characterize discrimination at the preattentive level. MMN responses arise to a rare acoustic event occurring amidst frequent ones and index a detection of change in either acoustic feature (e.g., frequency) or complex sound pattern (e.g., order of sounds in a sequence). MMNs often are also conceptualized as indices of sensory or perceptual memory (see Näätänen et al., 2001 for review). Corresponding to perceptual deficits present in various clinical populations, MMNs are also attenuated in these groups, as discussed below. Yet, it should be noted that, because MMN responses currently can only be reliably quantified at the group level (Dalebout & Fox, 2001; McGee, Kraus, & Nicol, 1997), and thus are a useful tool for the study of auditory processing in predefined groups, they are ill-suited for use as a diagnostic tool at the individual level.

Discrimination of Speech Sounds

Children with learning and reading problems often exhibit difficulties behaviorally discriminating minimal pairs of speech sounds (e.g., /da/ vs. /ga/). Reduced or absent MMN responses to these contrasts also often have been documented in individuals with various learning problems, suggesting that impaired physiologic processing at a preattentive, preconscious level may account for poor perception. Kraus et al. (1996) showed that children with LLD and children with

attention problems had reduced MMNs, especially when they had difficulties discriminating the /da/-/ga/ contrast used. In contrast, the same children had no difficulties perceiving a /ba/-/wa/ pair, and correspondingly had normal MMNs to this contrast. Similar findings were reported by Schulte-Korne, Deimel, Bartling, and Remschmidt (1998, 2001). Maurer, Bucher, Brem, and Brandeis (2003) studied the MMN response in children with familial risk for dyslexia compared to those of control children using a standard /ba/ and two deviants—/ta/ and /da/. They found that early positive mismatched responses (MMR) and late MMN responses were attenuated for the at-risk group. Children at risk had enhanced MMRs and reduced MMNs. Similar findings were obtained in a group of 6-month-old babies at risk for dyslexia (Leppanen et al., 2002).

More recently, researchers have looked at MMN in predefined subgroups of individuals with language-learning problems. Banai et al. (2005) compared MMNs in response to a deviant /da/ syllable in individuals with LD and normal and abnormal brainstem timing to the same speech syllable. MMN onsets were delayed in the latter group. Furthermore, individuals with abnormal brainstem timing were more likely to exhibit reduced MMN magnitude than individuals with normal brainstem timing. Lachmann, Berti, Kujala, and Schroger (2005) compared MMNs between diagnostic subgroups of dyslexia comparing subjects with deficits in nonword reading to those with deficits in common (frequent) word reading. They found that abnormal MMNs were characteristic of dyslexics with difficulties in reading frequent words, but not in those with difficulties specific to nonword reading. This was true for both a speech

(/ba/ vs. /da/) and a nonspeech (700 vs. 770 Hz) contrast. On the other hand, both dyslexic groups in this study had reduced N2 responses for both stimulus conditions. Similarly, in the population diagnosed with SLI, MMNs were absent in response to vowel deviants (/a/ standard, /i/ deviant) (Shafer, Morr, Datta, Kurtzberg, & Schwartz, 2005), yet when individual data were examined, no relationship was found between MMN and behavioral discrimination of the same speech contrast.

Discrimination of Acoustic Features (Frequency, Duration)

Because APD is associated with nonlinguistic deficits, and because a variety of nonverbal discrimination deficits have been observed in the LLD population, a review of the physiology of nonverbal discrimination deficits is relevant. Baldeweg, Richardson, Watkins, Foale, and Gruzelier (1999) recorded abnormal MMN responses to changes in frequency, but not to changes in the duration of a standard tone, a finding that coincides with the many reports of abnormal frequency discrimination in dyslexia (e.g., Ahissar et al., 2000; Baldeweg et al., 1999; Ben-Yehudah et al., 2004; McAnally & Stein, 1996). Similar findings were reported for at-risk 6-month-old infants and kindergarten children (Leppanen et al., 2002; Maurer et al., 2003, respectively) and for a subgroup of dyslexics with difficulties in frequent word reading (Lachmann et al., 2005). In contrast, other groups have reported that MMNs to frequency deviants did not differ between dyslexic and control subjects (Kujala, Belitz, Tervaniemi, & Näätänen, 2003; Schulte-Korne et al., 1998). Because

the frequency difference in Kujala et al.'s (2003) study was 250 Hz, as opposed to 50 to 70 Hz in studies that did report a group difference, it is possible that group differences emerge only when stimulus differences are smaller.

Abnormal MMNs typically are attributed to abnormal function of the auditory cortex; however, observed behavioral deficits likely involve an interaction between the physical characteristics of the stimulus and the required cognitive operation. Thus, Johnsrude, Penhune, and Zatorre, (2000) reported that patients with surgical excision of either the left or the right Heschl's gyrus (auditory cortex) could still adequately discriminate pitch, but patients with right hemisphere excisions could no longer discriminate the direction of pitch change (up or down) even though they could readily discriminate the two sounds as different. Similar findings were observed in the dyslexic population where the degree of deficit in frequency discrimination also depends on the type of discrimination required (Banai & Ahissar, 2006; France et al., 2002).

Backward Masking

One manifestation of abnormal temporal acuity in children with language problems is increased detection thresholds for backward masked signals (Wright et al., 1997). It has been suggested that for some children with LLD, difficulties in discrimination of consonant-vowel syllables arise from a masking effect of the steady-state vowel and the brief initial consonant (Tallal, Merzenich, Miller, & Jenkins, 1998). As explained above (see Temporal Processing), this perceptual deficit may be related to abnormal processing of backward masked signals at the level of the brainstem (Marler & Champlin, 2005). Another physiologic correlate of elevated backward masking thresholds is found, however, at the cortical level. Children with SLI exhibit delayed and smaller MMNs to backward masked signals (Marler et al., 2002). Similarly, in a group of participants with dyslexia, Kujala et al. (2003) found abnormal MMNs in response to sound order reversal within a tone pair when the pair was followed (i.e., backward masked) by an additional tone, but not when the pair was preceded by one (i.e., forward masked). In this study, no differences in MMN amplitude were observed to a simple frequency deviant or to an order reversal in a nonmasked condition as mentioned above.

The relationships between the MMN and brainstem abnormalities are not clear. Although in many cases deficits co-occur at both levels (Banai et al., 2005; Marler & Champlin, 2005), the causal direction is still not known. If one assumes that basic sensation is intact among children with LLD as evident from their basically normal responses to click-evoked ABR, their elevated backward masking thresholds may be attributed to an impairment of sensory memory (i.e., impaired cortical discrimination of sensory traces) (Kujala et al., 2003; Marler et al., 2002) or to other top-down influences.

Discrimination of Tonal Patterns

MMN responses can be elicited not only in response to a single-feature deviant, but also in response to deviations in tonal pattern or order. Several studies found abnormal MMNs in individuals with dyslexia in response to pattern deviations (Kujala et al., 2000; Kujala & Näätänen, 2001; Schulte-Korne, Deimel, Bartling, & Remschmidt, 1999). Schulte-Korne et al. (1999) reported reduced MMN among individuals with dyslexia in response to a violation of a sound pattern (i.e., the relative duration of two of the components in the pattern). Similarly, Kujala et al. (2000) reported reduced MMNs in a dyslexic group in response to rare tone sequences, but normal MMNs in response to rare tone pairs.

Available data imply that fine discrimination of small differences in acoustic features characterizes a subgroup of individuals diagnosed with LLD. Because MMNs are abnormal in response to both speech and nonspeech stimuli, these findings suggest that, when present, auditory discrimination deficits maybe of a general nature and probably not restricted to one type of stimulus. Future work will reveal if there are specific acoustic aspects, common to both speech and nonspeech signals that are deficiently perceived. For recent reviews of studies linking these auditory event related potentials (ERPs) to language-based learning problems see Lyytinen et al. (2005) and Heim and Keil (2004).

Binaural Processing

Binaural interaction is considered especially relevant to the diagnosis of APD, as binaural processing is thought to underlie deficits in both sound localization and listening in noise. Indeed, administration of behavioral tasks requiring the presence of binaural interaction is recommended in the report of the Consensus Conference on the Diagnosis of Auditory Processing Disorders (Jerger & Musiek, 2000). A physiologic measure of binaural interaction can be obtained from the binaural interaction component (BIC) of the brainstem evoked response. The BIC is computed as the difference between the sum of the responses to monaural stimulation and the response to binaural stimulation (Dobie & Berlin, 1979). The BIC may serve as an objective measure of binaural processing. See Chapter 11 in volume 1 of this Handbook for discussion of clinical measures of binaural interaction.

Children suspected of or diagnosed with APD showed a different BIC pattern compared to normal children (Delb, Strauss, Hohenberg, & Plinkert, 2003; Gopal & Pierel, 1999). However, because the amplitude and latency of the BIC is rather variable in the normal population and highly variable in the APD population, Delb et al. (2003) concluded that the BIC is of limited diagnostic value, especially given the time commitment to obtain the three sets of measurements required for its calculation.

Consistent with the presence of deficit in binaural processing, deficits in accurate perception that require integration of information from both ears such as sound localization and dichotic listening (Amitay et al., 2002; Ben-Artzi, Fostick, & Babkoff, 2005; Edwards et al., 2004) have been found, but little is known about the biological correlates of these deficits in the LLD population. The role of the auditory brainstem in binaural processing has been demonstrated in a rare case of a patient with a unilateral lesion of the inferior colliculus. In this patient, sound localization was impaired behaviorally and wave V of the ABR was delayed when evoked by stimulation of the contralateral ear (Litovsky, Fligor, & Tramo, 2002).

(How) Can Training Help Individuals with Auditory Processing Deficits?

Research on the outcomes of training aimed specifically at groups diagnosed with APD is limited, yet available data indicate that difficulties in speech perception in noise can be alleviated by training. Putter-Katz et al. (2002) studied a group of 20 children diagnosed with APD. All trained children had normal audiometric thresholds, good word recognition in ideal listening conditions, and normal click-ABR. Their most common complaint was difficulty understanding speech in noisy environments (e.g., the classroom). The children participated in 13 to 15 weekly remediation sessions over a period of 4 months. At the same time, classroom modifications were recommended and implemented. The goal of the remediation sessions was to improve auditory processing abilities in noisy environments. The sessions included listening comprehension activities in the presence of noise and competing stimuli and tasks of selective and divided attention. Noise levels or degree of stimulus competition increased progressively throughout the course of the program. In addition, children were coached in the use of compensatory strategies such as speech-reading and metacognitive awareness. In addition, the use of FM devices was demonstrated and tried by the participants. At the end of the program, significant improvements in processing speech in noise and understanding competing sentences (dichotic listening) were documented. Furthermore, parents and teachers reported improved listening behavior at home and in the classroom following training.

Another approach to training is based on commercially available computer-based listening training programs such as Fast ForWord® (FFW) (Merzenich et al., 1996; Tallal et al., 1996) and Earobics® (Diehl, 1999). These programs have gained increasing popularity in the years following the reports of improved speech perception, language comprehension, and phonological processing (Habib et al., 2002; Merzenich et al., 1996; Tallal et al., 1996). Despite differences between the programs, both emphasize improving speech perception and phonological processing through the use of acoustically modified speech and an adaptive training regimen. The rationale behind this approach is that in cases of severe temporal processing deficits, children (most notably with SLI) are not able to distinguish naturally produced speech sounds, but may be able to tell apart larger, artificially enhanced temporal differences (Tallal et al., 1996). Following improvement, these enhancements are reduced, with the expectation that by the end of training the child will learn to adequately discriminate natural speech. In addition, these programs include modules with specific training on phonological awareness, following oral instructions, and other tasks aimed at increasing the ability of the trainee to process language.

Although the benefits of such programs, compared with "traditional classroom instruction," seem obvious, independent assessments of their success have been rare. Several recent studies question training-related gains in reading and reading related skills (Agnew, Dorn, & Eden, 2004; Hook, Macaruso, & Jones, 2001), despite gains in nonverbal auditory discrimination (Agnew et al., 2004). In a randomized controlled trial, Cohen et al. (2005) compared outcome measures in children with severe SLI, all of whom continued their regular speech and language therapy in school, who participated either in home-based therapy with FFW or received home-based intervention using computer–based activities that did not employ modified speech. A third group received no additional intervention and served as the control. They found that each group made gains in language scores; however, FFW training resulted in gains in language skills that were no greater than that of the other computer intervention or the regular, school-based speech and language therapy.

In contrast to the disappointing gains in reading and reading-related skills reported in the Cohen et al. study, several studies have shown that commercial listening training may result in normalization of cortical function in children with LLD. Hayes Warrier, Nicol, Zecker, and Kraus (2003) have shown that cortical responses in quiet of LLD children trained with Earobics exhibited an accelerated pattern of maturation following training and that their cortical responses in noise were enhanced and became more resilient to the degrading effects of background noise. Warrier et al. (2004) found that the correlation between cortical responses in noise and in quiet increased following training, again suggesting increased reliability of cortical processing in noise following training. Moreover, Russo, Nicol, Zecker, Hayes, and Kraus (2005) showed that the FFR portion of the brainstem response to speech became more resilient to noise following training and that the magnitude of change was highly correlated with the degree of cortical change. The transient component of the speech-ABR appears to be unaffected by training

(Hayes et al., 2003; Russo, Nicol, Zecker, Hayes, & Kraus, 2005). Following FFW training, Temple et al. (2003) found increased activation in the left temporal parietal cortex and most notably in prefrontal cortex. *Taken together, these studies suggest that training serves to normalize brain function in trained children, although it does not necessarily result in immediate literacy-related changes. Yet, it is reasonable to hypothesize that normalized physiologic function may be a precondition to behavioral changes.*

Both Earobics and FFW have been criticized for the modest improvements in literacy related skills, which are typically stated as the reason for undertaking training. Remediation of LLD and APD remain, to date, an enormous challenge. Conventional phonologic-based intervention to reading problems does not always result in improved reading (Rivers & Lombardino, 1988), and in many cases reading remains abnormally slow (Wise, Ring, & Olson, 1999, 2000). Available data suggest that no single remediation is successful in all children with a variety of auditory-language disorders.

Another type of training that may enhance phonological processing in normal learning children is training on the discrimination of a wide array of phonemic contrasts (Moore, Rosenberg, & Coleman, 2005). An intriguing outcome of the Moore et al. study is that the literacy-related improvements were observed in the face of little or no improvement on the trained task. Although this type of training may be effective in the LLD population as well, it should be noted that the pattern of training-related gains (i.e., nonspecific generalization) likely reflect plasticity of higher order mechanisms (auditory attention, auditory memory)

rather than low-level sensory mechanisms (see Ahissar, 2001).

Moreover, because APD is associated with an auditory deficit that is not necessarily language-specific, it may be worthwhile referring to studies of nonverbal auditory training. In the general population, discrimination of many acoustic cues (e.g., pitch, duration) substantially improves with practice (Amitay, Hawkey, & Moore, 2005; Ari-Even Roth, Amir, Alaluf, Buchsenspanner, & Kishon-Rabin, 2003; Delhommeau, Micheyl, & Jouvent, 2005; Delhommeau, Micheyl, Jouvent, & Collet, 2002; Demany, 1985; Demany & Semal, 2002; Goldstone, 1998; Irvine, Martin, Klimkeit, & Smith, 2000; Wright, 2001; Wright et al., 1997) and training is accompanied by plastic neural changes in both humans (Atienza, Cantero, & Dominguez-Marin, 2002; Gottselig, Brandeis, Hofer-Tinguely, Borbely, & Achermann, 2004; Jancke, Gaab, Wustenberg, Scheich, & Heinze, 2001; Menning, Roberts, & Pantev, 2000) and other primates (E. Ahissar et al., 1992; Bao, Chang, Davis, Gobeske, & Merzenich, 2003; Beitel, Schreiner, Cheung, Wang, & Merzenich, 2003; Recanzone, Schreiner, & Merzenich, 1993), attesting to the plasticity of central auditory processing even in adulthood.

Studies of learning-impaired populations have been less common, but findings point to the potential of nonverbal auditory training. Kujala et al. (2001) trained 7-year-old children with reading impairment on an auditory-visual pattern matching task. Children heard a series of nonverbal sound patterns varying in pitch, duration, and intensity and were asked to match them to corresponding visual patterns. This training resulted in significant improvements in reading accuracy and speed and in a significant increase in the MMN response to tone-order reversals. Schaffler, Sonntag, Hartnegg, and Fischer (2004) trained a large group of dyslexic listeners on an array of five auditory tasks (i.e., intensity and frequency discrimination, gap detection, temporal order judgments, and lateralization). Up to 80% of trained individuals improved on any given task, reaching age-matched control levels. These perceptual gains were accompanied by significant improvements in phonemic discrimination and spelling. Preliminary evidence suggests that similar training on a wide array of auditory discrimination tasks in a group of teenagers with severe dyslexia accompanied by additional learning problems also resulted in improved speech perception and verbal working memory (Banai & Ahissar, 2003).

Finally, preliminary findings regarding the positive outcomes of music training are worth mentioning. Overy (2003) studied the effects of musical training in eight children with dyslexia. Children trained on a series of musical games designed to emphasize timing and rhythm skills for 20 minutes per session, three times a week for 15 weeks in small groups improved significantly on rapid auditory processing, rhythm copying, phonological processing, and spelling tests (although not on reading) compared to a 15-week pretraining waiting period.

Taken together with Moore et al.'s (2005) findings and with recent studies on the effects of prolonged musical experience on cognition (see Schellenberg, 2005) and verbal memory in both adults (Chan, Ho, & Cheung, 1998) and children (Ho, Cheung, & Chan, 2003), it seems that auditory training affects clusters of processes rather than the encoding of specific types of stimuli. *Importantly, these studies seem to suggest that effects of intensive training are not limited solely to the specific stimuli practiced, but rather extend to affect wider systems of the brain*, based on functional relationships with the trained processes, as would be suggested by theories regarding the hierarchy of perceptual processing (Hochstein & Ahissar, 2002). (See Chapter 4 in Volume II of this Handbook for additional review of the literature on auditory training and its use as treatment for APD.)

Summary

The findings reviewed in this chapter link different perceptual and cognitive manifestations of APD in the LLD population to different physiologic processes, as briefly summarized here. (1) Difficulties in *temporal processing* are linked to delays in neural timing at both the auditory brainstem and cortex, in response to speech and nonspeech sounds. (2) Abnormal *perception and cortical representation of speech in noise* similarly are linked with potential sources of deficit, as low as the brainstem. Furthermore, in individuals with LLD, cortical processing is more susceptible to the degrading effects of background noise compared to the normal population. (3) *Discrimination deficits* for both speech and nonspeech sounds are linked with abnormal cortical processing of fine stimulus differences (MMN). Furthermore, *auditory cortical processing* in infancy is predictive of later development of language and cognitive skills. (4) Little is known about the biological basis of abnormal *binaural processing* in LLD, although reduced binaural components, probably originating at the brainstem have been recorded in children with APD. (5) *Listening training* (with modified speech stimuli) has been shown to be effective in normalizing cortical function in children with LLD. Furthermore, training was found to improve the resilience of auditory pathway activity to noise at both brainstem and cortical levels. Additional research is required to create training regimens with sizeable effects on language and literacy and to determine who are the subgroups of LDs that are most aided by training.

APD is heterogeneous in nature. Different types of APD are present among subgroups of populations diagnosed with language-based learning problems, manifesting deficits spanning a wide range of stimuli (pure tones to speech syllables), and processing time frames (fractions of milliseconds to seconds). Although the causal relationships between the presence of an APD and the linguistic and cognitive deficits which form the crux of learning disabilities are still poorly understood, it is clear that in many cases (estimates range from 30 to 50% of diagnosed individuals) the presence of APD may serve as a marker of a language or learning problem. On the other hand, data on cases of APD without accompanying language or cognitive deficits are rare, possibly because individuals with an isolated deficit in one auditory process are not likely to detect it unless tested. Indeed, available perceptual data indicate that in the general population different auditory abilities are not correlated, whereas in the LLD population significant correlations exist (Banai & Ahissar, 2004). This suggests that, although sporadic symptoms of APD are in some cases present in the normal population,

they are unlikely to be diagnosed without the presence of additional pathology in the language or cognitive domain.

In addition to the variability in perceptual processing in the LLD population, the varied evoked response findings indicate that even among individuals with LLD with APD symptoms it is impossible to point to a single abnormal physiologic process. Thus, LLD subgroups exhibit abnormal processing at different levels of the auditory system, spanning the brainstem, the auditory cortex, or both. Additionally, individuals with LLD exhibit abnormal processing in areas outside what are considered classic auditory areas, such as prefrontal regions. In addition to the common bottom-up explanation for the role of auditory processing in literacy, a top-down account is thus also likely. Thus, it is possible that a deficient high-level process (e.g., attention, working memory) is manifested in literacy and language problems and in auditory processing deficits through feedback connections from higher to lower areas. It may be that these abnormalities, in turn, are accompanied by different behavioral manifestation of APD. Recent findings in animal models demonstrate how high-level influences shape auditory processing and plasticity (Fritz, Elhilali & Shamma, 2005; Polley, Steinberg & Merzenich, 2006). Thus, abnormal processing at the level of the lower and upper brainstem may be linked to difficulties in perception in noise, whereas cortical deficits may be more indicative of subtle discrimination deficits. Further research in well-defined groups is required to lend further support for this assertion.

In terms of etiology, numerous environmental and genetic mechanisms, as well as the interaction between genetics and environment, likely account for this large spectra of behavioral and physiologic findings. For example, following both a short period of anoxia and induced cortical microgyria (small cortical lesions), rats show evidence of abnormal auditory processing as well as deficient sound-evoked brainstem timing (Clark, Rosen, Tallal, & Fitch, 2000; Fitch, Tallal, Brown, Galaburda, & Rosen, 1994; Strata et al., 2005), reminiscent of temporal-processing deficits in persons with LLD. Although the functional significance of APD to the development of language and cognitive abilities and ultimately to success in school is still poorly understood, data from developmental studies certainly suggest a predictive link between auditory processing and later cognitive development.

Early diagnosis and treatment of auditory processing deficits is of potential importance in easing future learning problems and improving language development among children with LLD with APD-related symptoms. In recent years, several biological markers of auditory processing, literacy, and language have been proposed. These markers include delayed brainstem timing in response to speech syllables (see BioMAP; Johnson et al., 2005, for review) and a differential pattern of the cortical evoked response to speech syllables in newborns (see Lyytinen et al., 2005, for review). In the clinic, using these markers in addition to available test batteries can help inform the diagnosis and treatment recommendations of APD. Further studies are required to elucidate the relationships between these markers and behavioral diagnostic measures of APD, as well as their applicability to different subgroups and in different developmental stages. In addition, future research should look at possible separate markers, corresponding to the various APD observed, rather than a single universal marker. This biologically based approach may ultimately lead to improved understanding of a variety of clinical conditions that are still insufficiently understood.

Finally, because the preconscious encoding of sound at the cortical and subcortical levels and the perception of many acoustic features can be enhanced with training, auditory training regimens are promising tools for the amelioration of APD. However, in order for training to fulfill an important role in remediation, further research is required to create optimal training regimens for children and clinical populations; better understand the relationships between the behavioral outcomes of training and neural plasticity; and develop training procedures that will optimize the outcome in terms of generalization and transfer of learning.

References

Adlard, A., & Hazan, V. (1998). Speech perception in children with specific reading difficulties (dyslexia). *Quarterly Journal of Experimental Psychology A, 51*, 153–177.

Agnew, J. A., Dorn, C., & Eden, G. F. (2004). Effect of intensive training on auditory processing and reading skills. *Brain and Language, 88*(1), 21–25.

Ahissar, E., Vaadia, E., Ahissar, M., Bergman, H., Arieli, A., & Abeles, M. (1992). Dependence of cortical plasticity on correlated activity of single neurons and on behavioral context. *Science, 257*(5075), 1412–1415.

Ahissar, M. (2001). Perceptual training: A tool for both modifying the brain and exploring it. *Proceedings of the National Academy of Sciences, USA, 98*(21), 11842–11843.

Ahissar, M., Protopapas, A., Reid, M., & Merzenich, M. M. (2000). Auditory processing parallels reading abilities in adults. *Proceedings of the National Academy of Sciences, USA, 97*(12), 6832–6837.

Amitay, S., Ahissar, M., & Nelken, I. (2002). Auditory processing deficits in reading disabled adults. *Journal of the Association of Research in Otolaryngology, 3*(3), 302–320.

Amitay, S., Hawkey, D. J., & Moore, D. R. (2005). Auditory frequency discrimination learning is affected by stimulus variability. *Perception and Psychophysics, 67*(4), 691–698.

Ari-Even Roth, D., Amir, O., Alaluf, L., Buchsenspanner, S., & Kishon-Rabin, L. (2003). The effect of training on frequency discrimination: generalization to untrained frequencies and to the untrained ear. *Journal of Basic Clinical Physiology and Pharmacology, 14*(2), 137–150.

ASHA. (2005). *(Central) auditory processing disorders—the role of the audiologist.* Rockville, MD: Author.

Atienza, M., Cantero, J. L., & Dominguez-Marin, E. (2002). The time course of neural changes underlying auditory perceptual learning. *Learning and Memory, 9*(3), 138–150.

Baldeweg, T., Richardson, A., Watkins, S., Foale, C., & Gruzelier, J. (1999). Impaired auditory frequency discrimination in dyslexia detected with mismatch evoked potentials. *Annals of Neurology, 45*(4), 495–503.

Banai, K., & Ahissar, M. (2003). Perceptual training generalizes to verbal working memory. *Neural Plasticity, 10*(3), 182.

Banai, K., & Ahissar, M. (2004). Poor frequency discrimination probes dyslexics with particularly impaired working memory. *Audiology and Neuro-Otology, 9*(6), 328–340.

Banai, K., & Ahissar, M. (2006). Auditory processing deficits in dyslexia: task or stimulus related? *Cerebral Cortex.* Published on-line Jan 11 2006.

Banai, K., Nicol, T., Zecker, S. G., & Kraus, N. (2005). Brainstem timing: implications for

cortical processing and literacy. *Journal of Neuroscience, 25*(43), 9850–9857.

Bao, S., Chang, E. F., Davis, J. D., Gobeske, K. T., & Merzenich, M. M. (2003). Progressive degradation and subsequent refinement of acoustic representations in the adult auditory cortex. *Journal of Neuroscience, 23*(34), 10765–10775.

Beitel, R. E., Schreiner, C. E., Cheung, S. W., Wang, X., & Merzenich, M. M. (2003). Reward-dependent plasticity in the primary auditory cortex of adult monkeys trained to discriminate temporally modulated signals. *Proceedings of the National Academy of Sciences, USA, 100*(19), 11070–11075.

Ben-Artzi, E., Fostick, L., & Babkoff, H. (2005). Deficits in temporal-order judgments in dyslexia: evidence from diotic stimuli differing spectrally and from dichotic stimuli differing only by perceived location. *Neuropsychologia, 43*(5), 714–723.

Ben-Yehudah, G., Banai, K., & Ahissar, M. (2004). Patterns of deficit in auditory temporal processing among dyslexic adults. *NeuroReport, 15*(4), 627–631.

Bishop, D. V., & McArthur, G. M. (2004). Immature cortical responses to auditory stimuli in specific language impairment: Evidence from ERPs to rapid tone sequences. *Developmental Science, 7*(4), F11–18.

Breier, J. I., Fletcher, J. M., Denton, C., & Gray, L. C. (2004). Categorical perception of speech stimuli in children at risk for reading difficulty. *Journal of Experimental Child Psychology, 88*(2), 152–170.

Breier, J. I., Gray, L., Fletcher, J. M., Diehl, R. L., Klaas, P., Foorman, B. R., et al. (2001). Perception of voice and tone onset time continua in children with dyslexia with and without attention deficit/hyperactivity disorder. *Journal of Experimental Child Psychology, 80*(3), 245–270.

Cacace, A. T., McFarland, D. J., Ouimet, J. R., Schrieber, E. J., & Marro, P. (2000). Temporal processing deficits in remediation-resistant reading-impaired children. *Audiology and Neuro-Otology, 5*(2), 83–97.

Chan, A. S., Ho, Y. C., & Cheung, M. C. (1998). Music training improves verbal memory. *Nature, 396*(6707), 128.

Chermak, G. D., Hall, J. W., 3rd, & Musiek, F. E. (1999). Differential diagnosis and management of central auditory processing disorder and attention deficit hyperactivity disorder. *Journal of the American Academy of Audiology, 10*(6), 289–303.

Chermak, G. D., Tucker, E., & Seikel, J. A. (2002). Behavioral characteristics of auditory processing disorder and attention-deficit hyperactivity disorder: Predominantly inattentive type. *Journal of the American Academy of Audiology, 13*(6), 332–338.

Clark, M. G., Rosen, G. D., Tallal, P., & Fitch, R. H. (2000). Impaired processing of complex auditory stimuli in rats with induced cerebrocortical microgyria: An animal model of developmental language disabilities. *Journal of Cognitive Neuroscience, 12*(5), 828–839.

Cohen, W., Hodson, A., O'Hare, A., Boyle, J., Durrani, T., McCartney, E., et al. (2005). Effects of computer-based intervention through acoustically modified speech (Fast ForWord) in severe mixed receptive-expressive language impairment: Outcomes from a randomized controlled trial. *Journal of Speech, Language and Hearing Research, 48*(3), 715–729.

Collet, L., Kemp, D. T., Veuillet, E., Duclaux, R., Moulin, A., & Morgon, A. (1990). Effect of contralateral auditory stimuli on active cochlear micro-mechanical properties in human subjects. *Hearing Research, 43*(2–3), 251–261.

Cornelissen, P. L., Hansen, P. C., Bradley, L., & Stein, J. F. (1996). Analysis of perceptual confusions between nine sets of consonant-vowel sounds in normal and dyslexic adults. *Cognition, 59*(3), 275–306.

Cunningham, J., Nicol, T., Zecker, S., & Kraus, N. (2000). Speech-evoked neurophysiologic responses in children with learning problems: development and behavioral correlates of perception. *Ear and Hearing, 21*(6), 554–568.

Cunningham, J., Nicol, T., Zecker, S. G., Bradlow, A., & Kraus, N. (2001). Neurobiologic responses to speech in noise in children with learning problems: deficits and strategies for improvement. *Clinical Neurophysiology, 112*(5), 758–767.

Dalebout, S. D., & Fox, L. G. (2001). Reliability of the mismatch negativity in the responses of individual listeners. *Journal of the American Academy of Audiology, 12*(5), 245–253.

De Weirdt, W. (1988). Speech perception and frequency discrimination in good and poor readers. *Applied Psycholinguistics, 9*, 163–183.

Delb, W., Strauss, D. J., Hohenberg, G., & Plinkert, P. K. (2003). The binaural interaction component (BIC) in children with central auditory processing disorders (CAPD). *International Journal of Audiology, 42*(7), 401–412.

Delhommeau, K., Micheyl, C., & Jouvent, R. (2005). Generalization of frequency discrimination learning across frequencies and ears: Implications for underlying neural mechanisms in humans. *Journal of the Association of Research in Otolaryngology, 6*(2), 171–179.

Delhommeau, K., Micheyl, C., Jouvent, R., & Collet, L. (2002). Transfer of learning across durations and ears in auditory frequency discrimination. *Perception and Psychophysics, 64*(3), 426–436.

Demany, L. (1985). Perceptual learning in frequency discrimination. *Journal of the Acoustical Society of America, 78*(3), 1118–1120.

Demany, L., & Semal, C. (2002). Learning to perceive pitch differences. *Journal of the Acoustical Society of America, 111*(3), 1377–1388.

Diehl, S. (1999). Listen and learn? A software review of Earobics(R). *Language, Speech, and Hearing Services in Schools, 30*, 108–116.

Dobie, R. A., & Berlin, C. I. (1979). Binaural interaction in brainstem-evoked responses. *Archives of Otolaryngology, 105*(7), 391–398.

Duara, R., Kushch, A., Gross-Glenn, K., Barker, W. W., Jallad, B., Pascal, S., et al. (1991). Neuroanatomic differences between dyslexic and normal readers on magnetic resonance imaging scans. *Archives of Neurology, 48*(4), 410-416.

Edwards, V. T., Giaschi, D. E., Dougherty, R. F., Edgell, D., Bjornson, B. H., Lyons, C., et al. (2004). Psychophysical indexes of temporal processing abnormalities in children with developmental dyslexia. *Developmental Neuropsychology, 25*(3), 321-354.

Eggermont, J. J., & Ponton, C. W. (2002). The neurophysiology of auditory perception: from single units to evoked potentials. *Audiology and Neuro-Otology, 7*(2), 71-99.

Espy, K. A., Molfese, D. L., Molfese, V. J., & Modglin, A. (2004). Development of auditory event-related potentials in young children and relations to word-level reading abilities at age 8 years. *Annals of Dyslexia, 54*(1), 9-38.

Farmer, M. E., & Klein, R. M. (1995). The evidence for a temporal processing deficit linked to dyslexia: A review. *Psychonomic Bulletin and Review, 2*, 460-493.

Fischer, B., & Hartnegg, K. (2004). On the development of low-level auditory discrimination and deficits in dyslexia. *Dyslexia, 10*(2), 105-118.

Fitch, R. H., Tallal, P., Brown, C. P., Galaburda, A. M., & Rosen, G. D. (1994). Induced microgyria and auditory temporal processing in rats: A model for language impairment? *Cerebral Cortex, 4*(3), 260-270.

France, S. J., Rosner, B. S., Hansen, P. C., Calvin, C., Talcott, J. B., Richardson, A. J., et al. (2002). Auditory frequency discrimination in adult developmental dyslexics. *Perception and Psychophysics, 64*(2), 169-179.

Frisina, R. D. (2001). Subcortical neural coding mechanisms for auditory temporal processing. *Hearing Research, 158*(1-2), 1-27.

Fritz, J. Elhilali, M., & Shamma S. (2005). Active listening: task-dependent plasticity of spectrotemporal receptive fields in primary auditory cortex. *Hearing Research, 206*, 159-176.

Galbraith, G. C., Arbagey, P. W., Branski, R., Comerci, N., & Rector, P. M. (1995). Intelligible speech encoded in the human brain stem frequency-following response. *NeuroReport, 6*(17), 2363-2367.

Goldstone, R. L. (1998). Perceptual learning. *Annual Review of Psychology, 49*, 585-612.

Gopal, K. V., & Pierel, K. (1999). Binaural interaction component in children at risk for central auditory processing disorders. *Scandinavian Audiology, 28*(2), 77-84.

Gottselig, J. M., Brandeis, D., Hofer-Tinguely, G., Borbely, A. A., & Achermann, P. (2004). Human central auditory plasticity associated with tone sequence learning. *Learning and Memory, 11*(2), 162-171.

Griffiths, T. D., Uppenkamp, S., Johnsrude, I., Josephs, O., & Patterson, R. D. (2001). Encoding of the temporal regularity of sound in the human brainstem. *Nature Neuroscience, 4*(6), 633-637.

Griffiths, Y. M., Hill, N. I., Bailey, P. J., & Snowling, M. J. (2003). Auditory temporal order discrimination and backward recognition masking in adults with dyslexia. *Journal of Speech, Language and Hearing Research, 46*(6), 1352-1366.

Grontved, A., Walter, B., & Gronborg, A. (1988a). Auditory brain stem responses in dyslexic and normal children. A prospective clinical investigation. *Scandinavian Audiology, 17*(1), 53-54.

Grontved, A., Walter, B., & Gronborg, A. (1988b). Normal ABR's in dyslexic children. *Acta Otolaryngologica Supplement, 449*, 171-173.

Gross-Glenn, K., Duara, R., Barker, W. W., Loewenstein, D., Chang, J. Y., Yoshii, F., et al. (1991). Positron emission tomographic studies during serial word-reading by normal and dyslexic adults. *Journal of Clinical and Experimental Neuropsychology, 13*(4), 531-544.

Guttorm, T. K., Leppanen, P. H., Poikkeus, A. M., Eklund, K. M., Lyytinen, P., & Lyytinen, H. (2005). Brain event-related potentials (ERPs) measured at birth predict later language development in children with and without familial risk for dyslexia. *Cortex*, *41*(3), 291-303.

Guttorm, T. K., Leppanen, P. H. T., Richardson, U., & Lyytinen, H. (2001). Event-related potentials and consonant differentiation in newborns with familial risk for dyslexia. *Journal of Learning Disabilities*, *34*(6), 534-544.

Habib, M., Rey, V., Daffaure, V., Camps, R., Espesser, R., Joly-Pottuz, B., et al. (2002). Phonological training in children with dyslexia using temporally modified speech: a three-step pilot investigation. *International Journal of Language and Communication Disorders*, *37*(3), 289-308.

Hall, J. W. (1992). *Handbook of auditory evoked responses*. Needham Heights, MA: Allyn & Bacon.

Hayes, E. A., Warrier, C. M., Nicol, T. G., Zecker, S. G., & Kraus, N. (2003). Neural plasticity following auditory training in children with learning problems. *Clinical Neurophysiology*, *114*(4), 673-684.

Heath, S. M., Hogben, J. H., & Clark, C. D. (1999). Auditory temporal processing in disabled readers with and without oral language delay. *Journal of Child Psychology and Psychiatry*, *40*(4), 637-647.

Heim, S., Eulitz, C., & Elbert, T. (2003). Altered hemispheric asymmetry of auditory P100m in dyslexia. *European Journal of Neuroscience*, *17*(8), 1715-1722.

Heim, S., Eulitz, C., Kaufmann, J., Fuchter, I., Pantev, C., Lamprecht-Dinnesen, A., et al. (2000). Atypical organisation of the auditory cortex in dyslexia as revealed by MEG. *Neuropsychologia*, *38*(13), 1749-1759.

Heim, S., & Keil, A. (2004). Large-scale neural correlates of developmental dyslexia. *European Child and Adolescent Psychiatry*, *13*(3), 125-140.

Helenius, P., Salmelin, R., Richardson, U., Leinonen, S., & Lyytinen, H. (2002). Abnormal auditory cortical activation in dyslexia 100 msec after speech onset. *Journal of Cognitive Neuroscience*, *14*(4), 603-617.

Herdman, A. T., Lins, O., Van Roon, P., Stapells, D. R., Scherg, M., & Picton, T. W. (2002). Intracerebral sources of human auditory steady-state responses. *Brain Topography*, *15*(2), 69-86.

Ho, Y. C., Cheung, M. C., & Chan, A. S. (2003). Music training improves verbal but not visual memory: cross-sectional and longitudinal explorations in children. *Neuropsychology*, *17*(3), 439-450.

Hochstein, S., & Ahissar, M. (2002). View from the top: Hierarchies and reverse hierarchies in the visual system. *Neuron*, *36*(5), 791-804.

Hood, L. J. (1998). *Clinical applications of the auditory brainstem response*. San Diego, CA: Singular Publishing Group, Inc.

Hook, P. E., Macaruso, P., & Jones, S. (2001). Efficacy of Fast ForWord training on facilitating acquisition of reading skills by children with reading difficulties—A longitudinal study. *Annals of Dyslexia*, *51*, 75-96.

Irvine, D. R., Martin, R. L., Klimkeit, E., & Smith, R. (2000). Specificity of perceptual learning in a frequency discrimination task. *Journal of the Acoustical Society of America*, *108*(6), 2964-2968.

Jacobsen, J. (1985). *The auditory brainstem response*. San Diego, CA: College-Hill Press.

Jancke, L., Gaab, N., Wustenberg, T., Scheich, H., & Heinze, H. J. (2001). Short-term functional plasticity in the human auditory cortex: An fMRI study. *Brain Research Cognitive Brain Research*, *12*(3), 479-485.

Jerger, J., & Musiek, F. (2000). Report of the Consensus Conference on the Diagnosis of Auditory Processing Disorders in School-Aged Children. *Journal of the American Academy of Audiology*, *11*(9), 467-474.

Jerger, S., Martin, R. C., & Jerger, J. (1987). Specific auditory perceptual dysfunction in a learning disabled child. *Ear and Hearing*, *8*(2), 78-86.

Joanisse, M. F., Manis, F. R., Keating, P., & Seidenberg, M. S. (2000). Language deficits in dyslexic children: speech perception, phonology, and morphology. *Journal of Experimental Child Psychology*, *77*(1), 30-60.

Johnson, K. L., Nicol, T. G., & Kraus, N. (2005). Brain stem response to speech: A biological marker of auditory processing. *Ear and Hearing, 26*(5), 424-434.

Johnson, K.L., Nicol, T. G., Zecker, S. G., Wright, B. A., & Kraus, N. (2004). Brainstem timing in learning impaired children with excessive auditory backward masking [Abstract]. *Association for Research in Otolaryngology, 27,* 118.

Johnsrude, I. S., Penhune, V. B., & Zatorre, R. J. (2000). Functional specificity in the right human auditory cortex for perceiving pitch direction. *Brain, 123*(Pt. 1), 155-163.

King, C., Warrier, C. M., Hayes, E., & Kraus, N. (2002). Deficits in auditory brainstem pathway encoding of speech sounds in children with learning problems. *Neuroscience Letters, 319*(2), 111-115.

King, W. M., Lombardino, L. J., Crandell, C. C., & Leonard, C. M. (2003). Comorbid auditory processing disorder in developmental dyslexia. *Ear and Hearing, 24*(5), 448-456.

Kraus, N., & McGee, T. (1992). Electrophysiology of the human auditory system. In A. Poppler & R Fay (Eds.), *The mammalian auditory system* (Vol. II, pp. 335-404). New York: Springer-Verlag.

Kraus, N., McGee, T., Carrell, T., King, C., Littman, T., & Nicol, T. (1994). Discrimination of speech-like contrasts in the auditory thalamus and cortex. *Journal of the Acoustical Society of America, 96*(5, Pt. 1), 2758-2768.

Kraus, N., & Nicol, T. (2005). Brainstem origins for cortical "what" and "where" pathways in the auditory system. *Trends in Neurosciences, 28*(4), 176-181.

Krishnan, A. (2002). Human frequency-following responses: representation of steady-state synthetic vowels. *Hearing Research, 166*(1-2), 192-201.

Kujala, T., Belitz, S., Tervaniemi, M., & Näätänen, R. (2003). Auditory sensory memory disorder in dyslexic adults as indexed by the mismatch negativity. *European Journal of Neuroscience, 17*(6), 1323-1327.

Kujala, T., Karma, K., Ceponiene, R., Belitz, S., Turkkila, P., Tervaniemi, M., et al. (2001).

Plastic neural changes and reading improvement caused by audiovisual training in reading-impaired children. *Proceedings of the National Academy of Sciences, USA, 98*(18), 10509-10514.

Kujala, T., Myllyviita, K., Tervaniemi, M., Alho, K., Kallio, J., & Naatanen, R. (2000). Basic auditory dysfunction in dyslexia as demonstrated by brain activity measurements. *Psychophysiology, 37*(2), 262-266.

Kujala, T., & Näätänen, R. (2001). The mismatch negativity in evaluating central auditory dysfunction in dyslexia. *Neuroscience and Biobehavioral Reviews, 25*(6), 535-543.

Kuwada, S., Batra, R., & Maher, V. L. (1986). Scalp potentials of normal and hearing-impaired subjects in response to sinusoidally amplitude-modulated tones. *Hearing Research, 21*(2), 179-192.

Lachmann, T., Berti, S., Kujala, T., & Schroger, E. (2005). Diagnostic subgroups of developmental dyslexia have different deficits in neural processing of tones and phonemes. *International Journal of Psychophysiology, 56*(2), 105-120.

Lauter, J. L., & Wood, S. B. (1993). Auditory-brainstem synchronicity in dyslexia measured using the REPs/ABR protocol. *Annals of the New York Academy of Sciences, 682,* 377-379.

Leonard, C. M., Eckert, M. A., Lombardino, L. J., Oakland, T., Kranzler, J., Mohr, C. M., et al. (2001). Anatomical risk factors for phonological dyslexia. *Cerebral Cortex, 11*(2), 148-157.

Leppanen, P. H., Richardson, U., Pihko, E., Eklund, K. M., Guttorm, T. K., Aro, M., et al. (2002). Brain responses to changes in speech sound durations differ between infants with and without familial risk for dyslexia. *Developmental Neuropsychology, 22*(1), 407-422.

Litovsky, R. Y., Fligor, B. J., & Tramo, M. J. (2002). Functional role of the human inferior colliculus in binaural hearing. *Hearing Research, 165*(1-2), 177-188.

Lorenzi, C., Dumont, A., & Fullgrabe, C. (2000). Use of temporal envelope cues by children with developmental dyslexia. *Journal of Speech, Language and Hearing Research, 43*(6), 1367-1379.

Lyytinen, H., Guttorm, T. K., Huttunen, T., Hamalainen, J., Leppanen, P. H. T., Vesterinen, M., et al. (2005). Psychophysiology of developmental dyslexia: A review of findings including studies of children at risk for dyslexia. *Journal of Neurolinguistics, 18*(2), 167-195.

Marler, J. A., & Champlin, C. A. (2005). Sensory processing of backward-masking signals in children with language-learning impairment as assessed with the auditory brainstem response. *Journal of Speech, Language and Hearing Research, 48*(1), 189-203.

Marler, J. A., Champlin, C. A., & Gillam, R. B. (2002). Auditory memory for backward masking signals in children with language impairment. *Psychophysiology, 39*(6), 767-780.

Marsh, J. T., & Worden, F. G. (1968). Sound evoked frequency-following responses in the central auditory pathway. *Laryngoscope, 78*(7), 1149-1163.

Mason, S. M., & Mellor, D. H. (1984). Brainstem, middle latency and late cortical evoked potentials in children with speech and language disorders. *Electroencephalography and Clinical Neurophysiology, 59*(4), 297-309.

Maurer, U., Bucher, K., Brem, S., & Brandeis, D. (2003). Altered responses to tone and phoneme mismatch in kindergartners at familial dyslexia risk. *NeuroReport, 14*(17), 2245-2250.

McAnally, K. I., & Stein, J. F. (1996). Auditory temporal coding in dyslexia. *Philosophical Transactions of the Royal Society of London, B Biological Sciences, 263,* 961-965.

McAnally, K. I., & Stein, J. F. (1997). Scalp potentials evoked by amplitude-modulated tones in dyslexia. *Journal of Speech, Language and Hearing Research, 40*(4), 939-945.

McArthur, G. M., & Bishop, D. V. (2005). Speech and non-speech processing in people with specific language impairment: a behavioral and electrophysiologic study. *Brain and Language, 94*(3), 260-273.

McArthur, G. M., & Bishop, D. V. M. (2004). Which people with specific language impairment have auditory processing deficits? *Cognitive Neuropsychology, 21*(1), 79-94.

McGee, T., Kraus, N., & Nicol, T. (1997). Is it really a mismatch negativity? An assessment of methods for determining response validity in individual subjects. *Electroencephalography and Clinical Neurophysiology, 104*(4), 359-368.

Menell, P., McAnally, K. I., & Stein, J. F. (1999). Psychophysical sensitivity and physiologic response to amplitude modulation in adult dyslexic listeners. *Journal of Speech, Language and Hearing Research, 42*(4), 797-803.

Mengler, E. D., Hogben, J. H., Michie, P., & Bishop, D. V. (2005). Poor frequency discrimination is related to oral language disorder in children: A psychoacoustic study. *Dyslexia, 11*(3), 155-173.

Menning, H., Roberts, L. E., & Pantev, C. (2000). Plastic changes in the auditory cortex induced by intensive frequency discrimination training. *NeuroReport, 11*(4), 817-822.

Merzenich, M. M., Jenkins, W. M., Johnston, P., Schreiner, C., Miller, S. L., & Tallal, P. (1996). Temporal processing deficits of language-learning impaired children ameliorated by training. *Science, 271*(5245), 77-81.

Moisescu-Yiflach, T., & Pratt, H. (2005). Auditory event related potentials and source current density estimation in phonologic/auditory dyslexics. *Clinical Neurophysiology, 116*(11), 2632-2647.

Molfese, D. L. (2000). Predicting dyslexia at 8 years of age using neonatal brain responses. *Brain and Language, 72*(3), 238-245.

Molfese, D. L., & Molfese, V. J. (1985). Electrophysiologic indices of auditory discrimination in newborn infants: The bases for predicting later language development? *Infant Behavior and Development, 8*(2), 197-211.

Molfese, D. L., & Molfese, V. J. (1997). Discrimination of language skills at five years of age using event-related potentials recorded at birth. *Developmental Neuropsychology*, *13*(2), 135–156.

Moore, D. R., Rosenberg, J. F., & Coleman, J. S. (2005). Discrimination training of phonemic contrasts enhances phonological processing in mainstream school children. *Brain and Language*, *94*(1), 72–85.

Muchnik, C., Ari-Even Roth, D., Othman-Jebara, R., Putter-Katz, H., Shabtai, E. L., & Hildesheimer, M. (2004). Reduced medial olivocochlear bundle system function in children with auditory processing disorders. *Audiology and Neuro-Otology, 9*(2), 107–114.

Näätänen, R. (1992). *Attention and brain function*. Hillsdale, NJ: Lawrence Erlbaum.

Näätänen, R., Tervaniemi, M., Sussman, E., Paavilainen, P., & Winkler, I. (2001). "Primitive intelligence" in the auditory cortex. *Trends in Neurosciences*, *24*(5), 283–288.

Nagarajan, S., Mahncke, H., Salz, T., Tallal, P., Roberts, T., & Merzenich, M. M. (1999). Cortical auditory signal processing in poor readers. *Proceedings of the National Academy of Sciences, USA, 96*(11), 6483–6488.

Neville, H. J., Coffey, S. A., Holcomb, P. J., & Tallal, P. (1993). The neurobiology of sensory and language processing in language-impaired children. *Journal of Cognitive Neuroscience, 5*(2), 235–253.

Overy, K. (2003). Dyslexia and music. From timing deficits to musical intervention. *Annals of the New York Academy of Science, 999*, 497–505.

Phillips, D. P. (1995). Central auditory processing: A view from auditory neuroscience. *American Journal of Otology, 16*(3), 338–352.

Pinkerton, F., Watson, D. R., & McClelland, R. J. (1989). A neurophysiological study of children with reading, writing and spelling difficulties. *Developmental Medicine and Child Neurology, 31*(5), 569–581.

Poldrack, R. A., Temple, E., Protopapas, A., Nagarajan, S., Tallal, P., Merzenich, M., et al. (2001). Relations between the neural bases of dynamic auditory processing and phonological processing: evidence from fMRI. *Journal of Cognitive Neuroscience, 13*(5), 687–697.

Polley, D. B., Steinberg, E.E., & Merzenich, M. M. (2006). Perceptual learning directs auditory cortical map reorganization through top-down influences. *Journal of Neuroscience, 26*, 4970–4982.

Purdy, S. C., Kelly, A. S., & Davies, M. G. (2002). Auditory brainstem response, middle latency response, and late cortical evoked potentials in children with learning disabilities. *Journal of the American Academy of Audiology, 13*(7), 367–382.

Putter-Katz, H., Adi-Ben Said, L., Feldman, I., Miran, D., Kushnir, D., Muchnik, C., et al. (2002). Treatment and evaluation indices of auditory processing disorders. *Seminars in Hearing, 23*(4), 357–364.

Putter-Katz, H., Kishon-Rabin, L., Sachartov, E., Shabtai, E. L., Sadeh, M., Weiz, R., et al. (2005). Cortical activity of children with dyslexia during natural speech processing: evidence of auditory processing deficiency. *Journal of Basic Clinical Physiology and Pharmacology, 16*(2–3), 157–171.

Ramus, F. (2003). Developmental dyslexia: specific phonological deficit or general sensorimotor dysfunction? *Current Opinion in Neurobiology, 13*(2), 212–218.

Recanzone, G. H., Schreiner, C. E., & Merzenich, M. M. (1993). Plasticity in the frequency representation of primary auditory cortex following discrimination training in adult owl monkeys. *Journal of Neuroscience, 13*(1), 87–103.

Reed, M. A. (1989). Speech perception and the discrimination of brief auditory cues in reading disabled children. *Journal of Experimental Child Psychology, 48*(2), 270–292.

Rinne, T., Alho, K., Ilmoniemi, R. J., Virtanen, J., & Näätänen, R. (2000). Separate time behaviors of the temporal and frontal mismatch negativity sources. *Neuroimage, 12*(1), 14–19.

Rivers, K. O., & Lombardino, L. J. (1998). Generalization of early metalinguistic skills in a phonological decoding study with first-graders at risk for reading failure. *International Journal of Language and Communication Disorders, 33*, 369-391.

Rocheron, I., Lorenzi, C., Fullgrabe, C., & Dumont, A. (2002). Temporal envelope perception in dyslexic children. *Neuro-Report, 13*(13), 1683-1687.

Rosen, S. (1992). Temporal information in speech: acoustic, auditory and linguistic aspects. *Philosophical Transactions of the Royal Society of London, B Biological Sciences, 336*(1278), 367-373.

Rosen, S., & Manganari, E. (2001). Is there a relationship between speech and non-speech auditory processing in children with dyslexia? *Journal of Speech, Language and Hearing Research, 44*(4), 720-736.

Russo, N., Nicol, T., Musacchia, G., & Kraus, N. (2004). Brainstem responses to speech syllables. *Clinical Neurophysiology, 115*(9), 2021-2030.

Russo, N., Nicol, T. G., Zecker, S. G., Hayes, E. A., & Kraus, N. (2005). Auditory training improves neural timing in the human brainstem. *Behavioral Brain Research, 156*(1), 95-103.

Sams, M., Kaukoranta, E., Hamalainen, M., & Näätänen, R. (1991). Cortical activity elicited by changes in auditory stimuli: different sources for the magnetic N100m and mismatch responses. *Psychophysiology, 28*(1), 21-29.

Schaffler, T., Sonntag, J., Hartnegg, K., & Fischer, B. (2004). The effect of practice on low-level auditory discrimination, phonological skills, and spelling in dyslexia. *Dyslexia, 10*(2), 119-130.

Schellenberg, E. G. (2005). Music and cognitive abilities. *Current Directions in Psychological Science, 14*(6), 317-320.

Schulte-Korne, G., Deimel, W., Bartling, J., & Remschmidt, H. (1998). Auditory processing and dyslexia: Evidence for a specific speech processing deficit. *NeuroReport, 9*(2), 337-340.

Schulte-Korne, G., Deimel, W., Bartling, J., & Remschmidt, H. (1999). Pre-attentive pro-cessing of auditory patterns in dyslexic human subjects. *Neuroscience Letters, 276*(1), 41-44.

Schulte-Korne, G., Deimel, W., Bartling, J., & Remschmidt, H. (2001). Speech perception deficit in dyslexic adults as measured by mismatch negativity (MMN). *International Journal of Psychophysiology, 40*(1), 77-87.

Shafer, V. L., Morr, M. L., Datta, H., Kurtzberg, D., & Schwartz, R. G. (2005). Neurophysi-ological indexes of speech processing deficits in children with specific language impairment. *Journal of Cognitive Neuro-science, 17*(7), 1168-1180.

Sohmer, H., & Pratt, H. (1977). Identification and separation of acoustic frequency fol-lowing responses (FFRS) in man. *Electro-encephalography and Clinical Neuro-physiology, 42*(4), 493-500.

Song, J., Banai, K., Russo N. M., & Kraus, N. (2006). On the relationship between speech- and nonspeech-evoked auditory brainstem responses. *Audiology and Neuro-Otology, 11*(4), 233-241.

Strata, F., Deipolyi, A. R., Bonham, B. H., Chang, E. F., Liu, R. C., Nakahara, H., et al. (2005). Perinatal anoxia degrades auditory system function in rats. *Proceedings of the National Academy of Sciences, USA, 102*(52), 19156-19161.

Talcott, J. B., Gram, A., Van Ingelghem, M., Witton, C., Stein, J. F., & Toennessen, F. E. (2003). Impaired sensitivity to dynamic stimuli in poor readers of a regular orthog-raphy. *Brain and Language, 87*(2), 259-266.

Tallal, P. (1980). Auditory temporal perception, phonics, and reading disabilities in children. *Brain and Language, 9*, 182-198.

Tallal, P., Merzenich, M. M., Miller, S., & Jenk-ins, W. (1998). Language learning impair-ments: integrating basic science, technol-ogy, and remediation. *Experimental Brain Research, 123*(1-2), 210-219.

Tallal, P., Miller, S., & Fitch, R. H. (1993). Neurobiological basis of speech: A case for the preeminence of temporal process-ing. *Annals of the New York Academy of Sciences, USA, 682*, 27-47.

Tallal, P., Miller, S. L., Bedi, G., Byma, G., Wang, X., Nagarajan, S. S., et al. (1996). Language comprehension in language-learning impaired children improved with acoustically modified speech. *Science, 271*(5245), 81–84.

Tallal, P., & Piercy, M. (1973). Defects of non-verbal auditory perception in children with developmental aphasia. *Nature, 241*(5390), 468–469.

Temple, E., Deutsch, G. K., Poldrack, R. A., Miller, S. L., Tallal, P., Merzenich, M. M., et al. (2003). Neural deficits in children with dyslexia ameliorated by behavioral remediation: Evidence from functional MRI. *Proceedings of the National Academy of Sciences, USA, 100*(5), 2860–2865.

Temple, E., Poldrack, R. A., Protopapas, A., Nagarajan, S., Salz, T., Tallal, P., et al. (2000). Disruption of the neural response to rapid acoustic stimuli in dyslexia: evidence from functional MRI. *Proceedings of the National Academy of Sciences, USA, 97*(25), 13907–13912.

Walker, M. M., Shinn, J. B., Cranford, J. L., Givens, G. D., & Holbert, D. (2002). Auditory temporal processing performance of young adults with reading disorders. *Journal of Speech, Language and Hearing Research, 45*(3), 598–605.

Warrier, C. M., Johnson, K. L., Hayes, E. A., Nicol, T., & Kraus, N. (2004). Learning impaired children exhibit timing deficits and training-related improvements in auditory cortical responses to speech in noise. *Experimental Brain Research, 157*(4), 431–441.

Wible, B., Nicol, T., & Kraus, N. (2002). Abnormal neural encoding of repeated speech stimuli in noise in children with learning problems. *Clinical Neurophysiology, 113*(4), 485–494.

Wible, B., Nicol, T., & Kraus, N. (2004). Atypical brainstem representation of onset and formant structure of speech sounds in children with language-based learning problems. *Biological Psychology, 67*(3), 299–317.

Wible, B., Nicol, T., & Kraus, N. (2005). Correlation between brainstem and cortical auditory processes in normal and language-impaired children. *Brain, 128*(Pt. 2), 417–423.

Wise, B. W., Ring, J., & Olson, R. K. (1999). Training phonological awareness with and without explicit attention to articulation. *Journal of Experimental Child Psychology, 72*(4), 271–304.

Wise, B. W., Ring, J., & Olson, R. K. (2000). Individual differences in gains from computer-assisted remedial reading. *Journal of Experimental Child Psychology, 77*(3), 197–235.

Witton, C., Stein, J. F., Stoodley, C. J., Rosner, B. S., & Talcott, J. B. (2002). Separate influences of acoustic AM and FM sensitivity on the phonological decoding skills of impaired and normal readers. *Journal of Cognitive Neuroscience, 14*(6), 866–874.

Wright, B. A. (2001). Why and how we study human learning on basic auditory tasks. *Audiology and Neuro-Otology, 6*(4), 207–210.

Wright, B. A., Lombardino, L. J., King, W. M., Puranik, C. S., Leonard, C. M., & Merzenich, M. M. (1997). Deficits in auditory temporal and spectral resolution in language-impaired children. *Nature, 387*(6629), 176–178.

Ziegler, J. C., Pech-Georgel, C., George, F., Alario, F. X., & Lorenzi, C. (2005). Deficits in speech perception predict language learning impairment. *Proceedings of the National Academy of Sciences, USA, 102*(39), 14110–14115.

SECTION II

Diagnostic Principles and Procedures

CHAPTER 5

HISTORICAL FOUNDATIONS AND THE NATURE OF (CENTRAL) AUDITORY PROCESSING DISORDER

TERI JAMES BELLIS

Historically, there has been much debate among professionals in many disciplines regarding the nature of (central) auditory processing disorder ([C]APD) and the best means of diagnosing and treating the disorder. In recent years, professionals in the fields of audiology, speech-language pathology, education, and related fields have witnessed a dramatic upsurge in interest regarding (C)APD in both children and adults, and the demand for central auditory services has surged. As a result, it has become even more crucial that clinicians understand the fundamental principles underlying central auditory processing and its disorders.

The previous chapters in this volume have discussed the scientific bases of central auditory processing, both neuro-biologic and psychoacoustic, that inform our current conceptualization of the disorder. This chapter presents a historical overview of (C)APD to demonstrate how our understanding of this complex topic has evolved in recent years. Because an understanding of the fundamental nature of any disorder is critical to appropriate diagnosis and intervention, the current definition and nature of (C)APD is discussed, including how the disorder may lead to or be associated with difficulties in learning, language, communication, and related function. Finally, issues related to prevalence and etiology of (C)APD in children and adults are explored, and areas for future research in central auditory diagnosis and treatment are presented.

Historical Foundations of (C)APD

Interest in central auditory processing and its disorders has spanned more than five decades. In 1954, Helmer Myklebust discussed the importance of evaluating central auditory function in children suspected of communication disorders. Specifically, he emphasized the need to go beyond the audiogram alone when evaluating children presenting with what he termed *auditory imperception*, or hearing difficulties not attributable to peripheral auditory dysfunction. It was hypothesized that many of these children may have deficits in *how* they hear (i.e., higher-level auditory function) versus *what* they hear (i.e., simple auditory acuity) that lead to a variety of communication difficulties. Thus, Myklebust emphasized the importance of evaluating the entire auditory system, not just the auditory periphery, when assessing hearing in children. In an era when virtually all focus was on the audiogram, this was a truly revolutionary perspective, yet one that would eventually prove itself to be well founded.

During the same decade, diagnostic tests of central auditory function began to emerge. Bocca and colleagues (Bocca, Calearo, & Cassarini, 1954) demonstrated the sensitivity of psychophysical auditory paradigms in assessing "cortical hearing" in patients with temporal lobe lesions. Broadbent (1954) was the first to use a method of bilaterally competing digits to explore attention and memory function. Several years later, Kimura (1961a, 1961b) adapted Broadbent's technique to investigate hemispheric asymmetry and effects of unilateral lesions on audi-

tory function. Thus, Kimura generally is credited with the introduction of dichotic speech tests to the field of central auditory assessment and the development of a model of the physiologic mechanisms underlying dichotic listening. At the same time, Neff (1961) began to explore the mechanisms of selected auditory processes in the animal model.

These classic studies provided the bedrock upon which much of our current understanding of central auditory function has been built. The continued robustness of the concepts and paradigms first introduced in the 1950s for diagnosis of central auditory nervous system (CANS) dysfunction has been demonstrated repeatedly in the literature throughout the subsequent years (see Bellis, 2003 and Chermak & Musiek, 1997 for reviews). Similarly, although alternative, nonauditory explanations for the well-recognized right-ear advantage observed on dichotic listening tasks have been proposed (e.g., Efron, 1990; Sidtis, 1982; Speaks, Gray, Miller, & Rubens, 1975), a substantial amount of behavioral and electrophysiologic evidence has supported Kimura's theory of dichotic listening (e.g., Aiello et al., 1995; Hugdahl et al., 1999; Milner, Taylor, & Sperry, 1968; Musiek, Kibbe, & Baran, 1984; Sparks & Geschwind, 1968; Wioland, Rudolf, Metz-Lutz, Mutschler, & Marescaux, 1999). As a result, dichotic speech tests remain one of the mainstays of central auditory testing today. (See Chapter 7 for discussion of the central auditory test battery and Chapter 9 for discussion of dichotic tests in particular.)

Despite Myklebust's 1954 admonishment to clinicians on the importance of evaluating central auditory function in children, clinical interest in the diagnosis of (C)APD, especially in the pediatric population, did not begin to take hold until the 1970s. That decade witnessed a rise in research regarding clinical utility of diagnostic tests of central auditory function and the relationship between auditory perceptual deficits and learning difficulties in children, as well as the emergence of central auditory test batteries for the diagnosis of (C)APD (e.g., Jerger & Jerger, 1975; Katz & Ilmer, 1972; Keith, 1977; Willeford, 1977). In addition, the utility of electrophysiologic measures of central auditory function has led to growing use of auditory evoked and event-related potentials, in conjunction with psychophysical measures, for diagnosis of (C)APD (see Chapter 12). The auditory brainstem response (ABR) has long been a well-documented means of assessing brainstem function (see Hall, 1992 and Musiek, 1991 for reviews). Furthermore, the middle-latency and cortical evoked potentials have demonstrated sensitivity to cortical and subcortical dysfunction in the central auditory pathways, particularly when multiple electrode sites are used for recording (e.g., Knight, 1990; Kraus, Ozdamar, Hier, & Stein, 1982; Musiek, Charette, Kelly, Lee, & Musiek, 1999; see Cacace & McFarland, 2001 and Stapells, 2001 for reviews). More sophisticated paradigms using speech stimuli presented either monotically or dichotically have been reported recently, and appear to hold promise for the identification of atypical hemispheric asymmetries and abnormal neurophysiologic representation of phonemic segments that may give rise to auditory and related deficits (e.g., Banai, Nicol, Zecker, & Kraus, 2005; Bellis, Nicol, & Kraus, 2000; Greenwald & Jerger, 2003; Jerger & Lew, 2004; Jerger & Mar-

tin, 2004, 2005; Jerger, Martin, & McColl, 2004; Kraus, McGee, Carrell, Sharma, Micco, & Nicol, 1993; Kraus, McGee, Carrell, Zecker, Nicol, & Koch, 1996; Liasis, Bamiou, Campbell, Sirmanna, Boyd, & Towell, 2003; Moncrieff, Jerger, Wambacq, Greenwald, & Black, 2004; Tremblay, Friesen, Martin, & Wright, 2003; Wible, Nicol, & Kraus, 2005; see Chapter 4 for a review).

Due largely to the early lack of a concise definition of (C)APD, use of imprecise terms such as "auditory language learning disorder" or "auditory perceptual disorder" to describe (C)APD, and lack of precise diagnostic criteria, controversy arose regarding the very existence of a CANS deficit that could lead to or be associated with language and related difficulties (e.g., Bloom & Lahey, 1978; Rees, 1973). To some degree, elements of this controversy persist today (e.g., Cacace & McFarland, 1998, 2005; McFarland & Cacace, 1995; Watson & Kidd, 2002). However, as discussed later in this chapter, when one fully understands the nature and definition of (C)APD as presently conceptualized, a substantive body of literature supports both the existence of the disorder and the current methods of diagnosing and treating it (see ASHA, 2005a; Bellis 2002a, 2003; Chermak & Musiek, 1997; Musiek, Bellis, & Chermak, 2005, for reviews).

Since the 1970s, numerous conferences and committees have been convened to ponder the nature of (C)APD, psychophysical and electrophysiologic methods of diagnosing the disorder, intervention approaches, and the roles of various professionals in diagnosis and intervention (e.g., ASHA, 1992, 1996, 2005a, 2005b; Jerger & Musiek, 2000). Several full-length books and special issues of scholarly journals have been devoted to the subject, often with differing perspectives (e.g., Bellis, 1996, 1999, 2002b, 2003; Chalfant & Scheffelin, 1969; Chermak, 2002; Chermak & Musiek, 1997; Ferre, 1997; Katz, Stecker, & Henderson, 1992; Keith, 1977, 1981; Kelly, 1995; Lasky & Katz, 1983; Levinson & Sloan, 1980; Masters, Stecker, & Katz, 1998; Musiek, 2004; Musiek, Baran, & Pinheiro, 1994; Pinheiro & Musiek, 1985; Sloan, 1995; Sullivan, 1975; Willeford & Burleigh, 1985).

Just as our methods of diagnosing (C)APD have evolved, so too have our means of treating the disorder (see Wertz, Hall, & Davis, 2002, for a review). In addition to environmental modifications to improve signal-to-noise ratio within the listening environment, clinicians now have available to them a plethora of intervention strategies from which to choose when treating individuals with (C)APD. Some of these strategies have focused on top-down and/or multisensory stimulation to improve auditory perception and related skills (e.g., Lindamood & Lindamood, 1971). Others have focused in a bottom-up manner on discrimination of speech sounds and concomitant spelling and related abilities (e.g., Ferre, 1997; Sloan, 1995). More recently, intervention efforts for (C)APD have acknowledged the need for a combined bottom-up/top-down approach that addresses access to and perception of the auditory signal itself while, at the same time, strengthening and recruiting higher order metacognitive and metalinguistic central resources to facilitate attention to, comprehension of, and retention of auditorily presented information (e.g., ASHA, 2005a; Bellis, 2002c, 2003; Chermak & Musiek, 1997; Kelly, 1995). Furthermore, the importance of individualized, deficit-specific intervention that addresses a given individual's presenting deficits and functional

difficulties rather than the indiscriminate application of one-size-fits-all treatment approaches to all persons with (C)APD has been emphasized (e.g., ASHA, 2005a; Bellis, 2002b, 2002c, 2003; Bellis & Ferre, 1999). The recent development of computer-assisted therapy programs that allow for acoustically controlled presentation of auditory stimuli in an interesting and engaging format that encourages active participation and provides salient feedback (e.g., Cognitive Concepts, 1998; Scientific Learning, 1997) has been a significant addition to the clinician's armamentarium for treatment of (C)APD. (See Chapters 4, 5, and 7 in Volume II of the Hanbook for in-depth reviews of the primary approaches to intervention of (C)APD. Computer-assisted therapy programs are discussed in Chapters 4 and 6 of Volume II of the Handbook. Deficit-specific intervention is discussed in Chapter 10 of Volume II of the Handbook.)

A cumulative body of research in auditory and general neuroscience and neuroplasticity, cognitive science, neuropsychology, and related fields has informed our understanding of central auditory processing and its disorders, as well as the complex interrelationship among audition and listening, learning, language, communication, and related function. Our conceptualization of (C)APD has evolved continuously as new knowledge has accumulated; however, the roots of our current approaches continue to be embedded firmly in the early work of the 1950s. Most recently, ASHA (2005a, 2005b) presented a technical report and position statement that set forth current definitions and general principles of diagnosing, assessing, and treating (C)APD based upon an extensive review of the scientific literature to date. Nonetheless, as with all complex areas of inquiry, there is no doubt that our understanding of (C)APD will continue to evolve as new insights into central auditory function are attained.

The Nature of Central Auditory Processing and Its Disorders

The way in which a disorder is defined informs how it is diagnosed and treated, and by whom. Early definitions of (C)APD were rather amorphous and included processes and behaviors ranging the gamut from fundamental auditory skills to higher-order functions such as linguistic analysis, memory, and use of auditorily presented information (e.g, ASHA, 1992; Kelly, 1995). Because (C)APD can lead to or be associated with a variety of functional deficits in learning, language, and communication, as discussed subsequently in this chapter, professionals from a wide variety of disciplines including speech-language pathologists, audiologists, psychologists and neuropsychologists, educators and educational diagnosticians, physicians, and others began applying the label of (C)APD to their patients, often on the basis of symptoms alone and without benefit of any auditory testing whatsoever. As such, (C)APD became a "wastebasket term" used to describe any difficulty with auditory input or spoken language. This was a primary factor that led to the controversy surrounding the clinical utility of a diagnosis of (C)APD (e.g., Cacace & McFarland, 1998; McFarland & Cacace, 1995; Rees, 1973) because the disorder, as conceptualized by many, was virtually indistinguishable from a

host of other disorders with overlapping symptoms, including language disorder, attention deficit hyperactivity disorder (ADHD), and other higher order cognitive disorders, as well as many other impairments that may affect an individual's ability to listen to, comprehend, remember, or act upon auditory information.

In response, subsequent definitions of (C)APD were more concise and emphasized the auditory-specific nature of the disorder. Thus, many of these definitions either stated or strongly implied that a diagnosis of (C)APD should be made only when it could be demonstrated that the disorder is confined to the auditory modality and nowhere else; that is, that it be modality-specific (e.g., Jerger & Musiek, 2000; McFarland & Cacace, 1995). However, these definitions, too, were fraught with difficulty, as they failed to recognize the complex, nonmodular, and interactive nature of brain function with its proliferation of shared neuroanatomic substrates, multisensory neural interfaces, convergence and divergence of sensory "tracks," and interdependence of bottom-up and top-down factors.

Current definitions of (C)APD explicitly recognize both the auditory nature of the disorder and the inherent nonmodularity of the CANS (ASHA 2005a, 2005b; Bellis, 2002a, 2003; Musiek et al., 2005). ASHA (2005a) defines central auditory processing as "the perceptual (i.e., neural) processing of auditory information in the central nervous system (CNS) and the neurobiologic activity that gives rise to the electrophysiologic auditory potentials" (p. 2). It includes the neural mechanisms that underlie a variety of auditory behaviors, including localization/lateralization, performance with degraded or competing acoustic signals, temporal aspects of audition, auditory discrimination, and auditory pattern recognition (ASHA, 1996, 2005a, 2005b; Bellis, 2003; Chermak & Musiek, 1997). As elaborated by Musiek et al. (2005), several critical aspects of the current definition and conceptualization of (C)APD should be emphasized:

■ (C)APD is conceptualized as an *auditory* disorder of neurobiological origin. That is, in order for a diagnosis of (C)APD to be made, it must be demonstrated that a deficit exists in the CANS, using tests shown to be sensitive to dysfunction in the central auditory pathways.

■ Due to the interactive nature of brain function, (C)APD may coexist with other disorders (e.g., ADHD, language impairment, learning disability, deficits in other modalities); however, it *is not the result of* higher level global or multimodal dysfunction. For example, children with autism or mental retardation might have difficulty with listening and/or comprehending spoken language; however, their "auditory" difficulties are attributable to a higher-order, more global cognitive deficit and not to dysfunction in the CANS. Therefore, it would be inappropriate to apply the label of (C)APD in these cases.

■ Similarly, abilities such as phonologic awareness and analysis, auditory synthesis, spoken language comprehension, and attention to or memory for auditory information may rely in part upon the integrity of acoustic signal processing in the CANS. However, these are higher-order language- or cognitive-related abilities and are excluded from the definition of (C)APD (ASHA, 2005a).

■ Although the notion of *complete* modality-specificity of (C)APD is neurophysiologically untenable when one considers the complex nature of information processing in the brain, it is recognized that (C)APD is *primarily* an auditory disorder. Therefore, individuals with (C)APD present with difficulties, documentable deficits, and complaints that are more pronounced in the auditory modality and, in some cases, auditory-modality—specific findings may be demonstrated.

These factors hold significant implications for clinicians in terms of knowledge base required for engaging in central auditory processing service delivery, scopes of practice of the various professionals who work with individuals with central auditory dysfunction, and methods of diagnosing and treating (C)APD. Several of these topics are discussed in the ASHA (2005a, 2005b) documents and are summarized below.

Knowledge Base Required for Central Auditory Service Delivery

(C)APD cannot be viewed in a vacuum. Although (C)APD is an auditory disorder, the nonmodularity of the CANS and the complex nature of information processing in the CNS dictate that an understanding of the disorder requires familiarity with a wide variety of scientific topics. Research pertaining directly to (C)APD is not confined to the audiologic literature, but proliferates in numerous journals not typically read by those in the fields of hearing and speech/language. Moreover, our professional training programs generally have not addressed these areas adequately (Chermak, Traynham, Seikel, & Musiek, 1998). Many of the misconceptions that have surrounded (C)APD historically may be a result of this lack of education, leading to a unitary and overly simplistic view of auditory processing.

To understand the nature of central auditory processing and its disorders and, thereby, to assess, diagnose, and treat it appropriately, one should have at least a familiarity with, if not a working knowledge of, the current literature in those areas pertaining to brain structure and function and brain-behavior relationships, including general and auditory neuroscience, cognitive psychology and neuropsychology, neurophysiology, psychoacoustics, and other topics (ASHA 2005a, 2005b). This knowledge likely will need to be acquired through ongoing training and educational activities in addition to those obtained during the educational preparation process.

Finally, it is important to emphasize that new findings occur regularly in the clinical and scientific arenas that intersect with or underlie (C)APD. As our understanding of the scientific bases of central auditory processing increases, our views of the disorder must develop accordingly. Any theory of (C)APD, no matter how logical it appears on the surface or how long it has been accepted by popular consensus, cannot be accurate if it is inconsistent with the underlying scientific knowledge. A familiarity with the scientific bases of (C)APD will assist clinicians in evaluating the validity of theories, popular or new diagnostic and treatment tools, and anecdotal "evidence" pertaining to diagnosis or treatment of (C)APD and, thus, will result in better services to the patients who need them.

Scopes of Practice and (C)APD Diagnosis, Assessment, and Intervention

Because (C)APD has, in the past, often been used erroneously and inappropriately as an all-encompassing term to describe virtually anyone with difficulties listening to or understanding auditory information, it is not surprising that professionals from many different disciplines have assumed responsibility for diagnosing the disorder. Thus, the label of (C)APD has been applied to children and adults by audiologists, speech-language pathologists, psychologists, educators, physicians, and others. Further confounding this problem is the fact that many measures of listening, phonologic awareness, language processing, and related abilities use the term *auditory processing* in their titles.

By definition, (C)APD is an auditory disorder, and therefore, the responsibility for diagnosing (C)APD falls squarely within the audiologist's scope of practice (ASHA, 2005a, 2005b). Furthermore, the requirement for acoustical control for administration of central auditory tests and the specialized equipment necessary to diagnose (C)APD require administration by audiologists who typically have the appropriate education and training. Nonetheless, a multidisciplinary approach is needed to assess fully the presenting difficulties and the functional impact of the disorder. Multidisciplinary input also is critical for identifying the primary disorder, comorbid disorders, and overlapping and/or associated deficits (i.e., differential diagnosis). In this light, the speech-language pathologist is uniquely qualified to delineate the cognitive/communicative and language difficulties that may be associated with (C)APD (ASHA

2005a, 2005b, 2005c). Psychologists and neuropsychologists delineate cognitive capacities and brain-behavior relationships and, often in conjunction with educators and/or educational diagnosticians, assess academic function across domains. Other professionals may diagnose additional disorders that may affect the individual's ability to utilize auditory information. Collectively, all of this multimodal (and multidisciplinary) information is important in assessing fully the presenting complaints of a given individual and in differentiating a (C)APD from more global, higher order, or pan-sensory deficits that may mimic and/or coexist with (C)APD. With this information in hand, intervention can be implemented to target deficit areas.

It is important at this point to differentiate among *diagnosis*, *differential diagnosis*, and *assessment*. Assessment may be defined as a data-gathering process that may include both formal and informal procedures to document areas of strength and weakness (ASHA, 2005a). Diagnosis, on the other hand, refers to the actual identification and classification of a specific impairment (ASHA, 2005a). In this light, then, assessment of (C)APD is a multidisciplinary endeavor. Diagnosis of (C)APD, on the other hand, is the responsibility of the audiologist, using acoustically controlled diagnostic test tools that have been shown to be sensitive to dysfunction in the CANS. In contrast, comprehensive intervention for (C)APD may be undertaken by a team of professionals, whose composition depends on the specific needs of the individual. As elaborated in Volume II of this Handbook, intervention for (C)APD encompasses a variety of activities and methods and, as such, may involve audiologists, speech-language pathologists, edu-

cators, and others. Intervention, as well as assessment and differential diagnosis, most often requires a multidisciplinary effort to address the overall individual's presenting difficulties in a holistic and ecologically valid manner (ASHA, 2005a).

Etiology and Prevalence of (C)APD in Children and Adults

It has been estimated that as many as half of all children identified with a learning disorder (or 2–5% of the school-age population) exhibit (C)APD (e.g., Chermak & Musiek, 1997). Prevalence figures for (C)APD in the elderly population have ranged from as low as 2% to as high as 76% depending on the strictness of the criterion used for inclusion (e.g., Cooper & Gates, 1991; Golding, Carter, Mitchell, & Hood, 2004; see Chapter 13 in Volume II of the Handbook for a review). The lack of precise prevalence figures for (C)APD likely has arisen because of widely differing methods of defining and diagnosing the disorder. It is hoped that, with the advent of better guidance as to appropriate methods of defining and diagnosing (C)APD (e.g., ASHA 2005a), more accurate prevalence estimations will emerge.

Similarly, although the underlying etiology for central auditory dysfunction may be identified in some cases (e.g., head trauma, neurologic disorder or abnormality), in most cases, the cause of (C)APD remains unknown; however, poor or inefficient neurophysiologic representation of acoustic stimuli is suspected. Imprecise temporal processing and neural synchrony, atypical hemispheric asymmetry in the neural representation of auditory (especially speech) signals, and inefficient interhemispheric transfer of auditory information have been identified in many cases of (C)APD in both children and aging adults (e.g., Bellis, Nicol, & Kraus, 2000; Bellis & Wilber, 2001; Jerger et al., 2002; Kraus, McGee, Carrell, Zecker, Nicol, & Koch, 1996).

Relationships Among (C)APD and Language, Learning, Communication, and Related Difficulties

Not surprisingly, individuals with (C)APD typically present with auditory difficulties as their primary complaint (ASHA 2005a, 2005b; Bellis, 2003; Musiek et al., 2005). However, additional difficulties often are seen in other areas, especially in children. In some cases, and as discussed below, these additional difficulties may be related causally to central auditory deficits. In others, comorbidity of disorders may occur as a result of dysfunction in shared or closely adjacent neuroanatomic substrates. Even deceptively simple tasks, such as listening in noise, draw upon multiple brain regions and involve complex neurophysiologic interactions (e.g., Salvi et al., 2002).

The literature abounds with studies demonstrating, both behaviorally and electrophysiologically, relationships among central auditory deficits and disorders such as specific language impairment, learning disability, reading difficulties, and ADHD (e.g., Bellis & Ferre, 1999; Kraus et al., 1996; Moncrieff & Musiek, 2002; Riccio, Hynd, Cohen, & Gonzales, 1993; Riccio, Hynd, Cohen, & Molt, 1996; Tallal, Miller, & Fitch, 1993; Tillery, Katz,

& Keller, 2000; Wright, Lombardino, King, Puranik, Leonard, & Merzenich, 1997; see Chapters 4, 15, 16, and 17 in this Volume, for a review). Nonetheless, these linkages should not be taken as evidence that (C)APD should automatically be assumed as the underlying cause of learning, language, and related disorders. These higher order functions involve vast processes and mechanisms, only some of which may involve the auditory system.

It is important to recognize that (C)APD is a heterogeneous disorder, and the relative impact of a central auditory deficit on functional abilities will be the result of the unique confluence of an individual's bottom-up and top-down processing abilities and a host of other factors (Bellis, 2003). Similarly, language, learning, and related deficits are heterogeneous. Therefore, it is difficult to draw a clear one-to-one correspondence between deficits in central auditory processes and higher-order language, learning, communication, and related sequelae using large groups of subjects (ASHA, 2005a; Bellis, 2003). Indeed, the finding of a lack of correlation between fundamental auditory skills (e.g., temporal processing) and higher-order, learning-related outcomes (e.g., reading) in large subject groups has led some investigators to postulate that central auditory dysfunction does not result in a meaningful disability affecting learning or related function (e.g., Cacace & McFarland, 2005; Watson & Kidd, 2002).

Other studies, however, have demonstrated that the linkages among central auditory abilities and learning and related outcomes are affected differentially by the specific nature of the central auditory deficit(s) that is/are present and the type of learning or related difficulty with which the individual presents (e.g., Bellis & Ferre, 1999; Cestnick & Jerger,

2000; Heath, Hogben, & Clark, 1999). Furthermore, even when a direct causal relationship cannot be established or is unlikely, the presence of an auditory deficit certainly can be expected to exacerbate academic and related difficulties by requiring that more effort be expended toward processing the incoming acoustic signal, leaving fewer resources available upstream for comprehension, retention, and other higher order functions (e.g., McCoy et al., 2005; Pichora-Fuller, Schneider, & Daneman, 1995). This heterogeneity of disorders, combined with the complexity of interactions between bottom-up and top-down processing, further underscores the need for comprehensive, multidisciplinary assessment in delineating the full spectrum of difficulties exhibited by individuals with (C)APD.

Subprofiling (C)APD

Notwithstanding the heterogeneity of (C)APD and related disorders, an accumulated body of research in auditory neuroscience as well as in neuropsychology and related fields has demonstrated that dysfunction in various brain regions or processing levels can result in relatively predictable *patterns* of deficits across functional domains. These demonstrated brain-behavior relationships have allowed us, in recent years, to begin to develop functional deficit profiles, or subprofiles, of (C)APD that relate observed patterns of deficits on central auditory tests both to neurophysiologic underpinnings and to functional language, learning, communication, and related sequelae (e.g., Bellis & Ferre, 1999; see Bellis, 2002b, 2003 for review, and Chapter 10 of Volume II of the Handbook).

When considering subprofiling of (C)APD, three key caveats must be kept in mind. First, it is critical that any subprofiling method be consistent with what is known about the underlying neuroscience of the system and documented effects of CNS dysfunction on sensitized tests across domains (Bellis, 2003). As such, these theories must be dynamic and based upon solid neuroscience foundations. As the knowledge base regarding the neurophysiologic tenets of (C)APD and related disorders evolves, so too must the theoretical constructs evolve. No matter how logical a subprofiling theory may seem on the surface, or how well it appears to describe the functional difficulties exhibited by children and adults seen in the classroom or clinic, its validity should always be evaluated relative to the empirical evidence available in the auditory and cognitive neuroscience and related literature.

Second, subprofiling methods should never be viewed as "cookbook" methods of diagnosing or treating disorders. Perhaps the most immutable and predictable aspect of brain function is its very unpredictability. Despite the well-established documentation of certain fundamental brain-behavior relationships and deficit patterns arising from dysfunction in certain brain regions, information—including auditory—processing is too complex to assume homogeneity of functional deficits across individuals. Instead, subprofiling should be viewed as a guide to assist clinicians in identifying patterns of function across multimodal domains so that pansensory or global disorders may be ruled out and intervention efforts may be more focused and deficit-specific (Bellis, 2003). At all times, however, diagnosis and intervention should be individualized and based on the unique presentation of the child or adult in question, and one should never expect each individual to fit neatly into a predetermined and circumscribed "box."

Third, causality should not be assumed simply because of coexistence of functional deficits, although a causal relationship may be postulated in some cases. For example, deficits in the processing of rapid spectrotemporal acoustic changes, such as those involved in speech-sound (particularly stop-consonant) discrimination, mediated by the primary auditory cortex have been postulated to contribute causally to difficulties in reading and spelling decoding of those same poorly discriminated speech sounds. It has been suggested further that these same auditory processing deficits may lead to deficits in phonologic awareness, language, and articulation in much the same way that a hearing loss may cause similar difficulties in these domains (e.g., Bellis, 2002b, 2003; Bellis & Ferre, 1999; Kraus et al., 1996; Tallal et al., 1996). Treatment focused on speech-sound discrimination and speech-to-print skills, therefore, may be effective in improving the auditory component and also may have a beneficial effect on at least some of the related learning and language sequelae (e.g., Bellis, 2002b, 2002c, 2003; Sloan, 1995; Tallal et al., 1996).

In contrast, although individuals with central auditory findings indicative of deficient interhemispheric transfer of information also may exhibit increased visual-motor interhemispheric transfer time, subtle bimanual and/or bipedal deficits, and other interhemispheric difficulties (e.g., Bellis, 2002b, 2003; Bellis & Ferre, 1999; Bellis & Wilber, 2001), it would be unreasonable to assume that the auditory deficit *caused* the deficits in other

sensory systems. Instead, these likely represent *associated,* comorbid deficits resulting from dysfunction in shared neuroanatomic substrate (corpus callosum). In these cases, intervention may include activities that are auditory-specific, as well as activities that involve interhemispheric stimulation using other modalities (e.g., Bellis, 2002b, 2002c, 2003; Bellis & Ferre, 1999; Chermak & Musiek, 1997; Musiek & Chermak, 1995).

In still other cases, (C)APD may coexist with (albeit not in a causal manner) other, valid diagnoses (e.g., ADHD, multiple sclerosis, etc.) in much the same way that hearing loss and vision loss coexist in Usher's syndrome or auditory neuropathy/dys-synchrony may coexist with peripheral neuropathies in other sensory systems (Musiek et al., 2005). The presence of these comorbid conditions does not negate the existence of a central auditory deficit. It does, however, render it absolutely critical that the central auditory deficit be verified using tests validated for this purpose to establish that the source of the auditory difficulties derives from dysfunction in the CANS beyond any exacerbating auditory effects posed by the comorbid disorder. This is important both to rule out a more global, pansensory deficit as a causal factor for reported auditory difficulties, as well as for purposes of designing appropriate intervention.

In conclusion, the use of functional deficit profiling may provide a helpful guide for clinicians in identifying neurophysiologically tenable patterns of deficits across multidisciplinary test results. This may be useful both in differential diagnosis and for purposes of designing comprehensive, deficit-specific intervention plans that address the full spectrum of difficulties exhibited by the individual.

However, one should always keep in mind the complexity of the CNS and its function and never assume that any given categorization construct will describe adequately the vast range of difficulties exhibited by all individuals with (C)APD.

Future Research in the Diagnosis and Treatment of (C)APD

In recent years, the advent of functional neuroimaging and more advanced electrophysiologic and topographic mapping techniques have provided unique insights into neural processing of auditory stimuli. The degree to which these techniques ultimately will be transferable to the clinical arena has yet to be determined; however, these tools have advanced our understanding of central auditory processing and its disorders. By the same token, evidence indicating that neuroplasticity extends throughout the lifetime (Kolb, 1995) and that auditory training can facilitate stimulation-induced learning, thus decreasing or ameliorating central auditory dysfunction, has transformed our intervention for the disorder from a management-focused perspective to one that includes specific remediation (i.e., treatment) activities. Similarly, our accumulated knowledge of cognitive science and information processing, directs us to include top-down strategies, as well as bottom-up stimulation activities in intervention programs. Together, these bottom-up treatments and top-down, central resources strategy training have improved our ability to address (C)APD in a deficit-specific and individualized

manner. At the same time, the robustness of time-honored and well-established tools for diagnosis of and intervention for (C)APD has been demonstrated (e.g., dichotic listening tests, use of assistive listening devices and other environmental modifications, etc.), providing continued support for the use of these measures and paradigms in current practice.

As with any complex disorder involving the brain, future research will continue to affect our conceptualization, diagnosis, and treatment of (C)APD. Efficient means of screening for the disorder, as well as the development of additional sensitized diagnostic measures, are needed. Validation of models of central auditory processing, including those that involve subprofiling as discussed above, will assist in delineating further the relationship among central auditory processing and learning, language, and related functions. The clinical utility of electrophysiologic and neuroimaging techniques in diagnosis of and intervention for (C)APD has yet to be determined, as have the most efficient means to differentially diagnose (C)APD and other comorbid or multimodal disorders (ASHA, 2005a). Finally, in this era of evidence-based practice, treatment efficacy data supporting specific programs of remediation for (C)APD are needed. Nonetheless, we have come far since Myklebust's first description of children with "auditory imperception" and, at present, we have the tools available to us to diagnose and treat (C)APD in children and adults. (See Chapter 19 in this volume for discussion of future directions in diagnosis of (C)APD and Chapters 2 and 13 in Volume II for discussion of evidence-based practice and treatment efficacy, and future directions in intervention, respectively.

Summary

The past five decades have witnessed an evolution in the definition and conceptualization of (C)APD and in the methods of diagnosing, assessing, and treating the disorder. Current definitions of (C)APD emphasize its auditory, neurobiologic underpinnings while, at the same time, recognizing the complexity of CNS function and the interactive nature of information processing. Because (C)APD is an auditory disorder, the audiologist is the professional who, by education and professional scope of practice, is responsible for diagnosis; however, a multidisciplinary approach is essential to an appropriate differential diagnosis and comprehensive intervention. This is especially true when (C)APD coexists with or is linked, perhaps causally, to difficulties involving language, learning, communication, and related function. The development of functional deficit profiles of central auditory deficits, along with recent advances in diagnosis and treatment of (C)APD, likely will result in even more efficient means of serving patients with central auditory dysfunction in the future.

References

Aiello, I., Sotgiu, S., Sau, G. F., Manca, S., Conti, M., & Rosati, G. (1995). Long-latency evoked potentials in a case of corpus callosum agenesia. *Italian Journal of Neurological Sciences, 15,* 497–505.

American Speech-Language-Hearing Association. (1992). *Issues in central auditory processing disorders: A report from the ASHA ad hoc committee on central auditory processing.* Rockville, MD: Author.

American Speech-Language-Hearing Association. (1996). Central auditory processing: Current status of research and implications for clinical practice. *American Journal of Audiology, 5*(2): 41–54.

American Speech-Language-Hearing Association. (2005a). *(Central) auditory processing disorders* [Technical report]. Available at www.asha.org/members/deskref-journals/deskref/default

American Speech-Language-Hearing Association. (2005b). *(Central) auditory processing disorders—The role of the audiologist* [Position statement]. Available at http://www.asha.org/members/deskref-journals/deskref/default

American Speech-Language-Hearing Association. (2005c). *SLP preferred practice patterns.* Available at http://www.asha.org/members/deskref-journals/deskref/default

Banai, K., Nicol, T., Zecker, S. G., & Kraus, N. (2005). Brainstem timing: Implications for cortical processing and literacy. *Journal of Neuroscience, 25,* 9850–9857.

Bellis, T. J. (1996). *Assessment and management of central auditory processing disorders in the educational setting: From science to practice.* San Diego, CA: Singular Publishing Group.

Bellis, T. J. (Ed.). (1999). Auditory processing disorders in children. *Journal of the American Academy of Audiology (Special Issue), 10*(6).

Bellis, T. J. (2002a). Considerations in diagnosing auditory processing disorders in children. *American Speech-Language-Hearing Association Special Interest Division 9 (Hearing and Hearing Disorders in Children), 12,* 3–9.

Bellis, T. J. (2002b). *When the brain can't hear: Unraveling the mystery of auditory processing disorder.* New York: Pocket Books.

Bellis, T. J. (2002c). Developing deficit-specific intervention plans for individuals with auditory processing disorders. *Seminars in Hearing, 23*, 287–295.

Bellis, T. J. (2003). *Assessment and management of central auditory processing disorders in the educational setting: From science to practice* (2nd ed.). Clifton Park, NY: Thomson Learning.

Bellis, T. J., & Ferre, J. M. (1999). Multidimensional approach to the differential diagnosis of central auditory processing disorders in children. *Journal of the American Academy of Audiology, 10*, 319–328.

Bellis, T. J., Nicol, T., & Kraus, N. (2000). Aging affects hemispheric asymmetry in the neural representation of speech sounds. *Journal of Neuroscience, 20*, 791–797.

Bellis, T. J., & Wilber, L. A. (2001). Effects of aging and gender on interhemispheric function. *Journal of Speech, Language, and Hearing Research, 44*, 246–263.

Bloom, L., & Lahey, M. (1978). *Language development and language disorders.* New York: Wiley.

Bocca, E., Calearo, C., & Cassarini, V. (1954). A new method for testing hearing in temporal lobe tumors. *Acta Otolaryngologica (Stockholm), 44*, 219–221.

Broadbent, D. E. (1954). The role of auditory localization in attention and memory span. *Journal of Experimental Psychology, 47*, 191–196.

Cacace, A. T., & McFarland, D. J. (1998). Central auditory processing disorder in school-aged children: A critical review. *Journal of Speech, Language, and Hearing Research, 41*, 355–373.

Cacace, A. T., & McFarland, D. J. (2001). Middle-latency auditory evoked potentials: Basic issues and potential applications. In J. Katz (Ed.), *Handbook of clinical audiology* (5th ed., pp. 349–377). Baltimore: Lippincott, Williams & Wilkins.

Cacace, A. T., & McFarland, D. J. (2005). The importance of modality specificity in diagnosing central auditory processing disorder. *American Journal of Audiology, 14*, 112–123.

Cestnick, L., & Jerger, J. (2000). Auditory temporal processing and lexical/nonlexical reading in developmental dyslexia. *Journal of the American Academy of Audiology, 11*, 501–513.

Chalfant, J. C., & Scheffelin, M. A. (1969). *Central processing dysfunctions in children: A review of research.* National Institute of Neurological Diseases and Stroke Monograph No. 9. Bethesda, MD: U.S. Department of Health, Education, and Welfare.

Chermak, G. D. (Ed.). (2002). Management of auditory processing disorders. *Seminars in Hearing, 23*(4).

Chermak, G. D., & Musiek, F. E. (1997). *Central auditory processing disorders: New perspectives.* San Diego, CA: Singular Publishing Group.

Chermak, G. D., Traynham, W. A., Seikel, J. A., & Musiek, F. E. (1998). Professional education and assessment practices in central auditory processing. *Journal of the American Academy of Audiology, 9*, 452–465.

Cognitive Concepts. (1998). *Earobics™.* Evanston, IL: Cognitive Concepts, Inc.

Cooper, J. C., & Gates, G. A. (1991). Hearing in the elderly—the Framingham cohort, 1983–1985. Part II. Prevalence of central auditory processing disorders. *Ear and Hearing, 12*, 304–311.

Efron, R. (1990). *The decline and fall of hemispheric specialization.* Hillsdale, NJ: Lawrence Erlbaum.

Ferre, J. M. (1997). *Processing power: A guide to CAPD assessment and management.* San Antonio, TX: Communication Skill Builders.

Golding, M., Carter, N., Mitchell, P., & Hood, L. J. (2004). Prevalence of central auditory processing (CAP) abnormality in an older Australian population: The Blue Mountains hearing study. *Journal of the American Academy of Audiology, 15*, 633–642.

Greenwald, R. R., & Jerger, J. (2003). Neuroelectric correlates of hemispheric asymmetry: Spectral discrimination and stimulus competition. *Journal of the American Academy of Audiology, 14*, 434–443.

Hall, J. (1992). *Handbook of auditory evoked responses*. Boston: Allyn & Bacon.

Heath, S. M., Hogben, J. H., & Clark, C. D. (1999). Auditory temporal processing in disabled readers with and without oral language delay. *Journal of Child Psychology and Psychiatry, 40*, 637–647.

Hugdahl, K., Bronnick, K., Kyllingsback, S., Law, I., Gade, A., & Paulson, O. B. (1999). Brain activation during dichotic presentations of consonant-vowel and musical instrument stimuli: a 150-PET study. *Neuropsychologia, 37*, 431–440.

Jerger, J., & Jerger, S. (1975). Clinical validity of central auditory tests. *Scandinavian Audiology, 4*, 147–163.

Jerger, J., & Lew, H. L. (2004). Principles and clinical applications of auditory evoked potentials in the geriatric population. *Physical Medicine and Rehabilitation Clinics of North America, 15*, 235–250.

Jerger, J., & Martin, J. (2004). Hemispheric asymmetry of the right ear advantage in dichotic listening. *Hearing Research, 198*, 125–136.

Jerger, J., & Martin, J. (2005). Some effects of aging on event-related potentials during a linguistic monitoring task. *International Journal of Audiology, 44*, 321–330.

Jerger, J., Martin, J., & McColl, R. (2004). Interaural cross correlation of event-related potentials and diffusion tensor imaging in the evaluation of auditory processing disorder: A case study. *Journal of the American Academy of Audiology, 15*, 79–87.

Jerger, J., & Musiek, F. (2000). Report of the consensus conference on the diagnosis of auditory processing disorders in school-aged children. *Journal of the American Academy of Audiology, 11*, 467–474.

Jerger, J., Thibodeau, L., Martin, J., Mehta, J., Tillman, G., Greenwald, R., Britt, L., Scott, J., & Overson, G. (2002). Behavioral and electrophysiologic evidence of auditory processing disorder: A twin study. *Journal of the American Academy of Audiology, 13*, 438–460.

Katz, J., & Ilmer, R. (1972). Auditory perception in children with learning disabilities. In J. Katz (Ed.), *Handbook of clinical audiology* (pp. 540–563). Baltimore: Williams & Wilkins.

Katz, J., Stecker, N. A., & Henderson. D. (1992). *Central auditory processing: A transdisciplinary view*. St. Louis, MO: Mosby Year Book.

Keith, R. (Ed.). (1977). *Central auditory dysfunction*. New York: Grune & Stratton.

Keith, R. W. (Ed.). (1981). *Central auditory and language disorders in children*. San Diego, CA: College-Hill Press.

Kelly, D. A. (1995). *Central auditory processing disorder: Strategies for use with children and adolescents*. San Antonio, TX: Communication Skill Builders.

Kimura, D. (1961a). Some effects of temporal-lobe damage on auditory perception. *Canadian Journal of Psychology, 15*, 156–165.

Kimura, D. (1961b). Cerebral dominance and the perception of verbal stimuli. *Canadian Journal of Psychology, 15*, 166–171.

Knight, R. (1990). Neural mechanisms of event-related potentials: Evidence from human lesion studies. In J. Rorbaugh, R. Parasuraman, & R. Johnson, Jr. (Eds.), *Event-related brain potentials: Basic issues and applications* (pp. 3–18). New York: Oxford University Press.

Kolb, B. (1995). *Brain plasticity and behavior*. Mahwah, NJ: Lawrence Erlbaum Associates.

Kraus, N., McGee, T., Carrell, T., Sharma, A., Micco, A., & Nicol, T. (1993). Speech-evoked cortical potentials in children. *Journal of the American Academy of Audiology, 4*, 238–248.

Kraus, N., McGee, T. J., Carrell, T. D., Zecker, S. D., Nicol, T. G., & Koch, D. B. (1996). Auditory neurophysiologic responses and discrimination deficits in children with learning problems. *Science, 273*, 971–973.

Kraus, N., Ozdamar, O., Hier, D., & Stein, L. (1982). Auditory middle latency responses (MLRs) in patients with cortical lesions.

Electroencephalography and Clinical Neurophysiology, 54, 275-287.

Lasky, E. Z., & Katz, J. (1983). *Central auditory processing disorders: Problems of speech, language, and learning.* Baltimore: University Park Press.

Liaisis, A., Bamiou, D. E., Campbell, P., Sirimanna, T., Boyd, S., & Towell, A. (2003). Auditory event-related potentials in the assessment of auditory processing disorders: A pilot study. *Neuropediatrics, 34,* 23-29.

Levinson, P., & Sloan, C. (1980). *Auditory processing and language: Clinical and research perspectives.* New York: Grune & Stratton.

Lindamood, C., & Lindamood, P. (1971). *The Lindamood auditory test of conceptualization (LAC).* Boston: Teaching Resources.

Masters, M., Stecker, N., & Katz, J. (1998). *Central auditory processing disorders: Mostly management.* Boston: Allyn & Bacon.

McCoy, S. L., Tun, P. A., Cox, L. C., Colangelo, M., Stewart, R. A., & Wingfield, A. (2005). Hearing loss and perceptual effort: Downstream effects on older adults' memory for speech. *Journal of Experimental Psychology, 58*(1), 22-33.

McFarland, D. J., & Cacace, A. T. (1995). Modality specificity as a criterion for diagnosing central auditory processing disorders. *American Journal of Audiology, 4,* 36-48.

Milner, B., Taylor, S., & Sperry, R. (1968). Lateralized suppression of dichotically presented digits after commissural section in man. *Science, 161,* 184-185.

Moncrieff, D., Jerger, J., Wambacq, I., Greenwald, R., & Black, J. (2004). ERP evidence of a dichotic left-ear deficit in some dyslexic children. *Journal of the American Academy of Audiology, 15,* 518-534.

Moncrieff, D. & Musiek, F. (2002). Interaural asymmetries revealed by dichotic listening tests in normal and dyslexic children. *Journal of the American Academy of Audiology, 13,* 428-437.

Musiek, F. E. (1991). Auditory evoked responses in site of lesion assessment. In W. Rintelmann (Ed.), *Hearing assessment* (2nd ed., pp. 383-428). Boston: Allyn & Bacon.

Musiek, F. E. (Ed.). (2004). Hearing and the brain: Audiological consequences of neurological disorders. *Journal of the American Academy of Audiology [Special Issue], 15*(2).

Musiek, F. E., Baran, J. A., & Pinheiro, M. L. (1994). *Neuroaudiology case studies.* San Diego, CA: Singular Publishing Group.

Musiek, F. E., Bellis, T. J., & Chermak, G. D. (2005). Nonmodularity of the CANS: Implications for (central) auditory processing disorder. *American Journal of Audiology, 14,* 128-138.

Musiek, F., Charette, L., Kelly, T., Lee, W., & Musiek, E. (1999). Hit and false- positive rates for the middle latency response in patients with central nervous system involvement. *Journal American Academy of Audiology, 10*(3), 124-132.

Musiek, F. E., & Chermak, G. D. (1995). Three commonly asked questions about central auditory processing disorders: Management. *American Journal of Audiology, 4,* 15-18.

Musiek, F. E., Kibbe, K., & Baran, J. A. (1984). Neuroaudiological results from split-brain patients. *Seminars in Hearing, 5,* 219-229.

Myklebust, H. R. (1954). *Auditory disorders in children: A manual for differential diagnosis.* New York: Grune & Stratton.

Neff, W. (1961). Neural mechanisms of auditory discrimination. In W. Rosenblith (Ed.), *Century communication* (pp. 259-278). New York: Wiley & Sons.

Pichora-Fuller, M. K., Schneider, B. A., & Daneman, M. (1995). How young and old adults listen to and remember speech in noise. *Journal of the Acoustical Society of America, 97,* 593-608.

Pinheiro, M. L., & Musiek, F. E. (Eds.). (1985). *Assessment of central auditory dysfunction: Foundations and clinical correlates.* Baltimore: Williams & Wilkins.

Rees, N. S. (1973). Auditory processing factors in language disorders: The view from Procrustes' bed. *Journal of Speech and Hearing Disorders, 38*, 304–315.

Riccio, C. A., Hynd, G. W., Cohen, M. J., & Gonzalez, J. J. (1993). Neurological basis of attention deficit hyperactivity disorder. *Exceptional Children, 60*(2), 118–124.

Riccio, C. A., Hynd, G. W., Cohen, M. J., & Molt, L. (1996). The Staggered Spondaic Word Test: Performance of children with attention-deficit hyperactivity disorder. *American Journal of Audiology, 5*(2), 55–62.

Salvi, R. J., Lockwood, A. H., Frisina, R. D., Coad, M. L., Wack, D. S., & Frisina, D. R. (2002). PET imaging of the normal human auditory system: Responses to speech in quiet and in background noise. *Hearing Research, 170*, 96–106.

Scientific Learning Corporation. (1997). *Fast ForWord®*. Berkeley, CA: Author.

Sidtis, J. (1982). Predicting brain organization from dichotic listening performance: Cortical and subcortical functional asymmetries contribute to perceptual asymmetries. *Brain and Language, 17*, 287–300.

Sloan, C. (1995). *Treating auditory processing difficulties in children*. San Diego, CA: Singular Publishing Group.

Sparks, R., & Geschwind, N. (1968). Dichotic listening in man after section of neocortical commissures. *Cortex, 4*, 3–16.

Speaks, C, Gray, T., Miller, J., & Rubens, A. (1975). Central auditory deficits and temporal-lobe lesions. *Journal of Speech and Hearing Disorders, 40*, 192–205.

Stapells, D. R. (2001). Cortical event-related potentials to auditory stimuli. In J. Katz (Ed.), *Handbook of clinical audiology* (5th ed., pp. 378–406). Baltimore: Lippincott, Williams & Wilkins.

Sullivan, M. D. (Ed.). (1975). *Central auditory processing disorders: Proceedings of a symposium*. Lincoln: University of Nebraska Press.

Tallal, P., Miller, S. L., Bedi, G., Byma, G., Wang, X., Nagarajan, S. S., Schreiner, C., Jenkins, W. M., & Merzenich, M. (1996). Language comprehension in language-learning impaired children improved with acoustically modified speech. *Science, 271*, 81–84.

Tallal, P., Miller, S., & Fitch, R. H. (1993). Neurobiological basis of speech: A case for the preeminence of temporal processing. *Annals of the New York Academy of Sciences, 682*, 27–47.

Tillery, K. L., Katz, J., & Keller, W. D. (2000). Effects of methylphenidate (Ritalin) on auditory performance in children with attention and auditory processing disorders. *Journal of Speech, Language, and Hearing Research, 43*, 893–901.

Tremblay, K. L., Friesen, L., Martin, B. A., & Wright, R. (2003). Test-retest reliability of cortical evoked potentials using naturally produced speech sounds. *Ear and Hearing, 24*, 225–232.

Watson, C. S. & Kidd, G. R. (2002). On the lack of association between basic auditory abilities, speech processing, and other cognitive skills. *Seminars in Hearing, 23*, 83–93.

Wertz, D., Hall, J. W., & Davis, W. (2002). Auditory processing disorders: Management approaches past and present. *Seminars in Hearing, 23*, 277–285.

Wible, B., Nicol, T., & Kraus, N. (2004). Correlation between brainstem and cortical auditory processes in normal and language-impaired children. *Brain, 128* (Pt. 2), 417–423.

Wible, B., Nicol, T., & Kraus, N. (2005). Correlation between brainstem and cortical auditory processes in normal and language-impaired children. *Brain, 128*, 417–423.

Willeford, J. A. (1977). Assessing central auditory behavior in children: A test battery approach. In R. Keith, (Ed.), *Central auditory dysfunction* (pp. 43–72). New York: Grune & Stratton.

Willeford, J. A., & Burleigh, J. M. (1985). *Handbook of central auditory processing disorders in children*. New York: Grune & Stratton.

Wioland, N., Rudolf, G., Metz-Lutz, M. N., Mutchler, V., & Marescaux, C. (1999). Cerebral correlates of hemispheric lateralization during a pitch discrimination task: An ERP study in dichotic situation. *Clinical Neurophysiology, 110,* 516–523.

Wright, B. A., Lombardino, L. J., King, W. N., Puranik, C. S., Leonard, C. M., & Merzenich, M. M. (1997). Deficits in auditory temporal and spectral resolution in language-impaired children. *Nature, 387,* 176–178.

CHAPTER 6

SCREENING FOR (CENTRAL) AUDITORY PROCESSING DISORDER

RONALD L. SCHOW and J. ANTHONY SEIKEL

As will be discussed in Chapter 7, a thorough assessment includes a battery of behavioral and physiologic tests, often spanning multiple testing sessions. The intensity and complexity of the diagnostic process mandate the need for a screening instrument that will indicate individuals at risk for (central) auditory processing disorder ([C]APD) prior to initiation of assessment. The screening process proposed here uses behavioral tests for referral purposes for diagnostic testing. The tests reviewed as potential screening measures do not comprise an exhaustive list. All the measures reviewed have been selected because they represent three primary auditory processing domains reflected in recent conference and work group reports (ASHA, 2005; Jerger & Musiek, 2000) and almost all the

tests have been examined in at least one factor analysis study that demonstrated its loading on one of these domains. Other potentially useful screening measures that have not been involved in a factor analysis (e.g., Gaps-In-Noise; Musiek et al., 2005) have been omitted. This chapter reflects on the costs and benefits associated with screening, examines available screening tools, and makes recommendations based on the currently accepted theoretical model of (C)APD and recent recommendations from the Bruton Conference and ASHA (Jerger & Musiek, 2000; ASHA, 2005).

The following material addresses audiologic/speech-language screening for (C)APD, and accordingly is jointly written by an audiologist and a speech-language pathologist. This material represents a new, experimental hybrid screening approach that we believe holds promise for clinical use. Because (C)APD assessment should be within the context of a team of professionals (e.g., audiologist, speech-language pathologist, educator, psychologist, medical professional, parent, etc.), we assume that other professionals may have their own screening processes and that, at some point in the assessment process, this group of professionals would meet to discuss the audiologist's diagnosis of (C)APD, the need for further evaluation, and the plan for intervention. As part of the screening process, we discuss questionnaires that draw information from other key players, and we assume that the audiologist and/or speech-language pathologist involved in the screening process might use these questionnaires to gather information from psychologists, medical professionals, parents, teachers, and the individual of concern about potential comorbidities, such as attention deficit hyperactivity disorder (ADHD), learning disability (LD), reading problems, autistic spectrum disorder, and speech/language deficit (S/LD) as these disorders relate to behaviors suggesting (C)APD. This information becomes especially important if the child goes on to a full diagnostic workup.

Screening for children (or adults) at risk for (C)APD should be completed by the audiologist or speech-language pathologist in a manner similar to pure-tone screening in the school setting (probably at the third grade level) or, alternatively, may be completed following referral by teacher, parent, or other professional. Clearly, a screening protocol is important in helping to minimize the attendant problems for the individual with (C)APD, for parents, educators, and other involved professionals. Screening is important to allow timely intervention, which should minimize distress and maximize communicative, educational, and social function (Chermak, 1996; Musiek, Gollegly, Lamb & Lamb, 1990).

Costs and Benefits

Any discussion about the ability of a test to perform its function must be based on the knowledge that there is no *gold standard* behavioral assessment instrument, so this necessarily reduces the certainty with which sensitivity and specificity can be identified. Ultimately, the sensitivity and specificity of central auditory tests should be "derived from patients with known, anatomically confirmed central auditory dysfunction and used as a guide to identify the presence of central auditory dysfunction in children and adults suspected of (C)APD" (ASHA, 2005, p. 9). The above philosophical approach has been fundamental to the screening process recommended in this chapter in that from the beginning of our work we have followed the recommendations of Musiek and Chermak (1994), which were based on anatomically confirmed central auditory dysfunction. Table 6–1 illustrates issues related to sensitivity and specificity (Dawson & Trapp, 2004; Ingelfinger, Mosteller, Thibodeau & Ware, 1987).

Sensitivity is the ability of a test to identify the presence of a disorder when one is actually present. Note that this ability has no implicit relationship to misidentifying those who do not have the disorder. Thus, the perfectly sensitive test of (C)APD will never miss in diagnosing someone with (C)APD (true positive identification), but does not "care" about whether it is inadvertently misdiagnosing

Table 6–1. Outcomes Table for Screening C(APD)

Screening Outcome	(C)APD		
	Present	**Absent**	
Positive outcome	True positive identification: Presence of C(APD)in patient	False positive identification: Identified C(APD) when patient does not have C(APD)	Total positive findings (sum of true positives and false positives)
Negative outcome	False negative: Presence of C(APD)in patient is missed by screening	True negative: Absence of C(APD) in patient	Total negative findings (sum of false negatives and true negatives)
	Total with C(APD) (sum of true positives and false negatives)	Total absent of C(APD) (sum of false positives and true negatives)	

someone who does not have the disorder (false positive identification). That is, sensitivity is only related to positive outcome. By virtue of its highly sensitive nature, a test with high sensitivity will have a low false negative rate, where false negative is the group of people who have the disorder but are not identified by the test as having the disorder.

High sensitivity is a laudable goal in all cases, but comes at a cost. If one looks simply at economic outcome, overidentification of a disorder results in delivering services not only to those with the disorder but also to those for whom the services are unneeded. High sensitivity without regard for false positives is expensive in economic and human terms. However, high sensitivity is good even if specificity suffers a bit because if one uses a diagnostic test follow-up, the false positives will be detected and not passed on.

Specificity is the ability of a test to identify correctly those individuals who do not have the dysfunction. In this case, the test with perfect specificity will have no cases in the False Positive cell, because no one has been identified who does not have the disorder. Because of the test's cautionary approach to misidentification, the cost of this quality is that the number of true positives declines. A test with high specificity is conservative about identifying a disorder, whereas a test with high sensitivity is liberal in identifying the disorder. The perfectly specific test unerringly identifies all individuals who do not have (C)APD. It maximizes cases in the True Negative category without regard to the number of false negatives that will arise from its conservatism.

The reality, of course, is that both over- and underdiagnosis have their costs. Overdiagnosis (likely with high sensitivity) wastes resources by providing unneeded treatment, whereas underdiagnosis (likely with high specificity) incurs the risks related to the disorder itself: Underdiagnosing breast cancer at an early stage vastly increases the 5-year mortality for the disease, whereas underdiagnosing hay fever will have little impact on mortality. Overdiagnosing breast cancer will result in increases in the costs associated with lumpectomy or biopsy, which are traumatic but represent relatively small costs compared with loss of life. Overdiagnosing hay fever results in relatively small costs in medication incurred by the patient. Thus, the costs associated with the playoff between true positives and false positives are always associated with the risks of failure to identify (i.e., loss of health). The costs associated with true negatives and false negatives are similarly decided in terms of the costs associated with excessive diagnosis (e.g., loss of economic resources).

When the true outcome is knowable (such as in cancer assessment and diagnosis, where signs and symptoms will ultimately prove the accuracy of the diagnosis), one can calculate the sensitivity of a measure. This implies not only an agreed-upon definition of the disorder but a means of identifying the disorder accurately, both of which have been demonstrated for (C)APD with a reasonable degree of certainty in recent years (ASHA, 2005). A focused and neurobiologically anchored definition of (C)APD has been promulgated by the American Speech-Language-Hearing Association through an extensive peer-review process (ASHA, 2005). Furthermore, efficient behavioral and electrophysiologic tests and procedures are available to diagnose (C)APD in the case of known, identifiable lesions (Chermak & Musiek, 1997; Hendler,

Squires, & Emmerich, 1990; Jerger, Johnson, & Loiselle, 1988; Musiek, Shinn, Jirsa, Bamiou, Baran, & Zaidan, 2005; Rappaport Gulliver, Phillips, van Dorpe, Maxner, & Bhan, 1994). However, in the great majority of school children and in many adults who appear to have a form of (C)APD based on behavioral tests and questionnaires, there is no demonstrable lesion. Electrophysiologic and topographic mapping studies are revealing differences, however, in the neurophysiologic representation of auditory stimuli in the CANS of subjects with behaviorally diagnosed (C)APD and listening and learning problems (see, for example, Jerger et al., 2002; King, Warrier, Hayes, & Kraus, 2002; Musiek, Charette, Kelly, Lee, & Musiek, 1999; Purdy, Kelly, & Davies, 2002; Warrier, Johnson, Hayes, Nicol, & Kraus, 2004).

The difficulty of electrophysiologically tracking behavioral test changes and myelination changes was underscored in a study by Schochat and Musiek (2006). They examined the maturation course of the frequency and duration pattern tests and the middle latency response (MLR) in 150 normal participants ranging from 7 to 16 years of age. Results showed increased performance with increasing age for both behavioral tests up to age 12. However, there was no significant change across this age range for MLR on either latency or amplitude measures. Similarly, the P300 was inferior to two behavioral tests in identifying individuals with confirmed central nervous system lesions (Hurley & Musiek, 1997). In contrast, Musiek, Baran, and Pinheiro (1992) reported significant differences in P300 latency and amplitude between adults with confirmed CANS lesions and normal controls. Other studies also have demonstrated the ability of late evoked potentials to identify dysfunction in the central auditory nervous system. For example, Jerger et al. (2002) studied dizygotic (i.e., fraternal) twin girls, one presenting symptoms of (C)APD. They demonstrated that event-related potential activation patterns differentiated the twins better than the behavioral tests (i.e., dichotic listening within an oddball paradigm) performed concurrently, which showed essentially no performance difference between the girls. Similarly, Estes, Jerger, and Jacobson (2002) demonstrated the limitations of behavioral tests (i.e., auditory gap detection and auditory movement detection) relative to the capability of event-related potentials (i.e., N1-P2 and P300) in differentiating normal versus poor listeners.

Thus, it appears that, although there are accepted physiologic measures of (C)APD, and some may hold potential as screening measures, when it comes to school screening where advanced electrophysiological equipment will not be readily available, other screening tools must be used. Nonetheless, sensitivity and specificity of screening tests may be derived ultimately from patients with known, confirmed central auditory dysfunction (ASHA, 2005). Albeit with some reservations, it is our opinion that interim steps to estimate sensitivity and specificity may use performance outside normal limits on behavioral tests that are expected to have predictive power. (See Spaulding, Plante, and Farinella [2006] for discussion of the potential adverse consequences of such an approach.) These established behavioral tests will need to be used to estimate the efficiency (i.e., sensitivity and specificity) of screening procedures until a true gold standard—electrophysiologic or neuroimaging procedures—has demonstrated the efficiency of these behavioral tests with a large sample of school-aged children.

Sensitivity of a test is defined as the proportion of true positives that are identified (e.g., 5) compared with the total of those with the disorder (e.g., 7), yielding a percentage (e.g., 71 %). The specificity of a test is defined as the proportion of true negatives that are identified (e.g., 12) as compared with the total number who do not have the disorder (e.g., 48), yielding a percentage (e.g., 25%). A 71% hit rate is laudable, but a specificity of 25% is expensive. It is within this context of costs and benefits that we must enter the examination of screening instruments for (C)APD.

It is important to note that the prevalence of a disease or disorder influences a test's efficiency. If the disorder occurs rarely in the population (as does [C]APD estimated as 2–3% based on Chermak & Musiek, 1997), the chances of detecting it are low—even by a test with high sensitivity. In this same situation, the chances of persons passing the test would be high because most people do not have the disorder. Hence, this test's positive predictive value (defined as the ratio of those with the disorder who were identified by the test to the total number of those failing the test) would be low and its negative predictive value would be high. Clinicians must be aware of the approximate prevalence of a disorder in order to have some general idea of a test's positive and negative predictive values. (See Chapter 7 for further discussion of the concepts of test sensitivity and efficiency within the framework of clinical decision analysis.)

Sensitivity Versus Validity

Before leaving the topic of test sensitivity and specificity, it is important to note the relationship of these concepts to test validity. Ascertaining that a test is valid (i.e., measures what is purported to measure) does not imply that the test is sensitive (or specific) (see Chapter 1). In contrast to validity, sensitivity and specificity speak to the degree to which a valid measure of a domain reliably identifies a bivalent state—disease/nondiseased. (See Chapter 1 for additional discussion of this distinction.)

Screening Instruments for (C)APD

Screening instruments for (C)APD, therefore, should identify a high proportion of those with the disorder by use of a relatively brief and "inexpensive" procedure that is easy to administer and optimally, not influenced by hearing loss, language, cognition, culture or other nonauditory factors. The Bruton conference summary (Jerger & Musiek, 2000) suggested a 10-minute procedure. Our experimental hybrid screening procedure uses 2.5 times that much time, which we consider practical in a school situation where a mass screening might logically be used only once during the primary grades. Screening is "allowed" to have lower expectations concerning specificity than sensitivity. Indeed, as noted above, a high sensitivity rate, *at times*, takes its toll in reduced specificity; however, this is acceptable with a screening measure because the next step is to follow up with a more extensive diagnostic test battery. Hence, one must keep in mind that a screening procedure leads to an in-depth diagnostic assessment before a final diagnosis can be made. The cost of performing further diagnostic testing is low

relative to the cost of failure to identify. Thus, a screening test for (C)APD should err on the side of increased sensitivity even at the cost of diminished specificity.

The ASHA (1996, 2005) guidelines for (C)APD state that a diagnosis of (C)APD requires demonstration of a deficiency in one or more of the following areas: (a) auditory pattern recognition, (b) temporal processing (including temporal integration, discrimination, ordering, and masking), (c) auditory performance with degraded acoustic signals (monaural low redundancy), (d) auditory performance with competing acoustic signals (including dichotic listening), (e) auditory discrimination, and (f) localization and/or lateralization (binaural interaction). The guidelines do not differentiate verbal and nonverbal acoustic stimuli. A significant issue in using a screening measure for (C)APD is that the screener should be able to identify a "fail" in each of those categories to ensure inclusion, since a "true" fail in any *one* of those categories signals the presence of (C)APD (sensitivity). An alternative strategy is to use failure on one of the cardinal signs of (C)APD (e.g., temporal processing) as an indicator of the need for assessment in all domains. This alternative strategy assumes the interdependence across categories of central auditory processes (and their underlying neural substrate). Although such overlap might be anticipated, our research has suggested that these processes can in fact present independently; therefore, we consider a one-test screener inferior to the hybrid process described here. We recognize the downside of using a multiple-test screener: greater sensitivity may be achieved at the cost of poorer specificity.

We recommend behavioral strategies for screening (C)APD. The success of these behavioral tests is used to determine sensitivity and specificity. Following this, we suggest questionnaire surveys can be used successfully to provide good, functional information on an individual's everyday problems. Once a diagnosis is made, such questionnaire information can assist intervention planning, in counseling/collaborating with parents or other professionals, and even contribute as an outcome measure to monitor across the course of therapy. Physiologic tests are usually used in a more detailed assessment, but not in screening. The authors' hybrid strategy using behavioral tests is presented at the culmination of this review. The most widely used instrument for the behavioral approach to screening (C)APD is the *SCAN: A Screening Test for Auditory Processing Disorders* (Keith, 2000a, 2006b). The SCAN is discussed in a later section of this chapter.

Questionnaire surveys typically are presented to caregivers or teachers, and observable signs are identified that serve as indicators of disorder or dysfunction. Although questionnaires have advantages in sampling behaviors characteristic of (C)APD filtered through the eyes of someone familiar with the individual and revealing information that can be used to guide treatment decisions, they present limitations as well. Questionnaires are affected by the subjectivity and biases of the respondent. Questions can be unclear, misleading, too broad, or inappropriate. Also, questionnaires can be too lengthy, leading to inaccurate information due to respondent fatigue or lack of interest (Maxwell & Satake, 2006). The questionnaire described later in this chapter has items carefully selected to avoid many of these problems. Furthermore, all referrals are based on the behavioral test and not on the questionnaire, which is used

only to supplement and contextualize the behavioral test findings after a diagnostic battery confirms (C)APD.

Behavioral Tests

Instruments for screening and assessment should reflect the ASHA (1996, 2005) definition of (C)APD. Table 6–2 presents potential tests and subtests that reflect the seven ASHA (2005) test areas derived from the six central auditory processes identified above. These seven test areas are: auditory pattern/temporal tests, monaural low redundancy tests, binaural/dichotic speech tests, binaural interaction tests, auditory discrimination tests, electroacoustical tests, and electrophysiologic tests.

The SCAN seems to dominate clinical use as a screening instrument, although it only looks at two (i.e., binaural/dichotic tests and monaural low redundancy tests) of the seven test areas listed above. Several other tests and procedures have been proposed as screening tools for (C)APD including the Selective Auditory Attention Test (SAAT), dichotic digits, frequency patterns, gap detection, and so forth (Bellis, 2003; Cherry, 1980; Jerger & Musiek, 2000; Musiek, 1983). Some authors have proposed a requirement to isolate auditory from other sensory modalities in assessment of (C)APD (Cacace & McFarland, 1998). Nonetheless, indications are that no single test or procedure produces acceptable results on a sensitivity/specificity basis (in our work, sensitivity did not ever reach 50% with any of the screeners listed above including SCAN; Domitz & Schow, 2000), and, as stated in the ASHA (2005) *Position Statement on (C)APD*, completely separating sensory modalities is "neurophysiologically untenable" (p. 4).

Table 6–2. Auditory Domain, ASHA-Defined Area, and Potential Specific Test Instrument

Auditory Domain	ASHA (1996, 2005) Defined Area	Specific Test Instrument
Temporal (Auditory Pattern Temporal Ordering [APTO])	Auditory Temporal Processing and Patterning	**MAPA Pitch Pattern Test (temporal order) **MAPA TAP Test **MAPA Duration Patterns Test *Auditory Fusion Test-Revised **Dutch Duration Patterns†
Monaural (Monaural Separation Closure [MSC])	Monaural Low Redundancy Speech Tests	**MAPA M-SAAT **MAPA SINCA (Speech in Noise for Children & Adults) **SCAN Filtered Words **SCAN Auditory Figure Ground **Dutch Filtered Words and Auditory Figure Ground† QuickSIN Test Time-altered/compressed speech Performance-Intensity Functions (PI-PB) Speech In Noise (SPIN) Synthetic Sentence Identification (SSI-ICM)
Binaural (Binaural integration, Binaural separation [BIBS])	Dichotic Speech Tests	**MAPA Dichotic Digits **MAPA Competing Sentences **SCAN Competing Words **Staggered Spondaic Words (SSW) **Dutch Dichotic Digits†
	Binaural Interaction	Masking Level Difference Interaural Intensity Difference (IID) (binaural interaction) Sound Lateralization and Localization
	Auditory Discrimination Tests	Difference Limen for Frequency Difference Limen for Intensity Phoneme Discrimination
	Electroacoustic Measures	Otoacoustic Emissions (cochlear level screen) Acoustic Reflex Threshold Acoustic Reflex Decay

continues

Table 6–2. *(continued)*

Auditory Domain	ASHA (1996, 2005) Defined Area	Specific Test Instrument
	Physiologic Measures	Acoustic Reflex Decay (lower brainstem level screen)
		Auditory Brainstem Response
		Middle Latency Response
		N1, P2
		P300

*Through factor analysis it was found that this test does not load strongly on the APTO auditory domain.

**Through factor analysis these tests have been shown to load on the categorical auditory domain.

†Note that Dutch tests reported in this table are not discussed in this chapter in detail, but are included here because they support the factor findings on English tests (Neijenhuis, et al., 2000).

Note: MAPA = Multiple Auditory Processing Assessment (Schow, Chermak, Seikel, Brockett, & Whitaker, 2006).

It is the present authors' view that one cannot adequately screen without addressing each of the ASHA auditory test domains that have accepted, commonly used methods for testing, which therefore requires a screening battery. This was reinforced by Chermak (1996) who said in speaking of diagnostic testing " . . . given the complexity of the central auditory nervous system, it is unlikely that any one behavioral test can be considered the definitive test of central auditory function. Hence, a comprehensive pediatric central auditory evaluation requires a battery of tests . . . " (p. 211). For the same reasons we think screening requires a battery. Use of a battery runs somewhat counter to the definition of screening in terms of ease and time of administration, but we suggest it is justified and necessary in this case. Based on the Bruton Conference (Jerger & Musiek, 2000) and relevant discussions following that conference, we conclude there is

evidence that three commonly used test domains exist for (C)APD and that all three can and should be measured using behavioral tests (Chermak, 2001). These three, with recommended acronyms, are (a) auditory pattern/temporal ordering (APTO) tests, (b) monaural separation closure (MSC), (c) binaural integration/binaural separation (BIBS) tests (see "Auditory Domain" in Table 6-2). ASHA (2005) identified four other test areas (i.e., discrimination tests, binaural interaction tests, electroacoustical tests, electrophysiologic tests), but there are very few data to indicate the utility of screening in these areas for (C)APD, nor are there tools available in many of these areas that could be used in most screening settings, including the schools.

This chapter is organized to address the three generally accepted areas of measurement (i.e., APTO, MSC, and BIBS tests). If and when there are data to support additional areas, the same general strategy can be used to involve four, five, or more areas of concern. Below we summarize *representative* behavioral instruments based upon this categorization. Much of the material reported below in this three-pronged approach was developed from an initial recommendation by Musiek and Chermak (1994). They based their recommendations on the relationship between behavioral tests and known pathophysiology, although they also state that, in children, (C)APD is "usually a benign medical condition" (p. 24), The four tests suggested by Musiek and Chermak were focused on the three areas of measurement mentioned above, and formed the basis of MAPA. Using this framework, we have used their four recommended tests to develop normative data. The "outliers" from the normative data (i.e., those falling 2 SD below the mean) are identified as having (C)APD (i.e., our quasi behavioral *gold standard*). In short, this strategy has been used in a preliminary way to define children with (C)APD in an effort to develop a behavioral gold standard. This work involved a series of studies using factor analysis and careful test design strategies (Conlin 2003; Domitz & Schow, 2000; Schow et al., 2000, 2006; Schow & Chermak, 1999; Shiffman, 1999; Summers, 2003). In this process the Multiple Auditory Processing Assessment (MAPA) test battery was developed. Using one test (or one from the same domain in the case of the Selective Auditory Attention Test [SAAT]) recommended by Musiek and Chermak (1994) in each of three domains (SAAT, Pitch Patterns [PP], Dichotic Digits [DD]) and comparing these to the four test behavioral gold standard (which included Competing Sentences in addition to the SAAT, PP, and DD), we were able to obtain 90% sensitivity. In contrast, when using one test alone, we obtained no better than 40% sensitivity (obtained with the SAAT), with sensitivity of 30% obtained with the PP and 30% with the DD (Domitz & Schow, 2000). Inasmuch as (C)APD was here defined in terms of these four neurobiologically anchored behavioral tests, specificity was in all cases 100%.

Although the conclusions here are based on the behavioral test sensitivity and specificity of our work and on a behavioral quasi gold standard, we would argue that these findings underscore the need for a battery approach and are defensible as a measure of diagnostic accuracy. We simply have to start somewhere, and although a behavioral standard involves some assumptions, we think it is a reasonable approach and is similar to the approach used in language disorders. Swets (1988) has written some of the key articles on diagnostic accuracy and the gold standard. He explains that different diagnostic fields may use a variety of approaches and all have certain limitations, but by using the fundamental principles (sensitivity and specificity data) scientists in each field can work together (not in isolation) on defining the standards and test strategies and " . . . contribute mutually to their general refinement" (p. 1291). More details about the battery are summarized below as we contribute to this "general refinement." Because of the importance of factor analysis in test design nearly all the representative tests described below and in Table 6–2 have at least one study that supports the factor grouping.

APTO: (Auditory Pattern Temporal Ordering)

- MAPA Pitch Pattern Test
- MAPA TAP Test
- MAPA Duration Patterns
- MAPA Fusion Test

MAPA Pitch Pattern Test.

This test was modeled after the Frequency Patterns (FP) Test (Musiek & Pinheiro, 1987). The FP Test reflects the ASHA (1996, 2005) temporal component of auditory pattern recognition, and has been a staple for screening in (C)APD. The test consists of 120 test sequences, each made of three tones. Two of the tones are the same and one varies, and the subject is required to declare the pattern to the tester (verbally, by humming, or by pointing to a visual analog).

The MAPA Pitch Patterns Test (Schow, Chermak, Seikel, Brockett, & Whitaker, 2006) is derived from Pinheiro (1977). This test introduces high and low pitches binaurally in a four-tone series, and the subject identifies the pattern by verbalizing (e.g., high-high-low-high). The four-tone sequence was used instead of Pinheiro's original three-tone sequence because of a ceiling effect identified by Shiffman (1999) and Neijenhuis, Snik, Priester, van Kordenoordt, and van den Broek (2000). A four-tone pattern avoids the ceiling effect observed using the three-tone pattern and results in the same factor structure as the three-tone pattern test. Nonetheless, the additional tone is likely to exert greater demands on memory and reversals are scored correctly to avoid a floor effect.[1] Summers (2003) tested 119 children using the entire MAPA battery, and results were subjected to factor analysis.

This test loaded strongly (0.74) to the APTO domain).

MAPA TAP Test (Schow et al., 2006)

The MAPA TAP Test was developed upon the suggestion of Charles Berlin who has used it clinically for years and found it extremely useful (personal communication). It is purported to test temporal resolving dimensions of the auditory system. In this test, a series of tapping sounds is presented with an interval of 120 ms between taps. (Although the interstimulus interval is large in the context of temporal resolution, and may therefore burden working memory, the TAP Test factors strongly with at least one other test in the APTO domain.) Three series of taps are presented to the listener. After each series the listener must indicate the number of taps heard. The total number of test taps is 30, so that a raw score is based on the sum of the subject's estimate of number of taps. The test proved surprisingly sensitive to (C)APD, loading firmly (0.50) on the APTO domain (Summers, 2003). (Factor loadings on TAP were even larger, i.e., 0.75. when Duration Patterns and AFT-R were included in the tests factored.)

MAPA Durations Pattern Test (Schow et al., 2006).

This is based on the Musiek et al. (1990) three-tone Duration Patterns test, but in

---

[1]Factor analysis was reported in the development of the SCAN (Keith, 1986) and in the development of a Dutch (C)APD battery of tests (Neijenhuis et al., 2000). The obvious advantage of factor analysis is that the power of this statistical procedure allows many tests to be grouped in terms of the underlying factor that is being measured and similar tests can be grouped together. Through a series of five major studies, a strong, consistent, underlying factor structure has emerged supporting each of the two tests we used for the three domains, although in some tests a few minor factors were found. In the development of MAPA, both exploratory and confirmatory procedures were used that makes the test development even stronger (Domitz & Schow, 2000: Keith, 1986; Neijenhuis et al., 2000; Schow et al., 2000, 2006). It is important to note that a common factor loading does not imply comparable sensitivity or specificity among the tests grouped together.

this case groups of four-tone series are presented binaurally to the subject. Duration of the tones is randomly varied between short and long. The subject's task is to verbally report the series in the order that the tones were presented (e.g., "long-short-long-long"). Summers (2003) reported only a modest loading on APTO (0.36) based on 119 subjects. Accordingly, the Pitch Pattern and TAP Test were selected in the MAPA battery to measure the temporal domain because of their more favorable factor loading compared to Duration Patterns and Gap Detection (Fusion).

MAPA Fusion Test (Schow et al., 2006).

The Auditory Fusion Test-Revised (AFT-R) (McCroskey & Keith, 1996) purports to examine the resolving capacity of the auditory nervous system of listeners. It is actually a test of temporal resolution, as are gap detection tests. The AFT-R provides the listener with pairs of gated tonal stimuli that are separated by millisecond-level intervals of silence. Because the expected temporal resolution is 1 to 2 ms (Green, 1973), listeners who fail to recognize the gaps at smaller intervals are *assumed* to be at risk for (C)APD.

The RGDT is a revised version of the Auditory Fusion Test-Revised (AFT-R) (McCroskey & Keith, 1996). Keith (2001) notes that the purpose of the Random Gap Detection Test (RGDT) is to identify deficits related to temporal function of the auditory system as they relate to phonologic processing deficits, auditory discrimination, receptive language, and reading. Similar to the AFT-R, the RGDT measures temporal resolution through determination of the smallest time inter-

val between two temporally proximate stimuli. The listener attends to a series of paired stimuli as the silent interval between the pairs changes in duration. The task of the listener is to report whether the percept was of one or two tones. See Chermak and Lee (2005) for a comparison of tests of temporal resolution.

The MAPA Fusion Test (Schow et al., 2006) uses the final subtest of the RGDT, which utilizes click stimuli of 230 μsec duration followed by interstimulus intervals of 0 to 40 ms presented in random order. Each stimulus pair is separated by an interstimulus interval of 4.5 seconds. The clicks were derived from a 1-ms compression (positive) section of white noise (Keith, 2001). Temporal resolution was only weakly loaded on the MSC domain (−0.29) during exploratory analysis, and did not provide increased sensitivity in identification of children at risk for (C)APD (Summers, 2003). Although the Bruton Conference summary (Jerger & Musiek, 2000) recommended the use of either a gap detection test or dichotic digits for screening (C)APD, we have found only dichotic digits to be supported by factor findings in two school screening studies in tests on almost 200 children (Domitz & Schow, 2000; Summers, 2003). With reference to gap detection, the Bruton group did not specifically recommend any of the currently marketed versions (i.e., RGDT or AFT-R), about which questions were raised regarding validity and reliability.

MSC (Monaural Separation Closure)

- MAPA mSAAT
- MAPA SINCA (Speech in Noise for Children & Adults)

- SCAN Auditory Figure Ground (AFG) and Filtered Words (FW) subtests
- QuickSIN/BKB-SIN tests
- Performance-Intensity functions (PI-PB)

MAPA mSAAT: (MAPA Monaural Selective Auditory Attention Test; Schow et al., 2006)

The original SAAT (Cherry 1980, 1992) is normed for children between the ages of 4 and 9 years, and takes 8 minutes to administer. The test compares the ability of the patient to recognize monosyllabic words without competing background (speech recognition task) and embedded in background of competing high-interest speech. Both target and competition stimuli were recorded by the same speaker, thereby eliminating speaker recognition cues. The signal-to-competition ratio is 0 dB. Normative data provide evidence that it accurately screens in 90% of children who have been identified as having a learning disability, which Cherry claimed related to an underlying, but undiagnosed, (C)APD (Cherry, 1992).

The MAPA Monaural-SAAT (MAPA mSAAT; Schow et al., 2006) follows the construction of SAAT (Cherry, 1980, 1992). It requires the subject to listen for a word selected from the WIPI word list that is embedded in competing background noise of high-interest speech, recorded by the same speaker. This version utilizes only monaural stimulation, as a monaural low-redundancy test was needed more than a binaural test and dichotic stimulation did not improve the sensitivity of the test. This test loaded strongly (0.74) on the MSC domain in factor analysis (Summers, 2003).

MAPA Speech in Noise for Children and Adults (MAPA SINCA; Schow et al., 2006).

Monosyllabic PBK words were recorded and subjects were required to listen for the primary stimulus embedded in competing four-speaker babble background. With each stimulus the signal to noise ratio decreases, ultimately to 0 dB. This test loaded strongly (0.72) in the MSC domain in factor analysis (Summers, 2003).

Because the mSAAT and SINCA both load (i.e., the correlation between each variable and the various factors) strongly on the monaural factor (0.74 and 0.72, respectively) there is support for using these two tests to screen for the monaural domain. However, SCAN AFG and SCAN FW have been shown also to load strongly (0.68 and 0.55, respectively) with mSAAT (0.78 and 0.74 for left and right ear mSAAT; Domitz & Schow, 2000). It is presumed that QuickSIN/BKB-SIN, which are nearly identical to SINCA, would also load in the monaural domain. Thus, these four other tests should provide good backup for testing the MSC domain. This is helpful because form equivalency and test-retest reliability on mSAAT and SINCA need improvement, and until they are better in this area it would seem prudent to supplement mSAAT and SINCA with other tests. QuickSIN/BBK-SIN, fortunately have many equivalent forms and should have strong utility in the MSC domain.

SCAN AFG and FW (Keith, 1995, 2000a, 2000b)

The SCAN-C consists of four subtests (Auditory Figure-Ground [AFG], Filtered Words [FW], Competing Words [CW],

Competing Sentences [CS]) and represents two of the ASHA (1995, 2005) deficit areas, with AFG and FW falling into the MSC domain, and CW and CS being categorized as BIBS, based on factor studies (Domitz & Schow, 2000; Schow & Chermak, 1999). The purpose of the SCAN-C is to determine possible disorders of the central nervous system, to identify problems in auditory processing ability, and to identify children at risk for (C)APD (Keith, 1995, 2000).

The AFG subtest uses monosyllabic words with a competing multitalker babble to assist in identification of children who experience difficulty separating signal from noise. The FW subtest uses low-pass filtered (degraded) monosyllabic words in an attempt to identify children who are unable to re-create the missing information. The original SCAN was normed on 1,035 children in the schools (Keith, 1986), wherein a factor study was reported that supported AFG and FW as loading in the same domain (MSC). Neijenhuis et al. (2000) also found factor support for AFG and FW testing within an MSC domain.

The SCAN takes approximately 20 minutes to administer, but provides a reasonably deep level of screening, and is designed for use with children between the ages of 3 and 11 years. Test-retest reliability of the SCAN is relatively unstable (Amos & Humes, 1998), and administration of the SCAN is sensitive to the administration environment (Emerson, Crandall, Seikel & Chermak, 1997; but see Keith, 1998), but appears to be unbiased with reference to race of the individual being tested (Woods, Peña & Martin, 2004). Humes, Amos, and Wynne (1998) also noted weaknesses in that the SCAN does not have multiple forms. In addition, the SCAN uses internal consistency coeffi-

cients rather than test-retest coefficients to calculate confidence intervals, which results in artificially smaller standard errors of the mean and narrower confidence intervals, leading to classification of more scores as outside normal limits.

The SCAN is highly dependent upon verbal knowledge (Chermak & Musiek, 1997), and thus is limited to English-speaking children. Chermak, Styers, and Seikel (1995) found that the SAAT identified greater numbers of children as at-risk for (C)APD than did the SCAN.

QuickSIN test/BKB-SIN (QuickSIN Speech in Noise Test, Version 1.3; Etymotic Research, 2001, 2005)

The QuickSIN is designed to assess a subject's ability to listen within a background of noise. The BKB-SIN is a similar test which is appropriate and normed for children (Etymotic, 2005). These tests are designed to rapidly provide a reasonable estimate of the functional signal-to-noise ratio at which an individual can comprehend speech. QuickSIN/BKB-SIN are very similar to the MAPA SINCA and their use of noise to reduce redundancy places them in the MSC auditory domain category.

Performance-Intensity functions (PI-PB)

Performance-intensity functions for phonetically balanced words (PI-PB) have been proposed as a means of testing monaural low-redundancy processing (Humes, 2005). Theoretically, the performance-intensity function would improve dramatically as intensity increased, but could reveal deficits in individuals for whom greater redundancy is required. To date, only one study (Humes, 2005) has examined it with relation to auditory processing, and results were equivocal. Nonetheless, the ready ability to generate a PI-PB function through standard audiometric assessment speaks to the need to pursue this as a potential screening instrument.

BIBS (Binaural integration, Binaural separation)

- MAPA Dichotic Digits
- MAPA Competing Sentences
- SCAN Competing Words
- Staggered Spondaic Words (SSW)

MAPA Dichotic Digits

This test presents a different series of digits to each ear simultaneously, with the task being to identify as many numbers as possible. Instructions vary, including requiring correct order, identification of ear of presentation, or simply listing the numbers heard. Results rely on binaural integration, attention, and auditory memory.

The MAPA Dichotic Digits test (DD: Schow et al., 2006) is derived from Musiek (1983). The original formulation required that two number pairs be presented simultaneously to each ear of the listener, with the subject being required to repeat all four numbers. The MAPA DD employed number triplets presented dichotically, similar to that of Neijenhuis et al. (2000). The subject repeats items from the right ear first, then from the left, following Moncrieff and Musiek (2002). This test loaded strongly (0.67) on the BIBS auditory domain during factor analysis (Summers, 2003). Again, it is important to note that while loading on the same factor suggests that double-digit and triplet pairs both provide some measure of similar processes, the triplet MAPA DD probably involves memory to a greater extent than the double-digit DD.

MAPA Competing Sentences

Willeford (1985) introduced the Competing Sentences Test (CS), and Keith (2000) integrated competing sentences into the SCAN-A. In the MAPA Competing Sentences Test (Schow et al, 2006), two sentences are presented dichotically, and the subject repeats both sentences. This more difficult task was used because of a ceiling effect identified by Shiffman (1999) when only one sentence was repeated. Subjects are required to repeat either the right or the left ear first, and stimuli must be repeated with 100% accuracy to be considered correct. Subjects are not penalized for reversing the order of the sentences as repeated. Due to the greater difficulty of the modified task, 8- to 9-year-old subjects' mean performance was only 41% ($SD = 14$%), suggesting a floor effect. A passing score, therefore, may not carry the interpretive significance of scores falling more in the mid-range. This test loaded strongly (0.65) on the BIBS auditory domain during factor analysis. Besides the strong factor loading of DD and CS, the work of Domitz and Schow (2000) and Schow, Seikel, Chermak, and Berent (2000) recorded a 0.70 correlation between DD and CS, which strongly supports combining those two tests to derive a measure of the binaural domain (BIBS). DD is thought to involve binaural integration, and because subjects are asked to repeat competing sentences (CS) in a certain order, this appears to be a binaural separation task or some combination of binaural integration and separation.

SCAN CW Subtest (Keith, 2000a, 2000b).

The Competing Words subtest is a dichotic task in which words are presented simultaneously to both ears and the child is required to identify both words. Domitz and Schow (2000) reported that the CW subtest loaded onto the BIBS domain. Schow and Chermak (1999) compared results of SCAN CW and Staggered Spondaic Words (SSW: Katz, 1962), revealing that the SSW (left and right Competing SSW scores) were highly related to the CW subtests and all three load on the BIBS domain.

Staggered Spondaic Word Test (SSW; Katz, 1962)

The SSW is a dichotic task that requires the listener to simultaneously process information presented to both ears. The design of the stimuli is such that the second syllable of one spondee overlaps with the first syllable of its contralateral counterpart. As noted above, Schow and Chermak (1999) found that the SSW loads positively in the BIBS domain.

Binaural Interaction and Auditory Discrimination

Although masking level differences and interaural intensity and interaural time difference tests (i.e., localization/lateralization) have been proposed for testing in these domains, there are no known studies that have analyzed the factor structures of these tests or of auditory discrimination tests.

Questionnaires

Several questionnaires for (C)APD have been devised, based on the assumption that children and adults with the disorder have distinctive behavioral profiles that can provide useful screening information.

Fisher's Auditory Problems Checklist (Fisher, 1976)

This questionnaire itemizes behaviors such as failure to attend to instructions,

the need for repeated instructions, and easy distraction by auditory stimuli. Examination of the questionnaire reveals that the preponderance of items on the questionnaire relate to a language-based deficit (e.g., lack of comprehension of speech at age level). Several questions relate to discrimination ability, directly addressing the ASHA (1996, 2005) criteria, and one reflects degraded processing in a competing acoustic environment. Attentional and memory issues, not reflected in ASHA (1996; 2005), are relatively prominent elements of the questionnaire, as are language abilities.

Children's Auditory Processing Performance Scale (CHAPPS; Smoski, Brunt, & Tannahill, 1992)

The Children's Auditory Processing Performance Scale (CHAPPS) is a 25-item scale that allows the user to rate behaviors in multiple conditions. Parents and teachers can be used as informants. Smoski et al. (1992) reported variable listening performance for 64 children diagnosed with (C)APD on the basis of failing two or more of a four-test battery comprised of the Staggered Spondaic Word (SSW) Test, and versions of dichotic digits, competing sentences, and pitch patterns. Children with (C)APD demonstrated difficulties in quiet and ideal listening conditions, as well as in competing noise and stressful listening conditions.

Evaluation of Classroom Listening Behavior (ECLB; VanDyke, 1985)

The ECLB is a rating scale completed by the classroom teacher. It is designed to identify listening and academic problems in children. The listening behavior subtest focuses heavily on attention-based phenomena (e.g., paying attention to oral instruction; off-task behaviors; short attention span), but also includes more specific (C)APD elements, such as following oral instructions and distraction in background of noise. A specific Classroom Listening Behavior subscale elicits response differences based on environment (noise, group, quiet), presence of visual cues, complexity of directions, and distance from speaker. As such, it provides greater detail about specific classroom listening abilities related to (C)APD, and may be a useful broad-spectrum screen for the disorder. That having been said, no research has been identified relating results of ECLB and (C)APD testing.

Children's Home Inventory for Listening Difficulties (CHILD; Anderson & Smaldino, n.d.)

CHILD is a "family-centered" parent survey that allows parents to assess a child's listening behavior within the home environment. It may be used to assess listening skills in a child as young as 3 years old and as old as 12. The items focus on hearing difficulty and comprehension in quiet and noisy settings, rather than on specific (C)APD characteristics, but may serve as a broad screen for processing deficit.

Use of Questionnaires to Differentiate ADHD from (C)APD

Similarities between ADHD and (C)APD provide a source of ongoing unease within the educational and audiological communities. A diagnosis of ADHD is made based upon criteria put forward by the *Diagnostic and Statistical Manual* (DSM-IV), which provides the definition of ADHD. Within that framework, ADHD is

seen as a deficit resulting in inattention, hyperactivity, and/or impulsivity. Some characteristics provided by the DSM-IV guidelines include poor attention, poor listening skills, distraction, and forgetfulness, common characteristics ascribed to individuals with (C)APD. Chermak, Somers, and Seikel (1998) examined the overlap between characteristics ascribed to (C)APD and ADHD by the respective diagnosing professionals, and ferreted out discerning characteristics for each disorder that would serve as components of a questionnaire. See below how these findings in conjunction with other work have been used to create a new questionnaire. This new tool, therefore, provides discriminating elements used by professionals to differentiate the two disorders. See Chapter 15 for discussion of differential diagnosis of (C)APD and ADHD.

Scale of Auditory Behaviors (SAB) (See Appendix 6A; Conlin, 2003; Schow et al., 2006; Shiffman, 1999; Simpson, 1981; Summers, 2003)

The Teacher's Scale of Auditory Behaviors and the Parent's Scale of Auditory Behaviors (Simpson, 1981) were normed on 96 children, ages 4 to 6 years. Domitz and Schow (2000) validated the Teacher's Scale with the 81 participants in their study, including 17 who ultimately were identified as having (C)APD. Shiffman (1999) refined the instrument by identifying the most useful items to contrast the 7 children diagnosed with (C)APD versus the 12 children identified as not having (C)APD. Twelve of these items were found to be congruent with the recommendations of the Bruton group (Jerger & Musiek, 2000), as well as with the findings of Chermak, Somers, and Seikel (1998). These 12 items formed a new questionnaire called the Scale of Auditory Behaviors (SAB) (Conlin, 2006; Schow et al., 2006; Summers, 2003). Summers found that use of the SAB in conjunction with the MAPA provided a functional means of identification of children with auditory processing problems needing attention for (C)APD. In her study, she identified −1.5 SD as providing the best "fail" cutoff for identification of children with, or at risk for, (C)APD. Summers recommended using failure (−2 SD) of one or more subtests of the MAPA and a "fail" on the checklist as requiring follow-up/treatment for (C)APD.

Hybrid Screening Solution

Because the SCAN does not include all three auditory domains (APTO, BIBS, MSC), we think it cannot be proposed for screening without adding other tests. We have listed a series of tests in Table 6-2 that are within the three domains mentioned, and have indicated which of these have undergone factor analysis to determine the content validity (Chermak & Schow, 1997; Conlin, 2003; Domitz & Schow, 2000; Shiffman, 1999; Summers, 2003; Neijenhuis, et al, 2000). With Summers (2003) and Conlin (2003), and in our most recent work, the present authors have identified a set of six tests that represent each domain, with two tests per area that both strongly factor together, and are readily available as components of the Multiple Auditory Processing Assessment Battery (Schow et al., 2006). All six can be given in about 25 minutes and so we propose screening using all six tests. It is feasible that at some later time only one test will be used in each domain, which will cut the screening time in half.

Because the MAPA has not yet been tested on individuals with confirmed lesions in the CANS, we are unable at present to precisely define sensitivity and specificity in each of the three areas physiologically. This may eventually be possible and if the sensitivity is adequate in all three areas (and with reasonable specificity), this screening process can then be determined to be efficient in that manner. In the meantime, we have chosen to use outliers from normative data (a common method used to diagnose language disorders) on multiple tests in the same domain area as an interim step, recognizing the limitations of such an approach (e.g., see Spaulding et al., 2006).

Our strategy is to form a hypothesis about failure within each of the three domains based on the two tests and comparative norms for same-aged children. A (C)APD screening result will be based on the number of tests within the domain (1 or 2) for which there are reduced scores (two SDs below the mean) and the number of total domains (1, 2, 3) that show low scores. When the parent or teacher response (both types of input are recommended) of the SAB questionnaire reinforces the behavioral test findings, or there is comorbidity in ADHD, LD, reading, autism, or S/LD, we consider there is an increased urgency but the behavioral test scores alone are used as the basis for diagnostic referral. We recommend that those with "fail" questionnaire scores but no −2 SD behavioral test problem be followed and retested again in one year.

Normative Data for Behavioral and Questionnaire Instruments

Following Musiek and Chermak (1994), Domitz and Schow (2000) examined the utility of a four-test battery to screen for (C)APD, based upon the ASHA (1996) criteria for the disorder. The authors screened 81 children using two questionnaires, four behavioral tests (i.e., SAAT, PP, DD, and CS), the SCAN and the Auditory Fusion Test-Revised (1000 and 4000 Hz) (Keith, 2000a, 2000b). Seventeen of the 81 children failed the screening on at least one of the four tests and were on this basis assumed to have CAPD (this was our preliminary gold standard). Shiffman (1999) re-examined 7 of the original 17 students who failed using the same four tests, as well as 12 children identified as not having (C)APD. Shiffman's goal was to determine the degree to which the four-battery screener predicted later findings suggestive of (C)APD identified at retest two years later. This study supported the hybrid (behavioral test/questionnaire) approach and resulted in good agreement (83–85%) using the original findings as the standard. In the next phase of this work, the six-test MAPA was normed by Summers for the age groupings from 8 through 11 years, inclusive, and included 119 subjects. There were 14 (12%) found to have performance poorer than −2 SDs on one or more of these tests. Test-retest reliability of the MAPA for 19 children in the 8- to 11-year-old age range was also determined by Summers (2003) (PP = 0.91, CS = 0.86, TAP = 0.77, DD = 0.73, MSAT = 0.67, SINCA = 0.50) and preliminary norms for 12-year-olds and adults also were established. Two forms (A & B) of the MAPA are available (Conlin, 2003). Form equivalency ranged from moderate for the MSC tests (0.46) to high for the BIBS (0.81) and APTO tests (0.90). An overall correlation coefficient (for the three areas combined) of 0.79 revealed strong interform equivalency for the total battery. The SAB (Appendix A; Schow et al., 2006) was developed as a questionnaire to be used in conjunction with the behavioral screening process. Conlin provided norms (Appendix 6A). The questionnaire is used to support findings of the six-test battery. Thus, the questionnaire score can be used to determine the real-world impact of a potential deficit on an individual, and the behavioral test results can provide information about domain (APTO, MSC, BIBS) and severity (number of domains in which subject is deficient).

Summary and Conclusion

Although the ability to accurately identify children and adults who have (C)APD remains limited by the nature of the disorder, headway has been made in description of the disorder and in factor study of relevant tests (ASHA 1996, 2005; Chermak, 2001; Jerger & Musiek, 2000; Schow et al., 2006). In this chapter we have clarified the characteristics of (C)APD and condensed them into three currently useful domains, as supported by factor analysis results on over 300 children. We have provided summaries of some behavioral instruments used to screen these auditory domains, and using six of them in a hybrid approach we found a 12% referral rate on 119 school children. Finally, we have provided a questionnaire (SAB) that holds promise to contextualize the behavioral findings and to be used as an outcome measure, after the diagnostic process, if therapy is indicated and completed. These materials, although experimental, provide a basis for a battery screening approach until more basic and clinical research is completed.

References

American Speech-Language-Hearing Association. (1996). Central auditory processing: Current status of research and implications for clinical practice. *American Journal of Audiology, 5*(2), 41-54.

American Speech-Language-Hearing Association. (2005). (Central) auditory processing disorders—The role of the audiologist. Position Statement of the Working Group on Auditory Processing Disorders of the American Speech-Language-Hearing Association. Rockville, MD: Author.

Amos, N. E., & Hume, L. E. (1998). SCAN test-retest reliability for first- and third-grade children. *Journal of Speech and Hearing Research, 41*(4), 834-846.

Anderson, K. L. (1989). *Screening Instrument for Targeting Educational Risk.* Upper Saddle River, NJ: Interstate Printers and Publishers.

Anderson, K. L., & Smaldino, J. (n.d.). *Children's Home Inventory for Learning Difficulties (CHILD).* Stäfa, Switzerland: Phonak Hearing Systems, http://www.phonak.com.

Bellis, T. J. (2003). *Central auditory processing disorders in the educational setting: From science to practice* (2nd ed.). Clifton Park, NY: Thomson-Delmar Learning.

Cacace, A. T., & McFarland, D. J. (1998). Central auditory processing in school age children: A critical review. *Journal of Speech-Language-Hearing Research, 41*, 355-373.

Chermak, G. D. (1996). Central testing. In S. E. Gerber (Ed.), *The handbook of pediatric audiology* (pp. 206-253). Washington, DC: Gallaudet University Press.

Chermak, G. D. (2001). Auditory processing disorder: An overview for the clinician. *The Hearing Journal, 54*(7), 10-21.

Chermak, G. D., & Lee, J. (2005). Comparison of children's performance on four tests of temporal resolution. *Journal of the American Academy of Audiology, 16*(8), 554-563.

Chermak, G. D., & Musiek, F. E. (1997). *Central auditory processing disorders: New perspectives.* San Diego: Singular Publishing Group, Inc.

Chermak, G. D., Somers, E. K., & Seikel, J. A. (1998). Behavioral signs of central auditory processing disorder and attention deficit hyperactivity disorder. *Journal of the American Academy of Audiology, 9*(1), 78-84.

Chermak, G. D., Styers, S. A., & Seikel, J. A. (1995). Study compares screening tests of central auditory processing. *The Hearing Journal, 48*(5), 29-33.

Cherry, R. (1980). *Selective Auditory Attention Test (SAAT).* St. Louis, MO: Auditec of St. Louis.

Cherry, R. (1992). Screening and evaluation of central auditory processing disorders in young children. In J. Katz, N. Stecker, & D. Henderson (Eds.), *Central auditory processing: A transdisciplinary view* (pp. 129-140). St. Louis, MO: Mosby Year Book.

Conlin, L. (2003). *Form equivalency on the Beta III version of Multiple Auditory Processing Assessment (MAPA).* Master's thesis, Idaho State University, Pocatello.

Dawson, B., & Trapp, R. G. (2004). *Basic and clinical biostatistics* (4th ed.). New York: Lange Medical Books.

Domitz, D. M., & Schow, R. L. (2000). A new CAPD battery–Multiple auditory processing assessment: Factor analysis and comparisons with SCAN. *American Journal of Audiology, 9*, 101-111.

Emerson, M. F., Crandall, K. K., Seikel, J. A., & Chermak, G. D. (1997). Observations on use of the SCAN administered in a school setting to identify central auditory processing disorders in children. *Language, Speech and Hearing Services in Schools, 28*, 43-49.

Estes, R. I., Jerger, J., & Jacobson, G. (2002). Reversal of hemispheric asymmetry on auditory tasks in children who are poor listeners. *Journal of the American Academy of Audiology, 13*, 59-71.

Etymotic Research. (2001). *QuickSIN Speech-in-Noise Test*. Elk Grove Village, IL: Etymotic Research.

Etymotic Research. (2005). *BBK-SIN Speech-in-Noise Test*. Elk Grove Village, IL: Etymotic Research.

Fisher, L. (1976). *Fisher's auditory problems checklist*. Bemidji, MN: Life Products.

Green, D. M. (1973). Temporal acuity as a function of frequency. *Journal of the Acoustic Society of America, 54*, 373-379.

Hall, J. W., & Keske, C. (1994, March). *Clinical experience with central auditory processing disorders (CAPD)*. Presented at the Annual Convention of the American Academy of Audiology, Richmond, VA.

Hendler, T., Squires, N. K., & Emmerich, D. S. (1990). Psychophysical measures of central auditory dysfunction in multiple sclerosis: Neurophysiological and neuroanatomical correlates. *Ear and Hearing, 11*(6), 403-416.

Humes, L. E. (2005). Do "auditory processing" tests measure auditory processing in the elderly? *Ear and Hearing, 26*(2), 109-119.

Humes, L., Amos, N., & Wynne, M. (1998). Issues in the assessment of central auditory processing disorders. In F. Bess (Ed.), *Children with hearing impairment* (pp. 127-136). Memphis, TN: Bill Wilkerson Center Press.

Hurley, R., & Musiek, F. (1997). Effectiveness of three central auditory processing tests in identifying cerebral lesions. *Journal of the American Academy of Audiology, 8*, 257-262.

Ingelfinger, J. A., Mosteller, F., Thibodeau, L. A., & Ware, J. H. (1987). *Biostatistics in clinical medicine* (2nd ed.). New York: Macmillan Publishing Co., Inc.

Jerger, S., Johnson, K., & Loiselle, L. (1988). Pediatric central auditory dysfunction. Comparison of children with confirmed lesions versus suspected processing disorders. *American Journal of Otology, 9*(Suppl), 63-71.

Jerger, J., & Musiek, F. (2000). Report of the Consensus Conference on the Diagnosis of Auditory Processing Disorders in School-Age Children. *Journal of the American Academy of Audiology, 11*(9), 467-474.

Jerger, J., Thibodeau, L., Martin, J., Mehta, J., Tillman, G., Greenwald, R., Britt, L., Scott, J., & Overson, G. (2002). Behavioral and electrophysiologic evidence of auditory processing disorder: A twin study. *Journal of the American Academy of Audiology, 13*(8), 438-460.

Katz, J. (1962). The use of staggered spondaic words for assessing the integrity of the central auditory nervous system. *Journal of Auditory Research, 2*, 327-337.

Keith, R. W. (1986). *SCAN: A Screening Test for Auditory Processing Disorders*. San Antonio: The Psychological Corporation.

Keith, R. W. (1995). Development and standardization of SCAN-A: A test of auditory processing disorders in adolescents and adults. *Journal of the American Academy of Audiology, 6*(4), 286-292.

Keith, R. (1998). Comments on "The Use of SCAN to Identify Children at Risk for CAPD" by Emerson et al. (1997). *Language, Speech, and Hearing Services in Schools, 29*(2), 117-118.

Keith, R. W. (2000a). Development and standardization of the SCAN-C test for auditory processing disorders in children. *Journal of the American Academy of Audiology, 11*(8), 438-445.

Keith, R. W. (2000b). *SCAN-C: Test for Auditory Processing Disorders in Children-Revised*. San Antonio, TX: Psychological Corporation.

Keith, R. W. (2001). *Random Gap Detection Test Manual*. St. Louis, MO: Auditec.

King, C., Warrrier, C. M., Hayes, E., & Kraus. N. (2002). Deficits in auditory brainstem encoding of speech sounds in children with learning problems. *Neuroscience Letters, 319*, 111-115.

Maxwell, D., & Satake, E. (2006). *Research and statistical methods in communication sciences and disorders*. Clifton Park, NY: Thomson-Delmar Learning.

McCroskey, R. L., & Keith, R. W. (1996). *Auditory Fusion Test–Revised (AFT-R)*. St. Louis, MO: Auditec.

Moncrieff, D. E., & Musiek, F. E. (2002). Interaural asymmetries revealed by dichotic listening tests in normal and dyslexic children. *Journal of the American Academy of Audiology*, *13*, 428–437.

Musiek, F. E. (1983). Assessment of central auditory dysfunction: The dichotic digit test revisited. *Ear and Hearing*, *4*(2), 79–83.

Musiek, F. E., Baran, J. A., & Pinheiro, M. L. (1992). P300 results in patients with lesions of the auditory areas of the cerebrum. *Journal of the American Academy of Audiology*, *3*(1), 5–15.

Musiek, F. E., Charette, L., Kelly, T., Lee, W., & Musiek, E. (1999). Hit and false-positive rates for the middle latency response in patients with central nervous system involvement. *Journal of the American Academy of Audiology*, *10*, 124–132.

Musiek, F. E., & Chermak, G. D. (1994). Three commonly asked questions about central auditory processing disorders: Assessment. *American Journal of Audiology*, *3*(3), 23–26.

Musiek, F. E., Gollegly, K. M., Lamb, L. E., & Lamb, P. (1990). Selected issues in screening for central auditory processing dysfunction. *Seminars in Hearing*, *11*, 372–384.

Musiek, F. E., Shinn, J. B., Jirsa, R., Bamiou, D. E., Baran, J. A., & Zaidan, E. (2005). GIN (Gaps-In-Noise) test performance in subjects with confirmed central auditory nervous system involvement. *Ear and Hearing*, *26*(6), 608–618

Neijenhuis, K. A. M., Snik, A., Priester, G., van Kordenoordt, S., van den Broek, P. (2000). Age effects and normative data on a Dutch test battery for auditory processing disorders. *International Journal of Audiology*, *41*, 334–346.

Oelschlaeger, M. L., & Orchik, D. (1977). Time-compressed speech discrimination in central auditory disorder: a pediatric case study. *Journal of Speech and Hearing Disorders*, *42*(4), 483–486.

Pinheiro, M. (1977). Tests of central auditory function in children with learning disabilities. In R. Keith (Ed.), *Central auditory dysfunction* (pp. 223–256). New York: Grune & Stratton.

Purdy, S., Kelly, A., & Davies, M. (2002). Auditory brainstem response, middle latency response, and late cortical evoked potentials in children with learning disabilities. *Journal of the American Academy of Audiology*, *13*, 367–382.

Rappaport, J. M., Gilliver, J. M., Phillips, D. P. Van Dorpe, R. A., Maxner, C. E., & Bhan, V. (1994). Auditory temporal resolution in multiple sclerosis. *Journal of Otolaryngology*, *23*(5), 307–324.

Schochat, E., & Musiek, F. E. (2006). Maturation of outcomes of behavioral and electrophysiologic tests of central auditory function. *Journal of Communication Disorders*, *39*(1), 78–92.

Schow, R. L., & Chermak, G. D. (1999). Implications from factor analysis for central auditory processing disorders. *American Journal of Audiology*, *8*(2), 137–142.

Schow, R. L., Chermak, G. D., Seikel, J. A., Brockett, J. E., & Whitaker, M. M. (2006). *Multiple auditory processing assessment*. St. Louis, MO: Auditec.

Schow, R. L., Seikel, J. A., Chermak, G. D., & Berent, M. (2000). Central auditory processes and test measures: ASHA 1996 revisited. *American Journal of Audiology*, *9*, 63–68.

Shiffman, J. M. (1999). *Accuracy of CAPD screening: A longitudinal study*. Master's thesis, Idaho State University, Pocatello.

Simpson, J. G. (1981). *A comparison of two behavioral screening scales for children with auditory processing disorders*. Master's thesis, Idaho State University, Pocatello.

Smoski, W. J., Brunt, M. A., & Tannahill, J. C. (1992). Listening characteristics of children with central auditory processing disorders. *Language, Speech and Hearing Services in Schools*, *23*, 145–152.

Spaulding, T. J., Plante, E., & Farinella, K. A. (2006). Eligibility criteria for language impairment: Is the low end of normal always appropriate*? Language, Speech, and Hearing Services in Schools, 37*, 61–72.

Summers, S. A. (2003). *Factor structure, correlations, and mean data on Form A of the Beta III version of Multiple Auditory Processing Assessment (MAPA)*. Master's thesis, Idaho State University, Pocatello.

Swets, J. A. (1988). Measuring the accuracy of diagnostic systems. *Science, 240*, 1285–1293.

VanDyke, J. (1985). Evaluation of classroom listening behaviors. *Rocky Mountain Journal of Communication Disorders, 1*.

Warrier, C. M., Johnson, K. L., Hayes, E. A., Nicol, T., & Kraus, N. (2004). Learning impaired children exhibit timing deficits and training-related improvements in auditory cortical responses to speech in noise. *Experimental Brain Research, 157*, 431–441.

Willeford, J. (1976). Differential diagnosis of central auditory dysfunction. In L. Bradford (Ed.), *Audiology: An audio journal for continuing education, 2*. New York: Grune & Stratton.

Willeford, J. A. (1985). Assessment of central auditory disorders in children. In M. L. Pinheiro & F. E. Musiek (Eds.), *Assessment of central auditory dysfunction: Foundations and clinical correlates* (pp. 239–255). Los Angeles: Williams & Wilkins.

Woods, A. G., Peña, E. D., & Martin, F. N. (2004). Exploring possible socio-cultural bias on the SCAN. *American Journal of Audiology, 13*(2), 173–184.

Appendix 6A

Scale of Auditory Behaviors (SAB)
(Conlin, 2003; Schow et al., 2006; Shiffman, 1999; Simpson, 1981; Summers, 2003)

Please rate each item by circling a number that best fits the behavior of the child you are rating. At the top of the column of numbers there is a term indicating the frequency with which the behavior is observed. Please consider these terms carefully when rating each possible behavior. A child may or may not display one or more of these behaviors. A high rating in one or more of the areas does not indicate any particular pattern. If you are undecided about the rating of an item, use your best judgment.

Name: _____ Age: _____ Grade: _____ Today's Date: _____

Teacher: _____ School: _____

	ITEMS	Frequent	Often	Sometimes	Seldom	Never
1.	Difficulty hearing or understanding in background noise	1	2	3	4	5
2.	Misunderstands, especially with rapid or muffled speech	1	2	3	4	5
3.	Difficulty following oral instructions	1	2	3	4	5
4.	Difficulty in discriminating and identifying speech sounds	1	2	3	4	5
5.	Inconsistent responses to auditory information	1	2	3	4	5
6.	Poor listening skills	1	2	3	4	5
7.	Asks for things to be repeated	1	2	3	4	5
8.	Easily distracted	1	2	3	4	5
9.	Learning or academic difficulties	1	2	3	4	5
10.	Short attention span	1	2	3	4	5
11.	Daydreams, inattentive	1	2	3	4	5
12.	Disorganized	1	2	3	4	5

Score: _____ (sum of circled items)

Means and Standard Deviations for the Scale of Auditory Behavior, from Summers (2003). Summers recommended use of −1.5 *S.D.* (<30) as the fail point for the questionnaire.

	Scale of Auditory Behaviors Score	
	Parent (n = 117)	**Teacher (n = 120)**
8- to 9-year-olds	MN 45.6	MN 43.5
	SD 9.6	SD 10.7
10- to 11-year-olds	MN 46.8	MN 47.4
	SD 11.5	SD 9.6
Total	MN 46.1	MN 45.3
	SD 10.4	SD 10.3
	Concern 1 SD = 35	Concern 1 SD = 35
	Concern 1.5 SD = 30	Concern 1.5 SD = 30

CHAPTER 7

TEST BATTERY CONSIDERATIONS

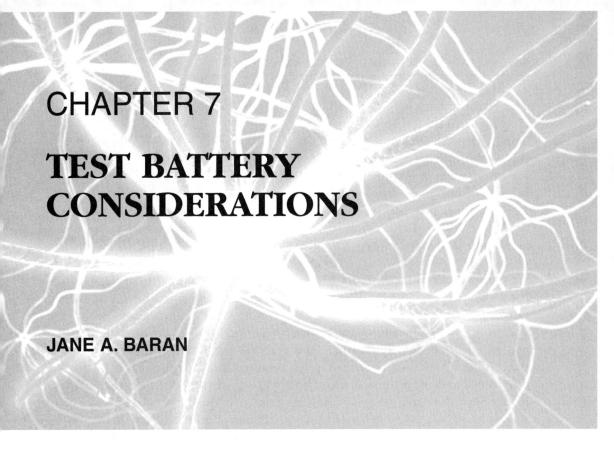

JANE A. BARAN

Introduction

As one prepares to undertake the assessment of an individual at risk for a (central) auditory processing disorder ([C]APD), a number of important variables and factors should be given serious consideration. Failure to do so may result in an incomplete assessment of the extent of the individual's auditory deficits, or the misdiagnosis of a nonauditory deficit (e.g., a cognitive disorder, such as attention deficit or a working memory dis-order, or a language disorder, such as specific language impairment) as an auditory deficit.

The audiologist who is involved in the evaluation and management of (C)APD should be well grounded in the anatomy and physiology of the auditory system.

The central auditory nervous system (CANS) is a complex system of neural pathways whose function underlies a number of different auditory processes that serve as the foundation for normal auditory processing. This system extends from the cochlear nucleus complex in the region of the low brainstem on each side of the brain to the primary auditory reception areas of the temporal lobes in each hemisphere. The auditory pathways then course from the primary auditory cortices of each hemisphere to other regions of the brain in the same hemisphere (e.g., association areas) as well as to both homolateral and heterolateral areas of the brain in the opposite hemisphere. As sensory information travels within this system via both ipsilateral and contralateral pathways, the signal undergoes several levels of processing.

This processing occurs in both a hierarchical or serial fashion, as well as an overlapping or parallel manner. The result of this combined serial and parallel processing of information is a highly efficient, but redundant, system (Baran & Musiek, 1999; Chermak & Musiek, 1997; Musiek & Baran, 2007). In addition to the ascending pathways, there are also descending pathways, which can moderate the response of the auditory system to an incoming acoustic signal or signals (Musiek & Baran, 2007).

Due to the complexity of the CANS and its intricate neural networks, the processing of auditory information is not a single unitary process that can be readily identified and assessed using a single test. In fact, the processing of auditory information involves a number of subprocesses that are necessary for the normal and efficient processing of an auditory signal to occur. Although a number of definitions of central auditory processing have been offered, most of these definitions identify a number of specific component skills or subprocesses that underlie normal auditory processing (e.g., ASHA, 1996, 2005; Baran & Musiek, 1999, 2003; Bellis, 2003; Chermak & Musiek, 1997). For example, a recent task force convened by the American Speech-Language-Hearing Association (ASHA, 2005) has offered the following definition of (central) auditory processing:

> (C)AP [(Central) Auditory Processing] includes the auditory mechanisms that underlie the following abilities or skills: sound localization and lateralization; auditory discrimination; auditory pattern recognition; temporal aspects of audition, including temporal integration, temporal discrimination (e.g., temporal gap detection), temporal ordering, and

temporal masking; auditory performance in competing acoustic signals (including dichotic listening); and auditory performance with degraded acoustic signals (ASHA, 2005, p. 2).

As readily can be seen as one considers this definition, normal auditory processing involves a number of distinct subprocesses or skills. A breakdown or deficit in any one of these skills or subprocesses is possible and it is not necessary that all subprocesses, or even a majority of these processes be affected for a (C)APD to be present. In fact, it is unusual that an individual with (C)APD will experience a deficit in each of these areas. Therefore, the selection of a comprehensive and valid test battery is an important clinical skill that the audiologist must master. If a test battery does not include an assessment of a particular subprocess or skill and that subprocess or skill is a deficit area for a given individual, then the presence of a (C)APD may go undiagnosed, even if a test battery approach is utilized.

In addition to the considerations mentioned above, there are a number of test principles and features that are important to consider when one is selecting tests for inclusion in a test battery. What specific auditory process (or processes) is (are) being assessed by the test? What other nonauditory influences might there be on test performance? If these influences exist, what are the potential effects of these nonauditory influences on test performance? Are the test materials appropriate to the age, linguistic, and/or cognitive abilities of the individual being tested? Are there normative data available, and if so, are these appropriate for the individual being tested? How have these norms been derived and are they valid for the purpose they are being used? How efficient is the test (or the battery of tests) in differentiating the presence versus the absence of a (C)APD? What are the effects of comorbid conditions on the auditory tests being administered? Are some tests less resistant to the potential confounding effects of a comorbid condition, and therefore are they better choices for inclusion in a test battery? What does the patient's case history and presenting symptomatology tell the audiologist about his or her patient's auditory processing abilities, and how can this information be used to inform the development of a test battery to assess the individual's auditory processing abilities?

It is essential, therefore, that each of these factors and influences (specific auditory deficits, comorbid disorders or disabilities, age, native language and/or general language ability, motivation, fatigue, general malaise, task/test demands, and so forth) be taken into consideration when designing an evaluation protocol for an individual considered to be at risk for (C)APD. Failure to do so is likely to result in the development of an assessment battery that will not meet with optimal diagnostic success and may lead to an inaccurate diagnosis.

Case History

A comprehensive and carefully elicited case history is central to the planning, conduct, and interpretation of a central auditory test battery. The information obtained during this process can provide invaluable information that can help the clinician begin to form clinical hypotheses about the nature and extent of the disorder, its potential etiology, and the presence of other comorbid conditions that can seriously affect the test processes and/or confound the test interpretation. It can also provide critical information about the functional implications of the disorder and the impact of the behavioral deficits on the individual's everyday functioning. At a minimum, the history should include information on the patient's personal and familial medical history, including known or potential genetic abnormalities, the individual's prenatal, perinatal, and postnatal history and development, the patient's general health status, including the presence of any significant medical conditions or psychological factors, the individual's communication, listening, and auditory skills and behaviors, his or her social development and linguistic and cultural background, and any prior therapies and/or current treatments. This information can be obtained by direct interview of the individual, his or her parents, or other family members, or from another informant who is responsible for the individual. In addition, important information can be obtained through direct observation techniques; that is, an audiologist who is a good observer of patient behavior is likely to be a good diagnostician as insights gained from observation of the patient during the interview process or in some other context that can be arranged can help inform test battery selection, the need for modifications of test procedures, and so forth. Another method of gaining at least some of this information is through the use of self-assessment tools or behavioral checklists. A number of such tools are available and these can provide valuable insights into the individual's behaviors and functional deficits. The behavioral checklists or self-assessment instruments can be completed by the patient's parents, his or her teachers, or by the patient him- or herself, depending upon the nature of the checklist or assessment tool and the ability of the individual to complete the requirements associated with reviewing and completing the self-assessment forms or behavioral checklists. (See Chapter 6 for a discussion of the use of behavioral checklists with individuals at risk for [C]APD.)

Case history information is more efficiently elicited if the interviewer has some knowledge of the etiologic bases of the disorder for which the individual is seeking evaluation and its presenting symptomatology and behavioral manifestations. Equipped with this knowledge the interviewer can carefully probe relevant medical, educational, and behavioral areas that could reveal important insights into the individual's history and deficits.

Research on children and adults with (C)APD has revealed a number of etiologic bases for the auditory deficits experienced by patients with (C)APD. In some patients, the deficits can be linked to frank neurologic lesions or disease processes which compromise the integrity and function of the CANS, such as trauma, neoplasms, degenerative disorders, metabolic dysfunction (including neonatal hyperbilirubinemia), neurotoxicity, viral infections, and surgical lesions (Musiek, Baran, & Pinheiro, 1994). In other individuals, the deficits are related to benign CANS dysfunction. These etiologic bases include delays in the neuromaturational development of the CANS (Musiek, Gollegly, & Baran, 1984), cerebromorphological abnormalities of the CANS (Musiek, Gollegly, & Ross, 1985),

and age-related changes within the CANS (Baran & Musiek, 1999). For a more exhaustive review of the etiologic bases of (C)APD, the reader is referred to Baran and Musiek (1999, 2003), Bellis (2003), Chermak and Musiek (1997), Musiek, Baran, and Pinheiro (1994), and Chapter 5 of this Handbook.

There are also a number of behavioral characteristics that are commonly noted in individuals with (C)APD. Some of the more commonly reported symptoms include: (1) difficulty hearing spoken messages in the presence of other competing speech messages or in noisy or reverberant environments, (2) difficulty localizing the source of a signal, (3) difficulty learning a foreign language or other novel speech materials, such as technical language, (4) frequent requests for repetition, (5) difficulty processing rapid speech, (6) inconsistent or inappropriate responding to verbal stimuli, (7) inability to detect humor or sarcasm that is signaled by subtle changes in prosody, (8) being easily distracted by external stimuli, (9) difficulty maintaining attention, (10) difficulty following directions, (11) poor musical ability, and (12) reading, spelling, and/or learning problems. The above listing of symptoms also presents a quick overview of many of the items that appear on some of the more commonly used behavioral checklists of listening and related behaviors (see Chapter 6).

As readily seen by reviewing this list of symptoms or behavioral characteristics, many if not most of these symptoms are not unique to individuals with (C)APD. In fact, there is considerable overlap with the symptoms commonly noted in a variety of other disorders, including but not limited to learning disabilities, attention deficit disorder with or without hyperactivity, language disorder, difference or delay, disorders on the autism spectrum, other cognitive and/or behavioral disorders, and peripheral hearing loss (Baran & Musiek, 1999, 2003; Bellis, 2003; Chermak & Musiek, 1997). Therefore, the presence of any of these behavioral characteristics should not be interpreted as evidence that the individual has a (C)APD, but rather as an indication that further diagnostic testing is warranted.

Test Principles

There are a number of test principles that should be considered when an auditory test battery is being developed. Many of these are simply good test principles that should be applied whenever any type of audiologic assessment is being undertaken, whereas others are test principles that are unique considerations for the development of a central auditory test battery. It is important to note at the outset that central auditory testing should not commence until a comprehensive audiologic evaluation has been completed. The test principles are enumerated below.

1. It is important that the individual who is administering and interpreting a test battery do so in an ethical and efficient manner. The audiologist who is going to undertake central auditory assessments must have the requisite knowledge, preparation, and skills necessary for the administration and interpretation of the central auditory tests to be administered.

2. As (C)APD represents a heterogeneous group of auditory deficits, it is important that a test battery approach be used so that different underlying processes, as well as different levels of functioning within the CANS, can be assessed. Reliance on a single test or a limited battery of tests may fail to uncover an existing auditory deficit if the deficit is in an area not tapped by the selected test procedure or procedures. Likewise the use of a single test or a battery of tests that assesses CANS function only at one level of the auditory system or within a limited region of the auditory system may fail to uncover compromise within the CANS.

3. The test battery used with any given patient should be individualized as the presenting complaints and auditory behaviors that the individual experiences can be, and often are, quite diverse. A single test battery approach, which is test driven, will not result in the most comprehensive and sensitive assessment of every patient who presents in the clinic as at risk for (C)APD.

4. There are numerous tests of central auditory processing that have been developed over the past 50 years. However, not all of these tests are equal in their ability to identify auditory processing disorders. It is important that tests chosen for inclusion in a test battery be valid and reliable measures of the auditory processing skill and/or level of CANS functioning that the test purports to assess. Selection of tests to be included in a test battery should be based on a

consideration of the test's sensitivity, specificity, and overall efficiency. (see Clinical Decision Analysis below for more extensive discussion of this principle.)

5 Test batteries should include a variety of test stimuli, as well as test procedures. It is strongly recommended that test batteries include both verbal and nonverbal test stimuli to explore different auditory processing skills, and it is also advisable that the test battery include both behavioral as well as electrophysiologic test measures as these different assessment protocols can be useful in elucidating the nature and the extent of the disorder. Additionally, tests should be carefully selected for inclusion in a test battery based on a consideration of their potential value in differential diagnosis of (C)APD from cognitive and/or language disorders, which often can masquerade as auditory-based problems. (see Interpreting Test Results below.)

6. It is important that any tests included in the test battery are appropriate to the individual's age, background, level of intellectual functioning, and peripheral hearing status. It is important, therefore, to take into consideration the patient's developmental age, cognitive abilities, level of language functioning, motivation, level of alertness and potential for fatigability during testing, cultural background, native language, and hearing sensitivity when selecting tests for administration as part of a test battery.

7. Related to the previous principle, it is important to be sure that if a patient has a cognitive and/or behav-

ioral problem for which he or she is being medicated, that the individual be appropriately medicated during testing. If not, the chances of a non-auditory problem significantly influencing the test results are greatly increased.

8. As fatigue and motivation can affect many, if not most, of the tests to be administered in a central auditory test battery, it is important to employ a test strategy that will provide the greatest amount of information in the most time-efficient manner. Careful monitoring of the patient's alertness, energy level, and motivation throughout the test session is essential. Tests that require considerable attention and mental effort should be administered early in the test session, whereas tests that are not likely to be affected by these variables, or only minimally affected by these variables, should be positioned toward the end of the battery. Frequent breaks may be needed to maintain attention and motivation in some individuals. In others it may be necessary to bring the patient back for a second testing session to complete the testing, if this is possible. If this is not possible, then it becomes even more important that the audiologist administer the tests in a carefully planned sequence in order to maximize the amount of information available at the conclusion of testing so that he or she can make as comprehensive an assessment as possible given the testing limitations.

9. The audiologist must carefully review the recommended testing procedures, normative data, and back-

ground information that accompany the tests and use only the test procedures that were recommended by the test developer when administering tests. Any modifications to test procedures, or use of a test with populations other than those on which the test was normed, will limit the applicability of the test findings and may lead to an inappropriate diagnosis. Often the audiologist will be faced with the pressure to assess auditory processing in young children. However, when testing children younger than 7 years (developmental age), task difficulty, response demands, and performance variability will severely limit the utility of these test measures for assessment purposes. There are a limited number of tests that have been specifically developed for use with young children (e.g., Pediatric Speech Intelligibility [PSI] Test [Jerger & Jerger, 1984]; Test for Auditory Processing Disorders in Children-Revised [SCAN-C] [Keith, 2000]). In addition, there are some other tests that were not specifically developed for use with children that can be used with young children due to the simplicity of the tasks involved (e.g., Gaps-In-Noise [GIN] test) (Chermak & Lee, 2005; Musiek, Shinn, Jirsa, Bamiou, Baran, & Zaidan, 2005). Unfortunately, the limited number of tests appropriate for use with young children restricts the number and variety of auditory processing skills that can be assessed reliably in this population. In the absence of diagnostic tests to test certain auditory processes, the audiologist will have to rely on more informal assessments of auditory processing skills in young children. Behavioral checklists that can be completed by parents and/or teachers, behavioral observations by the audiologist or another adult observer, and some screening procedures may be used to identify a child who is "at risk" for a (C)APD. However, a definitive diagnosis of a (C)APD should be withheld until such time as appropriate and comprehensive testing can be completed. With this caveat in place, it is strongly recommended that periodic follow-up and monitoring of the young child's auditory performance be maintained so that an appropriate diagnosis can be rendered as early as is clinically feasible.

10. As there is a high comorbidity of other cognitive and linguistic disorders in individuals with (C)APD, it is important to involve other professionals (i.e., multidisciplinary team approach) in the assessment of individuals considered to be at risk for (C)APD, especially when case history information, behavioral observations during the test session, or test results obtained during the (C)APD evaluation point to potential speech and/or language delays, deficits, or disorders, intellectual, behavioral or psychological disorders, or academic or learning deficits or problems. Generally, if these types of assessments can be completed prior to the central auditory assessment, the interpretation of the central test results can be made with appropriate levels of caution, and this is likely to result in the accurate interpretation of the test results. If not, then it will be important that a cautionary

note be included in the clinical report indicating the limitations of the diagnostic assessment and the potential that some other cognitive or linguistic deficit may be contributing to the test results noted and the diagnosis rendered. In some cases, the existence of significant cormorbid conditions (e.g., severe to profound hearing loss, severe developmental delay) may pre-empt central auditory assessment altogether.

11. Finally, it is important to realize that the assessment of auditory processing abilities in a clinical setting assesses auditory function in only one context, and that context is often ideal; that is, testing occurs in a sound-treated booth with minimal extraneous distractions. Also, the individual who is coming in for testing typically comes in well rested, on appropriate medications, and so forth. Therefore, the test results, which are derived under such favorable test conditions, may not fully reveal the effects of the auditory processing disorder on the individual's ability to function in everyday conditions. It is therefore strongly recommended that assessment not be limited to formal diagnostic testing, but should include behavioral and systematic observation of the individual's performance in daily activities, whenever feasible. This type of information can be used to corroborate test findings and to assist in management planning. (See Chapters 8 and 9 in Volume II of this Handbook for additional information on observation techniques in everyday settings, and see ASHA [2005] for additional discussion of test principles.)

Types of Behavioral and Electrophysiologic Tests

Interest in the assessment of central auditory processing deficits associated with compromise of the CANS can be traced back to the mid-1950s when a group of Italian physicians (Bocca, Calearo, & Cassinari, 1954; Bocca, Calearo, Cassinari, & Migliavacca, 1954) used a distorted speech test (i.e., low-pass filtered speech test) to assess auditory performance in patients with confirmed temporal lobe lesions. These physicians noted the failure of routine peripheral hearing tests to uncover the auditory difficulties being experienced by their patients and the ability of a low-pass filtered speech test to document the presence of auditory deficits in many of these individuals. Since the initial efforts of these Italian physicians to develop a test that would be sensitive to the auditory difficulties of patients with CANS compromise, a number of other tests have been developed or utilized for this purpose. These tests have included both behavioral and electrophysiologic tests. (See Baran & Musiek, 1999, for a comprehensive review of this history.)

Since the mid-1950s there have been a number of central auditory tests developed. These tests differ in terms of the auditory processes that they assess, the types of stimuli used in the tests, the test procedures employed, and the level of CANS that is being evaluated. In an effort to categorize these tests, a number of classification approaches have been used. However, for the purposes of the present discussion (as well as for the organization of this Handbook), a five-category classification system will be used. These categories include binaural interaction tests, dichotic speech tests, monaural low-redundancy speech tests, temporal patterning and processing tests, and electroacoustic and electrophysiologic procedures. Following a brief review of each of these test categories, the reader will be referred to the pertinent chapters in this Handbook for additional coverage of the various tests and test procedures that fall within each of the test categories introduced here.

The following overview provides a description of the properties of the test categories, a brief discussion of a representative test within each of the categories, and information regarding the sensitivity of the tests to CANS dysfunction at various levels within the CANS. This latter information is also summarized for the reader in Table 7–1, and additional information can be found in a number of other sources (Baran, 1997; Baran & Musiek, 1999, 2003; Bellis, 2003; Chermak & Musiek, 1997).

Binaural Interaction Tests

Binaural interaction tests include those tests that require the efficient integration of acoustic information from both ears in order to mediate the fusion or synthesis of acoustic information that differs in time, intensity, or frequency between the two ears. Test stimuli used in binaural interaction tests include both speech stimuli and tonal stimuli.

The tests in this category are designed to assess the ability of the CANS to take disparate information presented to the two ears and to unify this information into a single perceptual event. This unification of the disparate auditory information being presented to two ears is presumed to occur in the brainstem. For this

reason, tests that fall into this category are believed to be sensitive to brainstem pathology. They can, however, also be affected by cerebral lesions, although the probability of an abnormal finding with lesions above the level of the low brainstem is quite low (as in the case for masking level differences discussed below) (Lynn, Gilroy, Taylor, & Leiser, 1981). Due to the nature of the tests in this category, a "binaural" deficit is expected—however, as the ears are not tested independently, it is not possible to differentiate the performance of one ear versus the other (Table 7–1) (Baran & Musiek, 1999).

One of the more sensitive tests in this category is the *masking level difference* (MLD) test. This test involves the presentation of a stimulus, either spondee words or pulsed pure tones, to both ears at the same time that a broad-band masking noise is delivered to the two ears (Licklider, 1948). The patient is tested under two conditions—a homophasic and an antiphasic condition. In the homophasic condition the stimulus and the noise are presented in-phase to both ears (S_oN_o), whereas in the antiphasic condition one of the two signals is presented 180° out-of-phase while the other signal is maintained in-phase between the two ears. For example, in the $S_\pi N_o$ antiphasic condition, the noise is maintained in-phase between the two ears and the signal is presented 180° out-of-phase. Subtracting the threshold established in the homophasic condition from that found in either of the antiphasic conditions results in a difference score that is referred to as the masking level difference. In individuals with normal brainstem function, the threshold noted in the antiphasic condition is better (i.e., more sensitive) than the threshold obtained in the homophasic condition. This improvement in hearing

Table 7–1. Patterns of Central Test Results That May Be Observed in Patients with Lesions at Various Sites Along the CANS

Test Category	Low Brainstem	High Brainstem	Auditory Cortex	Interhemispheric Pathways
Binaural Interaction	Binaural deficit[a] (2)	Little or no deficit (3)	Little or no deficit (3)	Little or no deficit (3)
Phase Tests (e.g., MLD)	Binaural deficit[a] (2)	Little or no deficit (3)	Little or no deficit (3)	Little or no deficit (3)
Dichotic Speech	Ipsilateral ear deficit (2)	Contralateral ear deficit (2) Bilateral deficits (2) Ipsilateral ear deficit (2)	Contralateral ear deficit (3) Bilateral deficits (1)	Contralateral ear deficit (3)
Monaural Low-Redundancy Speech	Ipsilateral ear deficit (2)	Contralateral ear deficit (2) Bilateral deficits (2) Ipsilateral ear deficit (1)	Contralateral ear deficit (3)	No deficit (3)
Temporal Patterning	Ipsilateral ear deficit (1)	Contralateral ear deficit (1) Bilateral deficits (1) Ipsilateral ear deficit (1)	Bilateral deficits[b] (3)	Bilateral deficits[b] (3)
Auditory Brainstem Response[c]	Ipsilateral abnormality (3) Bilateral abnormalities (1) Contralateral abnormality (1)	Bilateral abnormalities (2) Ipsilateral abnormality (2) Contralateral abnormality (1)	No deficit (3)	No deficit (3)
Middle Latency Response[c]	Ipsilateral ear effect (1)	Contralateral ear effect (2) Bilateral effects (1) Ipsilateral effect (1)	Abnormality at electrode nearest pathology (2) Contralateral ear effect (2)	Little or no deficit (3)
Late Response (N1 and P2)[c]	Ipsilateral ear effect (1)	Contralateral ear effect (1) Bilateral ear effects (1) Ipsilateral ear effect (1)	Abnormality at electrode nearest lesion (2) Contralateral ear effect (2)	Little or no deficit (3)
Auditory Cognitive (P3)[c]	Same as late response	Same as late response	Nonlocalizing abnormality (2)	Little or no deficit (3)

Source: Central auditory processing disorders in children and adults (Baran & Musiek, 1995). Adapted with permission from Butterworth-Heinemann Medical Publishers.

Key: (3) high probability of occurrence, (2) moderate probability of occurrence, (1) low probability of occurrence.

[a] Binaural is used in this context as both ears are receiving segments of the stimulus and only one score is derived.

[b] Specified deficits would be predicted if the patient was asked to verbally describe the patterns perceived.

[c] Abnormal results may be noted for one or more of the indices derived during the electrophysiologic procedure (see Chapter 13). The use of the singular form in this context indicates that any abnormalities that exist are limited to one ear.

sensitivity in the antiphasic condition is considered to represent a "release from masking." This release from masking effect is considered to originate at the level of the CANS where information from the two ears is first integrated. (See Chapter 11 for discussion of clinical tests of binaural interaction and Chapter 2 for psychoacoustic considerations related to binaural interaction, including sound localization.)

Dichotic Speech Tests

Dichotic speech tests involve those tests in which different speech materials are presented to the two ears in a simultaneous or overlapping manner. Test stimuli used in these tests can involve any type of speech stimulus, for example, consonant-vowel combinations (CVs), digits, monosyllabic words, and sentences. Some of the tests in this category require patients to divide their attention (i.e., to repeat all stimuli heard in both ears), whereas others require patients to direct or focus their attention to a target ear (i.e., repeat only the stimuli perceived in the right ear or the left ear, as directed). Research findings suggest that when the CANS is presented with dichotic speech materials, the weaker ipsilateral pathways within the CANS tend to be suppressed, and the neural impulses travel up the pre-eminent contralateral pathways to reach the auditory reception areas of the cerebrum (Kimura, 1961a, 1961b).

Dichotic speech tests are particularly sensitive to lesions of the auditory cortex and the interhemispheric fibers, and to a lesser degree to auditory brainstem lesions (Baran & Musiek, 1999). Most typically contralateral ear effects are noted with lesions of the auditory cor-

tex, although binaural deficits can be noted if there is significant compromise of the left side of the brain. With lesions involving the corpus callosum and/or the interhemispheric pathways, left ear deficits are commonly noted. In cases of brainstem pathology, ipsilateral ear deficits are commonly observed in patients with extra-axial lesions (i.e., lesions originating from the periphery of the brainstem), whereas bilateral, contralateral, or ipsilateral ear effects may be observed with intra-axial lesions (i.e., lesions originating from within the brainstem) (Baran & Musiek, 1999).

One of the more commonly used tests in this category is the Dichotic Digits test (Musiek, 1983). For this test, two digit pairs (i.e., 4 digits) are presented to the patient at 50-dB SL (re: SRT), with one digit from each pair being delivered to each ear in an overlapping manner) and the patient is asked to repeat all digits perceived. The digits, which are carefully aligned in terms of their stimulus onsets, include all of the single syllable numbers from 1 to 10; the number 7 is not included as it is a two-syllable number. Patients are encouraged to guess if they are not sure as to the digits heard and they are informed that it is not necessary to repeat the digits in any particular order. A percent correct score is derived for each ear and compared to age-appropriate norms. (See Chapter 9 for further discussion of dichotic listening tests.)

Monaural Low-Redundancy Speech Tests

Monaural low-redundancy speech tests include tests in which speech stimuli have been degraded by modifying the frequency, temporal, or intensity characteristics of the undistorted signal. A common feature in all of these tests is the monaural presentation of a speech stimulus that has undergone some type of signal degradation.

Clinical research has demonstrated that these types of tests tap auditory closure abilities and that they are moderately sensitive to cortical lesions (see Table 7-1). With cortical lesions, contralateral ear deficits are most commonly noted (Lynn & Gilroy, 1977), although in some cases with extensive left hemisphere compromise, bilateral deficits may be noted (see Baran & Musiek, 1999). In these latter cases, it is likely that the auditory areas subserving speech recognition have been compromised. Monaural low-redundancy tests are less sensitive to brainstem lesions, and as was the case for the dichotic speech tests, the laterality effects noted are likely to differ with the specific location of the lesion. Finally, test performance on monaural low-redundancy speech tests is typically not affected in patients with interhemispheric pathway compromise (Baran & Musiek, 1999).

An example of a monaural low-redundancy speech test is the *Compressed Speech* test (Beasley, Forman, & Rintelmann, 1972; Beasley, Schwimmer, & Rintelmann, 1972). Some of the more commonly used versions of this test utilize monosyllabic words that have been compressed using time compression ratios of 60 or 65% (see Baran & Musiek, 1999). This time compression is achieved by removing brief segments of the original speech signal until either 60 or 65% of the original signal has been removed. The remaining segments of the original signal are then strung together to achieve a new speech signal that contains only 40 or 35% of the original signal. These com-

pressed stimuli are presented to each ear individually at 40 to 50-dB SL (re: SRT) and percent correct scores are derived for each ear. These scores are compared to age-appropriate norms, which differ for tests developed using computer waveform editing software in contrast to the older electromechanical compression techniques. (See Chapter 8 for further discussion of monaural low-redundancy speech tests.)

Temporal Patterning and Temporal Processing Tests

Temporal processing involves a number of subprocesses, as can readily be seen in the definition of central auditory processing that was presented earlier in this chapter. Until recently, most of the tests used clinically to assess temporal processing skills involved the use of temporal patterning tests. More recently, however, other temporal processing tests have found their way into the clinical assessment arena. These tests assess other temporal processes, such as temporal resolution (Musiek et al., 2005).

Temporal patterning tests assess feature detection abilities, frequency or duration discrimination, and acoustical pattern contour recognition. In addition, if the patient is asked to label the patterns perceived, then language processing also is required. Temporal patterning tests have been shown to be sensitive to compromise of the auditory cortex in the right hemisphere, which is the hemisphere responsible for the processing of the acoustical contour of the patterns (Musiek & Pinheiro, 1987) (see Table 7-1). In addition, if a verbal response is required, the test is sensitive to lesions in the left hemisphere (i.e., the hemisphere responsible for verbally labeling the patterns perceived) and/or the interhemispheric pathways (Musiek, Kibbe, & Baran, 1984). Deficits are less common in patients with brainstem lesions.

The *Frequency Pattern Sequences* test is one of the more popular tests within this category (Musiek & Pinheiro, 1987). It is composed of test sequences consisting of three tone-bursts. Two of the tone-bursts in each sequence are of the same frequency, whereas the third tone-burst is of a different frequency. The two tone-bursts used on commercially available frequency pattern sequence tests include a low-frequency tone (880 Hz) and a high-frequency tone (1122 Hz). Each tone-burst has a 10-ms rise/fall time and a total duration of 150 ms; there is a 200-ms interstimulus interval between successive tones in each sequence. Given these parameters, a total of 6 different sequences are possible: high-high-low, high-low-high, high-low-low, low-low-high, low-high-low, and low-high-high. Patients are typically asked to describe the sequences perceived using the words *high* and *low*. Thirty sequences are presented at 50-dB SL (re: SRT) to each ear individually and a percent correct score is derived for each ear. Clinical experience has shown, however, that ear differences are uncommon on this test. Therefore, it is possible to derive a single score (i.e., diotically under headphones or in the soundfield). In addition, if a patient is unable to describe the sequences, he or she may be asked to hum the acoustic patterns. If this is done, the test assesses primarily right hemisphere function. In either instance, test scores are compared to age-appropriate norms for the specific test procedure administered. (See Chapter 10 for further discussion of temporal patterning and temporal processing tests.)

Electrophysiologic and Electroacoustic Procedures

Electrophysiologic procedures can be used to evaluate function of the auditory pathways beginning with the cochlear nerve and progressing through the cortical levels of the CANS. Electroacoustic procedures (e.g., otoacoustic emissions, acoustic reflex thresholds, and acoustic reflex decay) are useful in identifying involvement of the low brainstem and in differentiating (C)APD from auditory neuropathy, as well as "central deafness" (i.e., hearing loss caused by significant and usually bihemispheric involvement of the CANS) from deafness or hearing loss of a peripheral origin (Baran & Musiek, 1999, 2003; Musiek, Charette, Morse, & Baran, 2004). The remainder of this section focuses on electrophysiologic procedures. The reader is referred to Chapters 12 and 14 for discussion of the use of electroacoustic procedures in the differential diagnosis of peripheral versus central compromise within the auditory system.

Electrophysiologic procedures provide objective measures of neural functioning, and as such, can serve as valuable adjuncts to the behavioral tests discussed above. The auditory brainstem response (ABR) is an early latency response that is frequently abnormal in patients with lesions of the cochlear nerve and/or caudal brainstem, whereas lesions in the thalamic regions and above are unlikely to result in abnormal ABR findings (see Table 7–1). Ipsilateral and bilateral deficits are common findings when utilizing the ABR; true contralateral findings are rare (Musiek, Gollegly, Kibbe, & Verkest, 1988).

The middle latency response (MLR) is sensitive to lesions located more rostrally within the CANS (thalamus and primary auditory projections), and the late auditory evoked response (LAER) and P300 assess cortical functions (Kileny, Paccioretti, & Wilson, 1987; Musiek, Baran, & Pinheiro, 1992) (Table 7-1). Abnormal findings for both of these procedures are more commonly noted with CANS compromise affecting the auditory cortex and subcortex, but deficits can be noted with lesions located more caudally within the CANS. With cortical lesions, deficits are more often noted from an electrode positioned over the compromised side of the brain, but contralateral ear abnormalities also are observed. In cases with compromise of the CANS in the high brainstem region, abnormalities are somewhat less frequently observed and no typical pattern of results is commonly observed. Contralateral, bilateral, and ipsilateral abnormalities can be noted. Finally, with compromise of the low brainstem, abnormalities on these electrophysiologic tests are relatively uncommon. When these are observed, the most common result is an ipsilateral abnormality (Kileny et al., 1987; Musiek, Baran, & Pinheiro, 1992).

Recently, interest has grown in the use of the mismatch negativity (MMN) response to assess an individual's ability to discriminate or selectively attend to certain stimuli. To date, however, the procedure has been used almost exclusively in research investigations. With continued research and development of the test procedures, this procedure may provide audiologists with another objective test that can be used to assess selected auditory subprocesses that are important for the normal and efficient processing of auditory information. The reader is referred to Hall (1992), Musiek

and Lee (1999), and Musiek et al. (1994), as well as to Chapter 12 for additional information on the use of electrophysiologic protocols in the assessment of (C)APD).

Assessment of (C)APD in Special Populations

As alluded to in the information presented above, there are certain populations of patients who present unique challenges for the audiologist who is attempting to assess their central auditory processing abilities. Young children may not have the linguistic and cognitive skills needed to meet the task demands associated with some of the (C)APD tests. As most of the behavioral central tests currently employed in the assessment arena were initially developed for use with adults, these tests may not be appropriate for use with young children because of the nature of the stimuli, the task demands associated with the test, and so forth. This situation may limit the test options that the audiologist has for use with this particular population of patients.

Many individuals who present for (C)APD assessments have other comorbid conditions (e.g., peripheral hearing loss, learning disabilities, autism spectrum disorder, speech and language disorders or delays, attention deficit disorder with or without hyperactivity, cognitive decline associated with aging, etc.). The presence of one or more these comorbid conditions in a given patient may well affect the individual's performance on many of the behavioral and/or electrophysiologic tests that the audiologist would like to include in the test battery as these comorbid conditions exist along a continuum of severity from mild to severe. In some cases, the conditions will be so severe as to preclude assessment. In other cases, however, the presence of the comorbid condition will not necessarily preclude assessment, but the administration and interpretation of test results will require particular diligence on the part of the audiologist. The reader is referred to Chapters 13, 14, 15, and 16 for an indepth discussion of differential diagnosis among these comorbid conditions.

Finally, with the changing demographics in the United States (Day, 1996), nonnative speakers of English (and to some extent, non-English speaking patients) are presenting at an ever increasing frequency in our audiology clinics for central auditory assessments. Clearly, these patients can present with unique testing challenges. Many of the behavioral tests used for central auditory assessments employ English words or sentences as test stimuli. This factor can severely limit the applicability of many of the commonly employed (C)APD tests for use with this population of patients—thus, leaving the audiologist with only a small subset of central auditory tests (e.g., electroacoustic and electrophysiologic procedures, nonverbal behavioral tests such as frequency pattern sequences or auditory duration patterns) that can be used to assess CANS function in nonnative English-speaking patients or in patients who do not speak English without running the risk that a patient's limited experience (or lack of experience) with English (i.e., knowledge and use) will negatively affect the test results. As was the situation when testing indi-

viduals with comorbid conditions, the testing of individuals for whom English is not the native language requires a deliberate and thoughtful approach to both test selection and the subsequent interpretation of test results.

Patients with Hearing Loss

The presence of a peripheral hearing loss in an individual being assessed for a potential (C)APD presents certain challenges for the audiologist. First, it must be recognized that peripheral auditory dysfunction can lead to central auditory dysfunction. Transynaptic degeneration of central auditory structures can occur subsequent to sensory deprivation (e.g., noise-induced or conductive hearing loss, longstanding peripheral hearing loss, or severely improverished auditory environments) (Hardie & Shepard, 1999; Schwaber, Garraghty, & Kaas, 1993; Webster & Webster, 1977). Moreover, comorbid peripheral hearing loss will affect an individual's performance on most central auditory tests, with few exceptions as noted below.

If a comorbid peripheral hearing loss is present in an individual being seen for a central auditory assessment, then one must question whether the findings noted during the testing are the result of compromise of the CANS or whether the performance deficits being noted are simply the manifestations of the peripheral hearing impairment. As cochlear distortion effects are common in individuals with peripheral hearing loss, the possibility exists that abnormal performance on a central auditory test is not reflecting a (C)APD, but rather that the auditory deficits being detected during central auditory testing are the result of distortion effects that are being introduced into the auditory system at the level of the periphery. The presence of distortion effects originating at the auditory periphery may well affect the performance of the individual with such compromise on many, if not all, of the central auditory tests to be administered. Clearly, if depressed scores are noted on routine speech audiometric procedures, then depressed scores would be anticipated for any central auditory test that requires the processing of speech stimuli. In these cases, it may not be possible to determine if a (C)APD actually coexists with the peripheral impairment, that is, unless some unique profiles of test results emerge (see discussion below). For many years, it was common practice for the audiologist to not administer any of the central auditory tests if a peripheral hearing loss was found to be present in an individual considered to be at risk for (C)APD. Although such a practice avoided the need to account for the potential contribution of the peripheral hearing loss to the central test results, it often failed to meet the needs of the patient who was denied testing, as a central hearing disorder may very well coexist with a peripheral hearing impairment and its identification may have important implications for management of the individual with hearing loss (Baran & Musiek, 1999, 2003; Musiek & Baran, 1996; Stach, 1990; Stach, Spretnjak, & Jerger, 1990).

A number of investigations have addressed the effects of peripheral hearing loss on central auditory test results. These investigations have shown that the presence of a peripheral hearing loss can negatively impact the results of a number of central auditory tests (Divenyi & Haupt, 1997a, 1997b; Fifer, Jerger, Berlin, Tobey, & Campbell, 1983; Grimes, Mueller, & Williams, 1984; Kurdziel, Noffsinger, & Olsen, 1976; Miltenberger, Dawson, & Raica, 1978; Musiek, Gollegly, Kibbe, & Verkest-Lenz, 1992; Noffsinger, 1982; Olsen, Noffsinger, & Carhart, 1976; Orchik & Burgess, 1977; Roeser, Johns, & Price 1976; Speaks, Niccum, & Van Tasell, 1985). However, in spite of these findings (i.e., that virtually all central auditory tests can be affected by peripheral hearing loss), some studies have shown that certain central tests may be more resistant to the confounding effects of peripheral hearing loss than others. Among the central tests that use speech recognition measures, both the dichotic digits test (Musiek, Gollegly, Kibbe, & Verkest-Lenz, 1991; Speaks, Niccum, & Van Tasell, 1985) and the dichotic sentence identification test (Fifer et al., 1983) appear to be less affected by the presence of mild to moderate hearing losses than the other speech-based (C)APD tests. However, it should be noted Humes et al. (1996) reported that the dichotic digits test (single digits version) and the dichotic sentence identification tests were among five central tests that were negatively affected by hearing loss in their investigation of the effects of hearing loss and aging on auditory test performance. In addition, the frequency pattern sequences test (Humes et al., 1996; Musiek & Pinheiro, 1987) and the auditory duration patterns test (Humes et al., 1996; Musiek, Baran, & Pinheiro, 1990) have been shown to be relatively resistant to the potentially confounding effect of mild to moderate peripheral hearing loss. Given these findings, these tests should be given serious consideration for administration whenever a central auditory assessment is being conducted on an individual with a peripheral hearing loss.

Despite the potential confounding effects of peripheral hearing loss and the limited number of tests that appear to be somewhat resistant to these effects, the assessment of central auditory function in individuals with mild to moderately severe peripheral hearing impairment should not be withheld. The presence of either normal or abnormal central auditory function can be implicated in a number of clinical situations and the identification of (C)APD or normal CANS function can lead to the more effective management of the individual with hearing loss. The situations in which a determination of the status of the CANS and the individual's auditory processing abilities can potentially be made include the following: (1) if hearing loss is present in one or both ears and the central test results fall within the normal range for both ears, then the presence of CANS compromise or a (C)APD can be ruled out, (2) if a bilaterally symmetrical hearing loss is present and the central test results are more depressed in one ear relative to the other ear, then the presence of a (C)APD and CANS dysfunction is implicated, (3) if a hearing loss is present, but it is a unilateral or asymmetrical loss and the "better ear" shows the poorer performance on central auditory testing, then (C)APD and CANS dysfunction is implicated, (4) if a symmetrical hearing loss is present and abnormal middle and/or late potentials are noted from electrodes positioned over one hemisphere versus the other (i.e., a significant electrode effect), CANS involvement should be suspected and as such

would implicate the presence of a (C)APD, (5) if a symmetrical hearing loss is present and an "ear effect" is noted during electrophysiologic testing, then the possibility of CANS involvement and a (C)APD should be entertained, and (6) if an asymmetrical hearing deficit is noted on a given test measure (such as word recognition or a MLR amplitude measure) and the binaural presentation of the acoustic stimulus results in a poorer performance or measure than that which is noted for the better ear for a monaural presentation condition (i.e., a binaural interference effect), then CANS compromise and a (C)APD is implicated. (Jerger, Silman, Lew, & Chmiel, 1993; Musiek & Baran, 1996). In these cases, a determination as to the presence or absence of a (C)APD can be made with a certain degree of confidence. However, for those individuals whose test results do not fit neatly into one of these categories or profiles, then the diagnosis of a (C)APD is difficult, if not impossible, to make. In spite of this significant limitation in the audiologist's ability to definitively diagnose the presence of (C)APD or CANS dysfunction in cases of coexisting peripheral hearing loss, the administration of central auditory testing may lead to the identification of auditory deficits, which if managed appropriately can significantly improve the quality of life for the patient with these auditory difficulties even though the etiologic basis for the deficits cannot be determined. Additional assessments outside the field of audiology, such as modern day neuroimaging, can often provide more definitive information about CANS involvement, when clinically necessary. (See Chapter 13 for a discussion of [C]APD and comorbid hearing loss in older adults and Chapter 19 for an overview of use of radiologic techniques in assessment of [C]APD.)

Young Children

There are a number of patient variables that are important to take into consideration when one is preparing to administer a central auditory test battery. One of these variables is patient age. As mentioned above, most of the tests that are currently available for clinical use were originally developed for use in the assessment of auditory processing abilities in adults. In fact, many of these tests were initially developed for clinical research purposes to assess auditory processing skills in adults with frank neurologic involvement of the CANS (Baran & Musiek, 1999). Following the initial clinical investigations of the auditory processing abilities in patients with documented lesions within the CANS, the tests were then used in the assessment of adults considered to be at risk for (C)APD, as the earlier research studies had established linkages between specific impairments of auditory function and various sites of compromise within the CANS. It was only after the application of some of these tests to the adult population of individuals considered to be at risk for (C)APD that much attention was directed toward the use of these tests with children. Initially these tests were administered to children with language and leaning disabilities, who were considered to be at risk for (C)APD (see Baran & Musiek, 1999). Available evidence on the development of the CANS suggests that this system does not reach the adult stage of maturity until the age of 10 to 11 years (Yakovlev & Lecours,

1967). Therefore, it is important that age-appropriate norms be available for any test that is to be administered to children below this age range. It is also advisable that the audiologist carefully scrutinize the tests to be administered to be sure that the test items are within the child's receptive vocabulary if the test involves speech recognition measures, and that the child being tested is capable of providing the type of response required by the test.

Other Populations

There are other populations for which the administration of central auditory testing will require special considerations. Space limitations preclude a detailed discussion of each of these populations; however, brief comments are offered in an effort to raise the audiologist's awareness of these populations and the need to consider the following: (1) whether central auditory testing is appropriate for a given individual from a special population, (2) whether modifications in test procedures are needed, and if they are, what are the implications of these modifications for test interpretation, and (3) whether there are methods and procedures available that will facilitate a differential diagnosis for individuals who may have comorbid conditions.

The audiologist who is involved in central auditory testing is likely to encounter the situation where he or she is being asked to assess an individual with a developmental delay. Several of the same considerations noted above when testing young children would apply for the development, execution, and interpretation of a test battery administered to an individual with a developmental delay. It will be important to verify that the tests to be administered are appropriate to the individual's level of cognitive and language functioning, and that the individual is capable of responding in the desired manner. Interpretation of the test results will also require special considerations. If the individual is developmentally delayed, then use of chronologically based age norms is not likely to be appropriate. In these cases, the audiologist may chose to use norms based upon mental age, language age, or some other measure of intellectual functioning. Even with such accommodations, diagnosis of a (C)APD must be rendered with due caution as any deficits noted during the testing may be reflecting nonauditory factors (attention, impaired intellectual functioning, etc.) rather than a true auditory deficit.

Similar considerations should be undertaken when testing individuals who are either at risk for or diagnosed with cognitive or behavioral deficits or disabilities (e.g., individuals with attention deficit disorders, learning disabilities, or the elderly, particularly the very old). In many cases, a diagnosis of these disorders or deficits will be known at the time of testing; however, in some cases, especially those with subtle deficits, these deficits may not be known to the patient and/or his or her family, and they may not be readily apparent even to the trained observer. These subtle deficits, however, may still negatively affect the individual's performance on an auditory test battery. In some instances when the existence of a comorbid condition is known, it may be possible for the audiologist to establish the existence of (C)APD in an individual with a comorbid condition. For example, if an individual with attention deficit hyperactivity disorder

(ADHD) shows significant deficits in one ear on a dichotic speech test, it is likely that the deficit is auditorily based and not simply a manifestation of the attention or behavioral regulation problem, as it would be expected that the attentional deficits noted in ADHD would affect performance in both ears. For additional information on the assessment of special populations, the reader is referred to Chapter 13 (the elderly), Chapters 15 and 17 (ADHD), and Chapter 16 (cognitive-communicative and language factors).

Clinical Decision Analysis

An important decision that the audiologist involved in central auditory assessments must make involves the decision as to which tests to include in a central auditory test battery. As discussed above (see section on Test Principles), the audiologist will want to include a variety of tests that assess various auditory processes and skills, as well as the efficiency of neural processing at various levels within the CANS. One potential strategy for developing a comprehensive test battery for central auditory testing would be to select one test from each of the test categories mentioned above. Although such a strategy for test selection may appear to be logical, it may in fact not necessarily result in the most efficient and valid test battery, as different tests have different test properties. Therefore, it will be important for the audiologist to carefully consider the individual test properties of the various tests within each test category to determine their individual test efficiencies prior to rendering a decision on the composition of a central auditory test battery.

Clinical decision analysis is a process which can be used by the audiologist to evaluate the performance of individual diagnostic tests, as well as various combinations of diagnostic tests, and to better understand the probabilistic uncertainties associated with the administration of these tests or test batteries (Turner, Robinette, & Bauch, 1999). Clinical decision analysis is based on the assumption that only two patient states or conditions are possible; that is, either the patient has the disorder or dysfunction or the patient does not have the disorder or dysfunction (Figure 7-1). Test outcomes are then compared to these two states or conditions to derive a number of measures of test performance. Take for example the information presented in Figure 7-1. On the left-hand side of the figure is information about the state or condition. There are only two options: a positive indicator (+) indicates that the state or condition is present, whereas a negative indicator (−) indicates that the state or condition is not present. Test results or outcomes are recorded in the columns of the table shown in Figure 7-1. In this figure, a positive indicator (+) as shown in the left-hand column signifies that the test result confirmed the existence of the state or condition and a negative indicator (−) as shown in the right-hand column indicates that the test results were not consistent with the presence of the state or condition. If one administers a test that is specifically designed to assess a given state or condition, and the test result obtained confirms the expected state or condition, then the test outcome is said to be a true positive (or a hit). If, however, on the other hand, the test does not result in the predicted outcome, then the test outcome is said to be a false negative. In an ideal situation, the test per-

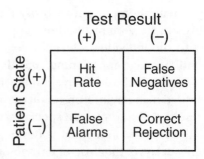

Figure 7-1. A decision matrix for diagnostic tests depicting the potential outcomes when a diagnostic test is administered to patients with and without a specific disease (defined as patient state in this figure; see text for additional discussion of the test outcome results shown in the four cells of this matrix). (Adapted with permisson from Turner et al., 1999.)

formance should be positive for every patient with the state or condition (often referred to as the hit rate), and negative for all individuals tested that do not have the condition (commonly referred to as the correct rejection rate). Unfortunately, such an ideal situation does not exist in our current testing protocols. What often occurs is that a patient with a given state or condition will perform differently from the expectation, rendering a negative finding in the presence of the state or condition (i.e., a false negative), and some individuals without the state or condition will test positive for the state or condition (i.e., a false positive or false alarm).

Several measures can be derived from the information presented in Figure 7-1, but two measures in particular are central to our discussion of test efficiency (i.e., test sensitivity and test specificity). Sensitivity, or hit rate (HR), refers to the percentage of patients with a given condition or pathology that the test accurately identifies as having the condition or pathology (see Eq. 7.1). For example, if a test is specifically designed to identify brainstem pathology, as would be the case for the MLD test, then the sensitivity measure provides an indication of how many patients in an experimental population of subjects with compromise at this level of the CANS actually performed abnormally on this test. A second measure that is important to consider when selecting a test for administration is the test's specificity or correct rejection rate (CR). Specificity refers to the percentage of individuals without the condition or pathology for which the test was designed to test who perform normally (or at least differently from the population of patients for whom the test was designed) (see Eq. 7.2).

$$(Eq.\ 7.1)\quad HR = tp/dp$$

$$(Eq.\ 7.2)\quad CR = tn/np$$

where HR = hit rate, tp = number of true positives, dp = number of diseased patients, CR = correction rejection rate, tn = number of true negatives, and np = number of nondiseased individuals (Turner et al., 1999).

The best tests for administration as part of a (C)APD test battery would be those tests that are high on both of these measures. However, for most tests there is a trade-off between the two measures. If a cutoff criterion on a given test is selected to increase one of these measures, the other measure generally suffers. For example, it may be possible to select a cutoff criterion that is so lax that any patient with a given condition, pathology, or disorder will fall outside the range of normal performance; however, as the criterion is relaxed the number of indi-

viduals without the condition who are inaccurately identified as having the condition, pathology, or disorder is likely to increase (i.e., the number of false alarms or false positives will increase). In these cases, the audiologist will be faced with the decision as to what type of error is more acceptable. Would it be better to identify more patients with the disorder, recognizing that this increase in the sensitivity of the test is likely to be accompanied by coincident decrease in the specificity of the test? Or would it be clinically preferable to limit the number of false alarms and accept the fact that some patients who would have been identified as having the disorder if an alternative criterion had been used would be missed? Obviously these are important decisions that can be made only following careful consideration of a number of factors, including the morbidity rate associated with the condition (if any), the financial and emotional costs of over-referrals, the potential long-term financial costs if intervention is delayed, and so forth.

As hit rates and false alarm rates vary significantly with the criterion used to differentiate normal versus abnormal performance, many researchers have begun to use the receiver operating characteristic (ROC) curve as a means for analyzing test performance. The ROC curve plots hit rate versus false alarm rate (i.e., 1–specificity, if proportional values are used, or 100–specificity, if percentages are used) for different cutoff criteria. A visual inspection of the data displayed in the ROC curve can lead to a decision regarding the best criterion to be used to maximize both the sensitivity and the specificity of the test. For example, the following function (Figure 7–2) was derived from gap detection

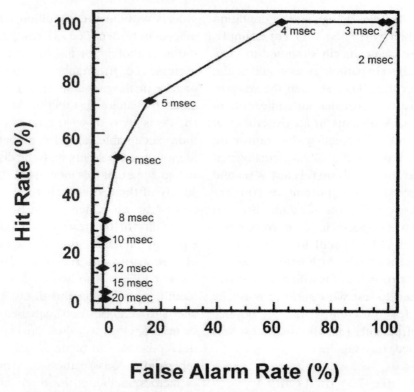

Figure 7–2. Receiver operating characteristic (ROC) curve for the approximate threshold (A.th.) measure derived during the administration of the Gaps-in-Noise (GIN) test. Hit rate (i.e., test sensitivity) is plotted on the y-axis and false alarm rate (100% minus the correct rejection rate or specificity) is plotted on the x-axis. (Adapted from Musiek et al., 2005, with permission.)

threshold data obtained by Musiek et al. (2005). Based on these data, the researchers concluded that a 5-msec cutoff criterion for a measure of a gap detection threshold resulted in a sensitivity of 73% and a specificity of 84%. In addition, the area under the curve can be calculated and can provide the investigator an indication of the "goodness" of the test. In the case of the ROC derived by Musiek et al. (2005), the area under the curve was 0.87. According to Hanley and McNeil (1982), an ROC curve with an area under the curve falling between 0.7 and 0.9 represents a "good" test. The use

of these types of analysis can help inform clinical decisions about the effectiveness and utility of any test that is subjected to such analysis. Space limitations preclude a detailed discussion of all of these test measures as well as other probability measures that can be derived using clinical decision analysis. The reader interested in a more in-depth discussion of clinical decision analysis is referred to Turner et al. (1999) and to Chapter 2 for discussion of both clinical decision analysis and signal detection theory.

Recently there have been an increasing number of clinical investigations that have attempted to determine test efficiency. Data are emerging that some tests are quite high on both sensitivity and specificity measures. For example, dichotic digits (Hurley & Musiek, 1997; Musiek, 1983), duration patterns (Hurley & Musiek, 1997; Musiek, Baran, & Pinheiro, 1990), frequency patterns (Musiek & Pinheiro, 1987), and MLR and P300 (Musiek, Baran, & Pinheiro, 1992; Musiek et al., 1999) have all been shown to perform quite well on both sensitivity and specificity measures. As more behavioral and electrophysiologic tests used in the assessment of (C)APD are subjected to these types of analysis, audiologists will be better equipped to make informed decisions regarding the selection of a given test or tests for each individual patient who is being seen for a (C)APD evaluation.

At this point in the discussion, a cautionary note appears to be in order. Inherent in the discussion offered above is the existence of a "gold standard" against which test performance can be measured to establish measures of test sensitivity, specificity, and efficiency (a combination of both sensitivity and specificity measures). Such a gold standard should be derived from a well-defined population of patients with the disorder, as well as from testing a population of subjects who can be documented as not having the disorder. Unfortunately, because of the variability in both the causes and the manifestations of (C)APD, such a gold standard does not readily exist, at least not in most clinical populations studied. Efforts to attempt to establish test efficiency measures (for the identification of [C]APD) based upon the presence or absence of a behavioral symptom (e.g., difficulty hearing in noise) are fraught with problems

as there is considerable overlap in the behavioral symptoms of many comorbid conditions. In the example given above (i.e., difficulty hearing in noise), there is no way to establish a priori that the origin of this behavioral symptom is (C)APD—the difficulty experienced may be due to a (C)APD, but it may also be related to other behavioral, psychological, and/or learning problems, and even peripheral hearing impairment. Therefore, the percentage of individuals in the group who performed abnormally on a test measure designed to assess speech recognition in noise does not reflect the percentage of individuals with (C)APD, but rather the percentage of individuals who have difficulty hearing in noise, regardless of the etiology of this problem. Likewise, the administration of a (C)APD test to a population of subjects with a comorbid condition (e.g., leaning disabilities or ADHD) cannot be used to definitively establish test performance measures for a (C)APD test for similar reasons—that is, there is no way to establish that each individual within the population of individuals with the cormobid condition being tested also exhibits (C)APD or has a CANS compromise. The best population for the establishment of these types of measures includes subject groups with confirmed lesions of the CANS as evidenced by radiologic findings. In these cases, sensitivity and specificity measures can be derived with a degree of confidence in the accuracy of the test measures, as it is possible to link site of pathology with test performance. Most of the available data on test efficiency have been derived from investigations of the performance of adults with confirmed lesions of the CANS on one or more of the (C)APD tests. In many cases, distinctive patterns of results have been observed in patients with confirmed lesions of the CANS, with similar patterns of results noted in other populations (e.g., children or adults) for whom confirmed CANS compromise is not available. By inference, if similar test results or patterns of results are seen in children and/or adults being seen for central auditory testing, then it may be reasonable to use sensitivity and specificity data derived from patients with known CANS lesions to guide test selection for individuals who are considered to be at risk for (C)APD, but for whom evidence of confirmed CANS involvement is lacking (ASHA, 2005; Baran & Musiek, 1999; Musiek, Gollegly, & Baran, 1984).

Interpreting Test Results

There are a number of different approaches that can be used to interpret the results of diagnostic tests used in the assessment of (C)APD. These include both norm-based (intersubject) approaches as well as a number of potential intrasubject (patient-referenced) comparisons. For norm-based approaches, the performance of the individual being tested is compared to the performance of a group of normal subjects who have served as the subjects for a normative study. Criterion for normal performance can be established by deriving a mean performance score or measure for the group and then adding and/or subtracting one or more standard deviations to or from the mean to establish a cutoff criterion or criteria for normal performance. For example, if a threshold measure or a latency measure is being derived, then typically the standard deviation measure (most often two standard

deviations) would be added to the value. If, on the other hand, a percent correct score is being derived, then the standard deviation measure would be subtracted from the mean. In some cases, there may be a range of normal performance in which the standard deviation measure is both added to and subtracted from the mean. This procedure is generally used if the normal performance on the measure is typically at or near 50% (as is the case of the dichotic rhyme test, Musiek, Kurdziel-Schwan, Kibbe, Gollegly, Baran, & Rintelmann, 1989). Another approach would be to establish a cutoff criterion based upon percentile ranks; that is, the test developer may establish a cutoff criterion value that is set to some percentile value.

Intrasubject analysis involves the comparison of an individual's performance relative to his or her own baseline performance. One such approach includes the comparison of an individual's performance on a given test under different conditions (e.g., interaural [ear] differences, interhemispheric differences, divided versus directed dichotic listening, multimodality differences). For example, on the MLR or LAER tests the amplitudes of the responses derived from an electrode or electrodes over one hemisphere are compared to those derived from an electrode or electrodes positioned over the other hemisphere. The assumption is that within an individual the size of the responses derived from the two sides of the brain should be approximately equal. Significant differences in the size of the response from one side of the brain compared to the other can signal CANS compromise. Other intrasubject assessment approaches can include an intertest comparison, which involves the comparison of trends across the test results obtained during the administration of a test battery, with the requirement that the pattern of test results be consistent with an anatomic site of lesion/dysfunction and neuroscience principles, or a *cross-discipline* analysis, which involves the comparison of test results obtained from the central auditory assessment and from related disciplinary assessments, such as speech and language, psychological, educational, and academic assessments. These sorts of intrasubject comparisons can also provide insights regarding differential diagnosis of comorbid conditions. For example, the finding of a greater deficit on a dichotic test administered in a divided attention mode relative to a focused or directed mode might indicate a nonauditory source of the problem, perhaps a cognitive deficit, rather than a (C)APD (See Chapter 15 for additional discussion of intrasubject strategies.)

As noted above, (C)APD is a heterogeneous disorder and there is no one pattern of results that will be seen in all patients with this disorder. Therefore, the diagnosis of (C)APD requires due diligence. Many professionals advocate that the diagnosis of a (C)APD be reserved for individuals who fail at least two (C)APD tests (i.e., with criterion of two standard deviations below the mean) (ASHA, 2005; Chermak & Musiek, 1997). Obviously, the greater the number of tests failed, especially if the tests assess diverse auditory processing abilities and neural functioning at different levels of the CANS, the more confident the audiologist can be in the diagnosis of a (C)APD. With limited evidence, the interpretation of the test results should always be made with caution. A below-normal performance on a single test may indicate the presence of some nonauditory deficit or subject-

variable effect (fatigue, boredom, malaise), but it may well be signaling that (C)APD is in fact present and in need of remediation. Although there may be some hesitancy on the part of the audiologist to diagnosis a (C)APD on the basis of a single abnormal test result, additional support for the presence of the deficit may be found in a careful analysis of the case history information. If the deficit noted is consistent with the behavioral complaint or complaints, then the audiologist can be more confident in rendering a diagnosis. Another strategy that the audiologist can use to increase his or her confidence in the test findings is to either readminister the failed test a second time or to administer a second test to the patient that assesses the same (or similar) underlying process(es). As noted above, there are several tests in each of the various test categories discussed in this chapter; therefore, the audiologist is not limited to the use of only one test to assess a given auditory process or a level of functioning within the CANS. The administration of an alternative test from within the same category of (C)APD tests is a reasonable approach to confirming central auditory deficits. Another strategy that has been advocated by the ASHA (2005) task force for diagnosing (C)APD under these conditions (i.e., failure on only one test or test measure) is to use a more stringent criterion for abnormal performance; for example, to use a cutoff criterion that is three standard deviations above or below the mean.

As there is considerable overlap in the behavioral manifestations of (C)APD and several other cognitive and learning disorders, it is important that the audiologist carefully observe the individual's performance throughout the test battery. Inconsistent behaviors or responding patterns are likely to signal a nonauditory problem or deficit rather than a (C)APD. Likewise, pervasive deficits noted on all tests within a central test battery may well signal a cognitive or supramodal deficit, such as an attention or memory deficit, or some other nonauditory influence on test performance, such as motivation, fatigue, boredom with the testing process, and so forth rather than a (C)APD.

Finally, it should be noted that although the identification of a (C)APD is one of the primary goals inherent in the evaluation of the individual at risk for (C)APD, a second and equally important goal is the identification of the auditory processes that are in need of remediation. Careful selection of the tests administered during a (C)APD test battery coupled with meticulous scrutiny of the test results can, and should, lead to the development of a comprehensive intervention plan. There are a number of resources that identify specific auditory processes, the diagnostic tests which assess these processes, and the intervention strategies that can be used if deficits are identified during the testing process (Musiek, 1999; Musiek, Baran, & Schochat, 1999; Musiek & Schochat, 1998). These resources can provide the audiologist with some guidance in terms of test selection and interpretation, and the subsequent development of a management plan, if a (C)APD is identified. In addition, a number of other authors have proposed classification systems that can be used to classify individuals diagnosed with (C)APD (Bellis, 2003, Bellis & Ferre, 1999; Katz, 1992). These classification systems were developed in an attempt to relate diagnostic test performance to both specific behavioral symptoms and performance difficulties, both auditory and nonaudi-

tory (e.g., communication difficulties, academic difficulties, difficulties in the workplace, etc.). Although these classification systems are not universally accepted at this time (ASHA, 2005), they may serve as guides to facilitate interpretation of test results and to develop deficit-specific interventions programs. (See Chapter 5 for discussion of [C]APD subprofiling.)

Concluding Comments

(C)APD represents a complex and heterogeneous group of auditory deficits that can result from a variety of etiologic bases and from dysfunction at multiple sites along the CANS. For this reason, it will be important that assessment of the individual considered to be at risk for (C)APD include a number of different behavioral, electroacoustic, and electrophysiologic tests specifically chosen to assess different auditory processes and skills, as well as CANS function at various levels within this system. One classification system for categorizing the available central auditory tests includes a five-category system. The five categories include binaural interaction tests, monaural low-redundancy speech tests, dichotic speech tests, temporal processing tests, and electrophysiologic and electroacoustic measures. Within each of these categories, there are a number of tests that can be selected for administration as part of a central auditory test battery, although not all tests within each of these categories are equal in terms of their test performance characteristics. A consideration of test performance measures, such as test efficiency, sensitivity, and specificity, can help inform the selection of tests, which when included in an individualized test battery should lead to the efficacious and comprehensive assessment of the patient's auditory processing abilities. Finally, a number of test principles that can affect the selection and the administration of the tests, as well as the interpretation of the test results, were discussed. Careful consideration of these principles will help ensure that an accurate and comprehensive assessment of an individual's central auditory processing skills and CANS functioning can be achieved. This, in turn, will help to inform the subsequent development of an efficacious management plan that will target the specific auditory deficits that were uncovered as part of the assessment process.

References

American Speech-Language-Hearing Association. (1996). Central auditory processing: Current status of research and implications for practice. *American Journal of Audiology*, *5*(2), 41–54.

American Speech-Language-Hearing Association. (2005). *(Central) auditory processing disorders*. Available at http://www.asha.org/members/deskref-journals/deskref/default

Baran, J. A. (1997). Speech perception test materials for central auditory processing assessment. In L. L. Mendel & J. L. Danhauer (Eds.), *Audiologic evaluation and management and speech perception assessment* (pp. 147–168). San Diego, CA: Singular Publishing Group.

Baran, J. A., & Musiek, F. E. (1995). Central auditory processing disorders in children and adults. In L.G. Wall (Ed.), *Hearing for the speech-language pathologist and health care professional* (pp. 415–440). Boston: Butterworth-Heinemann.

Baran, J. A., & Musiek, F. E. (1999). Behavioral assessment of the central auditory nervous system. In F. E. Musiek & W. F. Rintelmann (Eds.), *Contemporary perspectives in hearing assessment* (pp. 375–413). Boston: Allyn & Bacon.

Baran, J. A., & Musiek, F. E. (2003). Central auditory disorders. In L. Luxon, J. M. Furman, A. Matini, & D. Stephens (Eds.), *Textbook of audiological medicine: Clinical aspects of hearing and balance* (pp. 495–511). London: Martin Dunitz.

Beasley, D. S., Forman, B., & Rintelmann, W. F. (1972). Perception of time-compressed CNC monosyllables by normal listeners. *Journal of Auditory Research, 12,* 71–75.

Beasley, D. S., Schwimmer, S., & Rintelmann, W. F. (1972). Intelligibility of time-compressed CNC monosyllables. *Journal of Speech and Hearing Research, 15,* 340–350.

Bellis, T. J. (2003). *Assessment and management of central auditory processing disorders in the educational setting: From science to practice* (2nd ed.). Clifton Park, NY: Thomson Learning, Inc.

Bellis, T. J., & Ferris, J. M. (1999). Multidimensional approach to differential diagnosis of auditory processing disorders in children. *Journal of the American Academy of Audiology, 10,* 319–328.

Bocca, E., Calearo, C., & Cassinari, V. (1954). A new method for testing hearing in temporal lobe tumors. *Acta Otolaryngologica, 44,* 219–221.

Bocca, E., Calearo, C., & Cassinari, V., & Migliavacca, F. (1955). Testing "Cortical" hearing intemporal lobe tumors. *Acta Otolaryngologica, 45,* 289–304.

Chermak, G. D., & Lee, J. (2005). Comparison of children's performance on four tests of temporal resolution. *Journal of the American Academy of Audiology, 16,* 554–563.

Chermak, G. D., & Musiek, F. E. (1997). *Central auditory processing disorders: New perspectives.* San Diego, CA: Singular Publishing Group.

Day, J. C. (1996). *Population projections of the United States by age, sex, race, and Hispanic origin: 1995 to 2005* (U.S. Bureau of the Census, Current Population Reports, pp. 25-1130). Washington, DC: Government Printing Office.

Divenyi, P. L., & Haupt, R. M. (1997a). Audiological correlates of speech understanding in elderly listeners with mild-to-moderate hearing loss. I: Age and lateral asymmetry effects. *Ear and Hearing, 18,* 42-61.

Divenyi, P. L., & Haupt, R. M. (1997b). Audiological correlates of speech understanding in elderly listeners with mild-to-moderate hearing loss. III: Factor representation. *Ear and Hearing, 18,* 189-201.

Fifer, R. C., Jerger, J. F., Berlin, C. I., Tobey, E., & Campbell, J. (1983). Development of a dichotic sentence identification test for hearing impaired adults. *Ear and Hearing, 4,* 300-305.

Grimes, A. M., Mueller, H. G., & Williams, D. L. (1984). Clinical considerations in the use of time-compressed speech. *Ear and Hearing, 5,* 114-117.

Hall, J. W. (1992). *Handbook of auditory evoked responses.* Boston: Allyn & Bacon.

Hanley, J. A., & McNeil, B. J. (1982). The meaning and use of the area under the receiver operating characteristic curve (ROC). *Radiology, 143,* 29-36.

Hardie, N. A., & Shepherd, R. K. (1999). Sensorineural hearing loss during development: Morphological and physiological response of the cochlea and auditory brainstem. *Hearing Research, 128,* 147-165.

Humes, L. E., Coughlin, M., & Talley, L. (1996). Evaluation of the use of a new compact disk for auditory perceptual testing in the elderly. *Journal of the American Academy of Audiology, 7,* 419-427.

Hurley, R. E., & Musiek, F. E. (1997). Effectiveness of three central auditory processing (CAP) tests in identifying cerebral lesions. *Journal of the American Academy of Audiology, 8,* 257-262.

Jerger, J. F., & Jerger, S. W. (1974). Auditory findings in brainstem disorders. *Archives of Otolaryngology, 99,* 342-349.

Jerger, S., & Jerger, J. (1984). *Pediatric Speech Intelligibility Test: Manual for administration.* St. Louis, MO: Auditec.

Jerger, J., & Musiek, F. (2000). Report of the consensus conference on the diagnosis of auditory processing disorders in school-aged children. *Journal of the American Academy of Audiology, 11,* 467-474.

Jerger, J., Silman, S., Lew, H. L., & Chmiel, R. (1993). Case studies in binaural interference: Converging evidence from behavioral and electrophysiologic measures. *Journal of the American Academy of Audiology, 4,* 122-131.

Katz, J. (1992). Classification of central auditory processing disorders. In J. Katz, N. A. Stecker, & D. Henderson (Eds.), *Central auditory processing: A transdisciplinary view* (pp. 61-91). St. Louis, MO: Mosby Year Book.

Keith, R. W. (2000). *SCAN-C Test for Auditory Processing Disorders in Children—Revised.* San Antonio, TX: Psychological Corporation.

Kileny, P., Paccioretti, D., & Wilson, A. F. (1987). Effects of cortical lesions on middle latency evoked responses (MLR). *Electroencephalography and Clinical Neurophysiology, 66,* 108-120.

Kimura, D. (1961a). Cerebral dominance and the perception of verbal stimuli. *Canadian Journal of Psychology, 15,* 166-171.

Kimura, D. (1961b). Some effects of temporal lobe damage on auditory perception. *Canadian Journal of Psychology, 15,* 157-165.

Kurdziel, S., Noffsinger, D., & Olsen, W. (1976). Performance by cortical lesion patients on 40 and 60% time-compressed materials. *Journal of the Acoustical Society of America, 2,* 3-7.

Licklider, J. C. R. (1948). The influence of interaural phase relations upon the masking of speech by white noise. *Journal of the Acoustical Society of America, 20,* 150-159.

Lynn, G. E., & Gilroy, J. (1977). Evaluation of central auditory dysfunction in patients with neurological disorders. In R. W. Keith (Ed.), *Central auditory dysfunction* (pp. 177–221). New York: Grune & Stratton.

Lynn, G. E., Gilroy, J., Taylor, P. C., & Leiser, R. P. (1981). Binaural masking level differences in neurological disorders. *Archives of Otolaryngology, 107*, 357–362.

Miltenberger, G., Dawson, G., & Raica, A. (1978). Central testing with peripheral hearing loss. *Archives of Otolaryngology, 104*, 11–15.

Musiek, F. E. (1983). Assessment of central auditory dysfunction: The dichotic digit test revisited. *Ear and Hearing, 4*, 79–83.

Musiek, F. E. (1999). Habilitation and management of auditory processing disorders: Overview of selected procedures. *Journal of the American Academy of Audiology, 10*, 329–342.

Musiek, F. E., & Baran, J. A. (1996). Amplification and the central auditory nervous system. In M. Valente (Ed.), *Hearing aids: Standards, options, and limitations* (pp. 407–437). New York: Thieme Medical Publishers.

Musiek, F. E., & Baran, J. A. (2007). *The auditory system: Anatomy, physiology, and clinical correlates.* Boston: Allyn & Bacon.

Musiek, F. E., Baran, J. A., & Pinheiro, M. L. (1990). Duration pattern recognition in normal subjects and patients with cerebral and cochlear lesions. *Audiology, 29*, 304–313.

Musiek, F. E., Baran, J. A., & Pinheiro, M. L. (1992). P-300 results in patients with lesions of the auditory areas of the cerebrum. *Journal of the American Academy of Audiology, 3*, 5–15.

Musiek, F. E., Baran, J. A., & Pinheiro, M. L. (1994). *Neuroaudiology: Case studies.* San Diego: Singular Publishing Group.

Musiek, F. E., Baran, J. A., & Schochat, E. (1999). Selected management approaches to central auditory processing disorders. *Scandinavian Audiology, 28*(Suppl. 51), 63–76.

Musiek, F. E., Charette, L., Morse, D., & Baran, J. A. (2004). Central deafness associated with a mid brain lesion. *Journal of the American Academy of Audiology, 15*, 133–151.

Musiek, F. E., Gollegly, K. M., & Baran, J. A. (1984). Myelination of the corpus callosum in learning disabled children: Theoretical and clinical correlates. *Seminars in Hearing, 5*, 231–242.

Musiek, F. E., Gollegly, K. M., Kibbe, K. S., & Verkest, S. B. (1988). Current concepts on the use of ABR and auditory psychophysical tests in the evaluation of brain stem lesions. *American Journal of Otology, 9*(Suppl.), 25–35.

Musiek, F. E., Gollegly, K. M., Kibbe, K., & Verkest-Lenz, S. (1991). Proposed screening test for central auditory disorders: Follow-up on the dichotic digits test. *American Journal of Otolaryngology, 12*, 109–113.

Musiek, F. E., Gollegly, K. M., & Ross, M. K. (1985). Profiles of types of central auditory processing disorders in children with learning disabilities. *Journal of Childhood Communication Disorders, 9*, 43–61.

Musiek, F. E., Kibbe, K., & Baran, J. A. (1984). Neuroaudiological results from split-brain patients. *Seminars in Hearing, 5*, 219–229.

Musiek, F. E., Kurdziel-Schwan, S., Kibbe, K., Gollegy, K. M., Baran, J. A., & Rintelmann, W. F. (1989). The dichotic rhyme test: Results in split-brain patients. *Ear and Hearing, 10*, 33–39.

Musiek, F. E., & Lee, W. W. (1999). Auditory middle and late potentials. In F. E. Musiek & W. F. Rintelmann (Eds.), *Contemporary perspectives in hearing assessment* (pp. 243–272). Boston: Allyn & Bacon.

Musiek, F. E., & Pinheiro, M. L. (1987). Frequency patterns in cochlear, brainstem, and cerebral lesions. *Audiology, 26*, 79–88.

Musiek, F. E., Shinn, J. B., Jirsa, R., Bamiou, D-E., Baran, J. A., & Zaidan, E. (2005). GIN© (Gaps-in-Noise) test performance in subjects with confirmed central auditory nervous system involvement. *Ear and Hearing, 26*, 608–618.

Musiek, F. E., & Schochat, E. (1998). Auditory training and central auditory processing disorders. *Seminars in Hearing*, *19*, 357-365.

Noffsinger, D. (1982). Clinical applications of selected binaural effects. *Scandinavian Audiology*, *15*, 156-162.

Olsen, W. O., Noffsinger, D., & Carhart, R. (1976). Masking level differences encountered in clinical populations. *Audiology*, *15*, 287-301.

Orchik, D. J., & Burgess, T. (1977). Synthetic sentence identification as a function of the age of the listener. *Journal of the Acoustical Society of America*, *3*, 42-46.

Roeser, R., Johns, D., & Price L. (1976). Dichotic listening in adults with sensorineural hearing loss. *Journal of the American Auditory Society*, *2*, 19-25.

Schwaber, M. K., Garraghty, P. E., & Kaas, J. H. (1993). Neuroplasticity of the adult primate auditory cortex following cochlear hearing loss. *American Journal of Otology*, *14*, 252-258.

Speaks, C., Niccum, N., & Van Tasell, D. (1985). Effects of stimulus material on the dichotic listening performance of patients with sensorineural hearing loss. *Journal of Speech and Hearing Research*, *28*, 16-25.

Stach, B. A. (1990). Hearing aid amplification and central processing disorders. In R. E. Sandlin (Ed.), *Handbook of hearing aid amplification. Volume II: Clinical considerations and fitting practices* (pp. 87-111). Boston: College-Hill Press.

Stach, B. A., Spretnjak, M. L., & Jerger, J. F. (1990). The prevalence of central presbycusis in a clinical population. *Journal of the American Academy of Audiology*, *1*, 109-115.

Turner, R. G., Robinette, M. S., & Bauch, C. D. (1999). Clinical decisions. In F. E. Musiek & W. F. Rintelmann (Eds.). *Contemporary perspectives in hearing assessment* (pp. 437-463). Boston: Allyn & Bacon.

Webster, D. B., & Webster, M. (1977). Neonatal sound deprivation affects brain stem auditory nuclei. *Archives of Otolaryngology*, *103*, 392-396.

Yakovlev, P. I., & Lecours, A. R. (1967). Myelogentic cycles of regional maturation of the brain. In A. Minkiniwski (Ed.), *Regional development of the brain in early life* (pp. 3-70). Oxford: Blackwell Press.

CHAPTER 8

MONAURAL LOW-REDUNDANCY SPEECH TESTS

SRIDHAR KRISHNAMURTI

Introduction

Monaural low-redundancy speech tests are among the oldest tests used to assess the central auditory nervous system (CANS) (Bocca, Calearo, & Cassinari, 1954; Bocca, Calearo, Cassinari, & Migliavacca, 1955). These tests are administered monaurally using stimuli that have been degraded electroacoustically or digitally in the frequency/spectral, temporal, or intensity domain. Because the stimuli are degraded, the inherent redundancy of the signal is reduced and the tests are considered "sensitized" to detection of CANS pathology.

Redundancy facilitates auditory processing. Extrinsic redundancy is a characteristic of the speech signal itself. Extrinsic redundancy arises from multiple and overlapping acoustic (i.e., frequency, intensity, temporal) and linguistic cues inherent to speech and language (i.e., phonemic cues, prosodic cues, morphological cues, syntactic cues, and semantic cues) (Liberman, Cooper, Shankweiler, & Studdert-Kennedy, 1967; Sanders & Goodrich, 1971). Intrinsic redundancy is due to the structure and physiology of the auditory pathways whereby multiple and parallel pathways concurrently and sequentially transmit information across the CANS (Hall & Mueller, 1997).

The degree of redundancy associated with speech stimuli can exert significant effects on the performance of listeners in intelligibility tasks. Low-redundancy speech materials (e.g., nonsense syllables) are far less intelligible than high-redundancy speech materials (e.g., sentences). Miller, Heise, and Lichten (1951)

193

studied speech intelligibility in normally hearing listeners for words in sentences, digits 0 to 9, and nonsense syllables. Digits (a small, closed stimulus set) reached 100% intelligibility at signal-to-noise ratios (SNR) of −10 dB, whereas listeners required a SNR of 18 dB to achieve the same performance level for words in sentences. In contrast, listeners attained a maximum of only 70% intelligibility for low-redundancy nonsense syllables at the highest SNR of 18 dB.

Four behavioral domains have emerged from recent research employing the statistical approach of factor analysis to tests of central auditory processing: auditory pattern/temporal ordering (APTO); monaural separation/closure (MSC); binaural integration/binaural separation (BIBS); and binaural interaction (BI) (Domitz & Schow, 2000; Schow & Chermak, 1999). Monaural low-redundancy speech tests factor within the monaural separation/closure (MSC) category. Several factor analyses have demonstrated that tests involving auditory closure on the part of the listener and presumed to evaluate monaural auditory performance decrements due to degradation or competition (e.g., the Selective Auditory Attention Test, Auditory Figure-Ground, and Filtered Word subtests of the SCAN) load on the MSC factor (Domitz & Schow, 2000; Schow & Chermak, 1999).

Interaction Between Extrinsic Redundancy and Intrinsic Redundancy

Extrinsic redundancy has been most often degraded or reduced by: (a) altering the frequency or spectral aspects of speech (e.g., low-pass filtered speech tests), (b) adding background noise or speech to introduce competition (e.g., speech-in-noise tests), and (c) altering the temporal aspects of speech (e.g., time compressed speech tests). Less commonly, intensity alterations (e.g., low-sensation level speech tests) or other temporal alterations (e.g., interrupted speech) have been examined. Reduced intrinsic redundancy typically reflects a dysfunction in the CANS.

As seen in the first panel of Figure 8–1, when a listener with normal intrinsic redundancy (normal CANS) listens to unaltered speech with normal extrinsic redundancy, normal speech recognition performance is expected. Even when speech is degraded (i.e., extrinsic redundancy is reduced by filtering, adding competition, or altering temporal aspects), listeners with normal intrinsic redundancy can fill in the missing information by means of their auditory closure skills and achieve normal speech recognition performance (see panel 2 of Figure 8–1). When a listener with reduced intrinsic redundancy (CANS dysfunction) listens to unaltered speech with normal extrinsic redundancy, normal speech recognition performance is still expected. However, as shown in panel 3 of Figure 8–1, when speech is degraded (i.e., extrinsic redundancy is reduced), listeners with reduced intrinsic redundancy (due to CANS dysfunction) show a significant deficit in speech recognition performance (see panel 4 of Figure 8–1).

Not depicted in Figure 8–1 are the effects of peripheral hearing loss, which, like CANS dysfunction, also reduce the intrinsic redundancy of the auditory system. The presence of peripheral hearing loss reduces the ability of the auditory system to resolve spectral detail. Hence, central auditory tests employing stimuli placing significant demands on cochlear processing to resolve frequency and

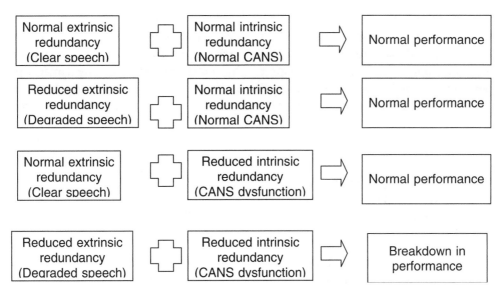

Figure 8–1. Interaction between intrinsic and extrinsic redundancy.

intensity transitions of the acoustic signal (e.g., consonant-vowel syllables, words) are subject to the potential confound of peripheral hearing loss (Chermak & Musiek, 1997). As all monaural low-redundancy tests are heavily dependent on resolution of rapid frequency-intensity interactions, the clinician should balance the value of these tests in the diagnostic battery against their potential to confound results. Results should be interpreted with caution when used as part of a central auditory test battery with individuals with known hearing loss (Baran & Musiek, 1999).

History of Monaural Low-Redundancy Speech Tests

Monaural low-redundancy speech tests (and central auditory tests in general) can historically be traced back to the pioneering work of Italian investigators (Bocca et al.) in the 1950s. They were the first to recognize that patients with temporal lobe lesions had normal pure tone audiograms and speech recognition but still complained of qualitative reduction of speech quality. Upon investigation with filtered speech tests, Bocca et al. (1955, 1958) found depressed scores in patients' ears contralateral to the affected hemisphere. Subsequently, speech-in-noise tests were subsequently introduced for detection of lesions in the CANS. Abnormal scores on speech-in-noise tests were reported for patients with temporal lobe lesions (Sinha, 1959) and also for patients with eighth nerve tumors and multiple sclerosis (Olsen, Noffsinger, & Kurdziel 1975). Time-compressed speech tests also have received attention since the normative studies by Beasley and his colleagues (Beasley, Schwimmer, & Rintelmann 1972). Normal listeners showed essentially normal performance for recognition of monosyllabic NU-6 words when lower time compression (30–60%) was applied; however, their performance broke down when a greater proportion of temporal segments were removed (i.e., 70% time compression). Kurdzeil, Noffsinger, and Olsen (1976) showed that patients with diffuse temporal lobe lesions exhibited poorer performance on time-compressed speech tests in the ear contralateral to the lesion at 40% and 60% time compression.

Classification of Monaural Low-Redundancy Speech Tests

Monaural low-redundancy speech tests continue to be one of the most widely used tests to evaluate central auditory function (Chermak, Traynham, Seikel, & Musiek, 1998). They continue to be used despite only moderate sensitivity to CANS lesions (Musiek & Baran, 2002) primarily because they: (1) have been incorporated into several popular clinical test batteries (Keith, 1986, 1994, 2000; Willeford, 1977), (2) are easy to administer, and (3) are easy to score and interpret. They also provide insight as to functional deficits (i.e., listening in noise and auditory closure problems) and therefore offer practical information for intervention (Bellis, 2003; Bellis & Ferre, 1999). Commercially available monaural low-redundancy speech tests currently used can be classified as: (1) low-pass filtered speech tests, (b) speech-in-noise tests, (c) speech-in-competition tests, and (d) time-compressed speech tests.

Low-Pass Filtered Speech Tests

The use of low-pass filtered speech (LPFS) can be traced historically to research by Bocca et al. (1954). They found that patients who were referred from neuro-logic wards presented normal hearing sensitivity (as revealed by pure-tone air conduction threshold testing); however, they exhibited temporal lobe damage. To probe their auditory function in more detail, Bocca et al. (1954) first devised tests for higher-order auditory processes. Bocca et al. (1954) reported reduced performance in the ear contralateral to the temporal lobe lesion for most patients.

Willeford (1977) proposed one of the earliest clinical test batteries to probe central auditory processing disorder [(C)APD] in children, aged 5 to 10 years. Included in his battery was a subtest composed of two, 50-item lists of filtered consonant-nucleus-consonant (CNC) words. The words were presented at 50 dB HL and filtered at a 500-Hz cutoff frequency at a rate of 18 dB per octave. A slight maturational effect, reflected by larger standard deviations and ranges for younger children, was reported; however, no major ear asymmetry was seen (in contrast to ear asymmetry seen on dichotic speech tasks) (Willeford, 1977). Despite sounding muffled due to the filtering, the CNC words are rather intelligible to listeners with normal peripheral and central auditory function (Bellis, 2003). In contrast, individuals with CANS dysfunction show evidence of considerable difficulty, reflecting deficits in auditory closure (Bellis, 2003).

Keith (1986, 1994, and 2000) developed several of the most widely used tools (SCAN, SCAN-A, SCAN-C) to probe auditory processing in children and adults (Emmanuel, 2002). One of the major advantages of these tests is that they look at multiple auditory processes (e.g., monaural auditory closure, monaural separation, and binaural integration). A second strength of these tests is that subtest raw scores are converted into standard scores, which facilitates objective interpretation of performance.

The Filtered Words (FW) subtest of the SCAN/SCAN-C is designed for children between 3.0 to 11.11 years. Children are required to repeat 20 monosyllabic words presented to each ear at 50 dB HL that have been low-pass filtered at 1000 Hz (roll-off of 32 dB/octave). In the FW subtest of SCAN-A (designed for ages 12–50 years), the difficulty level is slightly increased by low-pass filtering monosyllabic words with a 500 Hz cutoff frequency (roll-off = 32 dB/octave). For both the SCAN-C and SCAN-A, the raw scores are converted into standard scores (subtest mean standard score is 10 with a standard deviation of 3).

Clinicians should be aware of questions raised regarding the test-retest reliability of the SCAN. In a study that explored the test-retest reliability of SCAN in first-grade and third-grade schoolchildren, SCAN was administered to 25 first-graders and 22 third-graders (all between ages 6–9 years) and then retested after a 6 to 7 week interval (Amos & Humes, 1998). Results showed no significant differences in FW standard scores across first- and third-grade children; however, children obtained significantly higher scores on the retest condition relative to the first administration.

Another version of a low-pass filtered speech test is available on the Veterans Administration compact disk (*Tonal and Speech Materials for Auditory Perceptual Assessment*, 1992). The standardized version consists of two lists of low-pass filtered NU-6 words (lists 3C and 4C) with a filter cutoff of 1500 Hz. Standardization of this LPFS test was completed by playing recordings of the female talker version of monosyllabic NU-6 words at different filter cutoffs (800 Hz, 1200 Hz, 1500 Hz, and 1700 Hz) to eight young normal hearing adults (Bornstein et al., 1994). The target cut-off frequency which produced 70 to 80% correct word recognition performance at a comfortable listening level (50-dB HL) was found to be 1500 Hz, with normal young adults achieving on average 76.5% at this cutoff frequency (Bornstein et al., 1994).

Another version of a LFPS test is the Auditec recording of the filtered NU-6 words. According to Wilson & Mueller (1984), four low-pass filtered versions of this LPFS task (500 Hz, 700 Hz, 1000 Hz, and 1500 Hz) are available. Filtering using a 500 Hz cutoff frequency was found to pose difficulties even for listeners with normal peripheral and central auditory function and, therefore, is not recommended for clinical assessment of central auditory function (Wilson & Mueller, 1984). The 1000 Hz cutoff, male talker version has been recommended for clinical use (Wilson & Mueller, 1984), with norms available for NU-6 lists #1 to 4 (75%, 80%, 83%, and 78%, respectively) for normal-hearing young adults. Bellis (2003) reported pediatric norms for the Auditec recording (1000 Hz cutoff) at a presentation level of 50-dB HL: 62% (7-year-olds), 70% (8-year-olds), 68% (9-year-olds), 72% (10-year-olds), 75% (1-year-olds), and 78% or higher (12-year-olds to adult).

Limited sensitivity and specificity data for LFPS tests have been published; however, there is some evidence that these tests are more sensitive to temporal lobe lesions than interhemispheric and brainstem lesions. Lynn & Gilroy (1972, 1977) studied 34 patients with temporal lobe tumors and 27 patients with parietal lobe tumors. They found that 74% of patients with temporal lobe lesions showed expected contralateral deficits on LFPS, whereas 74% of patients with parietal lobe tumors presented normal performance on LFPS. Other studies reported similar outcomes, that is, lower scores in the ear contralateral to the temporal lobe lesion (Bocca et al., 1958; Jerger, 1960). Karlsson and Rosenhall (1995) reported that filtered speech tests showed modest sensitivity (62–64%) to brainstem lesions and slightly higher sensitivity (65–67%) to temporal lobe lesions.

In contrast to the findings in temporal lobe lesions, LFPS results have been found to be essentially normal in listeners with interhemispheric lesions (Baran, Musiek, & Reeves, 1986; Musiek, Wilson, & Pinheiro, 1979). In patients with brainstem lesions, LPFS findings vary considerably (Calearo & Antonelli, 1963; Musiek & Guerkink, 1982). Some of this variability may be due to size and location of the lesion. Large, diffuse lesions are likely to show bilateral deficits, lower brainstem lesions are likely to reveal ipsilateral deficits, and higher brainstem lesions may present with contralateral deficits (Musiek & Guerkink, 1982).

In summary, LPFS tests are moderately sensitive to lesions in the CANS, especially those located in the temporal lobe. In addition, some of these tests also can be useful to assess auditory processing skills of children suspected of (C)APD because they simulate listening in poor (degraded) listening conditions and, therefore, reveal functional deficits.

Speech-in-Noise Tests

In this category of tests, speech typically is embedded in a background of noise or speech competition. Early applications of these tests can be traced back to research by Sinha (1959) who reported deficits in the ear contralateral to cortical lesion in patients with CANS pathology. Subsequent studies also have shown speech-in-noise deficits contralateral to the hemisphere with auditory cortex involvement (Heilman, Hammer, & Wilder, 1973, Morales-Garcia & Poole, 1972). Other studies also have reported poor scores in patients with eighth nerve and extra-axial lesions (Dayal, Tarantino, & Swisher, 1966) and in patients with and intra-axial brainstem lesions (Morales-Garcia & Poole, 1972). Olsen, Noffsinger, & Kurdziel (1975) computed difference scores by subtracting NU-6 word recognition scores in noise from NU-6 word-correct scores in quiet. Significant differences (greater than 40%) between quiet and noise were seen for patients with eighth nerve lesions, Meniere's disease, and temporal lobe lesions. Many of the speech-in-noise tests discussed in the following paragraph have been standardized for use with children and adults suspected of (C)APD.

There are at least three standardized versions of speech-in-noise tests currently in clinical use: (1) Auditory Figure Ground (AFG) subtest of SCAN/SCAN-C/SCAN-A, (2) Synthetic Sentence Identification with Ipsilateral Competing Message (SSI-ICM) and (3) Pediatric Speech Intelligibility Test with Ipsilateral Competing Message (PSI-ICM). A key factor in using speech-in-noise tests is the SNR. Perhaps the most commonly used SNR is 0 dB which indicates that the sound pressure level of the speech is equal to the overall level of the noise (Rintelmann, 1985). The type of noise used in speech-in-noise tests can also vary considerably making comparisons among tests difficult. White noise, multitalker babble, and even competing discourse have been used in various speech-in-noise tests.

The AFG subtest of the SCAN-C (CD version) evaluates the child's ability to understand monosyllabic words in the presence of multitalker speech babble. Words are presented at 50 dB HL, with a message competition ratio (MCR) of +8 dB. Two practice items and 20 test words are presented to each ear. For the AFG subtest of the SCAN-A, 20 monosyllabic words are presented to each ear at levels of 50 dB HL with a 0 dB MCR.

In the SSI-ICM task, synthetic sentences are presented at 30 dB HL in competition with connected discourse (i.e., a story about Davy Crockett). The synthetic sentences are 10, third-order approximations of English sentences. The seven-word sentences are semantically meaningless. They were designed to reduce a listener's reliance on linguistic skills, while preserving the syntax and temporal feature of the English language (Jerger & Jerger, 1974). The SSI also can be presented with contralateral competition (SSI-CCM) (see Chapter 9). The SSI should only be administered to individuals with normal hearing sensitivity through 1000 Hz because the important audiometric frequency region underlying correct identification of sentence materials centers around 750 Hz (Hall & Mueller, 1997).

In the SSI-ICM task, the synthetic sentences are presented at a fixed level (i.e., 30 dB HL) and the level of the competition is varied to achieve varying MCR ratios (i.e., +10, 0, −10, −20). In contrast to the other tests reviewed above, the SSI requires that the listener be able to read the list of printed synthetic sentences. Also differentiating the SSI-ICM from the other tests reviewed above, the

SSI employs a closed message set (i.e., 10 sentences) and a closed response set (i.e., selection from among those same 10 sentences). Also, rather than repeating what is heard, the subject is asked to report the number of the sentence heard, thereby reducing the potential confounds of memory and language. Percentage correct scores are reported for each ear. Normative cutoffs for the SSI-ICM vary with MCR (e.g., +10 dB MCR: 100%, 0 dB MCR: 85%, −10 dB MCR: 70%, −20 dB MCR: 45%) (Jerger & Jerger, 1974).

The SSI-ICM test has been shown to be sensitive to lesions of the brainstem (Jerger & Jerger, 1974, 1975). Jerger and Jerger (1974) showed that all (11/11) patients with intra-axial lesions in their study showed SSI-ICM deficits. Jerger and Jerger (1975) also showed that the average SSI-ICM loss approximated about 40% in the ears contralateral to brainstem lesions in 10 patients with intra-axial brainstem lesions, whereas for patients with eighth nerve lesions, the average SSI-ICM loss approximated 50% in the ear ipsilateral to the lesion. In the same study (Jerger & Jerger, 1975), patients with eighth nerve lesions showed a loss for monosyllabic, phonetically balanced words for the ipsilateral ear, whereas patients with brainstem lesions showed a loss for monosyllabic, phonetically balanced words bilaterally, with greater loss in the contralateral ear.

The Pediatric Speech Intelligibility (PSI) test is an adaptation of the SSI test for the pediatric population (Jerger & Jerger, 1984). This test is appropriate for children aged 3 to 6 years. Like the SSI, the PSI allows for the construction of performance versus intensity functions (PI Fn) and message to competition functions. Moreover, the PSI constructs these functions based on the child's responses to both monosyllabic words (i.e., 20 simple nouns) and sentence stimuli (i.e., 10 simple sentences with animal agents). Twenty competing sentences also involve animal agents in simple contexts. Like the SSI, the PSI can be administered with competition in the contralateral ear (PSI-CCM- see Chapter 9.) The child is asked to point to the picture that is heard. In the competing conditions, the child is told to point to the picture said by "your man" and to ignore the "trick man." Like the SSI, the PSI employs a closed message set (i.e., 20 words and 10 sentences) and a closed response set (i.e., selection from among five pictures). The PSI closed response set requires the subject to point to the picture corresponding to the sentence heard, thereby reducing the potential confound of memory. The presentation level recommended for PSI-ICM is 30 dB HL with a 0 dB MCR for sentences and +4 dB MCR for words.

Based on norms reported in the test manual, SSI-ICM scores less than 80% fall outside the 95% confidence interval for normal-hearing children (Jerger & Jerger, 1984). Sensitivity and specificity data were not reported by Jerger and Jerger (1984); however, Jerger, Johnson, and Loiselle (1988) reported that children with suspected (C)APD presented deficits on the PSI similar to those demonstrated by children with confirmed temporal lobe lesions.

In summary, available data indicate that speech-in-noise tests may be marginally to moderately sensitive to a variety of CANS disorders (Jerger & Jerger, 1975; Morales-Garcia & Poole, 1972). Patients with low to mid-brainstem involvement, as well as cortical lesions, typically perform poorly on speech-in-noise tests.

Time-Compressed Speech Tests

Time-compressed speech tests employ speech that is compressed electronically by systematically sampling and discarding segments of the signal without distorting the frequency aspects of the signal. (Beasley & Maki, 1976; Beasley, Schwimmer, & Rintelmann, 1972) Time compression (TC) currently is accomplished using waveform-editing software that alters the rate of speech without altering the power spectrum or pitch. These tests assess the auditory system's capacity to process rapidly changing acoustic spectra. The amount of compression is expressed as a percentage of the original signal that is eliminated. TC of 45%, for example, indicates that the signal now occupies 55% of its original time frame, with 45% of signal having been removed. One big advantage of time compression is that while intervals between speech units are removed, the acoustical aspects (e.g., frequency, intensity) of the signal remain unaltered.

Time-compressed speech tests are sensitive to cortical lesions (Karlsson & Rosenhall, 1995; Kurdziel, Noffsinger, & Olsen, 1976), with performance typically reduced in the ear contralateral to the temporal lobe lesion (Calearo & Antonelli, 1973). Karlsson & Rosenhall (1995) studied the sensitivity of time-compressed speech in patients with brainstem lesions and temporal lobe lesions. Although time-compressed speech was only moderately sensitive to brainstem lesions (62–64%), its sensitivity was much higher (80%) for patients with temporal lobe lesions (Karlsson & Rosenhall, 1995). Kurdziel et al. (1976) studied the effects of several degrees of time compression (0%, 40%, and 60%) on speech recognition scores in 15 patients with diffuse cortical lesions and 16 patients with anterior temporal lobe surgical lesions. Patients with diffuse lesions showed a significant deterioration in speech recognition at 60% time compression in the ear contralateral to the lesion. In contrast, patients with discrete (i.e., anterior temporal lobe) lesions demonstrated essentially normal performance bilaterally.

Normative studies have explored the percentage of time compression that separates listeners with normal central auditory function from those with (C)APD. Wilson, Preece, Salamon, Sperry, & Bornstein (1994) studied time-compressed speech for NU-6 monosyllables at 45% and 65% time compression in young adults with normal hearing. They found that normal listeners showed difficulty at 65% time compression; however, they exhibited normal performance at 45% TC. In contrast, listeners with central auditory dysfunction demonstrate reduced performance at 45% TC (Wilson et al., 1994). Based on these studies, 45% TC is the recommended standard compression value used clinically (Bellis, 2003). To make time compression even more challenging, a 0.3 msec reverberation has been electronically added to the time-compressed speech on the VA CD (*Tonal and Speech Materials for Auditory Perceptual Assessment*, 1992).

These are at least two standardized recordings of time-compressed speech currently in clinical use. One recording is included on the VA CD (*Tonal and Speech Materials for Auditory Perceptual Assessment,* 1992). This recording consists of two lists of monosyllabic NU-6 words (lists 7A and 8A) administered at a level of 55 dB HL. Wilson et al. (1994) reported normative data (at 55 dB HL presentation level) with criterion values (i.e., two standard deviations below the

mean) for young normal-hearing adults (i.e., 45% TC = 86.5%; 45% TC plus reverberation = 34.9%). Bellis (2003) reported pediatric norms calculated at two standard deviations below the mean using the VA CD recording of 45% TC presented at 55 dB HL (i.e., 65% [9-year-olds]; 68% [10-year-olds]; 78% [11-year-olds]; and 85% [12-year-olds to adults]).

The second standardized recording of TC speech is the *Time Compressed Sentence Test* (TCST) for children ages 6 to 11 years developed by Keith (2002a). In this test, sentences are presented at 55 dB HL and compression rates are varied for subtests (0%, 40%, and 60% TC). All lists are composed of 10 sentences. In subtest 1 of the TCST, one list is presented at 0% (no) time compression; this easy baseline condition is used for practice and preliminary screening. Subtest 2 of the TCST is composed of two lists, each at 40% time compression, with one list presented to each of the two ears monotically. Subtest 3 is administered as is subtest 2 using 60% TC. Keith argued that sentences are more realistic and meaningful stimuli for children; however, sentence stimuli can increase the potential for language and memory confounds.

No sensitivity or specificity data have been published for the TCST; however, Keith (2002a) published normative data for children ages 6 years to 11 years. Based on published norms (Keith, 2002a), pediatric norms were calculated for right/left ears at two standard deviations below the mean for 40% TC presented at 55 dB HL (i.e., 75.6%/70.8% [6-year-olds]; 88.3%/89.3% [7-year-olds]; 87.5%/86.2% [8-year-olds], 86.8%/91.4% [9-year-olds]; and 96.9%/91.4% [10- and 11-year-olds]. For detailed norms on the TCST, the reader is referred to the manual (Keith, 2002b).

Comparison of Bellis' (2003) and Keith's (2002a) norms for children (ages 9–11 years) indicates that the children of the same age did relatively better on the TCST than on the TC NU-6 VA CD recording. These performance differences may be attributed to the considerable difference in the intrinsic redundancy of the stimuli (NU-6 monosyllables versus sentences), resulting in the TCST being an easier task for children to perform.

In summary, although time-compressed speech tests are only moderately sensitive to brainstem lesions, their sensitivity is much greater to diffuse lesions of the auditory cortex (Kurdziel et al., 1976) and temporal lobe lesions (Karlsson & Rosehall, 1995). Sensitivity and specificity data are not available for children with (C)APD and this is a need that must be addressed in future research.

Management Implications

As noted earlier, monaural low-redundancy test data provide information regarding real-life functional deficits and can be used to plan deficit-specific intervention. Poor performance on monaural low-redundancy speech tests implicates deficits in auditory closure and suggests that the listener could benefit from environmental noise reduction, signal enhancement, auditory training, and metalinguistic approaches discussed in this Handbook. (See Chapters 4, 5, and 7 in Volume II of this Handbook).

Summary

Monaural low-redundancy speech tests continue to be one of the most widely used types of tests for central auditory

dysfunction (Chermak et al., 1998; Chermak, Silva, & Musiek, personal communication), despite the rather limited number of published reports regarding these tests' sensitivity and specificity, especially with pediatric populations. As performance on monaural low-redundancy speech tests is not affected by interhemispheric involvement (i.e., corpus callosum), they are especially useful when used alongside dichotic tests or pattern tests which are sensitive to hemispheric as well as interhemispheric involvement (Musiek, Kibbe, & Baran, 1984). That is, a left ear deficit on a dichotic listening test coupled with normal left ear monaural low-redundancy performance suggests interhemispheric involvement. (A left ear deficit on a dichotic listening test coupled with abnormal left ear monaural low-redundancy performance suggests either right hemisphere involvement or possibly involvement of both the right hemisphere and interhemispheric transfer [Musiek et al., 1984]). In addition to assisting the audiologist in identifying the site/level of dysfunction, monaural low-redundancy tests are often included in the central auditory test battery because the test stimulates listening in poor (degraded) acoustic conditions, and, therefore reveals functional (i.e., auditory closure) deficits. Monaural low-redundancy speech tests can be useful, therefore, in assessing auditory processing skills of children suspected of (C)APD and in suggesting directions for deficit-focused intervention. (See Chapters 7, 9, and 10 for discussion of test battery interpretation.)

Available data suggest that LPFS tests are moderately sensitive to temporal lobe lesions (Lynn & Gilroy, 1977; Karlsson & Rosenhall, 1995). Speech-in-noise tests may be marginally-to-moderately sensitive to a variety of CANS disorders (Jerger

& Jerger, 1975; Morales-Garcia & Poole, 1972), including patients with low to mid-brainstem involvement, as well as cortical lesions. The PSI-ICM is a well-developed test that employs speech in competition to assess young children's ability to extract speech presented in background competition. At least one study suggests the PSI's sensitivity to CANS lesions or dysfunction (Jerger et al., 1988). Time-compressed speech tests appear to be sensitive to diffuse lesions of the auditory cortex (Kurdziel et al., 1976), and are also sensitive to temporal lobe lesions (Karlsson & Rosenhall, 1995).

Additional research is needed to determine the sensitivity of monaural low-redundancy speech tests to CANS lesions and (C)APD in children who do not present with evidence of lesions, but rather present more diffuse neurobiologic dysfunction. Additional normative data are needed as well for many of the tests reviewed in this chapter.

References

Amos, N. E., & Humes, L. E. (1998). SCAN test-retest reliability for first- and third-grade children. *Journal of Speech, Language, and Hearing Research, 41,* 834–845.

Baran, J., & Musiek, F. (1999). Behavioral Assessment of the Central Auditory System. In F. Musiek & W. Rintelmann (Eds.), *Contemporary perspectives on hearing assessment* (pp. 375–415). Boston: Allyn & Bacon.

Baran, J. A., Musiek, F. E., & Reeves, A. G. (1986). Central auditory function following anterior sectioning of corpus callosum. *Ear and Hearing, 7,* 359–362.

Beasley, D. S., & Maki, J. (1976). Time-and frequency-altered speech. In N. Lass (Ed.), *Contemporary issues in experimental*

phonetics (pp. 419–458). New York: Academic Press.

Beasley, D. S., Schwimmer, S., & Rintelmann, W. F. (1972). Intelligibility of time-compressed CNC monosyllable. *Journal of Speech and Hearing Research, 15,* 340–350.

Bellis, T. J. (2003). *Assessment and management of central auditory processing disorders in the educational setting: From science to practice.* Clifton Park, NY: Thomson-Delmar Learning.

Bellis, T. J., & Ferre, J. M. (1999). Multidimensional approach to the different diagnosis of central auditory processing disorders in children. *Journal of the American Academy of Audiology, 10,* 319–328.

Bocca, E. (1958). Clinical aspects of cortical deafness. *Laryngoscope, 68,* 301–309.

Bocca, E., Calearo, C., & Cassinari, V. (1954). A new method for testing hearing in temporal lobe tumors. *Acta Otolaryngologica (Stockholm), 44,* 219–221.

Bocca, E., Calearo, C., Cassinari, V., & Migliavacca, F. (1955). Testing "cortical" hearing in temporal lobe tumors. *Acta Otolaryngologica, 42,* 219–221.

Bornstein, S. P., Wilson, R. H., & Cambron, N. K. (1994). Low- and high-pass filtered Northwestern University Auditory Test No. 6 for monaural and binaural evaluation. *Journal of the American Academy of Audiology, 5,* 259–264.

Calearo, M. D., & Antonelli, A.R. (1973). *Disorders of the central auditory nervous system* (Vol. 2). Philadelphia: Saunders.

Chermak, G. D., & Musiek, F. E. (1997). *Central auditory processing disorders: New perspectives.* San Diego: Singular Publishing Group.

Chermak, G. D., Traynham, W. D., Seikel, A. J, & Musiek, F. E. (1998). Professional education and assessment practices in central auditory processing. *Journal of the American Academy of Audiology, 9,* 452–465.

Dayal, V. S., Taranito, L., & Swisher, L. P. (1966). Neuro-otologic studies in multiple sclerosis. *Laryngoscope, 76,* 1798–1809.

Domitz, D. M., & Schow, R. L. (2000). A new CAPD battery—Multiple auditory processing assessment (MAPA): Factor analysis and comparisons with SCAN. *American Journal of Audiology, 9*, 101–111.

Emmanuel D. C. (2002). The auditory processing battery: Survey of common practices. *Journal of the American Academy of Audiology, 13*, 93–117.

Hall, J. W. III, & Mueller, G. H. III. (1997). *Audiologists Desk Reference.* San Diego: Singular Publishing Group.

Heilman, K. M., Hammer, L. C., & Wilder, B. J. (1973). An audiometric defect in temporal lobe dysfunction. *Neurology, 23*, 384–386.

Jerger, J. (1960). Audiological manifestations of lesions in the auditory nervous system. *Laryngoscope 70*, 417–425.

Jerger J., & Jerger, S. (1974). Auditory findings in brainstem disorders. *Archives of Otolaryngology, 99*, 342–349.

Jerger J., & Jerger, S. (1975). Clinical validity of central auditory tests. *Scandinavian Audiology, 4*, 147–163.

Jerger, S., & Jerger, J. (1984). *Pediatric Speech Intelligibility Test: Manual for administration.* St. Louis, MO: Auditec.

Jerger, S., Johnson, K., & Loiselle, L. (1988). Pediatric central auditory dysfunction: Comparison of children with confirmed lesions versus suspected processing disorders. *American Journal of Otology,* (Suppl. 9), 63–71.

Karlsson, A., & Rosenhall, U. (1995). Clinical applications of distorted speech audiometry. *Scandinavian Audiology, 24*, 155–160.

Keith, R. W. (1986). *SCAN: A screening test for auditory processing disorders.* San Antonio, TX: The Psychological Corporation.

Keith, R. W. (1994). *SCAN-A: A test for auditory processing disorders in adolescents and adults.* San Antonio, TX: The Psychological Corporation.

Keith, R. W. (2000). *SCAN-C Test for Auditory Processing Disorders in Children—Revised.* San Antonio, TX: The Psychological Corporation.

Keith, R. W. (2002a). Standardization of the Time Compressed Sentence Test. *Journal of Educational Audiology, 10*, 15–20.

Keith, R. W. (2002b). Time Compressed Sentence Test, *Examiner's Manual.* St. Louis, MO: Auditec.

Korsan-Bengsten, M. (1973). Distorted speech audiometry: A methodological and clinical study. *Acta Otolaryngologica Supplement (Stockholm), 310*, 7–75.

Kurdziel, S., Noffsinger, D., & Olsen, W. (1976). Performance by cortical lesion patients on 40% and 60% time-compressed materials. *Journal of the American Audiological Society, 2*, 3–7.

Liberman, A. M., Cooper, F. S., Shankweiler, D., & Studdert-Kennedy, M. (1967). Perception of the speech code. *Psychological Review, 74*, 431–461.

Lynn, G. E, & Gilroy, J. (1972). Neuro-audiological abnormalities in patients with temporal lobe tumors. *Journal of Neurological Science, 17*, 167–184.

Lynn, G. E., & Gilroy, J. (1977). Evaluation of central auditory dysfunction in patients with neurological disorders. In R.W., Keith (Ed.), *Central auditory dysfunction* (pp. 177–221). New York: Gruen & Stratton.

Miller, G. A., Heise, G. A., & Lichten, W. (1951). The intelligibility of speech as a function of the context of the test materials. *Journal of Experimental Psychology, 4*, 329–335.

Morales-Garcia, C., & Poole, J. O. (1972). Masked speech audiometry in central deafness. *Acta Otolaryngologica, 74*, 307–316.

Musiek, F. E., & Baran, J. A. (2002). Central auditory evaluation of patients with neurological involvement. In J. Katz (Ed.), *Handbook of clinical audiology* (5th ed., pp. 532–544) Baltimore: Lippincott Williams and Wilkins.

Musiek, F. E., & Geurkink, N. A. (1982). Auditory brain response and central auditory test findings for patients with brain stem lesions: A preliminary report. *Laryngoscope, 92*, 891–990.

Musiek, F. E., Kibbe, K., & Baran, J. (1984). Neuroaudiological results from split-brain patients. *Seminars in Hearing, 5*(3), 219–229.

Musiek, F. E., Wilson, D. H., & Pinheiro, M. L. (1979). Audiological manifestations in "split-brain" patients. *Journal of the American Audiological Society, 5*, 25-29.

Olsen, W. O., Noffsinger, D., & Kurdziel, S. (1975). Speech discrimination in noise by patients with peripheral and central lesions. *Acta Otolaryngologica, 80*, 375-382.

Rintelmann, W. F. (1985). Monaural speech tests in the detection of central auditory disorders. In M. L. Pinheiro & F. E. Musiek (Eds.), *Assessment of central auditory dysfunction: Foundations and clinical correlates* (pp. 173-200). Baltimore: Williams & Wilkins.

Sanders, D., & Goodrich, S. (1971). Relative contribution of visual and auditory components of speech intelligibility as a function of three conditions of frequency distortion. *Journal of Speech and Hearing Research, 14*, 154-159.

Schow, R., & Chermak, G. D. (1999). Implications from factor analysis for central auditory processing disorders. *American Journal of Audiology, 8*(2), 137-142.

Sinha, S. O. (1959). *The role of the temporal lobe in hearing.* Unpublished master's thesis, McGill University, Montreal, Quebec.

Tonal and speech materials for auditory perceptual assessment. (1992). Long Beach, CA: Research and Development Service, Veterans' Administration Central Office.

Willeford, J. (1977). Assessing central auditory behavior in children: A test battery approach. In R. W. Keith (Ed.), *Central auditory dysfunction* (pp. 43-72). New York: Grune & Stratton.

Wilson, L., & Mueller, H. G. (1984). Performance on normal hearing individuals on Auditec filtered speech tests. *American Speech and Hearing Association, 27*, 189.

Wilson, R. H., Preece, J. P., Salamon, D. L., Sperry, J. L., & Bornstein, S. P. (1994). Effects of time compression and time compression plus reverberation on the intelligibility of Northwestern University Auditory Test No. 6. *Journal American Academy of Audiology, 5*(4), 269-277.

CHAPTER 9

DICHOTIC LISTENING TESTS

ROBERT W. KEITH and JILL ANDERSON

Dichotic listening tests are among the most powerful of the behavioral auditory processing test battery for the assessment of hemispheric function, interhemispheric transfer of information, development and maturation of the auditory nervous system, and the identification of lesions of the central auditory nervous system (CANS). Dichotic listening tests involve the simultaneous presentation of different acoustic stimuli to each of the two ears. Commonly used speech stimuli include consonant-vowel (CV) nonsense syllables, digits, words, spondees, and sentences. First introduced by Broadbent (Broadbent, 1954), the use of dichotic listening tests expanded after the landmark papers by Kimura (Kimura, 1961a, 1961b, 1967) who described their use in mea-

suring hemispheric asymmetry and brain dysfunction. Kimura's results showed that children of all ages recalled dichotic digits better from the right ear than the left ear. This finding was interpreted as indicating the language specialization of the left cerebral hemisphere, to which the right ear has relatively direct anatomic connection.

Interest in this test paradigm grew phenomenally; as early as 1976, Berlin and McNeil analyzed more than 300 studies on dichotic test studies (Berlin & McNeil, 1976). At present, there are thousands of research publications on studies that utilize or investigate dichotic listening. Recently, three major position papers (ASHA, 1996, 2005; Jerger & Musiek, 2000) have referenced the use of dichotic tests by audiologists in the diagnostic process, with the Jerger and Musiek (2000) report recommending dichotic tests as part of the minimum central auditory test battery.

Over the years, dichotic testing has been utilized in the study of human channel capacity, brain injury, structural lesions of the brain, hemispheric specialization, sustained attention, attention deficit disorders, and dyslexia (Jerger & Martin, in press). Dichotic tests are no longer as important to the identification of brainstem and cortical lesions with the advent of sophisticated imaging techniques such as magnetic resonance imaging (MRI). Dichotic test results still are used by audiologists, however, to describe maturation of the auditory nervous system in children and adolescents, specify the dominant hemisphere for language, assess short-term auditory memory storage and retrieval, and identify breakdowns in cortical auditory function for persons of all ages. The purpose of this chapter is to describe some of the diagnostic principles and procedures utilized with dichotic tests in the evaluation of individuals with CANS dysfunction, including those with auditory processing, language, learning, and reading disorders.

Dichotic Tests

Stimuli used in the assessment of the central auditory system using the dichotic paradigm include consonant-vowel (CV) syllables, digits, words, spondees, and sentences. Stimuli are presented simultaneously to opposite ears. Typically, dichotic tests require simultaneous onset and offset of the stimuli, although some dichotic CV tests used in the past incorporated 15- to 90-msec offset of stimulus onset.

Examples of specific dichotic tests include:

- Dichotic consonant-vowel (CV) test (Berlin, Lowe-Bell et al., 1973)
- Dichotic digits (Musiek, 1983)
- Competing words (Keith, 1998, 2000)
- Staggered spondaic word test (SSW) (Katz, 1962)
- Competing sentence tests (Keith, 1998; 2000; Willeford, 1997)
- Dichotic sentence identification test (DSI) (Fifer, Jerger, & Berlin, 1983)

In general, all of these tests require the subject to repeat the stimuli heard. One test, the DSI, was developed to evaluate central auditory function in adults with peripheral hearing loss. It requires subjects to read and identify sentences from a printed list. Given the cross-modality nature of the task (i.e., auditory to visual), the DSI is not an auditory-specific dichotic measure. Moreover, the DSI is inappropriate for individuals who cannot read and there are no normative data for children.

Each of these dichotic tests yields a higher percent of correct responses in the right than the left ear for younger subjects, although this ear difference is of smaller magnitude for adults. This finding is commonly called the right ear advantage (REA). The magnitude of the REA is dependent primarily on the instructions given to the subject and the linguistic content of the dichotic stimuli (i.e., as they move from CV syllables to sentences) (Hugdahl, 1988). (See also discussion of factors that affect dichotic test results below.)

Model of Dichotic Listening

Several authors have proposed models to explain perceptual asymmetries (i.e., contralateral and ipsilateral ear effects) obtained on tests of dichotic listening. (See Hugdahl, 1988 for a review.) Initial reports revealed that there was a slight right ear advantage in normal adults (Kimura, 1961a). A dichotic deficit was observed in the ear contralateral to the involved hemisphere in individuals with temporal lobe lesions (Kimura, 1961b). In the callosal relay model, Kimura (1967) proposed that the REA results from asymmetries in the pathways connecting the peripheral auditory system to the central auditory cortex. Information from the right ear is transferred directly to the language dominant left hemisphere; information to the left ear is transferred first to the nondominant right hemisphere and then crosses to the language dominant left hemisphere through the corpus callosum. Concurrently, the contralateral pathway suppresses information conducted through the ipsilateral pathway (see Figure 9-1). The callosal relay model is supported by studies using dichotic recall tasks on subjects with split-brains with disconnected hemispheres (i.e., created by commissurotomy of the corpus callosum) which revealed their inability to recognize stimuli presented to the left ear (Milner, Taylor, & Sperry, 1968; Sparks, & Geshwind, 1968). Consistent findings of improved left ear performance with normal maturation in children also supports this model, as the corpus callosum is known to be fully myelinated during adolescence, a period where REA reaches adult values.

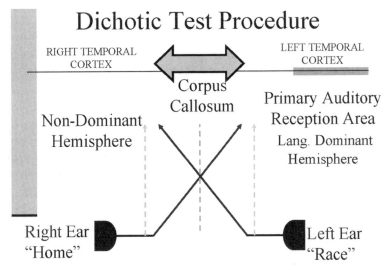

Figure 9-1. Model of the central auditory pathways showing transmission of the dichotic signal to the opposite hemisphere with interhemispheric transmission of information through the corpus callosum (J. Hall, personal communication).

Also supporting the callosal relay model are findings of a positive correlation between interhemispheric transfer times and the REA. In a study using dichotic monitoring of CV syllables, (Jancke, 2002) found that right ear auditory targets were detected more frequently and faster than left ear targets, supporting the callosal relay model. Various studies have consistently revealed that reaction times are 10 to 50 ms faster to right ear targets than to left ear targets (Geffen & Caudrey, 1981; Jancke & Steinmetz, 1994; Springer, 1971).

Kinsbourne (1970) originally suggested that directing attention to one ear or the other improves identification of verbal material in that ear and laterality of results also may shift to the directed ear. Directed attention during dichotic tests may result in enhanced right ear performance during directed right listening and improvement in left ear performance with directed left listening; however, there should be no overall change in the subject's total score (Obrzut, Boliek, & Obrzut, 1986). According to Obrzut et al. (1986) and Hynd, Cohen, and Obrzut (1983), children with learning disabilities demonstrate reversed ear advantage on directed right and left dichotic CV tests, whereas normal young children maintain a right ear advantage under both listening conditions.

The right ear advantage reflects left hemisphere dominance for language and is typically present regardless of handedness. According to Rasmussen and Milner (1975), approximately 96% of normal right-handed and 70% of left-handed persons have language represented in the left hemisphere. The remaining 4% of right-handed people display right hemisphere dominance, whereas equal percentages of left-handed persons exhibit bilateral (i.e., 15%) and right hemisphere dominance (i.e., 15%) for language. The implication of these findings is that it is unusual to find a substantial left ear advantage in a population of persons with normal reading and language ability. A left ear advantage (LEA) usually indicates mixed or reversed hemispheric dominance for language consistent with a neurologic basis for language and learning problems.

Administration of Dichotic Tests: Listener Instructions

In a review of dichotic listening tests, Jerger and Martin (in press) specified various modes of administration of dichotic tests, each of which is presumed to reflect disorders of the CANS. According to Jerger and Martin, there are seven distinct modes of administration: (1) divided attention, (2) divided attention with precued direction, (3) directed attention, (4) dichotic monitoring, (5) directed dichotic monitoring, (6) the ABX technique, and (7) four-interval choice. Each of the techniques is confounded by various factors including short-term memory, sequential memory, speed of mental processing, attention, and so on. The most commonly used modes in audiologic testing for (central) auditory processing disorder ([C]APD) include the following.

Divided Attention

In this mode, often referred to as "free recall" or "unfocused," the listener is instructed to report everything heard in both ears. This is the typical administration mode for dichotic digits tests: the listener must report all digits heard in both ears.

Divided Attention with Pre-cued Direction

In this mode, the listener is instructed to report what is heard in both ears, but is directed to report the stimuli heard in the pre-cued ear first. An example is the Competing Words subtest of the SCAN (Keith, 2000): the listener is instructed to report both words heard, but repeat the word heard in the pre-cued ear first. With these instructions, the REA is larger when the right side is pre-cued than when the left side is pre-cued. Indeed, it is often the case that the REA disappears altogether when the left side is pre-cued, and the ear differences are minimal. Nevertheless, substantial left ear advantages are not found in normal populations (Hugdahl & Andersson, 1986).

Directed Attention

In this mode, sometimes called "focused attention," the listener is instructed to report only what is heard in the pre-cued ear, and to disregard what is heard on the noncued ear (Bryden, Munhall, & Allard, 1983). Examples of this administration mode are the Competing Sentences test of the Willeford battery (Willeford & Burleigh, 1994) and the Competing Sentences subtest of SCAN (Keith, 2000).

Evolution of Terminology

It is interesting to note an evolution of terminology used in describing dichotic test paradigms, culminating in the modes used by Jerger and Martin (in press) in describing dichotic test instructions. In 1970, Carhart (p. 158) speaking at a symposium on speech audiometry proposed several principles that " . . . describe features of the normal flow and processing of incoming speech information within the central nervous system." He described the principle of channel separation where " . . . trains of speech are kept distinct from one another when the speech enters each ear separately." A second principle to which he referred involved the fusion into one message of an acoustically divided message when received binaurally. According to Carhart, this principle is most easily demonstrated by dividing the message into two dissimilar fractions and presenting one fraction to each ear (e.g., low-pass filtered speech to one ear and high-pass filtered speech to the other ear, or switching a speech signal rapidly back and forth between the two ears.)

The terminology introduced by Carhart, which was later expanded by Calearo and Antonelli (1973), suggests that binaural separation of dichotic signals is required to keep information at the two ears separate from each other and that binaural integration of incomplete message sets are fused at the brainstem level. According to Tobin (1985), alternating segments of sentences between ears (Cherry, 1953; Cherry & Taylor, 1954; Bocca & Calearo, 1963; Speaks & Jerger, 1965) and dividing a speech signal into two filtered portions (e.g., low- and high-frequency bands) presented with only one band to each of the two ears (Matzker, 1959) are examples of binaural integration of signals.

More recently, audiologists began using different terminology to describe dichotic listening tasks. For example, Musiek and Pinheiro (1985) described binaural separation tasks as occurring "when the subject responds only to the word presented to a designated ear and ignores the other words in the opposite ear" (p. 203). They described binaural integration tasks as those that require the subject to respond to the stimuli presented to both ears. According to Musiek and Pinheiro, dichotic CVs, digits, words, and the SSW are examples of binaural integration tasks (referred to as divided attention by Jerger and Martin [in press], as noted above). Musiek and Pinheiro consider competing sentence tests and the Synthetic Sentence Identification (SSI) test with contralateral competing messages to be examples of binaural separation tasks (referred to as directed attention by Jerger and Martin [in press], as noted above). Medwetsky (2002) described integration as "the ability to integrate acoustic or linguistic information across different processing regions or modalities" (p. 506). His definition characterizes integration as "the efficient transfer of information between hemispheres across the corpus callosum" (p. 506).

Based on this review of terminology, it appears that some authors maintain that all dichotic tests involve binaural separation of information presented to the two ears (e.g., Calearo & Antonelli, 1973), but others separate dichotic tests into those that involve separation of information presented at the two ears and those that involve integration of information across the corpus callosum (Medwetsky, 2002;

Musiek & Pinheiro, 1985). It is important to note this evolution in order to understand that authors may have different meanings for the same terms.

Effects of Central Auditory Lesions on Dichotic Test Results

Lesion studies have proved to be a foundation for interpretation of dichotic test outcomes. As has been reported consistently, the most common lesion effect is that of deficit dichotic performance in the ear opposite the involved hemisphere (i.e., the contralateral effect) (Hugdahl, 1988; Musiek & Pinheiro, 1985). Also documented has been what is termed the *paradoxical* left ear ipsilateral effect: the finding of reduced dichotic performance in the ear ipsilateral to the lesion. This left ear deficit occurs when the corpus callosal fibers are compromised in the left hemisphere, thereby impeding the neural signal before it reaches the auditory cortex of the left hemisphere. Bilaterally reduced scores on dichotic listening are also seen. Obviously, when there is dysfunction in both hemispheres, bilateral deficits can be observed on dichotic tests. Bilateral reduction can also result, however, from compromise of only one hemisphere (i.e., the left auditory cortex), when accompanied by involvement of callosal fibers. In this case, the left ear deficit occurs because of callosal involvement and the right ear deficit results from the classic contralateral ear effect (Musiek & Pinhero, 1985). Lesions in the more rostral brainstem usually show contralateral effects, whereas compromise of the more caudal brainstem yields ipsilateral deficits on dichotic listening. Due to the small distances and compressed structure of the brainstem, both ipsilateral and contralateral pathways can be impacted by one lesion in either pathway; therefore, bilateral dichotic deficits also are a common finding in cases of brainstem lesions (Musiek & Pinheiro, 1985).

Noncentral Auditory Factors That Affect Dichotic Test Results

There are multiple factors that may affect dichotic test results beyond the status of the CANS, including acoustic features of the signal, linguistic content of the signal, listener instructions, symmetry of a subject's peripheral hearing, and a subject's age, memory span, motivation, and cognitive abilities (Denckla, 1989; Silman, Silverman, & Emmer, 2000). Other factors of equal importance are those related to the test materials, such as the stimulus complexities and scoring method. Tests that seek to assess auditory processing should minimize the confounding effects of language, speech production, and sensorimotor and motor learning problems. This can be achieved by controlling linguistic variables by using stimuli with minimal linguistic demands or those with systematically manipulated linguistic variables, minimizing memory load, and employing a simple response mode (Jerger & Musiek, 2000).

Some time ago, Matkin and Hook (1983) reported that dichotic sentence testing requiring the repetition of both sentences had the highest hit rate for identifying children with auditory processing disorders than any other single measure. Of course, requiring a child to repeat two sentences presented dichotically presents a tremendous challenge to binaural separation (and binaural integration), short-term and working memory, and linguistic sequencing. The presence of these confounding nonauditory factors indicates that, although repetition of both sentences may yield valuable diagnostic information, it is not an auditory specific task.

Effect of Stimulus Intensity on Dichotic Test Results

In general, dichotic speech tests are presented at equal intensity to the two ears. In an early study, Cullen et al. (1974) found that signals must be at least 30 to 50-dB SL to assure maximum performance. When testing normal hearing subjects, 50-dB HL or the subject's most comfortable listening level (MCL) is commonly used (Silman, Silverman, & Emmer, 2000). It should be noted that the level at which the stimulus should be presented to achieve maximum performance is dependent on the stimulus type. For example, digits and words for the W-22 lists can be presented at lower levels than CVs (Berlin & Cullen, 1977). Few data are available on the effects of small interaural intensity differences on dichotic outcomes; however, Berlin and Cullen (1977) reported that interaural differences between 5 and 10 dB produced response decrements in the test ear when the signal to the opposite ear was of higher intensity and the overall presentation level was about 50-dB HL.

Effect of Peripheral Hearing Loss

Peripheral hearing loss is known to affect central auditory processing test results, with some tests being more influenced than others. Accordingly, many studies have been conducted to examine the robustness of various dichotic test materials to hearing loss. In general the findings suggest that dichotic digit test materials are not significantly affected by mild to moderate cochlear hearing loss (Musiek, 1983; Musiek, Gollegly, Kibbe, & Verkest-Lenz, 1991; Speaks, Niccum, & Van Tassel, 1985; Strouse & Wilson, 2000). Different cutoff points have been suggested, however, to identify (C)APD in patients with normal hearing (90%) and in those with mild to moderate hearing loss (80%) (Musiek, 1983; Musiek et al., 1991).

Speaks, Niccum, and Van Tassell (1985) compared the effect of stimulus material on dichotic listening performance in patients with sensorineural hearing loss. Their findings revealed digit material to be least affected by hearing loss compared to monosyllables that emphasized either low-frequency vowel sounds (e.g., car, bow, and boy) or high-frequency consonant sounds (e.g., pan, fan, and coat). CV syllables were seen to be most affected by peripheral hearing loss. CV syllables vulnerability to the effects of peripheral hearing loss is due to the fact that CV recognition depends on the fast resolution of intensity and frequency transitions (Chermak, 2001). Stimuli with greater complexity of intensity and frequency interactions, especially over a restricted time period, place a greater demand on cochlear processing and therefore will be influenced more by peripheral hearing loss (Chermak & Musiek, 1997).

Effect of Age on Dichotic Listening Tests

Studies of the effect of developmental age on dichotic listening have generally shown a greater REA in younger age groups that tends to become smaller with age. Berlin and colleagues (Berlin, Lowe-Bell, Cullen, Thompson, & Loovis, 1973) tested dichotic listening in children aged 5 to 13 years old using dichotic CVs. They noted that developmental effects were seen only when subjects were required to repeat both stimulus pairs, and proposed this finding to be attributed to increased channel capacity with increasing age. Normative data for the SSW test (Katz & Wilde (1994) indicate that the REA is pronounced in children age 6 years and decreases with age until approximately 11 years where the ear differences are minimal (see Figure 9–2). A similar finding is reported for the REA in the competing words and competing sentences subtests of SCAN-C (Keith, 1998). The decreasing REA as a function of age is probably related to the maturational course of the corpus callosum, which becomes fully myelinated at approximately 11 years of age (Obrzut, Hynd, & Pirozzolo 1981). However, Obrzut et al. (1981) also reported persistent minimal REAs in all listening modes including directed left.

An example of changes in ear advantage with increasing age (and as a function of linguistic complexity) is shown in Figure 9–3. In Figure 9–3A, this 6-year-old child shows a slight REA for dichotic CVs, with generally increasing REA for stimuli with higher linguistic content. Also seen in Figure 9–3A is the overall improvement in performance from competing words to spondees to sentences,

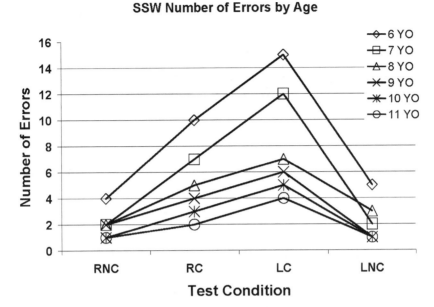

Figure 9–2. Changes in ear advantage with age on the Staggered Spondaic Word (SSW) test.

demonstrating the benefits of context and reduced message set (in the case of spondees). At age 11 years (Figure 9–3B), the dichotic CV performance has changed little from age 6 years while overall improvement is found for all the other tests. Minimal REA is observed at this age.

Studies on elderly adult subjects generally reveal a decreased REA with increasing age. This deterioration or breakdown in binaural processing has been attributed to two factors: cognitive processing deficits, such as selective attention and or short-term memory deficits (Craig, 1965; Inglis & Caird, 1963), and the reduced efficiency of the auditory system to process dichotically presented stimuli secondary to degenerative changes in the CANS (Kirikae, Sao, & Shitara., 1963). Martin and Cranford (1991) correlated the dichotic digit tests results of 40 female subjects aged 20 to 80 years old with their late auditory evoked potentials (LAEP).

Their study revealed a decline in ability to perform the free recall dichotic task with advancing age; however, there was no correlation between this behavioral deficit and the LAEPs. They concluded that impairment of central auditory processing was not the only explanation of decreased dichotic test scores in elderly subjects. They argued that decreased dichotic performance might be expected in older adults due to degenerative changes from aging processes and that these changes are likely to affect all systems rather than affecting a particular organ or system in isolation.

Differentiating CANS and Cognitive Dysfunction

Hallgren, Larsby, Lyxell, and Arlinger (2001) reported a left ear deficit to CV stimuli that increased with age. The authors related this asymmetry to cognitive

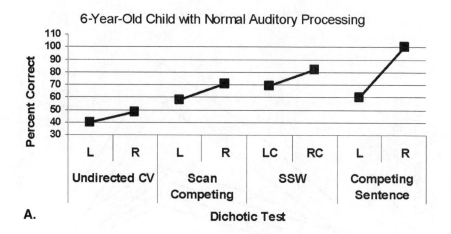

A.

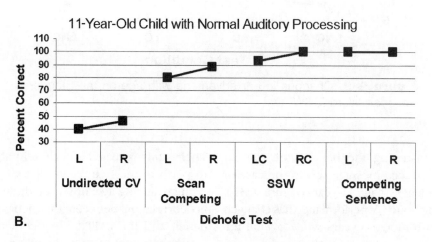

B.

Figure 9–3. A. and **B.** Mean results of dichotic testing for children ages 6 and 11 years showing overall improvement in performance and decreasing right ear advantage (REA) in older children.

processing dysfunction. Their findings correspond to those of an earlier study by Jerger, Chmiel, Allen, and Wilson (1994) that showed a correlation between an increasing left ear deficit on dichotic listening with increasing age, particularly for individuals over 80 years of age. Chmiel and Jerger (1996) proposed a method to differentiate cognitive from central auditory processing effects on dichotic listening. The differentiation is accomplished by comparing performances in the free recall dichotic mode to the directed attention mode. Subjects with cognitive deficit are expected to score more poorly in the free recall mode than in the directed listening mode, whereas subjects with auditory processing difficulty should score poorly in both free recall and directed recall modes.

Summary Comments on the Interpretation of Dichotic Test Results

The following are some general principles for interpreting ear advantage scores in children and adults:

- An REA within normative values indicates that language is appropriately established in the left cerebral hemisphere.
- An atypical LEA indicates that the individual may have right hemisphere or mixed dominance for language.
- An atypical REA in a directed right-ear first task and an atypical LEA in a directed left ear first task is an abnormal finding associated with neurologically based language and learning disabilities (Obrzut, Hynd, & Pirozzolo, 1981).
- The finding of an atypically large REA (i.e., left-ear deficit) as children approach 11 or 12 years, or in an adolescent, indicates a possible developmental delay in maturation of the CANS.
- It is necessary to retest the child annually for two to four years in order to determine if auditory maturation is occurring or the neurologic pathways are changing (e.g., through plasticity),
- When individuals have a strong LEA for all dichotic tests, and no evidence of specific lesion of the left hemisphere or corpus callosum, there is behavioral test evidence of a neurologically based language/learning disorder.
- Failure to show improvement in overall performance and/or failure to show improvement in the left ear score, as shown on repeated testing over several years, indicates an auditory system that has experienced developmental delay or damage to the central auditory system that is not improving.
- Individuals who show decreasing performance on dichotic tests (or any central auditory test) over a series of repeated administrations should be referred for medical/neurologic evaluation.
- Lesion effects include contralateral deficits, paradoxical left ear deficits, and bilateral deficits, depending on the specific site of involvement. Hemispheric, callosal, and brainstem involvement all can yield deficits in dichotic listening.

The author's experience suggests that children who do not show improvement in overall performance or who have substantial and persistent abnormalities on dichotic tests will likely have a long remediation course, and probably experience residual deficits into adulthood. The question of whether subjects who have abnormalities on dichotic tests should be referred for neurologic evaluation is a complex issue, depending on many factors. The fact is that the majority of individuals with developmental disorders and abnormal dichotic test results will have negative findings on neurologic evaluation including MRI exams. However, they may show abnormal findings on functional magnetic resonance imaging (fMRI) testing as discussed below.

Dichotic Test Abnormalities in Subjects with Language, Learning, and Reading Disorders

Enhanced left ear performance compared to the right ear is a frequently observed dichotic test outcome in children with phonologic, reading, and language disorders. This left ear advantage (LEA) is considered abnormal in subjects of any age. Another abnormal finding is the child or adult with a strong right ear advantage (REA) on directed ear testing with the right ear first, and a strong left ear advantage (LEA) on directed ear testing with the left ear first. A switch in ear advantage on directed ear testing is found in children with specific learning disabilities (Obrzut, Hynd, & Pirozzolo, 1981). As indicated in previous paragraphs, the typically developing child has an REA with better performance in the right than the left ear and the size of the REA is a function of the linguistic content of the signal and the age of the subject.

The finding of an LEA can be the result of several factors, including presence of a lesion of the auditory reception areas of the dominant left hemisphere, lack of typical left hemisheric dominance for language in a child or adult, or mixed dominance for language in the right and left hemispheres. An example of the latter scenario is illustrated in a 6-year-old boy with a history of developmental delays in language and reading. The child's birth, motor, and cognitive development were normal. There was no history of head injury at birth or during childhood; his peripheral hearing was normal and there was no history of early middle-ear disease. This was a normal healthy boy with a language and reading disorder. Tests of auditory processing included filtered words, auditory figure ground, competing words, and competing sentence subtests of SCAN-C (Keith, 2000) and the SSW (Katz, 1962). Test findings indicated a left ear advantage for all subtests including the monaural degraded speech tests, as well as dichotic words and sentences, and the SSW (see Figures 9–4A and 9–4B). The typically developing 6-year-old child will not show ear differences on monaural tests of degraded speech, but will show a substantial right ear advantage on all dichotic speech tests. The findings on this child and others like him indicate that the left hemisphere is not the dominant hemisphere for language, and that there is minimally mixed dominance for language or abnormal right hemisphere dominance for language. In this case magnetic resonance imaging (MRI) studies were conducted upon recommendation from his pediatrician due to the significance of the auditory processing test results and the medical history of one of this child's siblings. Nonetheless, the MRI findings were completely normal confirming that there was no lesion of the left or right hemisphere or the corpus callosum.

The finding of substantial left ear advantage in typically developing children is unusual and is considered abnormal. For example, normative data on the competing words subtest of SCAN-C (Keith, 2000) indicate that 95% of 10-year-old children (as an example) have a left ear advantage of only 6% or less with directed ear instructions with the right ear first and only 10% or less advantage on directed left ear first. There are no data available for the number of normal children showing a left ear advantage on

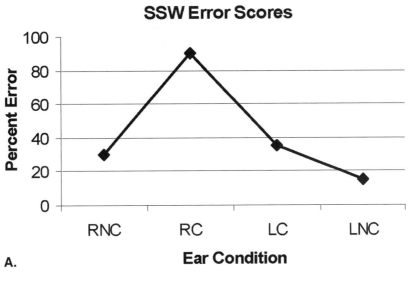

A.

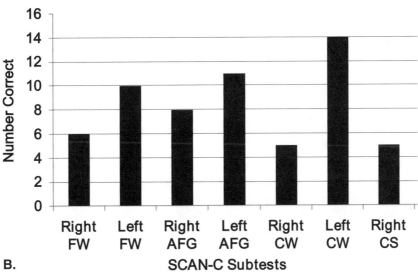

B.

Figure 9–4. A. and **B.** Abnormal central auditory test performance showing left ear advantage in a 6-year-old boy with reading and language disorder on the Staggered Spondaic Word (SSW) test, and the Filtered Words (FW), Auditory-Figure Ground (AFG), Competing Words (CW), and Competing Sentences (CS) subtests of the SCAN-C.

the SSW; however, an LEA of any magnitude is considered abnormal on that test. The present authors have never examined a child with normal language and reading abilities who has a substantial LEA on any dichotic speech test, and every child examined by the authors who has reversed dominance for language as indicated by substantial LEAs on dichotic digits, words, spondees, or sentences has had language and/or reading problems. Many studies confirm that children and adults with substantial reversed dominance for language have related language, learning, and reading problems.

The basis of the language and reading disorders resulting from reversed hemispheric dominance for language can be attributed to inefficiency of information processing when areas of the brain not designed to manage language or phonologic processing are involved in those tasks (Breznitz, 2006). Neuropsychological models (Gazzaniga, Ivry, & Mangun, 2002; Josse & Tzourio-Mazoyer, 2003; Kandel, Schwartz, & Jessel, 2000) attribute traits associated with the left side of the brain to include:

- Linear cognitive processing: from part to whole, straightforward, logical
- Sequential cognitive processing: from first to last
- Symbolic cognitive processing: symbols as pictures; likes to use letters, words, mathematical symbols
- Logical cognitive processing: information processed piece by piece using logic to solve problem
- Verbal cognitive processing: processes thoughts and ideas with words
- Reality-based cognitive processing: based on reality; focused on rules and regulations;

Whereas traits associated with the right side of the brain include:

- Holistic cognitive processing: from whole to parts; sees big picture first, not details

- Random cognitive processing: changes from one task to another before completing the first (or completed out of order)
- Concrete cognitive processing: needs to see, feel, or touch to understand; hands-on
- Intuitive cognitive processing: knows the answer but not sure how one "got it"
- Nonverbal cognitive processing: knows what you mean but has trouble expressing it; visual
- Fantasy-oriented cognitive processing: tries to change environment rather than adjusting to it; makes up rules rather than follows them

Simplistically, the left hemisphere has a superior ability to process verbal information, and the right hemisphere is specialized for the processing of spatially structured information (Springer & Deutsch, 1981). The left hemisphere has specialized mechanisms for rapid sensory integration within the tens of milliseconds range. Tallal, Miller, and Fitch (1993) speculated that the left hemisphere specializes in linguistic processing because of the temporal specialization of that hemisphere. Lesions of the speech areas of the left hemisphere or developmental abnormalities in which language is processed in the right hemisphere lead to inefficient information processing. This inefficiency results in decreased speed and accuracy of information processing, ultimately resulting in auditory processing disorders, phonologic disorders, language impairments, and reading impairments (Breznitz, 2006). These impairments, therefore, are neurobiologically related such that individuals with reversed dominance for language, shown by abnormalities in dichotic listening tests, exhibit slower and less accurate processing of information, slower acquisition of information, and residual deficits into adulthood.

Relationships Among Electrophysiologic and Imaging Measures and Dichotic Tests of Auditory Processing

In addition to behavioral measures of auditory processing abilities, the use of advanced electrophysiologic measures and neuroimaging techniques of the central auditory system are steadily uncovering the *what, where*, and *how* the brain processes auditory information. Several investigations have been and are currently underway utilizing each technique in isolation. However, an increasing trend in more recent investigations is the use of a combination of two or more of these methods to obtain a more thorough understanding of both the structure and function of the CANS. The electrophysiologic examination gives a more accurate assessment of the speed of cognitive processes and neuroimaging gives a more accurate spatial assessment (Demonet, Tjoerru, & Cardebat, 2005).

Functional Magnetic Resonance Imaging

With new advancements in functional magnetic resonance imaging (fMRI) technology, imaging techniques are not only providing data on the hemodynamic or BOLD (blood oxygenation level dependent) responses of the cortical auditory areas of the brain, but are also beginning to provide similar data on the responses of the lower subcortical auditory pathways as well (Yetkin, Roland, Mendelsohn, & Purdy, 2004). The first reported study to show activation of the lower subcortical auditory areas of the brain (medial geniculate body, inferior colliculus, lateral lemniscus, superior olivary complex, and cochlear nucleus) during pure tone auditory stimulation was conducted at the University of Texas Southwestern Medical Center (Yetkin et al., 2004). The findings of this initial study suggest that in-depth examination of the entire auditory neural pathways from cochlear nuclei to auditory cortex is now possible. This study creates an impetus for subsequent investigation of the auditory neural pathways employing appreciably more complex auditory stimuli.

Even with significant advancements in auditory research with fMRI technology, obstacles still remain. The most significant challenge in conducting auditory studies with fMRI techniques has been to create and maintain an appropriate acoustic environment in which to conduct these investigations. "The acoustic scanner noise that is generated by rapid gradient switching in echo planar imaging (EPI) is an important confounding factor in auditory fMRI" (Schwarzbauer, Davis, Rodd, & Johnsrude, 2006, p. 774). The acoustic scanner noise may often reach in excess of 120-dB SPL (Schwarzbauer et al., 2006). Many such investigations report this confounding variable as a contribution to unexplained or inconclusive results. However, with the introduction and reported success of silent fMRI technology, it seems probable that future auditory investigations may be able to eliminate or at least diminish this interference (Schwarzbauer et al., 2006; Yetkin et al., 2004).

Currently, most fMRI data on both normal and abnormal auditory function have been derived from investigations conducted in adult populations. Equivalent data on the auditory function of children are presently limited due in part to the challenges of keeping young children immobile during fMRI examination. Sedation measures in this population are typically utilized when examinations using structural imaging are medically necessary; however, the precise effects of sedation on higher cortical functional processes still remain uncertain. An investigation performed by Altman and Bernal (2001) examined brain activation patterns of sedated children during functional auditory and visual stimulation (Altman & Bernal, 2001). They concluded that "visual and auditory cortices can be activated in children who have been sedated. Auditory activation is seen in temporal and frontal lobes" (p. 56).

In addition to the limitations of immobilizing infants and young children for fMRI evaluation, problems also exist in the interpretation of the data once obtained, as the brains of infants and very young children differ considerably from adult brains (Demonet, Thierry, & Cardebat, 2005). These differences may be related to myelination, vascularization, and metabolic factors. Despite these differences, a few researchers have forged ahead in investigating this population and have reported successful outcomes in conducting functional neuroimaging assessments of speech perception in nonsedated neonates and infants (Dehaene-Lambertz, Dehaene, & Hertz-Pannier, 2002; Dehaene-Lambertz & Gliga, 2004).

fMRI and Brain Lesion Studies

fMRI examinations of brain activation patterns to auditory stimuli in normal-hearing subjects have provided greater understanding of the nature and function of the mechanisms of the human auditory system. Auditory studies conducted with fMRI have examined hemodynamic brain activation patterns related to the psychoacoustic phenomena of pitch, loudness, and duration judgments using simple auditory stimuli (Lasota et al., 2003). Because data are more readily available on subjects from young and relatively healthy individuals who have experienced acute brain lesions, most of our understanding of how the auditory system works has been derived from these subjects. Functional images obtained from individuals with brain lesions in conjunction with behavioral auditory test results are providing more insight into the specific functions of individual components of the auditory neural pathways and, ultimately, their specific contributions to overall human auditory processing abilities.

One such contribution was derived from a case report that involved the sudden onset of acute cortical deafness experience by a 21-year-old male (Musiek, Charette, Morse, & Baran, 2004). Because central deafness is a rare occurrence, this case has shed light on the significance that bilateral lesions of the inferior colliculi play in higher auditory functions. The young man reported in this case study experienced cortical deafness from bilateral lesions of the inferior colliculi as a complication of meningitis. Documentation of the recovery of his hearing was made through audiologic evaluations from very near the initial onset through approximately a 10-month aural rehabilitation program (Musiek et al., 2004). The gradual recovery of near-normal auditory function beginning with the processing of simple acoustic stimuli to more complex auditory stimuli over a

10-month period may be attributed to either the plasticity from spontaneous recovery, intervention measures, or a combination of both.

Many other brain lesion studies also have revealed data on the functions of the components of the auditory neural pathways. One unusual case study that has helped decipher the functions of discrete unilateral lesions on the lower auditory system was reported by Cho et al. (2005). This case study involved a 32-year-old right-handed woman with an isolated unilateral lesion of the lateral lemniscus. Although the subject complained of tinnitus and hearing impairment contralateral to the lesion, she was found audiometrically normal for pure tone and speech tests bilaterally. However, further evaluation with dichotic listening tests showed no response in the ear contralateral to the lesion (Cho et al., 2005). Overall, this case study illustrates the importance of implementing more complex and taxing dichotic listening tests to expose central auditory pathway pathology in the presence of normal speech and pure tone results.

Dichotic Listening and fMRI

fMRI in conjunction with dichotic listening tasks are helping determine hemispheric lateralization of language through the observation of brain activation patterns during the processing of simple and complex speech stimuli. Comparison of adult brain activation patterns during binaural and dichotic testing reveals that dichotic speech stimuli cause brain activation patterns different from binaural stimuli (Thomsen, Rimol, Ersland, & Hugdahl (2004). These findings suggest that when the brain is required to employ tasks involving forced listening,

or to attend to stimuli presented to one ear while ignoring the stimuli presented to the other ear, the prefrontal cortex becomes active. However, for the binaural condition, activation was only observed in the auditory areas of the brain with no observation of prefrontal participation. This study suggests that the prefrontal cortex is involved in more complex dichotic auditory tasks that require increased or "forced" attention to the auditory stimuli.

Other investigations in this area (Thomsen et al., 2004) examined the role of attention in dichotic listening tasks between younger and older subjects. Because the area of the prefrontal cortex is believed to assist in activities that are involved in attention, this study was conducted to observe the effects that aging may have on dichotic or forced listening tasks. Older subjects in the study appeared to have less activation in the attention areas (prefrontal cortex) of the brain than the younger subjects.

Dichotic Listening and Epilepsy

Dichotic listening tasks in conjunction with fMRI evaluation have been crucial in helping to determine cerebral hemispheric language lateralization in severe epileptic children who are presurgical candidates for temporal lobectomies. The Wada test (or the intracarotid amorbarbital procedure) has been the primary means of determining hemispheric lateralization since its introduction in 1949 (Meador & Loring, 2005). The Wada test involves the anesthetization of one brain hemisphere while requiring the subject to respond to subjective tests of language from the nonanesthetized hemisphere. This technique is very accurate in determining hemisphere lateralization for language but is a very invasive procedure with multiple high risks.

Due to the risks of the Wada test, Fernandes, Smith, Logan, Crawley, and McAndrews (2006) explored a reliable noninvasive alternative procedure to determine language lateralization in presurgical patients. They examined brain activation patterns through fMRI evaluation while subjects were given a dichotic listening test (i.e., Forced Dichotic Word Test [FDWT]). The language lateralization scores obtain with the (FDWT) test were compared with the hemodynamic brain response observed using fMRI. Agreement between fMRI and FDWT was greater for patients with left language lateralization compared to bilateral language representation on the FDWT; however, overall, the dichotic listening test provided a valid estimate of language lateralization in children who were required to undergo temporal lobe resection to eliminate seizure activity.

Dichotic Listening and Electrophysiology

Electrophysiologic measures or auditory evoked potentials (AEPs) are an additional objective means of assessing the auditory function of the brain by recording the electrical responses of neuronal synaptic activity measured at the scalp. In addition, magnetoencephalography (MEG), or event-related fields, are also a measure of cortical neuronal activity. MEG responses are the small magnetic fields that are produced by active neurons. Advanced brain mapping technology utilizing multiple-channel recordings for both cortical AEPs and MEGs are revealing the electrical or magnetic responses of the brain over the entire surface of the head. Through the use of both brain mapping measures, more data have been reported on the activity of the whole brain response to auditory stimulation as well as from the primary auditory and adjacent areas in the temporal lobes.

Many AEP studies have been conducted with the intent to establish an objective physiologic means of identifying children with (C)APD. AEP studies have been utilized to determine the presence of lower subcortical auditory pathway dysfunction all the way up to the higher cortical responses at or near the primary auditory cortices. As the coding of auditory information is believed to be performed at the lower subcortical levels, many studies have been interested in the early brainstem response activity as a potential source of dysfunction in children with (C)APD.

Delb, Strauss, Hohenberg, and Plinkert (2003) were interested in examining the binaural interaction component (BIC) of the brainstem through auditory brainstem response (ABR) testing. Hypothesizing that dysfunction at the brainstem level may be an etiology of a subtype of (C)APD in children, they sought to determine if a correlation between the BIC and dichotic tests of brainstem function could be found. If a correlation between BIC and dichotic tests were established, the BIC could possibly provide the basis for an objective means of screening for (C)APD in children. Their results, however, yielded overall efficiency of only 76% between the measures; therefore, based on this outcome, they concluded that the BIC may be only of some diagnostic value in identifying various types of (C)APD (Delb et al., 2003).

The majority of electrophysiologic studies of auditory processing abilities have focused on the later auditory responses or cortical evoked potentials. Eichele, Nordby, Rimol, and Hugdahl (2005) investigated interhemispheric differences in N1 latencies in 12 normal college students. They compared these latencies to the subjects' behavioral dichotic results to determine whether a correlation existed between hemispheric latencies and ear advantage. Eichele et al. (2005) reported an overall group effect of an REA. They also reported that the corresponding N1 latencies measured from the left temporal lobe were approximately 15 msec earlier than corresponding latencies from the right temporal lobe responses. The overall results from this study suggest that the left hemisphere, or dominant hemisphere, responds more quickly to auditory stimuli than the right hemisphere or nondominant hemisphere.

Moncrieff, Jerger, Wambacq, Greenwald, and Black (2004) also examined cortical evoked potential latencies and amplitudes in a group of 10 children with dyslexia and 10 control subjects while they listened to quasi-dichotic auditory stimuli (i.e., a familiar fairy tale). The children classified as dyslexic were found to have a left ear deficit (LED) on the Competing Words subtest of the SCAN-C (Keith, 2000), while the control group scored within normal limits. The children with dyslexia (and LEDs) had reduced peak amplitudes and longer latencies for the P800 response than the control group. These findings suggest slower synaptic activity and slower interhemispheric transfer of information among the children with dyslexia than those in the normal group.

A study utilizing a combination of dichotic listening, electrophysiology measures, and neuroimaging techniques to investigate an auditory processing dis-

order was conducted by Jerger, Martin, and McColl (2004). This case study was conducted on 10-year-old twin girls, one (twin E), who was suspected of having an auditory processing disorder due to electrophysiologic abnormalities during a dichotic listening, paradigm and one (twin C), who showed normal responses. Jerger et al. (2004) hypothesized that the difference between the brains of the twins may be due to reduced myelination of the corpus callosum of twin E, leading to the inhibition of normal interhemispheric transfer. Each twin underwent diffusion tensor magnetic imaging specifically utilized for analysis of the white matter of the brain. The results from the neuroimaging study revealed that twin E had reduced myelination of the corpus callosum compared to twin C. This finding led the researchers to conclude that reduced or incomplete myelination of the corpus callosum may be an underlying factor contributing to some auditory processing disorders in children.

Summary

In the opening paragraph of this chapter we noted that dichotic listening tests are among the most powerful of the behavioral auditory processing test battery for the assessment of hemispheric function, interhemispheric transfer of information, development and maturation of the auditory nervous system, and the identification of lesions of the auditory nervous system. Abnormal findings on dichotic tests are found in individuals with various developmental language, reading, and learning disorders and indicate a neurobiologic basis for their problems. In addition, recent studies correlating findings of electrophysiologic and fMRI findings with dichotic test results lend further understanding to the nature and function of the mechanisms of the human auditory system.

Acknowledgement. The authors wish to acknowledge Siti Zamratol-Mai Sarah Mukari who contributed to portions of this chapter.

References

Altman, N. R., & Bernal, B. (2001). Brain activation in sedated children: Auditory and visual functional MR imaging. *Radiology*, *221*, 56–63.

American Speech-Language-Hearing Association. (1996). Central auditory processing: Current status of research and implications for clinical practice. *American Journal of Audiology*, *5*, 51–55.

American Speech-Language-Hearing Association. (2005). (Central) auditory processing disorders—The role of the audiologist [Position statement]. Available at: http://www.asha.org/members/deskref-journals/deskref/default.

Berlin, C. I., & Cullen, J. K., Jr. (1977). Acoustic problems in dichotic listening tasks. In S. Segalowitz & F. Gruber (Eds.), *Language development and neurological theory* (pp. 75–88). New York: Academic Press.

Berlin, C., Lowe-Bell, S., Cullen, J., Thompson, C., & Loovis, C. (1973). Dichotic speech perception: An interpretation of right ear advantage and temporal offset effects. *Journal of the Acoustical Society of America*, *53*, 699–709.

Berlin, C. I., & McNeil, M. R. (Eds.). (1976). *Dichotic listening*. New York: Academic Press.

Berlin C. I., Porter, R. J., Jr., Lowe-Bell, S. S., Berlin, H. L., Thompson, C. L., & Hughes, L. F. (1973). Dichotic signs of the recognition of speech elements in normals, temporal lobectomees, and hemispherectomees. *IEEE Transactions on Audio and Electroacoustics, AU-21*, 189–195.

Bocca, E., & Calearo, C. (1963). Central hearing processes. In J. Jerger (Ed.), *Modern developments in audiology* (pp. 337–370). New York: Academic Press.

Breznitz, Z. (2006). *Fluency in reading: Synchronization of processes*. Mahwah, NJ: Lawrence Erlbaum Associates.

Broadbent, D. (1954). The role of auditory localization in attention and memory span. *Journal of Experimental Psychology*, *47*, 191–196.

Bryden, N., Munhall, K., Allard, F. (1983). Attentional biases for the right-ear effect in dichotic listening. *Brain and Language*, *18*, 236–248.

Calearo, M. D., & Antonelli, A. R. (1973). Disorders of the central auditory nervous system. In M. Paparella & D. Shumrick (Eds.), *Otolaryngology* (pp. 407–425). Philadelphia: Saunders.

Carhart, R. (Ed.). (1970). *Neurological implications of the capacity for message separation*. Odense, Denmark: Andelsbortrykkeriet.

Chermak, G. D. (2001), Auditory processing disorder: An overview for the clinician. *The Hearing Journal*, *54*, 10–26.

Chermak, G. D., & Musiek F. E. (1997). *Central auditory processing disorders: New perspectives*. San Diego, CA: Singular Publishing Group.

Cherry, E. C. (1953). Some experiments on the recognition of speech with one and with two ears. *Journal of the Acoustical Society of America*, *25*, 975–979.

Cherry, E. C., & Taylor, W. K. (1954). Some further experiments upon the recognition of speech, with one and with two ears. *Journal of the Acoustical Society of America*, *26*, 554–559.

Chmiel, R., & Jerger, J. (1996). Hearing aid use, central auditory disorder, and hearing handicap in elderly persons. *Journal of* the *American Academy of Audiology*, *17*, 190-202.

Cho, T. H., Fischer, C., Nighoghossian, N., Hermier, M., Sindou, M., & Mauguiere, F. (2005). Auditory and electrophysiological patterns of a unilateral lesion of the lateral lemniscus. *Audiology and Neuro-Otology*, *10*, 153-158.

Clark, L. E., & Knowl, J. B. (1973). Age differences in dichotic listening performance. *Journal of Gerontology*, *28*, 173-178.

Craig, F. (1965). Age differences in dichotic listening. *Quarterly Journal of Experimental Psychology*, *17*, 227-240.

Cullen, J. K., Jr., Thompson, C. L., Hughes, L. F., Berlin C. I., & Samson, D. (1974). The effects of varied acoustic parameters on performance in dichotic speech perception tasks. *Brain and Language*, *1*, 307-322.

Dehaene-Lambertz, G., Dehaene, S., & Hertz-Pannier, L. (2002). Functional neuroimaging of speech perception in infants. *Science*, *298*, 2013-2015.

Dehaene-Lambertz, G., & Gliga T. (2004). Common neural basis for phoneme processing in infants and adults. *Journal of Cognitive Neuroscience*, *16*, 1375-1387.

Delb, W., Strauss, D. J., Hohenberg, G., & Plinkert , P. K. (2003). The binaural interaction component (BIC) in children with central auditory processing disorders (CAPD). *International Journal of Audiology*, *42*, 401-412.

Demonet, J. F., Thierry, G., & Cardebat, D. (2005). Renewal of the neurophysiology of language: Functional neuroimaging. *Physiology Review*, *85*, 49-95.

Denckla, M. B. (1989). Executive function, the overlap zone between attention deficit hyperactivity disorder and learning disabilities. *International Pediatrics*, *4*, 155-160.

Eichele, T., Nordby, H., Rimol, L. M., & Hugdahl, K. (2005). Asymmetry of evoked potential latency to speech sounds predicts the ear advantage in dichotic listening. *Brain Research and Cognitive Brain Research*, *24*, 405-412.

Fernandes, M.A, Smith, M. L., Logan, W., Crawley, A., & McAndrews, M. P. (2006). Comparing language lateralization determined by dichotic listening and fMRI activation in frontal and temporal lobes in children with epilepsy. *Brain and Language*, *96*, 106-114.

Fifer, R., Jerger, J., Berlin, C., Tobey, E., & Campbell, J. (1983). Development of a dichotic sentence identification test for hearing-impaired adults. *Ear and Hearing*, *4*, 300-305.

Gazzaniga, M. S., Ivry, R., & Mangun, G. R. (2002). *Fundamentals of cognitive neuroscience* (2nd ed.). New York: W.W. Norton.

Geffen, G.,& Caudrey, D. (1981). Reliability and validity of the dichotic monitoring test for language laterality. *Neuropsychologia*, *19*, 413-423.

Gelfand, S. A., Hoffman, S., Waltzman, S.B., & Piper, N. (1980). Dichotic CV recognition at various interaural temporal onset asynchronies. Effect of age. *Journal of the Acoustical Society of America*, *68*, 1258-1261.

Hallgren, M., Larsby, B, Lyxell, B., & Arlinger S. (2001). Cognitive effects in dichotic speech testing in elderly persons. *Ear and Hearing*, *22*, 120-129.

Hugdahl, K. (1988). *Handbook of dichotic listening: Theory, methods and research*. Cichester, England: John Wiley & Sons

Hugdahl, K., & Andersson, L. (1986). The "forced attention paradigm" in dichotic listening to CV-syllables: A comparison between adults and children. *Cortex*, *22*, 417-432.

Hynd, G., Cohen, M., Obrzut, J. (1983). Dichotic consonant-vowel testing in the diagnosis of learning disabilities in children. *Ear and Hearing*, *4*, 283-286.

Inglis, J., & Caird, W. K. (1963). Age differences in successful responses to simultaneous stimulation. *Canadian Journal of Psychology*, *17*, 98-105.

Jancke, L. (2002). Does "callosal relay" explain ear advantage in dichotic monitoring? *Laterality*, *7*, 309-320.

Jancke, L., & Steinmetz , H. (1994). Interhemispheric transfer time and corpus callosum size. *NeuroReport, 5*, 2385-2388.

Jerger, J., Chimel, R., Allen, J., & Wilson A. (1994). Effects of age and gender on dichotic sentence identification. *Ear and Hearing, 15*, 274-286.

Jerger, J., & Martin, J. (in press). Dichotic listening tests in the assessment of auditory processing disorders. *Audiological Medicine.*

Jerger, J., Martin, J., & McColl, R. (2004). Interaural cross correlation of event-related potentials and diffusion tensor imaging in the evaluation of auditory processing disorder: A case study. *Journal of the American Academy of Audiology, 15*, 79-87.

Jerger, J., & Musiek, F.E. (2000). Report of the consensus conference on the diagnosis of auditory processing disorders in school-aged children. *Journal of the American Academy of Audiology, 11*, 467-474.

Josse, G., & Tzourio-Mazoyer, N. (2003). Review: Hemispheric specialization for language. *Brain Research Reviews, 44*, 1-12.

Kandel, E., Schwartz, J., & Jessel, T. (2000). *Principles of neural science* (4th ed.). New York: McGraw-Hill.

Katz, J. (1962). The use of staggered spondaic words for assessing the integrity of the central auditory nervous system. *Journal of Auditory Research, 2*, 327.

Katz, J., & Wilde, L. (1994). Auditory processing disorders. In J. Katz (Ed.), *Handbook of clinical audiology* (4th ed., pp. 490-502). Baltimore: Williams & Wilkins.

Keith, R. W. (1998). Re: "Development of SCAN-A: test of auditory processing disorders in adolescents and adults" *(Journal of the American Academy of Audiology. 1996, 6*, 286-292). *Journal of the American Academy of Audiology, 9*, 311.

Keith, R. W. (2000). Development and standardization of SCAN-C: Test for auditory processing disorders in children—revised. *Journal of the American Academy of Audiology, 11*, 438-445.

Kimura, D. (1961a). Some effects of temporal lobe damage on auditory perception. *Canadian Journal of Psychology, 15*, 156-165.

Kimura, D. (1961b). Cerebral dominance and the perception of verbal stimuli. *Canadian Journal of Psychology, 15*, 166-171.

Kimura, D. (1967). Functional asymmetry of the brain in dichotic listening. *Cortex, 22*, 163-178.

Kinsbourne, M. (1970). The cerebral basis of lateral asymmetries in attention. *Acta Psychologica, 33*, 193-201.

Kirikae, I., Sato, T., & Shitara T. (1963). A study of hearing in advance age. *Laryngoscope, 73*, 205-220.

Lasota, K. J., Ulmer, J. L., Firszt, J. B., Biswal, B. B., Daniels, D. L., & Prost R. W. (2003). Intensity-dependent activation of the primary auditory cortex in functional magnetic resonance imaging. *Journal of Computer Assisted Tomography, 27*, 213-218.

Markin, J., & Hook, P. (Eds.). (1983). *A multidisciplinary approach to central auditory evaluations.* Baltimore: University Park Press.

Martin, D. R., & Cranford J. L. (1991). Age-related changes in binaural processing: II. Behavioral findings. *American Journal of Otology, 12*, 365-369.

Matzker, J. J. (1959). Two new methods for the assessment of central auditory function in cases of brain disease. *Annals of Otology, 68*, 1185.

Meador, K. J., & Loring, D. W. (2005), The Wada test for language and memory lateralization. *Neurology, 65*, 659.

Medwetsky, L. (2002). Central auditory processing. In J. Katz (Ed.), *Handbook of clinical audiology* (5th ed., pp. 495-531). Baltimore: Williams & Wilkins.

Milner, B., Taylor, L., & Sperry, R. W. (1968). Lateralized suppression of dichotically presented digits after commissural section in man. *Science, 161*, 184-186.

Moncrieff, D., Jerger, J., Wambacq, I., Greenwald, R., & Black J. (2004). ERP evidence of a dichotic left-ear deficit in some dyslexic children. *Journal of the American Academy of Audiology, 15*, 518-534.

Musiek, F. E. (1983). Assessment of central auditory dysfunction: the dichotic digit test revisited. *Ear and Hearing, 4,* 79-83.

Musiek , F. E., Charette, L., Morse, D., & Baran, J. A. (2004). Central deafness associated with a midbrain lesion. *Journal of the American Academy of Audiology, 15,* 133-151.

Musiek, F. E., Gollegly, K. M., Kibbe, K. S., & Verkest-Lenz S. B. (1991) Proposed screening test for central auditory disorders: Follow-up on the dichotic digits test. *American Journal of Otology, 12,* 109-113.

Musiek, F., & Pinheiro, M. (1985). Dichotic speech tests in the detection of central auditory function. In F. Musiek & M. Pinheiro (Eds.), *Assessment of central auditory dysfunction: Foundations and clinical correlates* (pp. 201-218). Baltimore: Williams & Wilkins.

Obrzut, J. G., Boliek, C. , & Obrzut, A. (1986). The effect of stimulus type and directed attention on dichotic listening with children. *Journal of Experimental Psychology, 41,* 198-209.

Obrzut, J. G., &, Pirozzolo, F. (1981). Effects of directed attention on cerebral asymmetry in normal and learning disabled children. *Developmental Psychology, 17,* 118-125.

Rasmussen, T., & Milner, B. (1975). Clinical and surgical studies of the cerebral speech areas in man. In K. J. Zülch, O. Creutzfeldt, & G. C. Galbraith (Eds.), *Cerebral localization* (238-255). New York: Springer-Verlag.

Schwarzbauer. C., Davis, M. H., Rodd, J. M., & Johnsrude, I. (2006). Interleaved silent steady state (ISSS) imaging: A new sparse imaging method applied to auditory fMRI. *Neuroimage, 29,* 774-782.

Silman, S., Silverman, C. A., & Emmer, M. B. (2000). Central auditory processing disorders and reduced motivation. *Journal of the American Academy of Audiology, 11,* 57-63.

Sparks, R., & Geshwind, N. (1968). Dichotic listening in man after section of neocortical commisure. *Cortex, 4,* 249-260.

Speaks, C., & Jerger, J. (1965). Method for measurement of speech identification. *Journal of Speech and Hearing Research, 8,* 185-194.

Speaks, C., Niccum, N., & Van Tassel, D. (1985). Effects of stimulus material on the dichotic listening performance of patients with sensorineural hearing loss. *Journal of Speech and Hearing Research, 28,* 16-25.

Springer, S. P. (1971). Ear asymmetry in a dichotic listening task. *Perception and Psychophysics, 10,* 239-241.

Springer, S. P., & Deutsch, G. (1981). *Left brain right brain*. San Francisco: W. H. Freeman.

Strouse, A. C., & Wilson, R. H. (2000). The effect of filtering and interdigit interval on the recognition of dichotic digits. *Journal of Rehabilitation Research and Development, 37,* 599-606.

Tallal, P., Miller, S., & Fitch, R. (1993). Neurobiological basis of speech: A case for the preeminence of temporal processing. In P. Tallal, A. M. Galaburda, R. R. Llinas, & C. von Euler (Eds.), *Temporal information processing in the nervous system: Special reference to dyslexia and dysphasia* (pp. 27-47). New York: Annals of the New York Academy of Sciences (Vol. 682).

Thomsen, T., Rimol, L. M., Ersland, L., & Hugdahl K. (2004). Dichotic listening reveals functional specificity in prefrontal cortex: An fMRI study. *Neuroimage, 21,* 211-218.

Thomsen, T., Specht, K., Rimol, L. M., Hammar, A., Nyttingnes, J., Ersland, L., & Hugdahl, K. (2004). Brain localization of attentional control in different age groups by combining functional and structural MRI. *Neuroimage, 22,* 912-919.

Tobin, H. (1985). Binaural interaction tests. In F. E. Musiek & M. Pinheiro (Eds.), *Assessment of central auditory dysfunction: Foundations and clinical correlates* (pp. 155-172). Baltimore: Williams & Wilkins.

Willeford, J. (1977). Assessing central auditory behavior in children: A test battery approach. In R. W. Keith (Ed.), *Central auditory dysfunction* (pp. 43-72). New York: Grune & Stratton.

Willeford, J., & Burleigh, J. (Eds.). (1994) Sentence procedures in central testing. In J. Katz (Ed.), *Handbook of clinical audiology* (4th ed., pp. 256–270). Baltimore: Williams & Wilkins.

Yetkin, F. Z., Roland, P. S., Mendelsohn, D. B., & Purdy, P. D. (2004). Functional magnetic resonance imaging of activation in subcortical auditory pathway. *Laryngoscope, 114,* 96–101.

CHAPTER 10

TEMPORAL PROCESSING AND TEMPORAL PATTERNING TESTS

JENNIFER BROOKE SHINN

Introduction

Auditory temporal processing can be defined as the perception of sound or the alteration of sound within a restricted or defined time domain (Musiek, Shinn, Jirsa, Bamiou, Baran, & Zaiden, 2005). One could argue that temporal processing is the fundamental component of most auditory processing capabilities. This is strongly supported by the fact that many, if not all, characteristics encompassing auditory information are in some way influenced by time (Pinheiro & Musiek, 1985). Temporal processing can be observed at many levels, ranging from the most basic level of neural timing in the auditory nerve to cortical processing for binaural hearing and speech perception (e.g., voice onset time to prosodic detail).

In diagnosing (central) auditory processing disorder ([C]APD), specifically with respect to temporal processing, there are two key knowledge domains with which clinicians should be conversant. First, one should possess a thorough understanding of temporal processing and its four subcomponents: (1) temporal ordering or sequencing, (2) temporal resolution or discrimination, (3) temporal integration or summation, and (4) temporal masking. In addition, one must be keenly aware of the diagnostic tools available, as well as the limitations of current diagnostic techniques.

The purpose of this chapter is to review: (1) clinical behavioral tests which assess the ability to analyze acoustic events over time, (2) the contribution of temporal tests to differential diagnosis, (3) the functional impact of temporal processing deficits, and (4) primary treatment strategies for temporal processing deficits. The reader is referred to Chapter 2 for elaboration of some of the psychoacoustic principles underlying aspects of temporal processing, to Chapter 11 for a review of tests of binaural interaction, and to Chapter 12 for a review of electrophysiologic measures of central auditory nervous system (CANS) timing.

Categories of Temporal Processing and Their Clinical Assessment

The underlying neural mechanisms of temporal processing are not well understood. We do know, however, that although brainstem and subcortical mechanisms support efficient processing, temporal processing appears dependent primarily on cerebral and interhemispheric processing (Pinherio & Musiek, 1985). Before discussing how best to evaluate temporal processing, it is necessary to review the types of temporal processes and their components. (See Chapter 3 for discussion of timing in the CANS.)

Generally, there are four categories of temporal processing of auditory signals that are critical to central auditory processing abilities. These include: (1) temporal ordering or sequencing, (2) temporal resolution or discrimination, (3) temporal integration or summation, and (4) temporal masking. Although auditory temporal processing has been studied extensively in the research arena, there is a paucity of information on clinical applications. Clinical measures of temporal ordering and temporal resolution are available; however, there are no clinically feasible

measures of temporal integration (i.e., summation), or of temporal masking. As discussed below, thorough evaluation of multiple temporal processes is important not only for proper diagnosis, but for targeted intervention designed to improve specific temporal processing deficit(s).

Temporal Ordering or Sequencing

Temporal ordering, or sequencing, refers to the processing of two or more auditory stimuli in their order of occurrence in time (Pinheiro & Musiek, 1985). This has been a highly investigated phenomenon, particularly because of its importance in speech perception (Fu, 2002; Hirsh, 1967; Neff, 1961; Pichora-Fuller & Souza, 2003). Accurate temporal ordering requires that both the left and right hemispheres be anatomically and physiologically intact. In the animal model, it has been demonstrated that following bilateral ablations of the auditory cortex, auditory pattern recognition is severely impaired (Colavita, Szelgio & Zimmer, 1974; Colavita & Weisberg, 1977; Diamond & Neff, 1957). It also has been demonstrated by Musiek and colleagues (1980, 1987, 1990) that both split-brain patients (i.e., patients with a surgically sectioned corpus callosum) and patients with cerebral lesions demonstrate significant deficits on frequency and duration pattern tests. The effect of cochlear hearing loss also has been investigated for both types of patterning tests (Musiek et al., 1987, 1990). Interestingly, the Duration Pattern Test seems relatively resistant to the effects of cochlear lesions because it is not highly dependent on good frequency discrimination (Musiek, Baran, & Pinheiro, 1990).

The ability to properly recognize, identify, and sequence auditory patterns involves several perceptual and cognitive processes (Pinheiro & Musiek, 1985). These processes are not restricted to one hemisphere alone, but rather require integration of information from both hemispheres across the corpus callosum (Musiek, Pinheiro, & Wilson, 1980). Until the split-brain study by Musiek and colleagues (1980), it was assumed that the temporal lobe of the left hemisphere was primarily responsible for temporal sequencing (Efron, 1963; Halperin, Nachshon, & Carmon, 1973). We now know that neither hemisphere alone can adequately process temporal patterns. Hence, pattern tests are sensitive to hemispheric lesions, as well as interhemispheric dysfunction (Musiek & Pinheiro, 1987; Musiek et al., 1990).

Figure 10–1 illustrates the responsibility of each ear, each hemisphere, and the corpus callosum with respect to processing of tonal stimuli. Information regarding contour recognition must be processed in the right hemisphere and then passed via the corpus callosum to the left hemisphere where the linguistic label is applied to the signal. In cases where poor verbal responses are produced in the presence of normal hummed responses, a perceptual auditory deficit cannot be assumed. Rather, an individual who can

Temporal Patterning Physiology

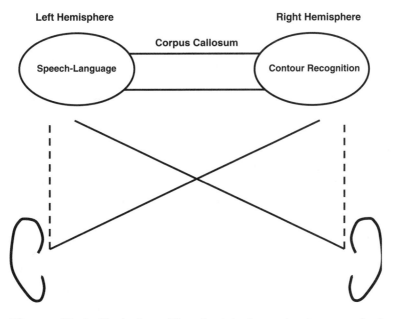

Figure 10–1. Illustration of the physiologic mechanisms required for temporal patterning. Contour recognition occurs in the right hemisphere and information is transferred across the corpus callosum to the left hemisphere where the linguistic process occurs.

hum, but not verbally label tonal patterns most likely suffers from dysfunction in interhemispheric transfer to the left hemisphere, or dysfunction in the left hemisphere, the presumed site of the speech processor (Pinherio & Musiek, 1985). Swisher and Hirsh (1972) reported evidence that the auditory cortex is responsible for not only the organization of neural events, but also for maintaining the proper sequence of the acoustic stimuli. In their study, individuals with left temporal lobe lesions needed a much greater onset time difference to identify the order of two rapidly presented acoustic stimuli.

The ability to properly sequence auditory information also is affected by subject and stimulus variables including: (1) subject training, (2) type of stimuli, (3) number of stimuli, (4) duration of stimuli, and (4) rate and manner of stimulus presentation (Pinheiro & Musiek, 1985). All are critical variables that should be taken into account when developing and administering pattern tests. For example, anyone who has ever administered temporal pattern tests is aware of the important effect of subject training. Efron (1963) demonstrated a significant difference in test performance between naïve and trained listeners. (This is true for almost all temporal processing tasks, as these are highly trainable processes.) Additionally, the type of stimuli presented is of importance. Stimuli used to date have included noise, tones, clicks, and speech. Also, as the number of components within the stimulus increases, so does the complexity of the task (i.e., three-component patterns are more difficult to process accurately than two-component patterns). Perhaps one of the most critical considerations is the effect of temporal integration, as reflected in

the duration of the components. If components of less than 200 msec duration are used, then subjects will perform more poorly than for those components greater than 200 msec (Warren & Obusek, 1972). This also holds true for the rate of presentation, where shorter interstimulus intervals result in poorer performance.

Evidence dating back to the early 1960s (Milner, 1962) suggests that individuals with temporal lobe lesions demonstrate poor performance when asked to identify differences in sequences of tones. Swisher and Hirsh (1972) identified a deficit in the ability of subjects with damage to the cerebrum to order tones with respect to their occurrence in time. A number of additional studies also demonstrated temporal ordering deficits in patients with lesions of the cerebrum (Belmont & Handler, 1971; De Renzi, Faglioni, & Villa, 1977; Karaseva, 1972).

Undoubtedly the most widely used clinical tests of temporal ordering are the Frequency Pattern Test and Duration Pattern Test (Emanuel, 2002). The Frequency Pattern Test was first introduced by Pinheiro and Ptacek in 1971. Patients are asked to verbalize the order of a series of three tones (Musiek, 1994). Due to their ease of administration and their efficiency (i.e., sensitivity and specificity), the pattern tests have gained rather widespread clinical acceptance (Emanuel, 2002). They are both sensitive (86%) and specific (92%) with respect to cerebral lesions of the CANS; however, their sensitivity to brainstem lesions is weaker (Musiek et al., 1987, 1990). Additionally, the Frequency Pattern Test bas been established as an excellent tool to use with young children, ages 8 and older (Musiek, 1994).

The Frequency Pattern Test is composed of three 200-msec tones, each with a 10-msec rise-fall time and a 150-msec interval between tones. The tones are 880 Hz and 1122 Hz, which allows for both a "low" and a "high" pitch representation. A 200-msec intertone interval is used. As seen in Figure 10–2, there are three tones presented in each token or trial with two frequencies per token, yielding six possible combinations (LLH, LHL, LHH, HLH, HLL, HHL). The Duration Pattern Test, developed by Dr. Frank Musiek, (Figure 10–3) also is composed of three pure tones per token. Each tone is 1000 Hz and is either 250 msec (short) or 500 msec (long) in duration. A 300-msec intertone interval is used for this test. Again, there are six randomizations that occur (LLS, LSL, LSS, SLS, SLL, SSL).

Duration Patterns

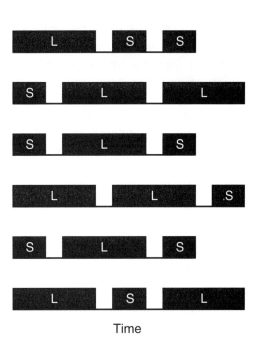

Time

Figure 10–3. The six duration patterns with time represented on the x-axis and amplitude on the y-axis. (L = long, 500 msec.; S = short, 280 msec.)

Both pattern tests utilize a 6 second interpattern interval.

It is recommended that each test be administered at approximately 50-dB SL in reference to either the speech recognition threshold or the pure-tone average. As there is little effect of intensity on performance on these tests, they can be presented at levels as low as 10-dB SL and yield essentially the same results (Musiek, 1994). This makes the pattern tests particularly useful in the assessment of central auditory processing in individuals with peripheral hearing loss.

Subjects are instructed that they will hear three tones that vary in either pitch (for the Frequency Pattern Test) or duration (for the Duration Pattern Test). The subject is asked to repeat the pattern that

Frequency (Pitch) Patterns

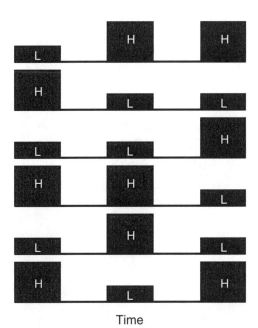

Time

Figure 10–2. The six frequency patterns with time represented on the x-axis and amplitude on the y-axis. (L = low frequency, 880 Hz; H = high frequency, 1122 Hz.)

they hear by verbally indicating either "high or low" or "long or short." It is recommended that the examiner train the patient by first using visual cues (such as finger pointing) in conjunction with the auditory stimuli. Once this has been mastered, then the visual cues should be removed and the examiner should ensure that the patient is able to complete the task in the auditory-only condition. Individuals should be encouraged to guess if they are unsure. Both pattern tests are scored in percent correct.

Temporal Resolution or Discrimination

Temporal resolution or discrimination refers to the shortest duration of time in which an individual can discriminate between two auditory signals (Gelfand, 1998). For brief sounds, this is generally about 2 to 3 msec (Phillips, 1999). The threshold for temporal resolution is known as *temporal auditory acuity* or *minimum integration time* (Greene, 1971).

Temporal resolution can be assessed utilizing a variety of methodologies. Historically, this has been achieved by determining the temporal modulation transfer function (TMTF) or gap detection threshold. TMTF assesses one's ability to detect amplitude modulation (see Figure 10–4). Gap detection tasks require subjects to indicate whenever they hear a "silent" interval embedded in an ongoing sound or noise burst (see Figure 10–5). The interstimulus interval is varied and the gap detection threshold (GDT) is defined as the shortest interval in a stimulus a lis-

Temporal Resolution
TMTF

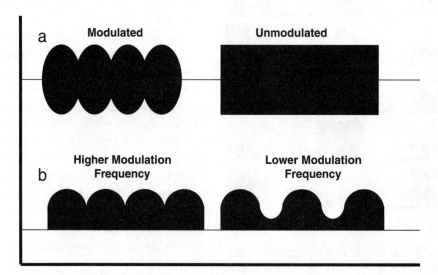

Figure 10–4. Illustration of lower and higher modulation frequency versus no modulation sounds used to determine temporal modulation transfer function.

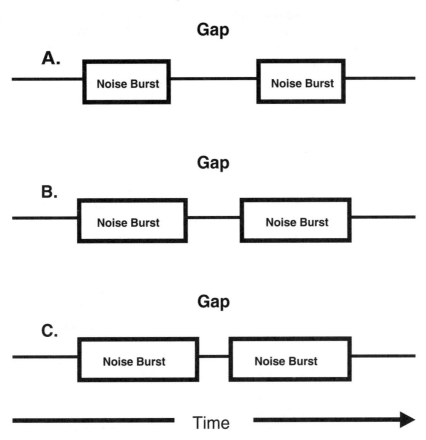

Figure 10–5. An example of gap detection. The progression from **A.** to **C.** demonstrates larger to smaller gap representations.

tener is able to detect (Lister, Besing, & Koehnke, 2002). As there are no clinically available tests using TMTFs, the following discussion focuses on clinical measures of gap detection.

One of the issues surrounding the incorporation of temporal resolution measures into clinical practice is that the assessment of temporal resolution abilities has traditionally been accomplished with classic psychoacoustic gap detection (GD) procedures. Such measures often are not feasible in a clinical setting

for a variety of reasons, which include the fact that they are often time consuming, making them difficult to use within a test battery for patients or children who cannot tolerate long periods of testing. Additionally, clinicians may find they do not have the instrumentation necessary to run these classic GD paradigms in the standard audiology clinic.

The investigation of temporal resolution through the use of GD paradigms is not a novel approach, but can actually be traced back to Garner in 1947. Numerous researchers since have investigated the phenomenon of temporal resolution through the use of GD using many different stimuli. Many investigators have explored the effects of a variety of variables (e.g., age, hearing impairment) on temporal resolution abilities. However, as there are some controversies regarding the effects of certain variables, further research is still required. For example, it has been demonstrated that older subjects may present with increased GDTs in comparison to younger control subjects (Bertoli, Smurzynski, & Probst, 2002; He, Horwitz, Dubno & Mills, 1999; Snell, 1997; Strouse, Ashmead, Ohde & Grantham, 1998). Other studies, however, have placed in question whether GDT measures are affected by age (Moore, Peters, & Glasberg, 1992). Differences in stimulus and procedural variables may underlie differences in findings across studies. A broad-band stimulus may be the best stimulus for use in GDT paradigms, as it is less likely to lead to variability across different age groups or as a function of peripheral hearing status (Musiek et al., 2005).

Until recently, the application of GD paradigms with pediatric populations had received little attention. Although gap detection research with pediatric participants is somewhat limited, one study reported a maturational effect for GD tasks in normal children (Trehub, Schneider, & Henderson, 1995). It also appears that children with learning disabilities demonstrate abnormal temporal resolution abilities based on GD procedures (Hautus, Setchell, Waldie, & Kirk, 2003). Taken together, these findings suggest that GD procedures should be a useful component of central auditory processing test batteries with pediatric populations.

A commercially available and frequently used test of temporal resolution is the Random Gap Detection Test (RGDT), a revision of the Auditory Fusion Test—Revised, developed by Keith (2000). The subject is asked to indicate whether or not he or she has heard one or two tones or clicks either verbally or by raising one or two fingers (i.e., nonverbally). The tones are 15 msec in duration with a 1.5-msec rise-fall time. The clicks are 1 msec of white noise. One advantage of using tonal stimuli is that it allows the clinician to obtain frequency-specific information regarding temporal resolution skills. There are four subtests, each of which uses nine interpulse intervals ranging from 2 to 40 msec. The RGDT is presented binaurally at 55-dB HL. Normative values for the RGDT tonal stimuli range from 6.0 to 7.8 msec. Currently, to the author's knowledge, there are no published normative values for the click stimuli. Test administration requires approximately 10 minutes. Unfortunately there is only one list available which limits the ability to retest patients.

The Gaps-In-Noises (GIN©) test is a relatively new test of temporal resolution (Musiek et al., 2005). It is composed of a series of 6-sec segments of broad-band noise. Each segment contains 0 to 3 silent intervals or "gaps" per noise segment. The interstimulus interval between successive noise tokens (segments) is 5 seconds and the gap durations presented are 2, 3, 4, 5, 6, 8, 10, 12, 15, and 20 msec. Ten practice items precede the administration of the test items. There are six tokens of each gap duration within each list. Additionally, there are four lists available for testing which allows for test-retest comparisons. Although the test is administered through one channel, the second channel is used by the examiner to monitor and score the responses. Two measures are derived from the GIN. The approximate threshold (A.th.) for the GIN is defined as the shortest gap duration for which there are at least 4 of 6 correct identifications. This is an "approximate" threshold because the exact gap detection threshold is not determined in this procedure, in contrast to traditional psychoacoustic procedures. In addition to the A.th., the percentage of correct responses out of the total number of gaps (i.e., 36 out of 60 would be equal to 60% correct) can be computed for each ear.

The GIN is one of the few measures of temporal processing that has published data regarding sensitivity and specificity to CANS lesions. Specifically, the sensitivity of the GIN is on the order of 72% and the specificity is 94% (Musiek et al., 2005). The GIN appears to be more sensitive to cortical compromise as opposed to brainstem involvement (Musiek et al., 2005). This sensitivity is similar to the patterning tests, which suggests that temporal processing is primarily mediated in the cerebrum (Pinheiro & Musiek, 1985). In addition, test-retest and interlist consistency are high for the GIN test (Musiek et al., 2005). Finally, there are four available lists which demonstrate interlist equivalence (Musiek et al., 2005). This is important because equivalency across lists allows for comparisons for follow-up testing, various types of monitoring, and for assessing treatment effectiveness.

Mean thresholds for the GIN are slightly longer than traditional psychoacoustic gap detection thresholds. Most gap detection in noise thresholds with humans have been reported on the order of 2 to 3 msec (Moore, 2003; Phillips, 1999). The mean A.ths. for the GIN are 4.8 and 4.9 msec for the left and right ears, respectively (Musiek et al., 2005). Differences in gap detection thresholds likely result from a number of procedural differences including less training for subjects participating in the normative data collection for the GIN, and the use of somewhat larger gap intervals in the GIN than those used in many traditional psychoacoustic experiments.

The RGDT and the GIN are essentially the only two true measures of temporal resolution available for clinical application. Although these are both measures of temporal resolution, clinicians should be aware of the differences between these temporal tests. These differences include stimulus variables (tones versus noise), presentation mode (binaural versus monaural), response mode (verbal versus motoric), range of interpulse intervals, gap durations, normative values, and test time (Chermak & Lee, 2005). Most important, the GIN is a true measure of gap detection, whereas the author views the RGDT and the Auditory Fusion Test—Revised (often mistaken as tests of gap detection) as fusion tasks. Given the importance of temporal discrimination to auditory processing, clinicians should include a gap detection measure in their behavioral test batteries.

Temporal Integration

Temporal integration results from the summation or aggregation of neuronal activity as a function of the additional duration of sound energy (Gelfand, 1998). This summation results in threshold improvements as duration increases up to about 200 msec in normal hearing populations (Durrant & Lovrinic, 1995). As duration is decreased by a factor of 10 (i.e., one-tenth of its original duration), a decrease of approximately 10 dB in threshold is observed. This relationship is referred to as a "time-intensity trade off." A similar trade-off is needed to maintain the stimulus at a constant loudness. That is to say, that as duration of a brief signal is increased at suprathreshold levels, the signal is perceived as being "louder." As depicted in Figure 10–6, temporal summation approaches an asymptote at about 200 msec such that further increases in duration have no affect on threshold.

The primary pathologic population on which temporal integration has been studied is individuals with cochlear involvement (Buss, Florentine, & Poulsen, 1999; Carlyon, Buss, & Florentine, 1990; Garnier, Micheyl, Berger-Vachon, & Collett, 1999; Moore, 1996; Papsin & Abel, 1988); however, several investigations have studied populations with CANS involvement (Baru & Karaseva, 1972; Cranford, 1984; Cranford, Stream, Rye, & Slade, 1982). Temporal integration has been found to be impaired in individuals with temporal lobe lesions. Specifically, subjects with temporal lesions demonstrated elevated frequency difference limens for short-duration tones in the ear contralateral to the lesion (Cranford et al., 1982). The finding of a contralateral

deficit in temporal integration in cases of temporal lobe lesions has been demonstrated by several investigators.

When considering differential diagnosis in patients with suspected temporal integration deficits, it is the length of the stimulus tone that is a critical factor. Baru and Karaseva (1972) investigated a large group of patients with various pathologic factors affecting the temporal lobe. They demonstrated that for long intensity-tones of 1200 msec there is no significant difference between the control and the pathologic groups; however, brief tones of only 1 msec yielded large differences between the two groups. These patients also demonstrated differences between the ipsilateral and contralateral condition on the order of 3 to 23 dB suggesting that in addition to using large-group normative value comparisons, individual patients may also serve as their own controls. It has been suggested that if patients demonstrate threshold differences of greater than

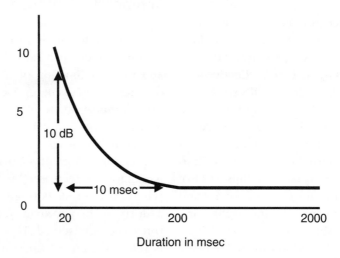

Figure 10–6. Illustration of a temporal integration function demonstrating the time-intensity tradeoff.

15 dB for two tones differing in duration, temporal lobe dysfunction should be suspected (Wright, 1978).

It is important to note that absolute thresholds often are undisturbed in cases of CANS involvement (Bocca & Calearo, 1963). This is because stimuli such as pure tones are simple and static. However, dynamic stimuli (i.e., patterns, numbers and speech), such as those used in traditional psychoacoustic assessments of temporal integration are more sensitive to cerebral lesions. Clinicians should keep in mind that patients often exhibit CANS lesions despite normal pure-tone findings, underscoring the need for inclusion of central auditory tests in audiologic batteries. At this time, there is no means by which audiologists can easily measure temporal integration in the clinic. Unfortunately, brief tone audiometry which was once used to examine temporal integration is no longer used clinically.

Temporal Masking

Temporal masking refers to masking that occurs when the threshold of one sound shifts due to the presence of another sound which precedes or follows it. Backward masking occurs when the masker follows the signal, and forward masking takes place when the masker precedes the signal (see Figure 10-7). Interest in temporal masking dates back to the early 1950s, and although the literature clearly demonstrates the effects of temporal masking, the exact mecha-

Temporal Masking

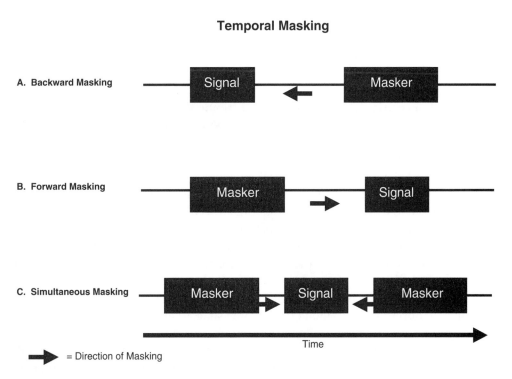

Figure 10–7. Illustration of masking: **A.** Backward masking. **B.** Forward masking. **C.** Simultaneous masking.

nisms underlying this phenomenon are unclear (Durrant & Lovrinic, 1995). Temporal masking may reflect a difference in latencies of neural timing within the CANS; however, this has never been fully confirmed.

There are several major parameters surrounding temporal masking that deserve attention. These include the time interval between the masker and signal, masker level, masker duration, and the acoustic similarity between the masker and the signal. With respect to the time interval between the masker and the signal, assuming that all else is equal, temporal masking drastically decreases as the time interval between the masker and the signal increases. In the case of forward masking, when the time interval between the masker and the signal reaches or exceeds 200 msec, essentially no masking occurs (Durrant & Lovrinic, 1995). Interestingly, as noted above, this is the same duration required for temporal integration to reach its minimum threshold. In backward masking, we see a reduction in masking effects at about 25 msec of separation (Durrant & Lovrinic, 1995).

In a classic study in 1962, Elliott demonstrated several key principles of temporal masking. Elliot found that backward masking is more effective than forward masking: given the same time interval between maskers, more masking occurs when the masker follows the signal. Masking is more effective when the stimuli are delivered monotically as opposed to dichotically (with masker and signal presented to opposite ears). Elliott (1967) later demonstrated that the duration of the masker influences forward, but not backward, masking. Another important variable is the frequency relationship between masker and the signal. The greatest degree of masking occurs when the masker and signal are identical, with the amount of masking decreasing as spectral differences increase between the masker and signal (Elliott, 1967). This means that there will be more masking when a click is used for the masker and the stimulus, than say a click and pure tone. The amount of masking increases as the level of the masker increases, although the relationship between the intensity of the masker and the amount of masking observed is nonlinear. Generally, a 10-dB increase in masking level may only result in a threshold shift of approximately 3 dB (Gelfand, 1998). The simultaneous masking condition always produces greater masking than either backward or forward masking if all parameters other than temporal distance between signal and masker are held constant (Wilson & Carhart, 1971).

Children appear more susceptible to the effects of backward masking than adults (Buss, Hall, Grose, & Dev, 1999; Hartley et al., 2000). Some researchers attribute these finding to children's poor temporal resolution abilities (Irwin et al., 1985; Wrightman et al., 1989). Others attribute the findings to processing "inefficiency" in children (i.e., a deficiency in their ability to extract information) (Hill et al., 2002).

Unlike temporal ordering and temporal resolution, few studies have examined the effects of CANS lesions on temporal masking in children; however, children with language impairments have been investigated (Wright, Lombardino, King, Puranik, Leonard, & Merzenich, 1997). Wright and colleagues reported that children diagnosed with specific language impairment demonstrate a severe temporal processing deficit with respect to their ability to separate one sound that is rapidly followed by another sound (backward masking). They concluded that this deficit may indeed degrade the "perception of brief acoustic elements of speech" (Wright et al., 1997).

The evidence that children with language and speech perception deficits demonstrate abnormal temporal masking skills is not surprising when one considers the potential influence of coarticulation for speech perception. Coarticulation, an aspect of speech production resulting from the concurrent movement of multiple articulators, leads to parallel transmission of acoustic information across neighboring phonemes and, therefore, to the potential for temporal masking. This linkage suggests that it is reasonable to hypothesize that speech and language impairments may co-occur with temporal masking deficits. This linkage also underscores the importance of studying temporal masking as it is a process that may affect our basic communication function. Unfortunately, like temporal integration, there are no clinically available tests of temporal masking. We hope, in the near future, clinical researchers will recognize the need for clinical measures of temporal masking and begin to develop feasible tests to assist in the differential diagnosis of temporal processing disorders.

Clinical Considerations in Test Administration and Interpretation

In the following section, we pose and respond to several key questions which continue to arise with respect to administering and interpreting temporal processing tests as part of a central auditory processing test battery.

Which Temporal Tests Do Clinicians Administer as Part of Their (Central) Auditory Processing Battery?

There is a clear divide between what is occurring in the research arena in comparison to clinical practices. Emanuel (2002) surveyed a large group of audiologists to determine auditory processing practices using an open-ended questionnaire. With regard to temporal processing tests, she found the most commonly reported test administered is the Frequency (Pitch) Pattern Test (76% of respondents) followed by the Duration Pattern Test (44% of respondents). The Duration Pattern Test may be used less frequently because no normative values have been published for the pediatric population. With respect to temporal resolution, 28% of respondents reported use of the Auditory Fusion Test—Revised. With the recent development of the GIN test, there most likely will be a significant increase in the number of clinicians including temporal resolution tests in their test batteries.

Audiologists are beginning to have choices among tests of temporal processing. In comparing several older and more recent temporal resolution tests, Chermak and Lee (2005) concluded that for the pediatric population there do not appear to be any statistically significant differences among temporal gap detection and temporal fusion test means, and that all tests demonstrated high specificity. They noted, however, that the RGDT is quick and easy to administer; however, it is limited by the number of trials, therefore, influencing the test's reliability. The GIN test, although initially a bit more challenging to administer and score, yields strong face validity and reliability, good sensitivity, and excellent specificity (Musiek et al., 2005).

Is Reversal Considered Correct on the Pattern Tests?

Reversals are not considered correct on either the Frequency Pattern Test or the Duration Pattern Test. Reversals should be considered errors and marked as such. It is recommended, however, that clinicians keep track of the number of reversals and consider it in their interpretation. A significant number of reversals may be indicative of a larger, global perceptual deficit or gross neurologic insult.

What Should the Clinician Try Next if a Patient Cannot Linguistically Label the Frequency or Duration Patterns?

If a child or adult is experiencing significant difficulty labeling the tones as high or low or short or long, the clinician should ask the patient to perform the test in the "hummed" condition. This simply requires having the patient hum rather than label the response. Information derived from split-brain patients indicates that if an individual is unable to label the patterns, but performs within normal limits in the hummed condition, this localizes the deficit to the interhemi-

spheric pathways (i.e., corpus callosum), or possibly the left hemisphere (Baran & Musiek, 1999). As indicated above, the left hemisphere is responsible for one's ability to linguistically label the stimulus, whereas the right hemisphere supports resolution of acoustic contour and melody. Information must travel across the corpus callosum through the interhemispheric pathway to the left hemisphere in order for the listener to be able to accomplish the linguistic labeling process. By having the patient hum the response, the necessity for interhemispheric transfer and left hemisphere processing is eliminated.

Here is a useful clinical hint: Consider the use of kazoos to help children hum. Occasionally children will become shy when asked to hum the response, because it is a bit like singing and most do not like to sing. Using a kazoo offers children a fun and nonthreatening way to participate in the test and for you, the clinician, an opportunity to obtain meaningful test results.

Can I Administer Any of These Tests in the Sound Field?

Research has demonstrated that there are no significant ear differences on temporal patterning tests administered under headphones in either normal or pathologic populations suggesting that both the Frequency Pattern Test and the Duration Pattern Test may be administered in the sound field (Musiek & Pinheiro, 1987). If the patterning tests are administered in the sound field, then a total of only 45 items need be presented to the subject. This allows for a shorter test time without compromising sensitivity and specificity (Baran & Musiek, 1999).

Although the patterning tests may be administered in the sound field, this is not true for tests of temporal resolution. Ear differences have been observed on the GIN in neurologic populations; therefore, it is recommended that the GIN, be administered under headphones.

I Am Concerned About Attention and Fatigue. Must I Administer All 60 Items (30 to each ear) on the Pattern Tests?

As indicated above, if the pattern tests are administered in the sound field, then only 45 items total need be presented to the subject. Additionally, if a subject presents with 18 out of 20 either correct or incorrect responses under headphones or sound field, the test can be terminated. This allows for a shorter test time without compromising sensitivity and specificity. It should be noted that if a patient presents with 18 out of 20 incorrect responses, presenting the test in the hummed condition is *highly* recommended.

Why Are the Frequencies 880 Hz and 1122 Hz Employed for the Frequency Pattern Test?

This question makes a great graduate exam question. There is a simple and scientific reason why the frequencies of 880 Hz and 1122 Hz were chosen for the Frequency Pattern Test. If one examines the equal loudness contours (i.e., phon curves), it can be observed that these two frequencies are of equal loudness. This is important so as not to bias the test by introducing a loudness cue in addition to the pitch cue.

What Do I Do in Cases Where a Patient Is Referred for a Central Auditory Processing Evaluation but Presents with Hearing Loss?

There are several central auditory tests, including several temporal processing tests, which are relatively resistant to the effects of cochlear lesions. Of all the temporal processing tests, the Duration Pattern Test appears to be the most resistant to hearing loss (Musiek et al., 1990). In their 1990 study, Musiek and colleagues demonstrated that the performance of patients with cochlear hearing loss on the Duration Pattern Test was almost indistinguishable from those without hearing loss. In fact, over 90% of those individuals with hearing loss, including those with moderate degrees of hearing impairment, performed within normal limits, thus making the Duration Pattern Test an excellent test to use in the presence of cochlear pathology. Other tests of temporal processing, such as the Frequency Pattern Test, may be used with mild, relatively flat hearing losses; however, because there is a frequency or spectral element involved in this test, it may not be completely resistant to hearing loss (Musiek & Pinherio, 1987). Because the GIN incorporates a broad-band stimulus, it also appears promising for use with individuals with cochlear lesions.

There Are Several Tools Available Which Are Marketed as Temporal Processing Tests. Which Should I Use?

The answer to this question hinges on test sensitivity (i.e., the ability of a test to correctly detect a disease or disorder when it is truly present) and test specificity (i.e., the ability of a test to correctly identify an individual as normal when one does not present the disease or disorder). In a perfect world, all tests would yield sensitivities and specificities of 100%; however, this is nearly impossible to obtain because there is generally a trade-off between test sensitivity and specificity. That is to say, that as sensitivity increases, specificity decreases, and vice versa. (See Chapter 6 for discussion of sensitivity and specificity.)

With respect to tests of temporal resolution, the Duration Pattern Test demonstrates good sensitivity (86%) and specificity (92%) with adults (Musiek, Baran, & Pinheiro, 1990). No pediatric normative data have been published for the Duration Pattern Test. The Frequency Pattern Test demonstrates sensitivity and specificity of 83% for adults. Normative data for the pediatric population has been published for the Frequency Pattern Test. The clinician should be aware, however, that if language is of concern, the only essentially nonlinguistic test of temporal resolution available to date is the GIN. Although both the GIN and the RGDT employ nonverbal stimuli, only the GIN employs a nonverbal response mode. The GIN demonstrates sensitivity of approximately 72% for cortical lesions and high sensitivity of 94%. Unfortunately, limited data have been published for the RGDT with respect to validity, reliability, and efficiency data (Chermak & Lee, 2005). Ultimately, the clinician must use sound science and judgment based on the individual patient profile to determine which temporal processing test is most appropriate.

Should I Use More Than One Test to Assess Temporal Processing?

It may be beneficial to assess both temporal resolution and temporal patterning abilities during a (C)APD evaluation. If a deficit is identified in one area of temporal processing, if time allows, it would be beneficial to determine if a deficit also lies within other temporal processing areas as well. The related physiology for pattern perception and temporal resolution is different. It seems patterns require contour recognition and gestalt processing in the right hemisphere, appropriate transfer, and then sequencing for linguistic labeling in the left hemisphere (Musiek et al., 1980). Gap detection requires a synchronous offset and onset of auditory fibers consistent with the beginning and ending of the gap (Musiek et al., 2005). Information from several different types of temporal processing tests would be highly beneficial with respect to focusing intervention to specific deficits. Additionally, the use of multiple tests may yield information regarding different neurophysiologic processes.

How Can Clinicians Test Temporal Integration and Temporal Masking?

Unfortunately, clinically feasible measures of temporal processing are limited to temporal ordering and resolution. Although there are a number of paradigms reported in the literature for assessment of temporal integration and temporal masking, they are not clinically feasible due to the necessary equipment interfacing, as well as subject training and time requirements. Transfer of these paradigms from the lab to the clinic will require communication and cooperation between researchers and clinicians. (see Chapters 1 and 19).

Differential Diagnosis

Differential diagnosis cannot be made using one test alone. It is important that a battery of tests be employed to best determine an individual's overall auditory processing profile (Jerger & Musiek, 2000). Tests of temporal ordering and temporal resolution appear to be most sensitive to cerebral lesions and interhemispheric transfer via the corpus callosum (Musiek, Pinheiro & Wilson, 1980; Musiek & Pinheiro, 1987; Musiek et al., 1990). Typically, reduced scores on the patterning tests are seen bilaterally. As explained above, comparison of hummed versus labeled performance scores on the pattern tests provide considerable insight for differential diagnosis; however, other tests in the central auditory battery are necessary to contextualize temporal processing test results to accurately infer site or level of dysfunction as well as to identify the types of deficient central auditory processes and implications for function in everyday settings. Although the central auditory tests described in this chapter (i.e., temporal processing tests) are more sensitive to dysfunction at higher levels of the CANS, other central auditory tests provide more specific insight regarding the integrity of lower levels of the CANS (e.g., masking level differences [MLD] and auditory brainstem response [ABR]). In fact both the MLD and the ABR provide insight into timing

and temporal processing of the CANS (see Chapters 2, 11, and 12 in this volume).

The following case studies are intended to demonstrate how measures of temporal processing assist in the differential diagnosis of (C)APD.

Case 1. Traumatic Brain Injury

A 16-year-old male was involved in a motor vehicle accident. The radiologic report following the injury indicated a severe aneurysm affecting the pericallosal artery resulting in bleeding into the corpus callosum. Audiologic findings indicated pure-tone thresholds within the normal range bilaterally. The central auditory processing evaluation (Figure 10–8)

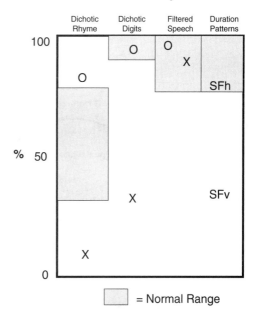

Figure 10–8. Behavioral central auditory processing profile for case study 1. (O = right ear; X = left ear; SFv = sound field verbal response; SFh = sound field hummed response.)

revealed a significant left ear deficit on dichotic listening. Duration Pattern Test performance in the sound field was reduced in the verbal condition, but was within the normal range in the hummed condition.

This is an interesting case study relative to the location of the lesion. The use of the dichotic listening data in conjunction with temporal pattern performance leads to the identification of the anatomic site of dysfunction. We see that there is a severe left ear deficit and reduced patterning scores for the labeling condition only. In order to process dichotic stimuli, as well as temporal patterns, information must be transferred across the corpus callosum to the left hemisphere. Figure 10-9 depicts the pathophysiology of this particular case. In this patient, the right

ear demonstrates normal scores for the dichotic measures because the right ear has direct access to the left hemisphere where digits and words are ultimately processed in the so-called speech processor. The left ear demonstrates a deficit because information is sent via the contralateral pathway (because it is stronger and contains greater neural substrate) to the right hemisphere (Pinheiro & Musiek, 1985). Although the stimuli may be processed in the right hemisphere, it cannot be transferred across the corpus callosum due to the lesion. The patterning results indicate that the right hemisphere and processing of contour recognition are intact because the patient was able to perform within normal limits in the hummed condition. The dichotic test results coupled with a significant deficit observed

Pathophysiology of
Case Study 1

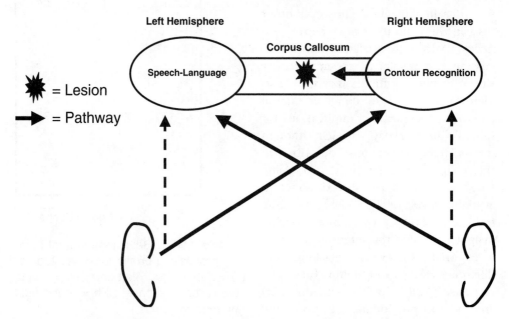

Figure 10–9. Proposed pathophysiology for case study 1.

in the verbal patterns condition point to disruption of information transfer across the corpus callosum, and hence difficulty in linguistic processing (as reflected in the depressed labeling condition).

Case 2. Auditory Cortical Involvement

Case study 2 involves a 56-year-old female who presented with grand mal seizures and neurologic symptoms. Radiologic findings indicated a large, right-sided glioma affecting the right temporal region. Audiologic findings indicated normal peripheral hearing sensitivity bilaterally. Central auditory processing evaluation revealed a severe left ear deficit on dichotic tests, as well as a severe temporal processing deficit as reflected on both the Frequency Pattern Test and the Duration Pattern Test, for both humming and labeling. A right ear deficit was also observed on the GIN (Figure 10–10).

This case provides an excellent example of what may happen in the presence of a right-sided lesion. (Figure 10–11). Similar to the previous case, there is a left ear deficit on the dichotic measures. Again, this is a result of the left's ear indirect access to the left hemisphere (where the digits and words are ultimately processed) via the corpus callosum. The left ear, demonstrates a deficit because information is sent via the contralateral pathway (because it is stronger and contains greater neural substrate) to the right ear where the lesion is located. Unlike the previous case, however, this patient

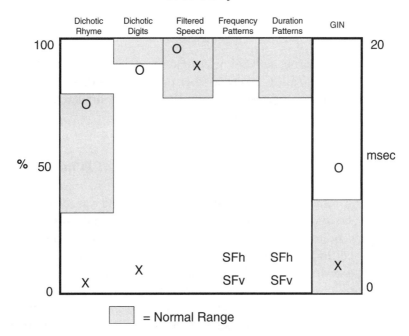

Figure 10–10. Behavioral central auditory processing profile for case study 2. (O = right ear; X = left ear; SFv = sound field verbal response; SFh = sound field hummed response.)

Pathophysiology of Case Study 2

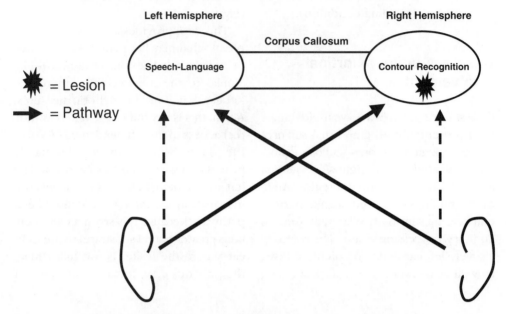

Figure 10–11. Proposed pathophysiology for case study 2.

is unable to either linguistically label or hum the pattern tests. This is likely a result of the fact that contour recognition necessary for processing of patterning elements is compromised due to the right-sided neurologic insult. Inability to recognize the melodic contour undermines the ability to hum the response. Labeling function remains intact in the left hemisphere; however, in the absence of the necessary auditory contour information processed in the right hemisphere, the left hemisphere is unable to label the pattern.

In this example, we also observe severely increased gap detection thresholds for the ear (right) ipsilateral to the lesion. Musiek et al. (2005) reported that gap detection deficits in cases of neuro-

logic insult can be reflected in any number of ways, including the ear ipsilateral to the insult, contralateral to the insult, or bilaterally.

Case 3. (C)APD in Children

A 7-year-old male was seen for a severe articulation deficit and a suspected (C)APD. This child presented a history of recurrent otitis media. In addition to the speech deficit, his parents also reported that he has difficulty with reading and spelling, and that there was a strong family history of learning disabilities. Although there were no concerns regarding hearing loss, the school's staff expressed concerns regarding his ability to hear in the presence of background noise and his poor musical skills. Audiologic evaluation confirmed normal peripheral hearing sensitivity bilaterally. The central auditory processing evaluation (Figure 10–12) revealed a right ear deficit on measures of binaural integration (i.e., Dichotic Digits Test and the Staggered Spondaic Word (SSW) Test), bilaterally reduced scores on low-pass filtered speech (LPFS), and severely depressed scores on two-tone frequency pattern tests in both the verbal and hummed conditions.

This child clearly presented with significant auditory processing deficits across several areas. Several recommendations were made, the first of which was to

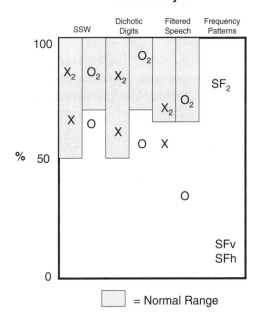

Case Study 3

Figure 10–12. Behavioral central auditory processing profile for case study 3. (O = right ear; X = left ear; O₂ = right ear following training; X₂ = right ear following training; SFv = sound field verbal response; SFh = sound field hummed response; SF₂ = sound field verbal response following training.)

implement the use of an FM system to improve the signal-to-noise ratio in the classroom. Improving access to the acoustic signal should lessen his auditory closure and discrimination difficulties (as revealed by his reduced LPFS scores), as well as his depressed auditory performance in competition (as reflected by depressed performance on the dichotic digits and SSW tests). In addition, vowel identification and discrimination training were recommended to address his reading and spelling deficits. Finally, the use of the SIMON game (see discussion below under Auditory Training) was recommended to improve his temporal processing skills.

Two months following a 6-week, 3 hour per week intervention program, the child returned for reassessment. His parents reported significant improvement in his reading and spelling abilities, and even resolution of his articulation deficits. As reflected in Figure 10–12, this child demonstrated significant improvements across all areas of auditory processing, with perhaps the greatest gains made in temporal processing.

Functional Implications of Temporal Deficits

Temporal processing deficits are associated with a range of functional deficits. Parents of children with temporal processing deficits often report that their children present poor musical skills, lack of prosody during speech and reading, poor emotional tone, difficulty understanding poetry, and difficulty understanding jokes. It is highly unlikely that you will find a concert pianist with poor temporal processing abilities because many of their skills require an ability to process the subtle timing elements of sound. Take, for example, temporal cueing as it refers to our ability to segment words. In the sentence "They saw the *snowdrift* by the window." There are actually two ways in which this sentence could be interpreted. First, it could be that "They saw the *snowdrift* by the window" or "They saw the *snow drift* by the window." Although these sentences are exactly the same with respect to the linguistic elements, their interpretation is entirely different depending upon where the individual places the temporal emphasis (Cole & Jakimik, 1980). Children and adults with temporal processing deficits often experience difficulty with such distinctions. Also of clinical significance is the overwhelming evidence of the frequently observed (as in Case 3) comorbid presentation of (C)APD and reading and spelling deficits. (Farmer & Klein, 1995; Hood & Conlon, 2004; Meng et al., 2005; Meyler & Breznitz, 2005; Putter-Katz et al., 2005; Tallal, 1980; Walker et al., 2002).

Primary Intervention Strategies

Many informal and formal training techniques, as well as a growing number of computer-assisted tools (e.g., Fast ForWord, Earobics, etc.) are available for auditory training. It has been our clinical experience that treatment programs are most successful when they are designed to address the specific deficits exhibited by the patient, as identified during the central auditory test battery. For example, many children in our clinic present with deficits in temporal ordering. For these children, we recommend auditory training focused on temporal skills. It is critical that training be directed to the specific area of weakness to maximize the ability of the CANS to undergo the plastic changes necessary to elicit improved auditory function. (See Chapter 1 of Volume II of this Handbook for discussion of neuroplasticity.) A brief overview of training techniques that parents, clinicians, and related professionals can implement with children and adults with temporal processing deficits is provided in the next section.

Auditory Training

Auditory training (AT) can be conducted as part of a home of school (re)habilitation program (i.e., informal AT) or within a clinic using highly structured stimuli and tasks (i.e., formal AT). Based on our clinical experience as well as reports in the scientific literature (Tremblay, Kraus, & McGee, 1998), training programs conducted for at least 4 to 6 weeks, for an average of 2 to 3 hours per week, can be highly effective in (re)training the brain with respect to auditory processing skills. Informal and formal training techniques to enhance temporal processing include: reading poetry with proper intonation (thereby exercising prosody), gap detection training, duration discrimination, sequencing tasks, heteronym differentiation, identifying word boundaries through temporal cues, and following auditory directives (Chermak & Musiek, 2002).

Perhaps one of the most inexpensive and engaging ways to train children's temporal processing skills is with the game SIMON, a hand-held computer game that has been available for over 25 years. The SIMON game uses sequences of sounds to build temporal ordering and concentration abilities. Visual cues should be removed by having the patient either turned away from the game or blindfolded. SIMON provides a variety of tasks of incremental difficulty, beginning with labeling simple pitch patterns, to counting tones, ultimately to identifying specific tone patterns. A maximum of three tones is used to maintain the focus on auditory skills rather than memory. Tone discrimination can also be exercised. (See Chapter 4 in Volume II of this Handbook for an in-depth discussion of auditory training.)

Summary

Temporal processing pervades all auditory processing abilities and is linked to many skills ranging from musical perception to speech perception to reading (Musiek et al., 2005) Clinicians must include tests of temporal processing in central auditory processing test batteries to fully examine the integrity of the CANS and to identify and corroborate associated functional deficits. Additional temporal processing tests with documented efficiency (i.e., sensitivity and specificity) that can be administered in the typical clinical setting are needed, especially in the areas of temporal integration and temporal masking.

References

Baran, J., & Musiek, F. (1999). Behavioral assessment of the central auditory nervous system. In F. Musiek & W. Rintlemann (Eds.), *Contemporary perspective in hearing assessment* (pp. 375-413). Boston: Allyn & Bacon.

Baru, A., & Karaseva, T. (1972). *The brain and hearing: Hearing disturbances associated with local brain lesions.* New York: Consultants Bureau.

Belmont, I., & Handler, A. (1971). Delayed information processing and judgment of temporal order following cerebral damage. *Journal of Nervous and Mental Disorders, 152,* 353-361.

Bertoli, S., Smurzynski, J., & Probst, R. (2002). Temporal resolution in young and elderly subjects as measured by mismatch negativity and a psychoacoustic gap detection task. *Clinical Neurophysiology, 113,* 396-406.

Bocca, E., & Calearo, C. (1963). Central hearing processes. In J. Jerger (Ed.), *Modern developments in audiology* (pp. 337-370). New York: Academic Press.

Buss, E., Hall., J., Grose, J., & Dev., M. (1999). Development of adult-like performance in backward, simultaneous, and forward masking. *Journal of Speech, Language and Hearing Research, 42,* 844-849.

Carlyon, R., Buss, S., & Florentine, M. (1990). Temporal integration of trains of tone pulses by normal and by cochlearly impaired listeners. *Journal of the Acoustical Society of America, 87,* 260-268.

Chermak, G., & Lee, J. (2005). Comparison of children's performance on four tests of temporal resolution. *Journal of the American Academy of Audiology, 16,* 554-563.

Chermak, G., & Musiek, F. (2002). Auditory training: Principles and approaches for remediating and managing auditory processing disorders. *Seminars in Hearing, 23,* 297-308.

Colavita, F., Szelgio, F., & Zimmer, S. (1974). Temporal pattern discrimination in cats with insular-temporal lesions. *Brain Research, 79,* 153-156.

Colavita, F., & Weisberg, D. (1977). Spatio-temporal pattern discrimination in cats with insular-temporal lesions. *Brain Research Bulletin, 3,* 7-9.

Cole, R., & Jakimik, J. (1980). How are syllables used to recognize words? *Journal of the Acoustical Society of America*, *67*, 965–970.

Cranford, J. (1984). Brief tone detection and discrimination tests in clinical audiology with emphasis on their use in central nervous system lesions. *Seminars in Hearing*, *5*, 263–275.

Cranford, J., Stream, R., Rye, C., & Slade, T. (1982). Detection versus discrimination of brief duration tones: Findings in patients with temporal lobe damage. *Archives of Otolaryngology*, *108*, 350–356.

DeRenzi, E., Faglioni, P., & Villa, P. (1977). Sequential memory for figures in brain-damaged patients. *Neuropsychology*, *15*, 43–49.

Diamond, I., & Neff, W. (1957). Ablation of temporal cortex and discrimination of auditory patterns. *Journal of Neurophysiology*, *20*, 300–315.

Durrant, D., & Lovrinic, J. (Eds.). (1995). *Bases of hearing science.* Baltimore: Williams & Wilkins.

Efron, R. (1963). The effect of handedness on the perception of simultaneity and temporal order. *Brain Research*, *86*, 261–284.

Elliott, L. (1962a). Backward masking: Monotic and dichotic conditions. *Journal of the Acoustical Society of America*, *34*, 1108–1115.

Elliott, L. (1962b). Backward and forward masking of probe tones of different frequencies. *Journal of the Acoustical Society of America*, *34*, 1116–1117.

Elliott, L. (1967). Development of narrow-band frequency contours. *Journal of the Acoustical Society of America*, *42*, 143–153.

Emanuel, D. (2002). The auditory processing battery: survey of common practices. *Journal of the American Academy of Audiology*, *13*, 93–117.

Farmer, M., & Klein, R. (1995). The evidence for a temporal processing deficit linked to dyslexia: A review. *Psychometric Bulletin Review*, *2*, 460–493.

Fu, Q. (2002). Temporal processing and speech recognition in cochlear implant users. *NeuroReport*, *13*, 1635–1639.

Garner, W. (1947). The effect of frequency spectrum on temporal integration of energy at the ear. *Journal of the Acoustical Society of America*, *19*, 808–814.

Garnier, S., Micheyl, C., Arthaud, P., Berger-Vachon, C., & Collet, L. (1999). Temporal loudness integration and spectral loudness summation in normal-hearing and hearing-impaired listeners, *Acta Otolarngology*, *119*, 154–157.

Gelfand, S. (1998). *Hearing: An introduction to psychophysical and physiological acoustics* (3rd ed.). New York: Marcel Dekker.

Greene, D. (1971). Temporal auditory acuity. *Psychological Review*, *78*, 540–551.

Halperin, Y., Nachshon, I., & Carmon, A. (1973). Shift of ear superiority in dichotic listening of temporally patterned nonverbal stimuli. *Journal of the Acoustical Society of America*, *53*, 46–50.

Hartley, D., Wright, B., Hogan, S., & Moore, D. (2000). Age-related improvements in auditory backward and simultaneous masking in 6- to 10-year-old children. *Journal of Speech, Language and Hearing Research*, *43*, 1402–1415.

Hautus, M., Setchell, G., Waldie, K., & Kirk, I. (2003). Age-related improvements in auditory temporal resolution in reading-impaired children. *Dyslexia*, *9*, 37–45.

He, N., Horwitz, A., Dubno, J., & Mills, J. (1999). Psychometric functions for gap detection in noise measured from young and aged subjects. *Journal of the Acoustical Society of America*, *106*, 966–978.

Hill, P., Hartley, D., Glasberg, B., Moore, B., & Moore, D. (2002). Auditory processing efficiency and temporal resolution in children and adults. *Journal of Speech, Language and Hearing Research*, *47*, 1022–1029.

Hirsh, I. (1967). Information processing in input channels for speech and language: The significance of serial order on stimuli. In C. Milliman & F. Darley (Eds.), *Brain mechanisms underlying speech and language* (pp. 22–38). New York: Grune & Stratton.

Hood, M., & Conlon, E. (2004). Visual and auditory temporal processing and early reading development. *Dyslexia*, *10*, 234-252.

Irwin, R., Ball, A., Kay, N., Stillman, J., & Rosser, J. (1985). The development of auditory temporal acuity in children. *Child Development*, *56*, 614-620.

Jerger, J., & Musiek, F. (2000). Report of the consensus conference on the diagnosis of auditory processing disorders. *Journal of the American Academy of Audiology*, *11*, 467-474.

Karaseva, T. (1972). The role of temporal lobe in human auditory perception. *Neuropsychology*, *10*, 227-231.

Keith, B. (2000). *Random Gap Detection Test*. St. Louis, MO: Auditec.

Lister, J., Besing, J., & Koehnke, J. (2002). Effects of age and frequency disparity on gap discrimination. *Journal of the Acoustical Society of America*, *111*, 2793-2800.

Meng, X., Sai, X., Wang, C., Sha, S., & Zhou, X. (2005). Auditory and speech processing and reading development in Chinese school children: behavioral and ERP evidence. *Dyslexia*, *11*, 292-310.

Meyler, A., & Breznitz, A. (2005). Visual, auditory and cross-modal processing of linguistic and nonlinguistic temporal patterns among adult dyslexic readers. *Dyslexia*, *11*, 93-115.

Milner, B. (1962). Laterality effects in auditory. In V. Mountcastle (Ed.), *Interhemispheric relations and cerebral dominance*. Baltimore: John Hopkins Press.

Moore, B. (1996). Perceptual consequences of hearing loss and their implications for the design of hearing aids. *Ear and Hearing*, *17*, 133-161.

Moore, B. (2003). *An introduction to the psychology of hearing*. London: Academic Press.

Moore, B., Peters, R., & Glasberg, B. (1992). Detection of temporal gaps in sinusoids by elderly subjects with and without hearing loss. *Journal of the Acoustical Society of America*, *92*, 1923-1932.

Musiek, F. (1994). Frequency (pitch) and duration pattern tests. *Journal of the American Academy of Audiology*, *5*, 265-286.

Musiek, F., Baran, J., & Pinheiro, M. (1990). Duration pattern recognition in normal subjects and patients with cerebral and cochlear lesions. *Audiology*, *29*, 304-313.

Musiek, F., & Pinheiro, M. (1987). Frequency patterns in cochlear, brainstem and cerebral lesions. *Audiology*, *26*, 78-88.

Musiek, F., Pinheiro, M., & Wilson, D. (1980). Auditory pattern perception in "split brain" patients. *Archives of Otolaryngology*, *106*, 610-612.

Musiek, F., Shinn, J., Jirsa, R., Bamiou, D., Baran, J., & Zaiden, E. (2005). The GIN© (Gaps-in-Noise) Test performance in subjects with confirmed central auditory nervous system involvement. *Ear and Hearing*, *26*, 608-618.

Neff, W. (1961). Neural mechanisms of auditory discrimination. In W. Rosenblish (Ed.), *Sensory communication* (pp. 259-277). Cambridge, MA: MIT Press.

Papsin, B., & Abel, S. (1988). Temporal summation in hearing-impaired listeners. *Journal of Otolaryngology*, *17*, 93-100.

Phillips, D. (1999). Auditory gap detection, perceptual channels and temporal resolution in speech perception. *Journal of the American Academy of Audiology*, *10*, 343-354.

Pichora-Fuller, M., & Souza, P. (2003). Effects of aging on auditory processing of speech. *International Journal of Audiology*, *42*, 2S11-2S16.

Pinheiro, M., & Musiek, F. (1985). *Assessment of central auditory dysfunction: Foundations and clinical correlates*. Baltimore: Williams & Wilkins.

Pinheiro, M., & Ptacek, P. (1971). Reversals in the perception of noise and tone patterns. *Journal of the Acoustical Society of America*, *49*, 1178-1782.

Putter-Katz, H., Kishon-Rabin, L., Sachartov, E., Shabtai, E., Sadeh, M., Weiz, R., et al. (2005). Cortical activity of children with dyslexia during natural speech processing:

Evidence of auditory processing deficiency. *Journal of Basic and Clinical Physiology and Pharmacology, 16*, 157–171.

Snell, K. (1997). Age-related changes in temporal gap detection. *Journal of the Acoustical Society of America, 101*, 2214–2220.

Strouse, A., Ashmead, D., Ohde, R., & Grantham, D. (1998). Temporal processing in the aging auditory system. *Journal of the Acoustical Society of America, 104*, 2385–2399.

Swisher, L. & Hirsh, I. (1972). Brain damage and the ordering of two temporally successive stimuli. *Neuropsychology, 10*, 137–152.

Tallal, P. (1980). Auditory temporal perception, phonics and reading disabilities in children. *Brain and Language, 9*, 182–198.

Trehub, S. E., Schneider, B. A., & Henderson, J. L. (1995). Gap detection in infants, children, and adults. *Journal of the Acoustical Society of America, 98*(5), 2532–2541.

Tremblay, K., Kraus, N., & McGee, T. (1998). The time course of auditory perceptual learning: neurophysiological changes during speech-sound training. *NeuroReport, 9*, 3557–3560.

Walker, M., Shinn, J., Cranford, J., Given, G., & Holbert, D. (2002). Auditory temporal processing performance of young adults with reading disorders. *Journal of Speech, Language and Hearing Research, 45*, 598–605.

Warren, R., & Obusek, C. (1972). Identification of temporal order within auditory sequences. *Perceptual Psychophysiology, 12*, 86–90.

Wilson, R., & Carhart, R. (1971). Forward and backward masking: Interactions and additivity. *Journal of the Acoustical Society of America, 49*, 1254–1263.

Wright, B., Lombardino, L., King, W., Puranik, C., Leonard, C., & Merzenich, M. (1997). Deficits in auditory temporal and spectral resolution in language-impaired children. *Nature, 387*, 176–178.

Wright, H. (1978). Brief tone audiometry. In J. Katz (Ed.), *Handbook of clinical audiology* (pp. 218–232). Baltimore: Williams & Wilkins.

Wrightman, F., Allen, P., Dolan, T., Kistler, D., & Jamieson, D. (1989). Temporal resolution in children. *Child Development, 60*, 611–624.

CHAPTER 11

MEASURES OF BINAURAL INTERACTION

DORIS-EVA BAMIOU

Introduction

Hearing with two ears is better than hearing with one and leads to improved performance in several auditory tasks, such as sound localization and hearing in background noise, both in real life and in laboratory conditions. This happens because of binaural interaction (BI), which first occurs at the brainstem, and subsequently through processing at higher levels of the central auditory pathways. Binaural interaction mechanisms depend on balanced hearing input and are more sensitive to the effects of peripheral hearing loss over a longer developmental period than mechanisms underpinning monaural hearing. Following a brief review of the brainstem physiology that underpins binaural interaction, tests of binaural interaction and results in clinical populations are described. The reader is referred to Chapter 2 for psychoacoustic considerations related to binaural interaction underlying localization and to Chapter 3 for additional discussion of the neurobiology of binaural interaction.

Brainstem Pathways of Binaural Interaction

BI first occurs at the level of the superior olivary complex (SOC) in the lower brainstem and in two more rostral nuclei of the auditory brainstem, the nuclei of the lateral lemniscus (NLL) and the inferior colliculus (IC), both in parallel, as well as in hierarchical (i.e., serial) fashion relative to the SOC (Moore, 1991). The fibers of the auditory nerve bifurcate on entering the cochlear nucleus (CN), and synapse with morphologically different types of neurons in the different divisions of the CN. Some CN neurons project directly to the IC, whereas others project to the SOC via the medial nucleus of the trapezoid body (MNTB), as well as to the NLL, and from the NLL on to the IC (Figure 11–1). However, none of the cell populations in the CN will project to all brainstem targets, and none of the targets will receive inputs from all cell types (Cant & Benson, 2003). Projection of neurons to the IC are both highly convergent and divergent, and the central nucleus of the IC receives projections from 20 identified neuron types in ap-

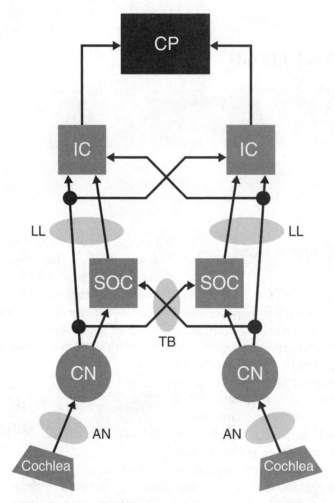

Figure 11–1. Schematic representation of the main brainstem nuclei of the auditory pathway and their main connections. AN—auditory nerve; CN—cochlear nucleus; SOC—superior olivary complex; LL—lateral lemniscus; IC—inferior colliculus; CP—central processor; TB—trapezoid body.

proximately 10 major brainstem nuclei (Irvine, 1992). These neuronal types have different functional properties due to the differing synaptic input received and intrinsic membrane properties, thus giving rise to distinct parallel pathways from the CN to the IC, which are responsible for the various aspects of binaural processing (Irvine, 1992).

Tonotopic Organization of the Brainstem

The CN is characterized by tonotopic organization and its projections maintain a topographic organization. This results in preservation of tonotopic organization throughout all major brainstem nuclei. A restricted region of the basilar membrane with a characteristic frequency (CF) is represented in the IC (and in other brainstem nuclei) as a sheet of neurons. The medial superior olivary nucleus (MSO) has an expanded representation of low frequencies, due to a major input from the large spherical bushy cell region of the anteroventral CN (Bourk, Mielcarz, & Norris, 1981). In contrast, the lateral superior olivary nucleus (LSO) and the medial nucleus

of the trapezoid body (MNTB) have a greater representation of high frequencies (Irvine, 1992).

Neurons Receiving Binaural Input

Eighty percent of central auditory neurons are influenced by stimulation of either ear. The binaural neurons at the SOC are classified on the basis of whether they exhibit a predominantly excitatory (E), inhibitory (I), or no effect (O) to ipsilateral and contralateral stimulation, thus leading to nine major categories (Goldberg & Brown, 1969) (Table 11-1). However, the effects of stimulation may not always be apparent in response to monaural stimulation.

The overwhelming majority of neurons at the MNTB are monaural. In the SOC, almost all LSO neurons receive inhibitory input in response to contralateral input and excititory input in response to ipsilateral input (i.e., IE input), except for a small proportion receiving OE input (i.e., no input in response to contralateral input and excitatory input in response to ipsilateral input), whereas about 60% of MSO neurons receive EE

Table 11-1. Classification of Binaural Neurons at the Level of Superior Olivary Complex (SOC) on the Basis of Predominant Effect of Monaural Stimulation of Either Ear

		Ipsilateral Stimulation		
		Excitation	Inhibition	No effect
Contralateral Stimulation	**Excitation**	EE	EI	EO
	Inhibition	IE	II	IO
	No effect	OE	OI	OO

input (i.e., excitatory input in response to both contralateral and ipsilateral input), with a smaller proportion receiving EO, EI, or IE input (Goldberg & Brown, 1968; Irvine, 1992). The difference in the responses characteristics of the MSO/LSO in combination with their biased frequency responses (low frequencies in the MSO versus high frequencies in the LSO) (Bourk, Mielcarz, & Norris, 1981; Irvine, 1992) result in a correlation between characteristic frequency and binaural response properties that is maintained throughout the central auditory pathway. Thus, in the central nucleus of the inferior colliculus (ICC), EE binaural input occurs more frequently in neurons with CF below 3 to 4 kHz, whereas EI and monaural (excitatory or inhibitory) input patterns occur more frequently in neurons with CF above this frequency range. There is also a remarkable segregation of neurons with respect to their binaural input properties within a frequency band (Irvine, 1992). It has thus been suggested that there is both functional and spatial segregation for different components of binaural function within the human auditory pathway, and this has been confirmed by several human lesion studies (See Tests of Binaural Interaction below for review).

Encoding Interaural Time Differences

If a sound is located at any other plane than at the median plane of a listener, the sound will have to travel a different path length to reach the two ears (as one ear will be nearer and one will be farther from the sound source). This will give rise to interaural time differences (ITDs), which help the listener localize sound. The ITD for a given azimuthal displacement will decrease with increasing stimulus frequency (Irvine, 1992) (i.e., ITDs will be larger for low-frequency sounds).

A large proportion of MSO neurons are sensitive to interaural time differences (ITDs). This has been attributed to simultaneous arrival at the MSO level of neural impulses from the two ears, with the variable path length from each anteroventral CN introducing an interaural delay, which compensates for the ITD in the real world (Moore, 1991). The predominance of IE neurons in the LSO suggests that this nucleus is responsible for the representation of interaural level (or intensity) differences (ILDs or IITs). However, LSO neurons may also be sensitive to ITDs.

There are two components of ITDs: (1) onset time difference (i.e., difference in the time of arrival of the first waveform at the two ears), and (2) ongoing time difference for sustained sounds (i.e., phase differences for pure tones, and in addition, differences in the envelope of the signal for ongoing complex stimuli). The MSO neurons are provided with precise phase-locked input by projections of the spherical bushy cells in the anterior part of the AVCN, which preserve auditory nerve discharge characteristics as a consequence of receiving input via the large axosomatic end-bulbs of Held. In the ascending auditory pathway, however, there is a progressive dramatic decrease in the number of neurons exhibiting phase-locking, as well as in the upper frequency limit for such phase-locking to occur. At the level of the auditory nerve, periodicity of sound is encoded by means of synchronized neural activity, termed as periodicity code. This is replaced by a rate code (i.e., distribution of discharge rate across the neural fibers) at the level of the ICC, with a large proportion of ICC neurons acting as temporal filters (Langner & Schreiner, 1988). For information encoded in terms of place/periodicity code at the periphery to be used by the central auditory nervous system, this information must be translated to a different code. This observation has led to the postulation of the existence of a "coincidence detector" in the brainstem (Jeffress, 1948), whose output is determined by the temporal correlation between the phase-locked input and a delayed replica of this input. Thus, brainstem neurons that process ITDs conduct a cross-correlation process (Yin, Chan, & Carney, 1987). Goldberg and Brown (1968, 1969) noted that the discharge at the most favorable delay of a neuron is greater than the sum of the monaural responses and the discharge at the least favorable delay is lesser than either monaural response (i.e., binaural facilitation takes place when the inputs arrive in phase and inhibition occurs when the inputs arrive out of phase). Most delay sensitive neurons have a characteristic delay (Rose, Geisler, & Hind, 1966).

In the SOC and ICC, neurons showing sensitivity to click ITDs receive EI or IE input, with maximal response when the stimulus from the ear from which they receive the excitatory input is leading and suppressed response when the stimulus to the inhibitory ear is leading (Irvine, 1992). Animal data indicate that for both the SOC and the ICC, there is topographic organization of the neuronal sensitivity to interaural time difference and thus for coincidence detection (Irvine, 1992).

Encoding Interaural Intensity Differences

Differences in the sound pressure level of an acoustic signal at the two ears (i.e., interaural intensity differences [IID]), produced by the head "shadow" effect and the directional amplifying effects of the pinna, provide the major cue for the azimuthal location of high-frequency sounds (Feddersen, Sandel, Teas, & Jeffress 1957; Rayleigh 1907). The major class of neurons that are sensitive to IIDs at the level of the SOC are concentrated at the LSO and receive IE binaural input, with excitatory input from the spherical bushy cells at the ipsilateral AVCN and inhibitory input from the principal neurons at the ipsilateral MNTB, which in turn receive input from bushy globular cells in the contralateral AVCN (Irvine, 1992). At higher brainstem levels, including the NLL and ICC, neurons sensitive to IIDs receive EI input (Irvine, 1986). Most of these neurons are affected by the base intensity in which IIDs are introduced. In addition, there is marked topographic organization of neuronal sensitivity to IIDs.

Binaural Hearing and Development

The neural connections subserving binaural processing are present at birth, but they are immature (Moore, 1985). The neural circuitry which underpins binaural hearing undergoes a structural reorganization after hearing onset (Kapfer, Seidl, Schweizer, & Grothe, 2002; Magnusson, Kapfer, Grothe, & Koch, 2005).

Postnatal maturation is experience dependent (Magnusson et al., 2005) and reduced or altered cochlear output during the early postnatal period may change the normal development of the central auditory nervous system (Kapfer et al., 2002; Moore, 1986).

Tests of Binaural Interaction

Binaural processing is assessed through two principal behavioral procedures. Tests of binaural integration/separation (generally referred to as dichotic listening tests) require the listener to integrate/separate different auditory stimuli presented to each ear simultaneously. Tests of binaural interaction, the subject of this chapter, assess the listener's ability to combine complementary input distributed between the ears. In binaural interaction tasks, the listener "synthesizes" intensity, time, or spectral differences of otherwise identical stimuli presented simultaneously at the two ears.

The 2005 American Speech-Language-Hearing Association (ASHA) technical report on (central) auditory processing disorder ([C]APD) identified binaural interaction as one of the main central processes that may need to be assessed as part of the evaluation for a (C)APD, particularly if the referring complaint or clinical information indicate that there may be a deficit in this domain. There are several tests that have been designed to assess binaural interaction. Binaural interaction can be assessed by means of tests which employ presentation of the stimulus in the sound field (e.g., sound localization) or under headphones (e.g.,

masking level differences). Binaural interaction tests are thought to be sensitive to brainstem pathology; however, the majority of these tests may also be affected by cortical pathology, as well as top-down processes (see each test description below for review). In addition, the presence of peripheral hearing loss may affect test results, which will need to be interpreted with caution. (See Chapter 9 for review of dichotic testing.)

Masking Level Difference

Theoretical Background

In the real world, when a tone and a noise arriving at the two ears of a listener are produced by sources separated in space, and thus the tone and noise arrive to the ears from different directions, the tone is more detectable than when the sound sources are in the same direction relative to the listener (Robinson & Jeffress, 1963). In general, the ability to detect a target signal in a background of masking noise when listening with two ears depends on: (1) the spectral and temporal characteristics of the target signal and the masker, as is true for the monaural listening condition, and (2) the interaural time differences between the target and masker, which enables binaural facilitation by activation of the coincidence detector in the brainstem (Jiang, McAlpine, & Palmer, 1997).

The original description of the binaural masking level difference phenomenon was provided independently by Hirsch (1948) for pure tones and by Licklider (1948) for speech signals. The masking level difference (MLD) refers to the difference in dB between signal detection thresholds in two binaural masking paradigms, which differ in phase attributes. The masking paradigms are termed as:

- Homophasic—when the signals in the two channels are in phase with one another (S_0) and the noise maskers in the two channels are also in phase with one another (N_0) (the 0 notation signifies that there is no phase difference). This condition is used as a reference condition, since masking is at its greatest, and the threshold for the signal is the poorest.

- Antiphasic—when either the signal (S_pN_0) or the noise masker (S_0N_p) are 180 degrees (p radians) out of phase. This is the condition which shows the greatest release of masking with a best threshold for the signal (see Figure 11–2).

The MLD is defined as the signal detection threshold in the S_0N_0 masking paradigm minus the signal detection threshold in the S_pN_0 masking paradigm or MLD = $S_0N_0 - S_pN_0$

When the N_0 broad-band masker is presented alone, the coincidence detector

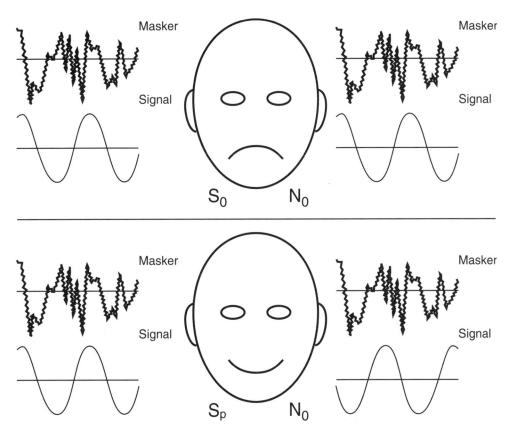

Figure 11–2. Illustration of the masking level difference paradigm. *Top panel*— homophasic condition; *bottom panel*—antiphasic condition leading to better threshold for signal detection.

will fire neural discharges of constant amplitude over a broad range of frequencies; therefore, introduction of the S_0 will have no effect on the pattern of coincidence-counting activity, as the interaural time difference of the target and masker are unchanged. However, introduction of the 500 Hz out-of-phase signal (S_p) cancels masker components at that frequency (Stern & Trahiotis, 1995), thus improving signal detection threshold. At intermediate values of phase-shift from 0° to 180°, the MLD shows a gradual decrease in size. Animal electrode recordings have shown that responses at the ICC are indeed consistent both with psychophysical data and with the current coincidence detection theory of binaural interaction models (Jiang et al., 1997). The MLD may thus provide a measure of our ability to segregate sounds on the basis of their location in space.

Test Description

MLDs can be obtained for either pure tones or speech. Several clinical audiometers are programmed for speech or tone MLDs. The MLD is usually obtained for a 500-Hz tone and a narrow-band masker which centers around that test frequency. A Békésy-type tracking method may be used to obtain the thresholds (see Noffsinger, Schaefer, & Martinez, 1985); however, test procedures may differ. The MLD used in the test battery currently developed at the Institute of Hearing Research for the evaluation of (C)APD in children employs a three-interval "oddball" paradigm (Moore, 2006). Each trial consists of 3 stimuli delivered sequentially (e.g., masker—masker + $S_{0\ or\ p}$—masker) and the child is asked to pick the odd one out.

Wilson, Zizz, and Sperry (1994) developed and evaluated an MLD paradigm for 10 spondaic words embedded in 2000-msec bursts of noise at 500 ms after the noise onset (recorded on Tonal and Speech Materials for Auditory Perceptual Assessment, track 2, left and right channels, 1998). Based on 60 normal-hearing subjects, they reported a 90th percentile MLD value of 5.5 dB (S_0N_0-S_pN_0) for both a 65-dB SPL and 85-dB SPL noise level, and suggested that an MLD <5.5 dB should be considered as abnormal. MLD paradigms for speech stimuli other than English also have been developed (e.g., Johansson & Arlinger, 2002) with reported MLD normative values broadly similar to those reported in the English literature. Test-retest reliability is reportedly less than 0.5 dB for both the S_0N_0 and S_pN_0 conditions for the MLD to a 500-Hz signal (Wilson, Moncrieff, Townsend, & Pilion, 2003).

Effects of Stimulus Parameters and Test Procedures

A range of stimulus parameters may affect the magnitude of the MLD. The MLD depends to a great extent on the frequency and type of target signal. For tone signals, the MLD will decrease as the frequency of the tone increases from 500 to 4000 Hz (Koehnke, Colburn, & Durlach 1986). The largest MLD is seen for the lower frequencies, with a maximum MLD of 15 dB at 500 Hz (Robinson & Jeffress, 1963). The smallest differences are seen for frequencies above 1000 to 2000 Hz, with an MLD of 3 dB for frequencies greater than 1500 Hz (Jiang et al., 1997). This frequency dependence may reflect reduced neural phase coding with increasing stimulus frequency (Durlach, 1964) and has been attributed to a decrease in the S_0N_0 threshold (Koehnke et al., 1986).

The MLD for speech target signals is smaller than for pure tones, and is, in general, larger for low-frequency than for high-frequency dominated words, similar to the frequency effect seen for pure tones (Wilson et al., 1994). In addition, the MLD for speech signals is larger for speech detection than for speech recognition tasks (Wilson et al., 1982). Wilson et al (1982) found a mean MLD (S_0N_0-S_pN_0) of 9.4 dB for a speech detection task versus 7.2 dB for a speech recognition task. The recognition MLDs for the individual spondaic words ranged from 4.4 dB (stairway) to 10.0 dB (oatmeal). In contrast, the duration of the stimulus does not appear to affect the MLD, as the masked threshold decreases with increasing stimulus duration in parallel for both masking conditions (Zwicker & Zwicker, 1984).

The masker level, masker bandwidth, envelope and fine structure (Eddins & Barber, 1998) do affect the MLD. The MLD increases in magnitude with increasing masker level and will reach a shallow maximum at bandwidths of the masker near 30 Hz (Henning & Zwicker, 1984). The interaural correlation of noise has a major effect on MLD, with the large MLD found under antiphasic conditions for a 500-Hz tone showing a rapid decrease as the interaural correlation for the noise is decreased slightly from a perfect value of 1. Further decreases in the correlation reduce the MLD further, but at a slower rate (Robinson & Jeffress, 1963).

Effects of Age

Although there is no reported effect of age per se on the MLD in adult listeners

(Kelly-Ballweber & Dobie, 1984; Wilson & Weakley, 2005), MLD values show some age-related changes in the first years of life. Nozza, Wagner, and Crandell (1988) compared MLDs in three subject groups. Nozza and colleagues obtained MLDs to speech signals (/ba/) using a computer-based head-turn with visual reinforcement procedure with infants 6 to 11 months old, a modified play audiometry task with preschoolers, and conventional testing procedures with adults, using the same apparatus as with the infants. After controlling for hearing threshold differences, they found a statistically significant difference between infants and adults, with lower MLD values in the infants. There were no significant differences between preschoolers and adults. These results indicate a possible developmental change in binaural hearing early in life, which may be underpinned by myelination-related synaptic efficiency and changes in neural firing synchrony.

To examine the development of the MLD as a function of age, Hall and Grose (1990) investigated the MLD for a 500-Hz pure-tone signal presented in a 300-Hz-wide masking noise centered on 500 Hz, where both interaural time and amplitude cues were present, and in 40-Hz-wide maskers centered on 500 Hz, where either amplitude (*MLD delta a*) or time (*MLD delta t*) cues were present, in children aged 3.9 to 9.5 years and in an adult control group. The MLDs of the children increased in magnitude up until the age of 5 or 6 years for the 300-Hz-wide masker, and was at that age still below adult values for the 40-Hz-wide maskers. They proposed two explanations for their findings: either the MLD is small in young listeners because the interaural time and amplitude cues underlying the MLD are coded with relatively poor precision, or that despite accurate peripheral encoding, more central auditory processes are relatively inefficient in extracting the interaural information. In a subsequent study, Hall, Buss, Grose, and Dev (2004) tested adults and children (aged 5 to 10 years) in an MLD paradigm in which detection of brief signals was compared for signal placement in masker envelope minima (and therefore a favorable signal-to-noise ratio) versus signal placement in masker envelope maxima. Maskers were 50-Hz-wide noise bands centered on 500 Hz, and the signals were S_0 or S_p 30-msec, 500-Hz tones. Hall et al. (2004) found that MLDs were greater for masker envelope minima placement than for masker envelope maxima placement and that the binaural advantage associated with the masker envelope minima increased with the age of the child. Adults may thus be able to take advantage of the brief albeit robust interaural decorrelations occurring when the S_p is presented in the masker envelope minima, whereas for young children the temporal window is relatively longer, indicating a developmental improvement in binaural temporal resolution over the age range tested.

Effects of Peripheral Hearing Loss

The presence of peripheral hearing loss will affect the MLD and the effects may persist even after the hearing loss has been corrected (e.g., Hall & Grose, 1993a, 1993b). This effect may be due to poorer encoding of temporal cues inherent to the signal at the periphery (Schoeny & Carhart, 1971). In addition, long-term deprivation or degradation of the acoustic signal at the periphery may lead to abnormal tuning at the brainstem level

(Miller & Knudsen, 2001), which may be responsible for the finding of abnormal MLD even after the resolution/correction of the hearing loss.

The effects of the hearing loss on MLD will depend not only on the frequencies affected by the hearing loss, but also on the age of onset and the duration of the hearing loss. In adults, the presence of high-frequency hearing loss does not affect the MLD for 500-Hz stimuli, although MLD to speech stimuli may be diminished (Olsen & Noffsinger, 1976). However, low-frequency hearing loss (e.g., the hearing loss observed in Meniere's disease) may lead to decreased MLDs for both 500 Hz and spondees (Olsen & Noffsinger, 1976).

Jerger, Brown, and Smith (1984) studied the MLD at 500 Hz in 651 subjects with conductive or sensorineural hearing loss and 270 normal controls. Consistent with Olsen and Noffsinger (1976), Jerger et al. also reported that hearing loss confined to 8000 Hz does not affect the magnitude of the MLD; however, if the hearing loss begins at 2000 or 4000 Hz, the MLD was reduced by 1 dB, and if the hearing loss started at 1000 Hz, the MLD was reduced by 3 dB. The reduced MLD was presumably due to the peripheral hearing loss resulting from deterioration in threshold in the antiphasic condition. The effect of symmetric conductive hearing loss at 500 Hz on the tonal MLD is remarkably similar to the effect of sensorineural hearing loss, with the MLD declining rapidly for a loss up to 30-dB HL and an abrupt reduction in MLD when the loss exceeded 30-dB HL (Jerger et al., 1984). The presence of asymmetric thresholds at 500 Hz between the two ears has a more pronounced effect on the MLD for a sensorineural, however, than for a conductive hearing loss.

Chronic conductive impairment in adults, due to otosclerosis, tympanic perforation, chronic middle ear infection, and cholesteotoma, may lead to reduced MLDs independent of hearing thresholds, due to central type changes, as reflected by changes in the auditory brainstem response (ABR) (Ferguson, Cook, Hall, Grose, & Pillsbury 1998). Subsequent restoration of hearing thresholds may lead to gradual recovery of the MLD over time, although not in all subjects. Hall and Grose (1993a) measured the masking-level difference in adults listeners with unilateral otosclerosis before stapedectomy surgery, one month following surgery, and one year following surgery. Their results indicated that the MLD in this group improved significantly over each of the sequential tests; however, two of their eight subjects did not show recovery to a normal MLD value over this time period. The authors postulated that a period of exposure to abnormal binaural auditory input can impair sensitivity to binaural cues. However, there appears to be a "plasticity" type readjustment or adaptation of the central auditory nervous system after restoration of normal hearing, such that binaural cues facilitation may return to a normal or near-normal level one year after the restoration of hearing. The efficiency and rate of readjustment of this process may differ among individuals.

In the pediatric population, the presence of conductive hearing loss such as in the presence of otitis media with effusion (OME) may have longer term effects on the MLD than in the case of adults with conductive type hearing loss. MLDs are often abnormally small in children with otitis media with effusion, and may sometimes remain abnormal after surgery for the placement of pressure equal-

ization tubes and after normal hearing sensitivity has returned (Pillsbury, Grose, & Hall, 1991). The MLD is more likely to be abnormally reduced if OME-related hearing loss is asymmetric between the two ears (Pillsbury et al., 1991). In general, children with a past history of OME have significantly lower MLDs than children without such history, and there is no correlation with the degree of the hearing loss (Moore, Hutchings, & Meyer, 1991). This reduction in MLD found in children with a history of OME has been attributed to abnormal brainstem processing, as reflected by the finding of concurrent abnormal ABR (Hall & Grose, 1993b). MLD appears to recover following restoration of normal hearing. Thus, the MLDs in a group of children with a past history of OME tested three years after middle ear surgery did not differ significantly from those of the normal control group (Hall et al., 1995), even though a small proportion of subjects with a history of OME continued to have MLDs smaller than normal limits.

Hogan, Meyer, and Moore (1996) reported restoration of normal MLD values in a group of teenagers (ages 12–18 years) with a past history of OME before their fifth birthday, who were found to have reduced MLDs when tested six years before this second study. Similarly, Stollman Snik, Schilder, and van den Broek (1996) assessed ABR, the binaural interaction component (BIC) in the ABR, the MLD, and the suppression of transient evoked otoacoustic emissions (OAEs) in five children with predominantly unilateral OME between the ages of 2 and 4 years who participated in the study at the age of 12 years. They reported that all these measures were within the normal range. Finally, the MLD of adults with a past history of persistent OME in childhood has not been found to be significantly different from the MLDs of normal controls (Stephenson, Higson, & Haggard, 1995).

Taken together these results suggest a slow recovery of binaural interaction, as reflected by normalization of MLD values in children with OME after restoration of normal hearing thresholds. However, this may not necessarily imply normal binaural hearing. Despite normal MLD values, adults with a past history of OME in childhood still complain of auditory disabilities in adulthood (Stephenson et al., 1995), and although the presence of OME in the first year of life does not appear to influence the MLD values in this age group (Hutchings et al., 1992), these children may demonstrate deficits during the first decade of life in some aspects of higher order auditory processing (Gravel, Wallace, & Ruben 1996), possibly due to the mild hearing loss experienced during an important period of early development.

MLD in Special Populations

In the presence of normal and symmetric hearing thresholds, MLDs are reported to be decreased to both 500-Hz tones and spondees in the presence of a variety of neurologic lesions affecting the lower brainstem (Olsen & Noffsinger, 1976) or the auditory nerve, but they remain unaffected by cortical lesions (Olsen et al., 1976). Lynn, Gilroy, Taylor & Leiser (1981) measured speech detection MLDs in 26 patients with cortical, subcortical, and brainstem lesions and in ten control subjects with normal hearing to assess the lesion's effects on the MLD. They reported that there were no significant differences between MLDs of normal subjects and of patients with cortical, subcortical, or rostral brainstem lesions. MLDs for patients with caudal

lesions of the brainstem showed significantly smaller MLDs when compared to the other groups. There is a close correspondence between the size of the MLD and the presence of ABR abnormalities, and with the integrity of wave III of the ABR in particular (Hanley et al., 1983). The MLD is frequently affected by the early stages of demyelinating disease (Noffsinger, Olsen, Carhart, Hart, & Sahgal,1972). Noffsinger and colleagues (1972) reported that almost half of 47 patients with multiple sclerosis (MS) gave abnormal MLDs at 500 Hz and 71% gave abnormal MLDs to spondees, whereas almost all these patients had normal hearing thresholds. The sensitivity of the MLD to detection of retrocochlear disease due to MS is comparable to that of ABR, and better than that provided by acoustic reflexes (Hendler, Squires, & Emmerich, 1990). Hendler et al. (1990) assessed central auditory function in 15 patients with MS by means of ABR, middle-latency responses (MLRs), and long-latency responses (LLRs), as well as by means of a gap-detection task and MLD. They found reduced MLDs in six patients with MS, similar to other reports (Olsen et al., 1976) and these were accompanied by abnormal ABRs and MLRs. They postulated that disrupted neural conduction as a result of demyelinated axons led to deficient processing of phase differences between the two ears.

Sweetow and Redell (1978) reported no difference in tonal or speech MLDs between a group of normal control children (N = 14, ages 4 to 12 years) and a group of normal adults (N = 11). They found significantly lower MLDs to pure tones, however, but not to speech stimuli in a subject group of children with suspected auditory processing deficits (N = 24, ages 4 to 12 years) versus the control group of normal children.

Interaural Timing and Lateralization/Localization Tests

Theoretical Background

A sound produced in an enclosed space reaches the listener's ears after numerous alterations to the wave's travel caused in large part by reflections of the wave from the hard surfaces of the enclosure. In a normal sized room, the original sound signal and its reflections will be perceived as a single "auditory image," and the apparent direction of this image will be determined by the interaural cues associated with the earlier-arriving direct sound, with suppression of the later-arriving reflections. This psychoacoustic phenomenon is known as "the precedence effect" (PE) (Wallach et al., 1949; Zurek, 1980).

The precedence effect is greatest when there is a short delay between the earlier and later arriving sound, whereas for longer delays, as occurs when the space is bigger and the reflecting surfaces are at a greater distance from each other, the listener may perceive an "echo." The precedence phenomenon has been reproduced in laboratory conditions, with the subject seated in an anechoic room between two loudspeakers, with one loudspeaker producing the leading sound and the other producing the lagging sound. For short delays, the listener will perceive a single sound, or "fused sound image," which originates on the side of the leading speaker, the exact position dependent upon the time delay and level differences (Freyman, Clifton, & Litovsky, 1991).

Different mechanisms may underpin localization/lateralization abilities for single-source sounds versus "precedence effect" paired stimuli. This is illustrated by the fact that 5-year-olds' single-source localization ability has already reached adult-level maturity, whereas "precedence effect" localization has not (Litovsky, 1997). These findings may indicate that whereas single-source sound localization requires more basic auditory abilities such as single-source discrimination, "PE" paired stimuli localization may require more sophisticated skills, such as accommodation of echoes and possibly other cognitive skills (Litovsky, 1997).

Test Description

Despite the inclusion of localization/lateralization processes among those that the clinician should consider in the evaluation of an individual suspected of (C)APD (ASHA, 2005), no such standard clinical test of localization/lateralization is currently available. The reader is referred to Chapter 19 for further discussion of developments in localization testing procedures and their application in the clinical setting. A summary of the main (experimental) test procedures that have been applied to clinical populations follows.

A sound localization test based on the precedence phenomenon was developed by Cranford et al. (1990a, 1990b). Subjects are presented with pairs of click stimuli of 100µ sec duration at a presentation level of 50-dB SL, with each click originating from one of two loudspeakers placed at 45° to the left and the right of the subject's midline (Figure 11–3). The time delay between the two clicks is varied, and the subjects are presented with three consecutive identical click pairs and asked whether the sound is perceived as originating in the midline, left, or right of the midline.

Aharonson, Furst, Levine, Chaigrecht, and Korczyn (1998) developed a locali-

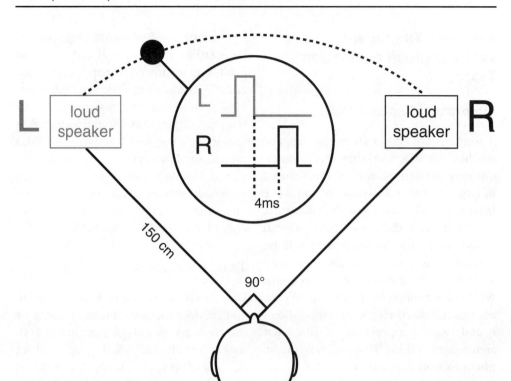

Figure 11–3. Illustration of the precedence effect. A subject presented with a pair of clicks, with each click originating from one of two loudspeakers placed at 45° to the left and right of the subject's midline, will perceive the sound as originating in the left of the midline if the left click precedes the right click by a certain time interval.

zation task presented to subjects under headphones (i.e., lateralization). The test procedure consists of the presentation of two successive short bursts for each trial, separated by an interval of 500 s. In the first trial, stimuli are presented binaurally and simultaneously; in the second trial, either the arrival time of the stimulus to one of the earphones is delayed (ITD trials), or the level is increased at one ear and decreased at the other ear by the same amount (ILD trials). The listener is required to indicate the position of the auditory image of the second burst by pushing one of nine equally spaced buttons on a keyboard.

Moore, Cranford, and Rahn (1990) developed a "dynamic" computerized auditory test, which requires pursuit auditory tracking of a moving fused auditory image (FAI) based on stimulus conditions that elicit the precedence effect. A pair of two clicks is presented, one each from two loudspeakers placed on opposite sides of the listener, as done in the "static" precedence effect localization task designed by Cranford et al. (1990a, 1990b). Movement of the FAI is simulated by incrementally varying the delay between the two clicks. Listeners are asked to direct a laser pointer to the perceived location of the FAI. Normal listeners are able to track the movement of the FAI accurately, and the perceived location of the FAI varies linearly with the interspeaker delay.

Besing and Koehnke (1995) evaluated a similar test of virtual auditory localization with speech signals presented via headphones and with presentation in nine simulated locations in the horizontal plane from −90° to +90°, in both (simulated) anechoic and reverberant listening conditions. A nine-alternative, forced-choice identification procedure was used to measure localization ability, and the outcome measures were the root-mean-square localization error in degrees and percent correct responses. The test, according to the authors, was both easy to administer and easy to perform, even for the children who performed more poorly in the tests than their peers. In addition, and of considerable interest for pediatric audiologists, young subjects found the test more interesting than the MLD.

Griffiths, Dean, Woods, Rees, and Green (2001) developed a test battery, the Newcastle Auditory Test Battery (NAB), which includes tests of static and dynamic lateralization for the psychoacoustic evaluation of neurologically impaired and other naive subjects. The battery contains two subtests for the measurement of binaural phase (subtest S1) and amplitude difference (S2) limens for the detection of the "static" lateralization of a 500-Hz tone toward the right or left. "Dynamic" lateralization is measured in another two tests (S3 and S4) in which the phase or amplitude of a 500-Hz tone is sinusoidally advanced at one ear and delayed at the other, thus resulting in perception by the listener of sinusoidal movement of a single sound between the two ears. In subtests S5 and S6, the phase (S5) or amplitude (S6) of a 500-Hz tone is linearly advanced at one ear and delayed at the other, and the listener perceives linear movement of a single sound from the midline toward either side. These tests measure the thresholds for

the detection of 600-ms phase or amplitude-graded changed (in radians and proportional amplitude change, respectively) ramp to the right or left. A full psychometric function can be plotted for each subtest for each subject. Griffiths and colleagues provide normative data for 30 naïve subjects in two age groups, 20 to 39 and 40 to 55 years.

Effects of Age and Peripheral Hearing Loss

Infants at the age of 2 months do not appear to localize precedence-effect sounds, whereas their ability to localize single source sounds is good (Clifton et al., 1984). By the age of 6 months, infants are reportedly able to localize precedence-effect stimuli as well as single-source stimuli (Clifton et al., 1984). Although the ability of 5-year-olds to localize a single-source sound has already reached adult-level maturity, their ability to localize "PE" paired stimuli is still significantly lower than that of adults (Litovsky, 1997).

Performance in more complex localization tasks shows a longer developmental course than for simpler tasks. Cranford et al. (Cranford & Morgan, 1993) tested normally developing children, aged 6 to 12 years of age, with both a "static" and "dynamic" FAI localization task. While children performed at normal adult levels with the stationary FAI test, a significant age-related trend was observed with the moving FAI test, with poorer tracking performance in the younger than in the older children. At the other end of the age spectrum, Cranford et al. (1990a) assessed the effects of aging on a localization task based on the precedence effect. Elderly listeners showed poorer performance with delay intervals below 0.7 ms (Cranford et al., 1990a; Cranford, Andres, et al., 1993).

Similarly, Griffiths et al. (2001) showed an age effect for their "dynamic" lateralization task. Thresholds for the detection of interaural phase modulation were lower than thresholds for the control binaural frequency modulation detection task by a factor of 6.6 for the age group 20 to 39 and a factor of 4.8 for the age group 40 to 59; thresholds for the frequency modulation task did not differ between the two age groups.

Localization tasks are adversely affected by the presence of hearing and it has been proposed that hearing loss may have a greater impact on the localization performance of elderly subjects than younger subjects (Cranford, Andres et al., 1993). A past history of OME may have long-term impact upon localization performance. Besing and Koehnke (1995) tested three groups of subjects with normal hearing sensitivity at the time of testing (adults, and children with and without history of OME) on a test of virtual auditory localization. Children with a past history of OME showed poorer and more variable performance in this test than children without OME history.

Localization Tests in Special Populations

As the precedence effect is underpinned by binaural interaction of disparate sound cues, a localization task based on the PE will be severely affected by brainstem pathology. Animal and human studies support this expectation. Results on the precedence effect localization task correlate with results in the synthetic sentence identification with ipsilateral competing message SSI-ICM (Cranford & Romereim, 1992), a test that is highly sensitive to brainstem pathology (Jerger & Jerger, 1974). Animal studies indicate that the inferior colliculus (IC) plays an important role in mediating the precedence effect, and inhibitory neural transmissions within this structure may account for the suppression of the lagging stimulus (Li & Yue, 2002).

Lesion studies employing localization tasks that are dependent upon ITD and ILD interaction support the existence of two separate pathways for ITD and ILD detection and sound lateralization. Griffiths et al. (1998) conducted detailed tests on a subject with multiple sclerosis affecting the brainstem, with a lesion in the region of the right superior olive and another lesion more dorsally placed in the pons. The patient experienced a total deficit in the detection of phase differences between the ears, although detection of interaural amplitude differences was preserved. Griffiths and colleagues interpreted these findings to indicate that interaural phase detection is subserved by a distinct mechanism to that for interaural amplitude difference detection. Also supporting dual pathways, Furst et al. (2000) reported that patients with multiple sclerosis (MS) with lesions restricted to the caudal pons showed lateralization of the sound to the side of the head for interaural level differences, but lateralization of the sound to the midline (i.e., more severe impairment) for interaural time differences. Patients with MS lesions rostral to the trapezoid body, however, showed side-oriented lateralization for both types of interaural differences. In addition, they reported that lesions at the trapezoid body and/or the superior olivary complex (SOC), were correlated to center-oriented lateralization performance, whereas lesions at the level of the lateral lemniscus (LL), and/or the IC were correlated to a side-oriented performance. Another study of patients with MS or stroke lesions (Aharonson & Furst, 2001) showed that most patients who had lesions below or at the SOC perceived all interaural differences in binaural stimuli as small, whereas most patients who had lesions above the SOC perceived all interaural differences as large.

Aharonson and Furst (2001) proposed that there is a two-level structure for the estimation of interaural differences in the brainstem, with an initial level at the SOC, and a second level at or above the IC. The first level is thought to detect differences between the left and right input, and if no difference is detected, the default decision is that the two inputs are similar, and, consequently, small interaural difference will be estimated. The second level at the IC is thought to assess for similarity between the left and right inputs, and if no similarity can be determined, the default decision is that the two inputs are different, and therefore large interaural differences will be estimated.

The auditory cortex appears to play an important role in discriminating both ITD and IID cues, but appears to be necessary for discriminating ITD, as patients with bilateral auditory cortex lesions are unable to detect ITDs (Yamada et al., 1996). Localization tests based on the precedence effect are affected by cortical lesions, with unilateral lesions resulting in greater difficulty localizing the paired sounds when the speaker contralateral to the lesion is leading (Cornelisse & Kelly, 1987; Cranford et al., 1990b). Moore et al. (1990) reported that two subjects with unilateral cortical lesions showed failure to track the FAI past the midline to the side contralateral to the lesion. Perception associated with the precedence effect may thus be underpinned by further processing in the ascending auditory pathway up to the cortex, which may contribute to the perception of the size of the acoustic space (Fitz-

patrick, Kuwada, Kim, Parham, & Batra 1999).

Sound lateralization/localization tasks using stimulus conditions known to elicit the precedence effect place greater demands on neural timing and integration than conventional (i.e., single-source) tests of localization, and may provide a more sensitive index of neural function (Moore et al., 1990). Cranford et al. (1990b) employed a sound localization test (see preceding Test Description section) as a behavioral measure of the neural instability resulting from demyelination in patients with multiple sclerosis (MS) and found that MS subjects exhibited problems with delays less than 1 ms and that the test had the greatest sensitivity in separating patients with MS from controls for delays from 0.3 to 0.7 ms. Aharonson et al. (1998) used a lateralization task (i.e., under headphones) using interaural time and intensity differences to test neurologic subjects with MS or stroke. They reported that lateralization tasks with high-frequency stimuli were more sensitive detectors of abnormality than just noticeable differences for any kind of stimulus, or for lateralization tasks using low-frequency stimuli or clicks.

Rapidly Alternating Speech Perception

Test Description

The Rapidly Alternating Speech Perception (RASP) test consists of segmented, continuous speech information, which is presented alternately and sequentially between the two ears. Synthesis of this information, which is necessary for the listener to perceive and report the complete speech signal, requires binaural interaction, which initially take places in the brainstem (Figure 11–4).

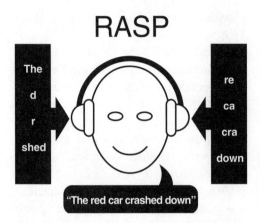

Figure 11–4. Illustration of the Rapidly Alternating Speech Perception (RASP) test.

Bocca and Calearo (1963) tested normal listeners with a test in which speech segments of 20 to 500-msec duration were presented alternately between the two ears, and found normal speech intelligibility. One of the best known tests in this category was developed by Willeford (1977) (Figure 11–4). In this test, segments of a sentence with approximately 7 words are presented alternately between the two ears, at a 300-ms alternation rate and at 40-dB sensation level (SL) referenced to the pure-tone average. Twenty sentences are presented in total, 10 with the right ear receiving the initial sentence segment first, and 10 with the left ear receiving the sentence segment first. It has been argued that as this test requires binaural interaction, a single score rather than separate left and right ear scores should suffice to identify deficits (Baran & Musiek, 1999).

RASP in Special Populations

Results of the RASP in different populations must be interpreted with caution as this test may also be affected by peripheral hearing loss (Miltenberg, Dawson,

& Raica, 1978). Moreover, although the RASP requires binaural interaction and is thus, in theory, dependent upon brainstem integrity, in practice it shows poor sensitivity to brainstem lesions. Lynn and Gilroy (1977) found the test to be abnormal only in patients with lower, but not upper brainstem lesions, and that the presence of cortical lesions also affected the test results to some extent. Musiek (1983) reported the RASP demonstrated a sensitivity of only 50% to brainstem lesions. Musiek and Geurkink (1980) used this test as part of a battery to assess five children with suspected (C)APD and found normal results in all their subjects, despite the fact that two of these children presented abnormal results in a binaural fusion task. Similarly, Willeford and Bilger (1978) reported that few children with (C)APD had difficulties with the RASP, even at a 30-dB SL. Welsh, Welsh, and Healy (1980) employed a RASP procedure described by Lynn and Gilroy (1972) to assess central auditory function in 77 students with dyslexia (age range 7–18 years). They found abnormal RASP results in only 13% of their population, although 75% of these students performed outside normal limits on a binaural fusion task. They noted that their sample had a wide range of scores, and that performance on the RASP improved in the 11 to 12 years age group. The RASP is seldom used clinically because of its marginal sensitivity to brainstem lesions.

Binaural Fusion Test

Test Description

The binaural fusion test (BFT) involves presentation of different segments of band-pass filtered speech to the two ears with a low bandpass filtered speech stimulus presented to one ear and a high-band pass filtered speech stimulus to the other ear. The patient should be able to fuse the information from each channel to report the word. Katz and Ivey (1994) proposed that these tests should be more aptly termed "binaural resynthesis," as the listener must combine simultaneous and complementary segments from the two ears into one composite item, rather than fuse or join equal signals into one midline image.

Probably the most well-known test of binaural fusion was included in Willeford's (1977) test battery. This BFT presented 20 spondees filtered though a low-band pass (500–700 Hz) filter and a high-band pass (1900–2100 Hz) filter at 30-dB SL referenced to the listener's 500-Hz threshold for the low band and to the listener's 2000 Hz threshold for the high band (Willeford, 1977) (Figure 11–5). The BFT test is difficult to calibrate due to differences in energy between the low-frequency and high frequency bands; therefore, it is difficult to equate the two ears without bias.

Matzker (1959) validated binaural fusion on more than 1,000 patients using a test similar to Willeford's. The patient groups included those with brain tumors, cerebral atrophy, multiple sclerosis, severe skull trauma, and patients with hypertension, as well as patients with psychosis. Using 41 words, Matzker presented the subjects with three conditions: (1) low-band pass segment presented to one ear (BF_lo); (2) high-band pass presented to one ear (BF_hi); and (3) simultaneous presentation of low-band pass to one ear and high-band pass to the other ear (BF_lohi). He reported that the scores in the binaural fusion condition (i.e., BF_lohi) were equal to or higher than the scores in the monaural conditions in high proportions of all the patient groups except the patients with psychosis. He interpreted the atypical finding of lower binaural fusion than monaural scores as evidence of a lack of auditory integration. Postmortem histopathology in some of the patient group with abnormal BFTs identified pathology in the brainstem, predominantly in the olivary region.

More recently, Wilson, Arcos, and Jones (1984) used consonant-vowel nucleus-consonant (CVC) words as stimuli for a BFT, with the consonant segments presented to one ear and the vowel segment presented to the other ear. Wilson and colleagues reasoned that if the spectral and temporal information is preserved despite the segmentation of the word, word recognition should be unaffected by monaural hearing loss. Using a 50-dB HL presentation level, normal hearing subjects achieved a 10% correct word recognition when the vowel segment or the consonant segments of the words were presented monaurally in isolation, and 90% correct word recognition in the binaural condition, (i.e., with the vowel segment presented to one ear and the consonant segments to the other ear). Neijenhuis, Stollman, Snik, and van den Broek (2001) reported reasonably good test-retest repeatability for their

Binaural fusion

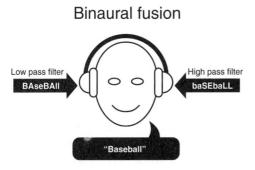

Low pass filter
BAseBAll

High pass filter
baSEbaLL

"Baseball"

Figure 11–5. Illustration of the binaural fusion paradigm.

version of the BFT, which used 22 mono-syllabic words (low-pass filter with cut-off frequency of 500 Hz and high-pass filter with a cutoff frequency of 3000 Hz, both with a slope of 60 dB per octave). However, they observed both ceiling effects and a small but significant improvement on retest. This may indicate that it would be more appropriate to conduct the BFT after a training session.

Effects of Stimulus Parameters and Test Procedures

Presentation level affects the low-band pass in a different manner relative to the high-band pass for the monaural condition, with a rapid rise in intelligibility of the high-band pass and a shallower slope for the low-band pass segment with increasing intensity (Katz & Ivey, 1994). A presentation level of 25 to 30-dB SL results in low intelligibility for the band-pass segments in the monaural condition, but high intelligibility for the binaural condition (i.e., the true measure of binaural fusion) (Katz & Ivey, 1994). Using his CVC BFT with 120 adults with normal-hearing sensitivity at various presentation levels, Wilson (1994) reported that with the monaural vowel segments there was minor improvement of about 8% when the presentation level was increased from 20 to 40-dB HL, and that the psychometric function was constant at 15 to 20% correct over the 20 to 70-dB HL range. Recognition performance improved substantially for the consonant segments in the monaural condition when the presentation level increased from 40 to 60-dB HL (from 17 to 67%), with the psychometric function approaching an asymptote around 65 to 70% over the 55 to 70-dB HL range. He attributed this improvement in performance to the rela-

tion between the presentation level and the level of energy in the segments of the words, with the low-frequency energy in the vowel speech spectrum peaking at 0-dB HL and the high-frequency energy in the consonant speech spectrum peaking at −30-dB HL.

Katz and Ivey (1994) noted that word familiarity also may affect BFT outcomes. Auditory closure appears to be a factor as well, as indicated by the correlation of BFT results to filtered-speech test results in principal component factor analysis (Neijenhusi et al., 2003). It has been suggested that children in particular should be familiarized with more difficult words (Windham et al., 1986) to eliminate the potential language confound.

Effects of Age and Peripheral Hearing Loss

In the adult population, aging per se does not affect BFT results, when peripheral hearing loss has been taken into account (Grady et al., 1984; Kelly-Ballweber et al., 1984). Not unlike other measures of speech recognition, the BFT is affected by the presence of peripheral hearing loss. Hearing-impaired subjects with a mild hearing loss and relatively flat audiometric configuration score significantly poorer on the BFT task than subjects with normal hearing, even though the test stimuli are presented at an adjusted level (i.e., SL), and even when scores are corrected on the basis of pure tone average by means of linear regression analysis (Neijenhuis et al., 2002). Similar to other binaural interaction tests, children with an early history of OME (at ages 2 to 4 years) present normal BFT performance when tested at a later age (age of 8 years) (Schilder Snik, Straatman, & van der Broek, 1994).

BFT in Special Populations

Smith and Resnick (1972) used monosyllabic words with a low band of 360 to 890 Hz and high band from 1750 to 2220 Hz using a procedure similar to Matzker (1959). Monaural word recognition for their normal hearing listeners hovered around 20% when either band pass was presented alone and at 65% when both the low-pass band and the high-pass bands were presented. They also compared scores for the task with the low-pass band presented to one ear and the high-pass band presented to the other ear to the task when both bands were presented to both ears in three patients with lesions of the temporal cortex. These patients demonstrated no difference between the presentations, similar to normal subjects and subjects with bilateral sensorineural hearing loss. Conversely, they found abnormal results (i.e. better performance for the condition in which both bands were presented to both ears by 18 to 34% for four patients with brainstem lesions, demonstrating abnormal binaural interaction. Noffsinger, Olsen, Carhart, Hart, and Sahgal (1972) reported abnormal BFT performance in 8 out of 36 subjects with multiple sclerosis; however, abnormal performance was more common in patients with lesions above the lower brainstem (i.e., above the binaural integrative mechanisms of the brainstem), and abnormalities were more frequently displayed for the task when both bands were presented to both ears, in contrast to the results of Smith and Resnick (1972).

Welsh, Welsh, and Healy (1980) employed the BFT designed by Matzker (1959) to assess central auditory function in 77 students with dyslexia (age range 7 to 18 years) and found abnormal results in three-quarters of this population. They interpreted their findings as indicative of the presence of a multifocal abnormality associated with dyslexia, also encompassing the brainstem. Stollman et al. (2003) used a Dutch BFT as part of a central auditory test battery to assess central auditory function in 20 six-year-old children with specific language impairment (SLI) and a group of 20 age-matched controls. The children with SLI obtained scores significantly lower than those of the control group, with an approximately zero difference between the binaural and summed monaural conditions for the SLI group, but significantly higher than zero differences in the normal control group. Stollman and colleagues interpreted these findings as strongly indicative of the presence of an auditory processing disorder as opposed to a language deficit. However, Neijenhuis et al. (2003) reported their BF task (described in Neijenhuis, Stollman, Snik, and van den Broek, 2001, see above for brief description) to have low sensitivity in identifying children and adults with (C)APD, with only 40% of their sample falling below the 25th percentile, which they attributed to the presence of a specific auditory decoding deficit in this subgroup of patients. The finding of abnormal BFT results in the presence of normal brainstem responses may be considered a false positive outcome or could result from the presence of an auditory decoding deficit (Musiek & Geurkink, 1982; Welsh et al., 1982).

Other Tests

The BFT developed by Musiek consists of a pair of noise clicks which are presented dichotically at 55-dB SL and separated by random interaural click intervals, ranging from 0 to 20 ms (Chermak & Lee, 2005). The listener reports whether one or two noise bursts were heard. A study on 10 normal children showed unexpectedly small thresholds (1 ms) for detection of two separate sounds, which was attributed to the large step sizes for the click interval, from 0 msec to 5 msec (Chermak & Lee, 2005).

Binaural interaction may also be assessed using the recently developed Listening in Spatialized Noise—Continuous Discourse Test (LISN-CD; Cameron, Dillon, & Newall, 2006), which requires special software for computerized administration under headphones. The test produces a virtual three-dimensional auditory environment. A target talker narrates a story while competing babble arrives from various directions in auditory space (0° and ±90°). The task requires the child to follow the story by the target talker, and the audiologist adaptively adjusts the signal-to-noise ratio to find the "just understandable" threshold. Cameron et al. propose that by comparing the thresholds for same talker versus different talkers, and for same direction versus different directions, a diagnosis can be made of the ability to use different cues to suppress noise. The authors report that nine of ten children presumed to have (C)APD on the basis of their presenting profiles failed the "spatial advantage" measure of the LISN-CD. Cameron and colleagues also reported good correlations with the MLD.

Consequences of Poor Binaural Interaction

Some of the most challenging acoustic environments are associated with multi-ple fluctuating sound sources (e.g., more than one simultaneous voice emanating from different speakers with additional degradation due to room reflections). In a normal-sized room, normal listeners will perceive the leading sound signal and its immediate reflections as a single fused "auditory image." The apparent direction of this image will be determined by the interaural cues associated with the earlier-arriving direct sound with suppression of the later-arriving reflections (Wallach et al., 1949; Zurek, 1980). In addition, the human brain has the remarkable ability to segregate the object of interest, such as the voice of an attended speaker, in a complex auditory scene, such as a cocktail party. If the different speakers are separated in space, it is easier for a listener to understand the target speech signal. This is due to both monaural advantages from improvements of speech-to-noise ratio at the better ear and to binaural advantage resulting from binaural unmasking of the low-frequency parts of the speech signal, which is facilitated by the ITD between the competing sources (Hawley et al., 2004). It has been proposed that some of the synapses involved in auditory sensory perception in complex auditory environments might be hardwired due to long-term evolution, thus reducing the time necessary for the complex brain computation (Chen, 2005). Binaural listening cues underpinned by interaural time and intensity differences, as well as other auditory processes (e.g., temporal processing, auditory discrimination) may be helpful in resolving the degraded signals in these degraded and challenging environments (Bronkhurst & Plomp, 1992; Chen, 2005).

Deficits in binaural interaction (e.g., in the presence of multiple sclerosis in adults or OME in children) result in listening difficulties in complex acoustic environments and manifest in deficits in at least two auditory processes: sound localization/lateralization and auditory performance in backgrounds of competing acoustic signals. Deficits in either or both of these processes would be consistent with the diagnosis of an (C)APD (ASHA, 2005). It has been proposed that, to some extent, age-related difficulties in understanding speech in reverberant environments can be attributed to a decreased ability to perceive the precedence effect (Cranford & Romereim, 1992). In addition, it has been suggested that small MLDs in children with OME may be reflected in difficulties detecting and attending to signals in noisy environments (Moore et al., 1991). Due to the long-term maturation of the various mechanisms which underpin binaural hearing, even normally developing children will have greater difficulties than adults in complex fluctuating auditory backgrounds (e.g., Hall, Buss, Grose, & Dev, 2004). This may be particularly relevant in the classroom environment where there may be multiple sources of noise, such as from a heating/ventilation unit, activity in an adjacent classroom or corridor, traffic or aircraft noise, student activity within the classroom, or any combination of these. Children with deficits in binaural interaction are at greater risk of having difficulties in localizing the voice of the teacher, and of having difficulties processing the speech signal of the teacher in background noise.

Primary Intervention Strategies

Human listeners may be trained to change their responses to cues of sound-source position by exposure to altered sound cues, and they may also improve their sound localization performance with training through the use of normal cues, although the degree of adaptation varies across subjects (Wright & Zhang, 2006). Indeed, practice during formal testing leads to improved test performance in both ITD and ILD discrimination tasks, although training results differ for the two tasks and depend on a number of factors, such as stimuli used for training, amount of training, and initial levels of performance, as well as increments of training (Linkehoker & Knudsen 2002; Wright & Fitzgerald, 2001; Wright & Zhang, 2006).

There is a substantial capacity for improvement of binaural interaction, both in animals and in humans (Linkehoker & Knudsen 2002; Wright & Fitzgerald, 2001; Wright & Zhang, 2006). Sound localization training in a reverberant room may lead to small, albeit significant improvements for a number of spatial judgments (Shinn-Cunningham, 2000), and these improvements are both stimulus and vision dependent (Abel & Paik, 2005). This processing plasticity may well be underpinned by the special properties of the SOC at a neurochemical level, as the SOC nuclei express molecules such as GAP-43 mRNA and subunits of integrin which are known to be involved in development, plasticity, and learning (Illing, Kraus, & Michler, 2000). For example, SOC neurons may respond to hearing impairment with the expression of these substances, indicating changes in neural connectivity (Illing, Kraus, & Michler, 2000). The reader is referred to Chapters 3 and 4 in Volume I of this Handbook and to Chapters 1 and 4 in Volume II for discussions of neuroplasticity.

Auditory training (AT) should lead to improved binaural interaction. Intervention for (C)APD should be deficit-focused;

therefore, if test results and functional deficits reveal a binaural interaction, deficit training should target that skills. Specific formal AT to improve binaural interaction could include: ITD and ILD detection or discrimination tasks, and localization and lateralization training in the sound field, both in quiet and in noise, and at various azimuths. Informal AT of binaural interaction also could be incorporated in everyday activities (e.g., taking a walk in the park) or could be exercised as part of a game such as "Blind Man's Bluff" and "Marco Polo." In addition to direct remediation, environmental adaptations to minimize reverberation in the classroom and provision of an FM system to improve signal-to-noise ratios would be of paramount importance for listeners with binaural interaction deficits. Central resources (compensatory) training might also relieve listening difficulties and might include auditory closure training (Bamiou et al., 2006; Musiek, 1999). The reader is referred to Volume II of this Handbook for extensive discussion of the range of treatment and management approaches, including auditory training for binaural interaction deficits.

Summary

Binaural interaction at the brainstem level underpins sound localization/lateralization and auditory performance in backgrounds of competing acoustic signals. Binaural interaction tests should therefore be included in the central auditory battery if the referring complaint (e.g., difficulties in localization or difficulties with understanding speech in noise), history (such as history of OME or multiple sclerosis), or the findings from other assessments (such as the binaural interaction component of the ABR) raise the suspicion that aspects of binaural hearing may be impaired or that maturation of this process is delayed in a specific individual. The currently available tests include various forms of the MLD and binaural fusion tests. It is hoped that localization/lateralization tasks will soon transfer into clinical practice, as they are easy and enjoyable to perform, and because these provide a measure of auditory performance in response to precisely controlled acoustic stimuli and may allow the clinician to make inferences for processing at different levels of the auditory system. In contrast, the RASP has not received much clinical acceptance because of the low sensitivity of this test in identifying patients with central auditory processing deficits, as well as in differentiating between different sites of brain pathology. In general, the clinician ought to be aware that, with the exception of the MLD, binaural interaction, tests can be affected by brain pathology outside the brainstem; thus poor scores in these tests may reflect deficits in higher-order processing. In addition, results ought to be interpreted with caution in the presence of hearing loss. However, correct application of these tests may help identify the auditory deficit(s) that need to be targeted by rehabilitation, and, in many cases, the level of the auditory pathway at which impaired processing occurs.

References

Abel, S. M., & Paik, S. (2005). Sound source identification with ANR earmuffs. *Noise and health*, 7, 1–10.

Aharonson, V., & Furst, M. (2001). A model for sound lateralization. *Journal of the Acoustical Society of America., 109,* 2840-2851.

Aharonson, V., Furst, M., Levine, R.A., Chaigrecht, M., & Korczyn, D. (1998). Lateralization and binaural discrimination of patients with pontine lesions. *Journal of the Acoustical Society of America, 103,* 2624-2633.

American Speech-Language Association (ASHA). (2005). *(Central) auditory processing disorders.* Available at http://www.asha.org/members/deskref-journals/deskref/default

Bamiou, D. E., Campbell, N., & Sirimanna T. (in press). Management of auditory processing disorders. *Journal of Audiological Medicine.*

Baran, J., & Musiek, F. M. (1999). Behavioural assessment of the central auditory nervous system. In F. E. Musiek & W. F. Rintelmann (Eds.), *Contemporary perspectives in hearing assessment* (pp. 375-413). Boston: Allyn & Bacon.

Besing, J. M., & Koehnke, J. (1995). A test of virtual auditory localization. *Ear and Hearing, 16,* 220-229.

Bocca, E., & Calearo, C. (1963). Central hearing processes. In J. Jerger (Ed.), *Modern developments in audiology* (pp. 337-370). New York: Academic Press.

Bourk, T. R., Mielcarz, J. P., & Norris, B. E. (1981). Tonotopic organization of the anteroventral cochlear nucleus of the cat. *Hearing Research, 4,* 215-241.

Bronkhorst, A. W., & Plomp, R. (1992). Effect of multiple speechlike maskers on binaural speech recognition in normal and impaired hearing. *Journal of the Acoustical Society of America, 92*(6): 3132-3139.

Cameron, S., Dillon, H., & Newall, P. (2006) The Listening in Spatialized Noise test: Normative data for children. *International Journal of Audiology, 45,* 99-108.

Cant, N. B., & Benson, C. G. (2003) Parallel auditory pathways: Projection patterns of the different neuronal populations in the dorsal and ventral cochlear nuclei. *Brain Research Bulletin, 60,* 457-474.

Chen, Z. (2005). Stochastic correlative firing for figure-ground segregation. *Biological Cybernetics, 92,* 192-198.

Chermak, G. D., & Lee, J. (2005). Comparison of children's performance on four tests of temporal resolution. *Journal of the American Academy of Audiology, 16,* 554-563.

Clifton, R. K., Morrongiello, B. A., & Dowd, J. M. (1984) A developmental look at an auditory illusion: The precedence effect. *Development Psychobiolgy, 17,* 519-536.

Cornelisse, L. E., & Kelly, J. B. (1987) The effect of cerebrovascular accident on the ability to localize sounds under conditions of the precedence effect. *Neuropsychologia, 25,* 449-452.

Cranford, J. L., Andres, M. A., Piatz, K. K., & Reissig, K. L. (1993). Influences of age and hearing loss on the precedence effect in sound localization. *Journal of Speech and Hearing Research, 36,* 437-441.

Cranford, J. L., Boose, M., & Moore, C. A. (1990a). Effects of aging on the precedence effect in sound localization. *Journal of Speech and Hearing Research 33,* 654-659.

Cranford, J. L., Boose, M., & Moore, C. A. (1990b). Tests of the precedence effect in sound localization reveal abnormalities in multiple sclerosis. *Ear and Hearing, 11,* 282-288.

Cranford, J. L., Morgan, M., Scudder, R., & Moore, C. (1993). Tracking of "moving" fused auditory images by children. *Journal of Speech and Hearing Research, 36,* 424-430.

Cranford, J. L., & Romereim, B. (1992). Precedence effect and speech understanding in elderly listeners. *Journal of the American Academy of Audiology 3,* 405-409.

Durlach, N. I. (1964). Note on binaural masking-level differences at high frequencies. *Journal of the Acoustical Society of America 36,* 576-581.

Eddins, D. A., & Barber, L. E. (1998). The influence of stimulus envelope and fine structure on the binaural masking level differ-ence. *Journal of the Acoustical Society of America, 103*, 2578-2589.

Feddersen, W., Sandel, T., Teas, D., & Jeffress L. A. (1957). Localization of high-frequency tones. *Journal of the Acoustical Society of America, 29*, 988-999.

Ferguson, M. O., Cook, R. D., Hall, J. W. 3rd, Grose, J. H., & Pillsbury, H. C. 3rd. (1998) Chronic conductive hearing loss in adults: Effects on the auditory brainstem response and masking-level difference. *Archives of Otolaryngology-Head and Neck Surgery 124*, 678-685.

Fitzpatrick, D. C., Kuwada, S., Kim, D. O., Parham, K., & Batra, R. (1999). Responses of neurons to click-pairs as simulated echoes: auditory nerve to auditory cortex. *Journal of the Acoustical Society of America, 106*, 3460-3472.

Freyman, R. L., Clifton, R. K., & Litovsjy, R. Y. (1991). Dynamic processes in the prece-dence effect. *Journal of the Acoustical Society of America, 90*, 874-884.

Furst, M., Aharonson ,V., Levine, A., Fullerton, B. C., Tadmor, R., Pratt, H., Polyakov, A., & Korczyn, A. D. (2000). Sound lateralization and interaural discrimination. Effects of brainstem infarcts and multiple sclerosis lesions. *Hearing Research 143*, 29-42.

Furst, M., Levine, R. A., Korczyn, A. D., Fuller-ton, B. C., Tadmor, R., & Algom, D. (1995). Brainstem lesions and click lateralization in patients with multiple sclerosis. *Hearing Research, 82*, 109-124.

Goldberg, J. M., & Brown, P. B. (1968). Func-tional organization of the dog superior olivary complex: An anatomical and elec-trophysiological study. *Journal of Neuro-physiology, 31*, 639-656.

Goldberg, J. M., & Brown, P. B. (1969). Response of binaural neurons of dog superior olivary complex to dichotic tonal stimuli: Some physiological mechanisms of sound localization. *Journal of Neuro-physiology, 32*, 613-636.

Grady, C. L., Grimes, A. M., Pilkus, A., Schwartz, M., Rapoport, S. I., & Cutler, N. R. (1984). Alterations in auditory pro-cessing of speech stimuli during aging in healthy subjects. *Cortex, 20*, 101-110.

Gravel, J. S., Wallace, I. F., & Ruben, R. J. (1996). Auditory consequences of early mild hearing loss associated with otitis media. *ACTA Oto-laryngologica, 116*, 219-221.

Griffiths, T. D., Dean, J. L., Woods, W., Rees, A., Green, G. G. (2001). The Newcastle Audi-tory Battery (NAB). A temporal and spatial test battery for use on adult naive sub-jects. *Hearing Research, 154*, 165-169.

Griffiths, T. D., Elliott, C., Coulthard, A., Cartlidge, N. E., & Green, G. G. (1998). A distinct low-level mechanism for interaural timing analysis in human hearing. *Neuro-Report, 9*, 3383-3386.

Hall, J. W., Buss, E., Grose, J. H., & Dev, M. B. (2004). Developmental effects in the masking-level difference. *Journal of Speech, Language and Hearing Research, 47*, 13-20.

Hall, J. W. III, & Grose J. H. (1990). The masking-level difference in children. *Jour-nal of the American Academy of Audiol-ogy, 1*, 81-88.

Hall, J. W., & Grose, J. H. (1993a). Short-term and long-term effects on the masking level difference following middle ear surgery. *Journal of the American Academy of Audiology, 4*, 307-312.

Hall, J. W., & Grose, J. H. (1993b). The effect of otitis media with effusion on the mask-ing-level difference and the auditory brain-stem response. *Journal of Speech and Hearing Research, 36*, 210-217.

Hall, J. W. III, Grose, J. H., & Pillsbury, H. C. (1995). Long-term effects of chronic otitis media on binaural hearing in children. *Archives of Otolaryngology-Head and Neck Surgery, 121*, 847-852.

Hanley, M., Jerger ,J. F., & Rivera, V. M. (1983). Relationships among auditory brain stem responses, masking level differences and the acoustic reflex in multiple sclerosis. *Audiology, 22*, 20-33.

Hawley, M. L., Litovsky, R. Y., & Culling, F. (2004). The benefit of binaural hearing in a cocktail party: effect of location and type of interferer. *Journal of the Acoustical Society of America, 115,* 833-843.

Hendler, T., Squires, N. K., & Emmerich, D. S. (1990). Psychophysical measures of central auditory dysfunction in multiple sclerosis: Neurophysiological and neuroanatomical correlates. *Ear and Hearing, 11,* 403-416.

Henning, G. B., & Zwicker, E. (1984). Effects of the bandwidth and level of noise and of the duration of the signal on binaural masking-level differences. *Hearing Research, 14,* 175-178.

Hirsch, I. J. (1948). The influence of interaural phase on interaural summation and inhibition. *Journal of the Acoustical Society of America, 20,* 536-544.

Hogan, S. C., Meyer, S. E., & Moore, D. R. (1996). Binaural unmasking returns to normal in teenagers who had otitis media in infancy. *Audiology and Neuro-Otology, 1,* 104-111.

Hutchings, M. E., Meyer, S. E., & Moore, D. R. (1992). Binaural masking level differences in infants with and without otitis media with effusion. *Hearing Research, 63,* 71-78.

Illing, R. B., Kraus, K. S., Michler, S. A. (2000). Plasticity of the superior olivary complex. *Microscopy Research and Technique, 51,* 364-381.

Irvine, D. R. F. (1986). The auditory brainstem: A review of the structure and function of auditory processing brainstem mechanisms. In D. Ottoson (Ed.), *Progress in sensory physiology* (Vol. 7, pp. 1-279). Berlin: Spinger-Verlag.

Irvine, D. R. F. (1992). Physiology of the auditory brainstem. In A. N. Popper & R. R. Fay (Eds.), *The mammalian auditory pathway: Neurophysiology* (pp. 153-223). New York: Spinger-Verlag.

Jeffress, L. A. (1948). A place theory of sound localization. *Journal of Comparative Physiology and Psychology, 41,* 35-39.

Jerger, J., Brown, D., & Smith, S. (1984). Effect of peripheral hearing loss on the masking level difference. *Archives of Otolaryngology, 110,* 290-296.

Jerger, J., & Jerger, S. (1974). Auditory findings in brain stem disorders. *Archives of Otolaryngology, 99,* 342-350.

Jiang, D., McAlpine, D., Palmer, A.R. (1997). Responses of neurons in the inferior colliculus to binaural masking level difference stimuli measured by rate versus level functions. *Journal of Neurophysiology, 77,* 3085-3106.

Johansson, M. S., & Arlinger, S. D. (2002). Binaural masking level difference for speech signals in noise. *International Journal of Audiology, 41,* 279-284.

Kapfer, C., Seidl, A. H., Schweizer, H., & Grothe, B. (2002). Experience-dependent refinement of inhibitory inputs to auditory coincidence-detector neurons. *Nature Neuroscience 5,* 247-253.

Katz, J., Ivey, R. G. (1994). Spondaic procedures in central testing. In J. Katz (Ed.), *Handbook of clinical audiology* (4th ed., pp. 239-255). Baltimore: Williams & Wilkins.

Kelly-Ballweber, D., & Dobie, R. A. (1984). Binaural interaction measured behaviorally and electrophysiologically in young and old adults. *Audiology, 23,* 181-194.

Koehnke, J., Colburn, H. S., & Durlach, N. I. (1986). Performance in several binaural-interaction experiments. *Journal of the Acoustical Society of America, 79,* 1558-1562.

Langner, G., & Schreiner, C. E. (1988). Periodicity coding in the inferior colliculus of the cat. I. Neuronal mechanisms. *Journal of Neurophysiology, 60,* 1799-1822.

Li, L., & Yue, Q. (2002). Auditory gating processes and binaural inhibition in the inferior colliculus. *Hearing Research, 168,* 98-109.

Licklider, J. C. R. (1948). The influence of interaural phase relations upon masking of speech by white noise. *Journal of the Acoustical Society of America, 20,* 150-159.

Linkehoker, B. A., & Knudsen, E. I. (2002). Incremental training increases the plasticity of the auditory space map in adult barn owls. *Nature, 419,* 293-296.

Litovsky, R. Y. (1997). Developmental changes in the precedence effect: estimates of minimum audible angle. *Journal of the Acoustical Society of America, 102,* 1739-1745.

Lynn, G. E., & Gillroy, J. (1972). Neuro-audiological abnormalities in patients with temporal lobe tumors. *Journal of the Neurological Sciences, 17,* 167-84.

Lynn, G. E., & Gillroy, J. (1977). Evaluation of central auditory dysfunction on patients with neurological disorders. In R. W. Keith (Ed.), *Central auditory dysfunction* (pp. 177-221). New York: Grune & Stratton.

Lynn, G. E., Gillroy, J., Taylor, P. C., & Leiser, P. C. (1981). Binaural masking-level differences in neurological disorders. *Archives of Otolaryngology, 107,* 357-362.

Magnusson, A. K., Kapfer, C., Grothe, B., & Koch, U. (2005). Maturation of glycinergic inhibition in the gerbil medial superior olive after hearing onset. *Journal of Physiology, 568,* 497-512.

Matzker, J. (1959). Two methods for the assessment of central auditory function in cases of brain disease. *Annals of Otology, Rhinology and Laryngology, 68,* 1185-1197.

Miller, G. L., & Knudsen, E. I. (2001). Early auditory experience induces frequency-specific, adaptive plasticity in the forebrain gaze fields of the barn owl. *Journal of Neurophysiology, 85,* 2184-2194.

Miltenberg, G. E., Dawson, G. J., & Raica, A. N. (1978). Central auditory testing with peripheral hearing loss. *Archives of Otolaryngology, 104,* 11-15.

Moore, C. A., Cranford, J. L., Rahn, A. E. (1990). Tracking of a "moving" fused auditory image under conditions that elicit the precedence effect. *Journal of Speech and Hearing Research, 33,* 141-148.

Moore, D. R. (1985). Postnatal development of the mammalian central auditory system and the neural consequences of auditory deprivation. *Acta Oto-laryngologica. Supplement, 421,* 19-30.

Moore, D. R. (1991). Anatomy and physiology of binaural hearing. *Audiology, 20,* 125-134.

Moore, D. R. (in press). Auditory processing disorders (APD): Definition, diagnosis, neural basis and intervention. *Journal of Audiological Medicine.*

Moore, D. R., Hutchings, M. E., & Meyer, S. E. (1991). Binaural masking level differences in children with a history of otitis media. *Audiology 30,* 91-101.

Musiek, F. E. (1983). The evaluation of brainstem disorders using ABR and central auditory tests. *Monographs in Contemporary Audiology, 4,* 1-24.

Musiek, F. E., Baran, J., Schochat, E. (1999). Selected management approaches to central auditory processing disorders. *Scandanavian Audiology Supplement, 51,* 63-76.

Musiek, F. E., & Geurkink, N. A. (1980). Auditory perceptual problems in children: considerations for the otolaryngologist and audiologist. *Laryngoscope, 90,* 962-971.

Musiek, F. E., & Geurkink, N. A. (1982). Auditory brain stem response and central auditory test findings for patients with brain stem lesions: A preliminary report. *Laryngoscope, 92,* 891-900.

Neijenhuis, K., Snik, A., Priester, G., van der Kordenoordt, S., & van den Broek, P. (2002). Age effects and normative data on a Dutch test battery for auditory processing disorders. *International Journal of Audiology, 41,* 334-346.

Neijenhuis, K., Snik, A., & van den Broek, P. (2003). Auditory processing disorders in adults and children: Evaluation of a test battery. *International Journal of Audiology, 42,* 391-400.

Neijenhuis, K., Stollman, M. H., Snik, A., & van den Broek, P. (2001). Development of a central auditory test battery for adults. *Audiology, 40,* 69-77.

Neijenhuis, K., Tschur, H., & Snik, A. (2004). The effect of mild hearing impairment on auditory processing tests. *Journal of the American Academy of Audiology, 15,* 6-16.

Noffsinger, D., Olsen, W. O., Carhart, R., Hart, C. W., & Sahgal, V. (1972). Auditory and vestibular aberrations in multiple sclerosis. *Acta Otolaryngologica Supplement 303*, 1-63.

Noffsinger, D., Schaefer, A. B., Martinez, C. D. (1985). Puretone techniques in evaluations of central auditory function. In J. Katz (Ed.), *Handbook of clinical audiology* (3rd ed., pp. 337-354). Baltimore: Williams & Wilkins.

Nozza, R. W., Wagner, E. F., Crandell, M. A. (1988). Binaural release from masking for a speech sound in infants, preschoolers, and adults. *Journal of Speech and Hearing Research, 31*, 212-218.

Olsen, W. O., & Noffsinger, D. (1976). Masking level differences for cochlear and brain stem lesions. *Annals of Otology, Rhinology and Laryngology, 85*, 820-825.

Olsen, W. O., Noffsinger, D., & Carhart, R. (1976). Masking level differences encountered in clinical populations. *Audiology, 15*, 287-301.

Pillsbury, H. C., Grose, J. H., & Hall, J. W. IIIrd. (1991) Otitis media with effusion in children. Binaural hearing before and after corrective surgery. *Archives of Otolaryngology-Head and Neck Surgery, 117*, 718-723.

Robinson, D. E., & Jeffress, L. A. (1963). Effect of varying the interaural noise correlation on the detectability of tonal signal. *Journal of the Acoustical Society of America, 35*, 1947-1952.

Rose, J. E., Geisler, C. D., & Hind, J. E. (1966). Some neural mechanisms in the inferior colliculus of the cat which may be relevant to localization of a sound source. *Journal of Neurophysiology, 29*, 288-314.

Schilder, A. G., Snik, A. F., Straatman, H., & van der Broek, P. (1994). The effect of otitis media with effusion at preschool age on some aspects of auditory perception at school age. *Ear and Hearing, 15*, 224-231.

Schoeny, Z. G., & Carhart R. (1971). Effects of unilateral Ménière's disease on masking-level differences. *Journal of the Acoustical Society of America, 50*, 1143-1150.

Shinn-Cunningham, B. (2000). *Learning reverberation: Considerations for spatial auditory displays* (pp. 126-134). International Conference on Auditory Display, Atlanta, GA.

Smith, B. B., & Resnick, D. M. (1972). An auditory test for assessing brain stem integrity: Preliminary report. *Laryngoscope, 82*, 414-424.

Stephenson, H., Higson, J., & Haggard, M. (1995). Binaural hearing in adults with histories of otitis media in childhood. *Audiology, 34*, 113-123.

Stern, R. M., & Trahiotis, C. (1995). Models of binaural interaction. In B.C Moore (Ed.), *Hearing* (2nd ed., pp. 347-385). London: Academic Press.

Stollman, M. H., Snik, A. F., Schilder, A. G., & van den Broek, P.(1996). Measures of binaural hearing in children with a history of asymmetric otitis media with effusion. *Audiology and Neuro-Otology, 1*, 175-185.

Stollman, M. H., van Velzen, E. C., Simkens, H. M., Snik, A., & van den Broek, P. (2003). Assessment of auditory processing in 6-year-old language-impaired children. *International Journal of Audiology, 42*, 303-311.

Sweetow, R. W., & Reddell, R. C. (1978). The use of masking level differences in the identification of children with perceptual problems. *Journal of the American Audiology Society, 4*, 52-56.

Tonal and speech materials for auditory perceptual assessment [compact disc 2.0]. (1998). Department of Veterans Affairs. Mountain Home, TN: VA Medical Center.

Wallach, H., Newman, E. B., & Rosenzweig, M. R. (1949). The precedence effect in sound localization. *American Journal of Psychology, 52*, 315-336.

Welsh, L. W., Welsh, J. J., & Healy, M. P. (1980). Central auditory testing and dyslexia. *Laryngoscope, 90*, 972-984.

Welsh, L. W., Welsh, J. J., Healy, M., & Cooper, B. (1982). Cortical, subcortical, and brainstem dysfunction: A correlation in dyslexic children. *Annals of Otology, Rhinology and Laryngology, 91,* 310–315.

Willeford, J. (1977). Assessing central auditory behavior in children. A test battery approach. In R. W. Keith (Ed.), *Central auditory dysfunction* (pp. 43–72). New York: Grune & Stratton.

Willeford, J. A., & Billger, J. M. (1978). Auditory perception in children with learning disabilities. In J. Katz, (Ed.) *Handbook of clinical audiology* (2nd ed., pp. 410–425). Baltimore: Williams & Wilkins.

Wilson, H., Zizz, C. A., & Sperry, J. L. (1994). Masking level difference for spondaic words in 2000 msec bursts of broadband noise. *Journal of the American Academy of Audiology, 5,* 236–242.

Wilson, R. H. (1994). Word recognition with segmented-alternated CVC words: Compact disc trials. *Journal of the American Academy of Audiology, 5,* 255–258.

Wilson, R. H., Arcos, J. T., & Jones, H. C. (1984). Word recognition with segmented-alternated CVC words: A preliminary report on listeners with normal hearing. *Journal of Speech and Hearing Research, 27,* 378–386.

Wilson, R. H., Hopkins, J. L., Mance, C. M., & Novak, R. E. (1982). Detection and recognition masking-level differences for the individual CID W-1 spondaic words. *Journal of Speech and Hearing Research, 25,* 235–242.

Wilson, R. H., Moncrieff, D. W., Townsend, E. A., & Pilion, A. L. (2003). Development of a 500-Hz masking-level difference protocol for clinic use. *Journal of the American Academy of Audiology, 14,* 1–8.

Wilson, R. H., & Weakley, D. G. (2005). The 500 Hz masking-level difference and word recognition in multitalker babble for 40- to 89-year-old listeners with symmetrical sensorineural hearing loss. *Journal of the American Academy of Audiology, 16,* 367–382.

Windham, R., Parks, M., & Mitchener-Colston, W. (1986) Central auditory processing in urban black children: A normative study. *Journal of Developmental and Behavioral Pediatrics, 7,* 8–13.

Wright, B. A. & Fitzgerald, M. B. (2001). Different patterns of human discrimination learning for two interaural cues to sound-source location. *Proceedings of the National Academy of Sciences of the United States of America, 98,* 12307–12312.

Wright, B. A., & Zhang, Y. (2006). A review of learning with normal and altered sound-localization cues in human adults. Submitted by invitation to IJA. *International Journal of Audiology.*

Yin, T. C., Chan, J. C., & Carney, L. H. (1987). Effects of interaural time delays of noise stimuli on low-frequency cells in the cat's inferior colliculus. III. Evidence for cross-correlation. *Journal of Neurophysiology, 58,* 562–583.

Zurek, P. M. (1980). The precedence effect and its possible role in the avoidance of interaural ambiguities. *Journal of the Acoustical Society of America, 67,* 953–964.

Zwicker, U. T., & Zwicker, E. (1984). Binaural masking-level difference as a function of masker and test-signal duration. *Hearing Research, 13,* 215–219.

CHAPTER 12

ELECTROACOUSTIC AND ELECTROPHYSIOLOGIC AUDITORY MEASURES IN THE ASSESSMENT OF (CENTRAL) AUDITORY PROCESSING DISORDER

JAMES W. HALL III AND KRISTIN JOHNSON

Introduction

The report of the Bruton Conference on auditory processing disorders (Jerger & Musiek, 2000) emphasized the importance and advantages of electroacoustic and electrophysiologic auditory measures in the clinical assessment of auditory processing disorder (APD). For example, the authors stated "Electrophysiologic and electroacoustic tests have the advantage of being less influenced by extraneous variables" (p. 470). The authors added "Many behavioral test paradigms can be incorporated within electrophysiologic procedures, thus providing both performance measures and gross site-specific information from the same test session" (p. 471). Participants in the Bruton Conference identified the following electroacoustic and electrophysiologic auditory mea-

sures, and the rationale for the inclusion of selected procedures in the clinical assessment of APD:

- Otoacoustic emissions (OAEs): "useful in ruling out inner ear disorders" (p. 471)
- Immittance audiometry: "essential to rule out middle ear disorder and to identify acoustic reflex abnormalities" (p. 471)
- Auditory brainstem response (ABR): measure of the status of auditory structures at the brainstem level
- Auditory middle latency response (AMLR): measure of the status of auditory structures at the cortical level
- Auditory late response (ALR)
- Mismatch negativity (MMN) response
- Event-related responses (ERPs).

In 2002, a number of well-respected audiologists published a summary of their concerns about the conclusions reached by participants at the Bruton conference (Katz et al., 2002). Katz and a dozen colleagues especially took issue with the role of electroacoustic and electrophysiologic measures in the assessment of APD, as described in detail in their paper entitled "Clinical and Research Concerns Regarding the 2000 APD Consensus Report and Recommendations." Katz et al. argued strongly against the inclusion of OAEs in the routine diagnostic test battery for APD. They also expressed a negative opinion regarding the role of auditory electrophysiologic measures, such as the ABR and AMLR, in the diagnostic assessment of APD. For example, Katz et al. stated that "because of the minimal contribution of auditory brainstem testing results and the added time and expense required for such measurements, it is our conclusion that ABR evaluation is inappropriate for the MTB (minimum test battery)" (p. 15). And, with regard to the AMLR, Katz and colleagues (2002) claimed that there is no research in support of the value of the response in APD diagnosis, citing several problems with AMLR measurement in children, including variability. In concluding their expressed concerns about the role of auditory electrophysiologic measurements, Katz and colleagues noted four alleged limitations of the AMLR, including problems recording the response from children under age 10 years, insensitivity of the AMLR to cortical lesions, the rare clinical application of the AMLR in pediatric audiology in general, and specifically for APD assessment, and the stated lack of an association between abnormal AMLR findings and recommendations for management.

Clinical experience confirms, however, that the practical advantages of electro-acoustic and electrophysiologic auditory measures in the assessment of APD are not trivial. Test time is relatively short for electroacoustic measures (typically less than 5 minutes for the assessment of both ears with both [OAEs and immittance] procedures). By definition, electroacoustic and electrophysiologic measures are objective and, therefore, not dependent on behavioral responses. Thus, the multiple subject factors often confounding conventional behavioral measures of auditory function, summarized in Table 12–1, have no influence on electrophysiologic or electroacoustic measures. In addition, aural immittance measures and OAEs provide information on very well-circumscribed portions of the auditory system, that is, they are highly site-specific. A few other features of each technique contribute to their clinical feasibility and popularity. Instrumentation for measurement of aural immittance and OAEs is readily available, and found in

Table 12–1. Factors Influencing Behavioral Measures of Auditory Processing Disorders (APD)

• Motivation
• Cognitive level
• Developmental age
• Attention
• State of arousal
• Motor skills, including oral motor (e.g., articulation) skills
• Native language
• The ability to understand verbal instructions
• Response strategies

Adapted from Jerger & Musiek (2000).

most audiology facilities. And, from a business perspective, current procedural terminology (CPT) codes exist for aural immittance measures (tympanometry and acoustic reflexes) and for both screening and diagnostic OAE techniques.

Clinical indications for the application of electroacoustic and electrophysiologic auditory measures in the clinical assessment of APD vary with the procedures. For example, as supported by data reported in the next section of this chapter, a strong case can be made for recording aural immittance measures and OAEs from all patients undergoing APD assessment. Evidence suggests that dysfunction in the peripheral auditory system can co-occur and exacerbate auditory processing disorders arising in the auditory nervous system (Kitzes, 1996; Recanzone, Schreiner, & Merzenich, 1993; Webster & Webster, 1977). Identification and quantification of peripheral auditory dysfunction is essential for complete description of APD, and for accurate analysis and interpretation of electrophysiologic and behavioral auditory responses arising from higher levels of the auditory nervous system. The remainder of this chapter presents research demonstrating the valuable role of electroacoustic and electrophysiologic measures in the comprehensive assessment of APD.

Electroacoustic Measures

Aural Immittance Measures

A detailed review of aural immittance measurement and analysis is beyond the scope of this chapter. Since the emergence of aural immittance measures as a valued component of the audiologic test battery in the early 1970s, hundreds of published papers, book chapters, and even entire books have been devoted to the topic. Classroom instruction on aural immittance principles and clinical practicum on aural immittance procedures, particularly tympanometry, is always found in the curricula of graduate audiology programs. The technique used for *tympanometry* in the assessment of APD is no different than that used in general pediatric audiologic assessment. A conventional low-frequency probe tone (e.g., 226 Hz) is appropriate for school-aged and older preschool-age children. Patient cooperation is rarely a problem in APD assessment. Measurement of the acoustic (stapedial) reflex should be performed immediately following tympanometry.

The protocol for measurement of *acoustic reflexes* in APD assessment departs somewhat from the approach taken often with general pediatric assessment. Specifically, the protocol should always include determination of acoustic reflex thresholds in four different measurement conditions, that is, measurement of ipsilaterally (uncrossed) and contralaterally (crossed) elicited acoustic reflexes for the right and left ears. Everyday application of acoustic reflexes in pediatric audiology often is limited to their measurement in either the ipsilateral or contralateral stimulus condition, but not both. Given the clinical and diagnostic importance of acoustic reflex measurement in the assessment of APD, a comprehensive review of the anatomy and physiology of the acoustic reflex arc is appropriate at this juncture.

Anatomy and Physiology of the Acoustic Reflex Arc

Seventy years ago, Lorente de Nó (1933) conducted careful neuroanatomic investigations of the acoustic stapedial reflex.

Information on the anatomy of the acoustic reflex arc is based largely on experimental studies in animals and clinical correlation of acoustic reflex abnormalities with sites of neuropathology, dating back to the 1970s (e.g., Borg, 1973). As illustrated schematically in Figure 12-1, the peripheral components of the arc include afferent portions—*the middle ear system*, the *cochlea*, and the *eighth (acoustic) cranial nerve*. The central components of the acoustic reflex arc, mediating activity between the afferent portion on one side and both left and right efferent portions, consist of direct and indirect pathways. The direct pathways consist of 3 or 4 neurons, including (1) sensory neurons of the eighth cranial nerve, that is, primary afferent fibers, (2) neurons from the ventral cochlear nucleus terminating in the vicinity of the ipsilateral motor facial nerve nucleus and in the ipsilateral and contralateral *medial superior olive* (MSO), (3) neurons from in or around the MSO and terminating on the ipsilateral or contralateral *region near the motor nucleus of the facial nerve,* and (4) motor neurons of the facial nerve arising from the area of the facial nerve motor nucleus and terminating on fiber(s) of the ipsilateral stapedius muscle. Thus, there are ipsilateral and contralateral acoustic reflex pathways, with the former involving afferent, brainstem intermediate, and efferent structures on the same side, and the latter involving afferents on one side, neurons which cross the caudal pontine brainstem midline, presumably via the trapezoid body, and efferent neurons on the opposite side.

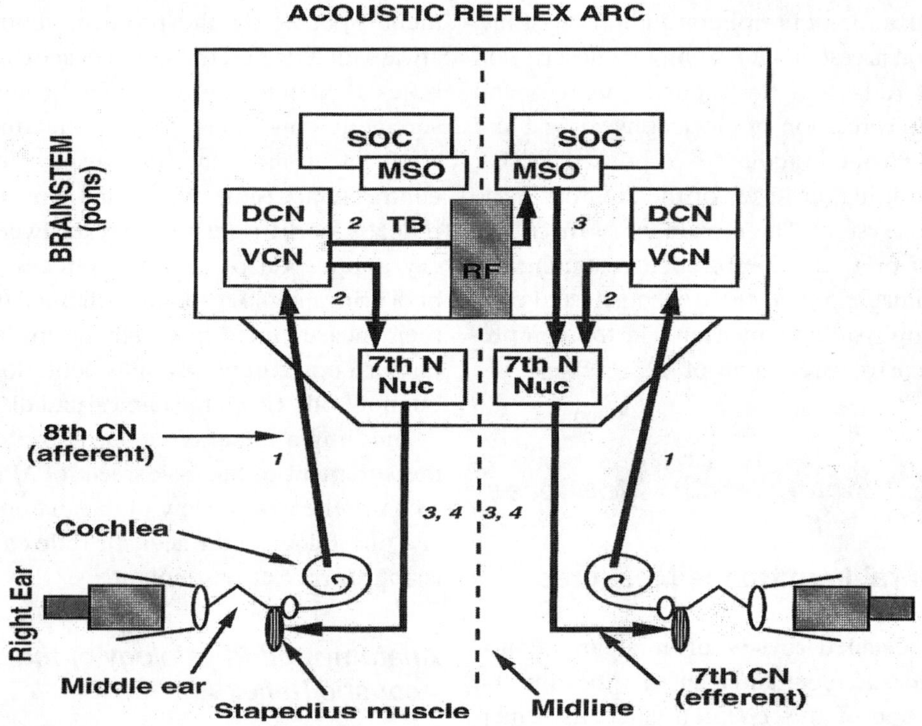

ACOUSTIC REFLEX ARC

Figure 12-1. Schematic diagram of the acoustic reflex pathways (described in the text).

The efferent portions of the acoustic reflex arc include the *seventh (facial) cranial nerve,* the *stapedius muscle and tendon,* and *the stapes.* The motor division of the facial nerve courses from its caudal pontine brainstem nucleus to the muscles of the face. After exiting the internal auditory canal at the stylomastoid foramen, it gives off a short branch of largely myelinated fibers (perhaps 10% of the entire motor division) to the stapedius muscle (Foley & DuBois, 1953). The stapedius is the smallest skeletal muscle in mammals. The stapedius muscle tendon emerges at the pyramidal eminence in the tympanic cavity (middle ear) to attach on the posterior aspect of the neck of the stapes.

An *indirect* acoustic reflex pathway clearly exists, although very little is known of its components in man or experimental animal. Borg (1973) speculated that this slower, polysynaptic pathway might involve the extrapyramidal motor system or the *reticular formation* (RF). The extreme sensitivity of the acoustic reflex to the influence of barbiturates (e.g., Hall, 1985a) supports the concept of an alternative, RF-mediated, pathway that may, in fact, predominate in man. Also, there are other, documented interactions between the traditional auditory structures and the RF (Brodal, 1981). Furthermore, the short- and long-latency components of the acoustically elicited stapedius muscle electromyography (EMG) show differential sensitivity to states of arousal and higher central nervous system (CNS) influences. The possible contribution of auditory cortical areas to acoustic reflex activity was also suggested in clinical reports (Downs & Crum, 1980; Jerger, 1980).

It is well known that contraction of the stapedius muscle occurs in response to high-intensity sound. The reflex is bilateral or consensual; that is, a sound presented to one ear produces contraction of the stapedius muscle on the same side (ipsilaterally) and on the opposite side (contralaterally). Normal stapedial muscle reflex activity in response to acoustic stimulation requires integrity of the afferent, brainstem, and efferent pathways. Acoustic reflex abnormalities are not, of course, typically a sign of neural dysfunction or central auditory dysfunction. More commonly in the clinical application of aural immittance measurement, detection of the acoustic reflex will be confounded or entirely precluded by middle ear dysfunction in the "probe ear," facial nerve dysfunction ipsilateral to the probe ear, and also moderate or severe conductive, sensory, or mixed hearing loss in the "stimulus ear."

The actual *physiologic basis* of the stapedial acoustic reflex remains unclear. Although the role of middle ear function in acoustic reflex measurements, at both the afferent and efferent extremes of arc, is well appreciated, the sensorineural and brainstem physiologic mechanisms underlying the acoustic reflex are not clearly defined. In normal hearers, at least, the acoustic reflex appears to be dependent in some way on loudness summation, that is, the perception of a sufficiently loud sound (Djupesland & Zwislocki, 1973; Flottorp, Djupesland, & Winther, 1971). Acoustic reflex activity also seems to be closely related to temporal summation (i.e., temporal integration) of acoustic energy, and interaction of stimulus duration and intensity (e.g., Djupesland, Sundby, & Flottorp, 1973). The reader is referred to Hall (1985b) for a more detailed review of the acoustic reflex arc and clinical applications of the acoustic reflex.

Clinical Application of Acoustic Reflex Measurement in APD

Acoustic reflex measurements are clinically useful in the identification and localization of peripheral and central auditory pathology. A simple schematic display of the pattern of acoustic reflex findings under the four measurement conditions (ipsilateral versus contralateral and right versus left ear) facilitates the differentiation among major types of auditory dyfunction, and also facial nerve dysfunction affecting the branch of the nerve that innervates the stapedius muscle. Three distinct patterns of acoustic reflex findings are depicted in the illustrations of the "faces" in Figures 12-2A, 12-2B, and 12-2C. The "vertical" abnormality pattern associated with middle ear or facial nerve dysfunction, that is, a peripheral or efferent dysfunction, is shown in Figure 12-2A. The acoustic reflex is abnormal whenever the measurement probe is in the involved ear. A "diagonal" abnormality pattern, depicted in Figure 12-2B, is found in persons with either severe/profound sensory hearing loss or retrocochlear auditory dysfunction. The acoustic reflex threshold is elevated, or the acoustic reflex is absent, whenever the stimulus is presented to the involved ear. The "horizontal" abnormality pattern (Figure 12-2C) is characteristic of persons with brainstem auditory dysfunction, and the pattern found most often in persons with APD. Acoustic reflex abnormalities are found in the contralateral (crossed) measurement condition, but not in the ipsilateral (uncrossed) condition.

Traditionally, one diagnostic role of acoustic reflexes is the differentiation of cochlear versus retrocochlear auditory dysfunction. Acoustic reflex threshold and decay are widely used as primary measures of eighth nerve functional integrity. Analysis of latency and amplitude parameters has further contributed to this diagnostic application of the acoustic reflex. Auditory abnormalities in intracanalicular eighth nerve lesions are ipsilateral, affecting peripheral afferent function exclusively. Griesen and Rasmussen (1970) first reported clinical evidence of contralateral (crossed) acoustic reflex abnormalities in brainstem pathology. Their observations were subsequently confirmed repeatedly with clinical and experimental investigations (e.g., Borg, 1971; Bosatra, 1977; Jerger & Jerger, 1974).

Three factors have contributed importantly to clinical application of acoustic reflexes in the assessment of central auditory dysfunction. First, Borg's (1973) correlations of acoustic reflex abnormalities with carefully defined experimental lesions of brainstem auditory nuclei and pathways in rabbits provided neuroanatomic information for meaningful interpretation of clinical reflex findings. Second, analysis and interpretation of the pattern of reflex findings for the four possible measurement conditions (ipsilateral and contralateral for the right and left ears) permits confident differentiation among afferent (sensorineural), efferent (middle ear or facial nerve), and central (brainstem) auditory dysfunction and substantially increases the specificity of reflex data. Clinical correlates of acoustic reflex patterns are described in detail in numerous publications, many by James and Susan Jerger, and colleagues (e.g., Jerger & Jerger, 1977; Jerger, Jerger, & Hall, 1979; Jerger & Jerger, 1981). Third, measurement of acoustic reflex amplitude, decay, and latency parameters augments threshold information and increases sensitivity of acoustic reflexes to brainstem pathology.

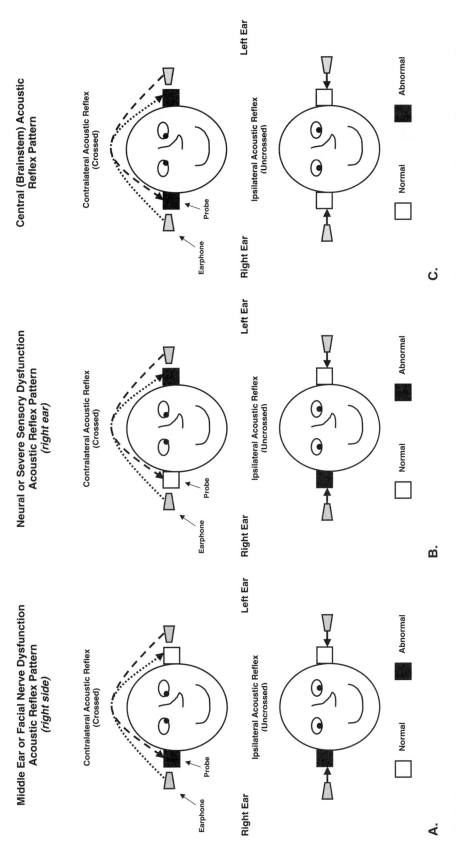

Figure 12–2. Typical patterns for acoustic reflex abnormalities including: **A.** the "vertical" pattern; **B.** the "diagonal" pattern; **C.** the "horizontal" pattern.

Amplitude decrements for crossed acoustic reflexes are reported in experimental and clinical brainstem auditory lesions that exert no apparent influence on acoustic reflex threshold levels (e.g., Borg, 1973; Bosatra, Russolo, & Poli, 1975; Hayes & Jerger, 1983; Jerger, Jerger, & Hall, 1979). There are also clinical reports of excessive decay of acoustic reflex amplitude in intra-axial brainstem pathology, in the absence of eighth nerve involvement and again without apparent acoustic reflex threshold abnormalities (Borg, 1982; Jerger & Jerger, 1977). Abnormally prolonged acoustic reflex latency may also be associated with brainstem pathology (Borg, 1973, 1982; Bosatra et al., 1975; Jerger & Jerger, 1977). Therefore, suprathreshold measures contribute to the diagnostic value of acoustic reflexes in the identification and localization of brainstem auditory pathology.

Scattered throughout the literature are reports of acoustic reflex findings in patients with diverse confirmed and suspected types of central auditory nervous system dysfunction. For example, Spitzer and Ventry (1980) found a significantly higher proportion of inexplicably absent acoustically measured reflexes in a group of chronic alcoholics than in an age-matched control group. Acoustic reflex threshold levels were equivalent for the two groups. The results of a diagnostic audiologic test battery, including these reflex findings, were consistent with brainstem auditory dysfunction. Acoustic reflex measurements may be clinically useful in patients with speech-language and voice problems of varied CNS etiologies, including autism, cerebral palsy, and mental retardation (Keith, Murphy, & Martin, 1977). Hall and colleagues (Hall & Jerger, 1976, 1978; Hall, 1981) observed acoustic reflex aberrations in two speech-voice disorders of unknown etiology. A reflex latency measure (rise time) was longer in a group of six patients with spastic dysphonia than an age- and sex-matched control group (Hall & Jerger, 1976). In a subsequent study, uncrossed reflex amplitude was curiously larger in a group of 12 subjects with spastic (spasmodic) dysphonia than in a control group, but crossed reflex amplitude showed no group differences. This deviant pattern (greater uncrossed reflex amplitude) had previously been associated with brainstem pathology (Bosatra & Russolo, 1976). In addition, reflex amplitude aberrations were reported in stuttering, again with reference to control data (Hall & Jerger, 1978).

In acutely and severely head-injured patients, acoustic reflexes are rarely observed, even in persons with normal middle ear function as determined by otologic examination and other acoustic immittance measures (Hall, Huangfu, & Gennarelli, 1982). Only 16% of a series of 25 patients showed evidence of any acoustic reflex activity within three days after a head injury defined as severe by the extent of coma. This high proportion of abnormal acoustic reflexes was probably related to their comatose state and neurosurgical management rather than to brainstem structural damage: severe head injury impairing consciousness presumably affects the brainstem reticular activating system. Barbiturate-induced coma, as noted earlier in the chapter, is sometimes employed therapeutically in management of brain pathophysiology secondary to head injury and was used in six of the above patients with no reflex activity. Both findings lend further support to the role of the reticular formation in the central acoustic reflex arc in man.

Acoustic Reflex Findings in APD

Given the clinical availability and feasibility of acoustic reflex measurement, and the potential for objective documentation of brainstem auditory dysfunction, there are surprisingly few formal studies of the acoustic reflex in APD. Over 20 years ago, Thomas, McMurry, and Pillsbury (1985) described ipsilateral and contralateral acoustic reflex findings in a rather heterogeneous series of 62 children with normal pure-tone hearing thresholds and tympanometry and "referred for suspected delays in development of language, learning disabilities, or disorders of auditory processing" (Thomas, McMurry, & Pillsbury, 1985, p. 811). Remarkably, 32% of the subjects showed acoustic reflex abnormalities in both the ipsilateral and contralateral signal conditions. According to the authors, there was no correlation between acoustic reflex abnormalities and patterns of language delay or disorder.

Expected abnormalities in acoustic reflex findings are elevated thresholds, reduced amplitudes, or total absence of the acoustic reflex. At the other extreme of the spectrum of abnormalities, Downs and Crum (1980) described in four children with APD, "hyperactive" acoustic reflexes, characterized by unusually low (better than expected) thresholds. The authors considered the pattern of findings as evidence of "decreased central inhibition of the peripheral auditory system" in some children with APD (p. 401). As reviewed in the next section of the chapter, Muchnik et al. (2004), in a study of minimal noise suppression effects on transient OAEs, also hypothesized decreased inhibitory auditory function in APD. Jerger, Jerger, and Loiselle (1988) reported a third category for

acoustic reflex findings, namely, normal acoustic reflex findings in a series of young children (ranging in age from 3 to 8 years) who had evidence of APD on dichotic listening tasks.

One possible explanation for the apparent discrepancy in findings among this small collection of studies of acoustic reflexes in APD is the difference in the patterns of abnormalities in auditory processing. For children diagnosed with APD on the basis of speech perception measures most sensitive to cortical and interhemispheric (e.g., corpus callosum) auditory dysfunction, abnormalities in the lower brainstem pathways involved in the acoustic reflex arc would be unlikely. On the other hand, an unselected group of children with suspected APD would by chance include some patients with dysfunction within more caudal regions of the central auditory nervous system, including abnormalities in excitatory (afferent) pathways (e.g., elevated, diminished, or absent acoustic reflexes) or, at the other end of the abnormality spectrum, unusually brisk reflexes with less intense stimuli.

Otoacoustic Emissions

Otoacoustic emissions (OAEs) were included among the auditory procedures in the test battery recommended by the participants at the Bruton Conference on APD (Jerger & Musiek, 2000). As noted above, Katz and colleagues took issue with the routine application of OAEs in the assessment of APD. For example, Katz et al. (2002) stated "We can find no research that children with APD have a high risk or incidence of inner-ear pathology. In fact, for general purposes, pure tone thresholds reflect cochlear pathology at lower hearing levels than OAEs" (p. 15). The authors went on to note, "Because OAEs offer little information for assisting children with their auditory processing deficit, the recommendations for OAEs as part of the MTB (minimal test battery) appears to be without merit" (p. 15).

In a follow-up response to the concerns, the clinical application of OAEs in the assessment of APD was vigorously defended by Jerger and Musiek (2002), as reflected by the following statement: "One important dimension in the differential diagnosis of APD is to differentiate APD from speech understanding problems due to malfunction at either the auditory periphery or the low brainstem level." "We know that a pure-tone audiogram within 'normal limits' does not guarantee normality at the auditory periphery. Before you can say that a child's listening problems are due to a disorder in the processing of auditory information at a relatively high level in the central auditory system, it is essential to rule out peripheral disorders at the hair cell level. The best, and virtually only, technique we currently have available for excluding this possibility is evoked OAEs" (p. 20).

There are three clinically important reasons for detecting and quantifying peripheral auditory dysfunction in the comprehensive, diagnostic assessment of APD. First of all, peripheral auditory dysfunction can lead to central auditory dysfunction. Transynaptic degeneration affecting central auditory structures can occur secondary to sensory deprivation (e.g., noise-induced or conductive hearing loss; longstanding peripheral hearing loss) (Hardie & Shepard, 1999; Schwaber, Garraghty, & Kaas, 1993; Webster & Webster, 1977). In other words,

the diagnostic assessment of APD is insufficient without careful measurement of even the most peripheral of auditory structures and functions. Secondly, peripheral auditory dysfunction, in isolation or in combination with central auditory dysfunction, certainly can affect speech perception in different listening conditions (e.g., quiet to noisy), the acquisition of other communication skills (e.g., phonemic awareness skills essential for reading) and academic performance. Audiologic management decisions for children with APD may depend in part on the status of the peripheral auditory system. Finally, the status of peripheral auditory function must be taken into account in the analysis and interpretation of diagnostic measures of central auditory processing. The possible impact of conductive and/or sensory hearing loss on clinical tests of auditory processing has been appreciated for many years. Recently, Neijenhuis, Tschur, and Snik (2004) confirmed that children with even mild sensorineural hearing loss performed significantly poorer on a variety of commonly used auditory processing tests, including sentences in noise, frequency and duration pattern tests, dichotic digits tests, filtered-speech test, and the binaural-fusion test.

Experimental and clinical evidence consistently supports the sensitivity and specificity of OAEs in the diagnosis of cochlear auditory dysfunction (see Hall [2000] for review). Virtually any insult to the cochlea is likely to affect outer hair cell function, including hypoxic/ischemic events, ototoxicity, and exposure to high-intensity sounds. As the generation of otoacoustic emissions is entirely dependent on the integrity of outer hair cell function, OAEs are exquisitely sensitive to even subtle cochlear abnormalities, including those most commonly encountered clinically. The close link between OAE findings and underlying integrity of the cochlea (specifically outer hair cells) is the basis for reliance on OAEs in newborn hearing screening. OAEs are a quick and objective technique for identification of most forms of peripheral auditory dysfunction. Considering the demonstrated value of OAEs in early detection of peripheral auditory dysfunction in newborn infants, it seems imminently logical to apply them likewise in the early detection of auditory disorders at the level of the cochlea. In addition, as noted at the outset of the chapter, and summarized in Table 12-2, OAEs offer multiple advantages for clinical assessment of APD, in addition to their sensitivity to subtle cochlear dysfunction.

Clinical Applications in APD

Our clinical experience confirms the value of OAEs in detecting peripheral auditory dysfunction in children undergoing assessment for APD. We analyzed audiolologic records for a series of 65 children (ages 5-20 years; M = 9 years) referred consecutively for assessment of APD in the Speech and Hearing Center at the University of Florida Health Science Center. Consistent with the opinions expressed by Katz and colleagues (2002), professionals or parents referring these children to the Center for auditory processing assessment generally presumed that hearing sensitivity was normal. For example, rarely were concerns about a hearing loss raised in the formal physician referral process or by the children's

Table 12-2. Advantages of Otoacoustic Emissions in the Diagnostic Assessment of Auditory Processing Disorders (APD)

- Very site specific, that is, to cochlear (outer hair cell) dysfunction

- Highly sensitive to auditory dysfunction, for example, abnormal OAEs may be recorded in persons with normal audiogram

- Frequency specific findings for multiple interoctave frequencies

- Brief test time, that is, usually <2 minutes/ear

- OAE abnormalities related experimentally to deficits in peripheral auditory processing, for example, deficits in frequency selectivity (e.g., abnormal tuning curves)

- As a nonbehavioral technique, OAEs are independent of listener variables, for example,
    - Age (chronologic and developmental)
    - State of arousal
    - Fatigue
    - Attention
    - Motivation
    - Cognition
    - Language

parents in the survey that each completed prior to the assessment. As an aside, however, a history of one or more basic hearing tests (e.g., "audiograms") was reported for over 80% of the children undergoing APD assessment, suggesting prior concern about auditory status by parents, physicians, and/or school personnel.

Distortion product otoacoustic emissions (DPOAEs) were recorded with a rather typical diagnostic test protocol using a clinical device (GSI 60). DPOAEs were recorded for f2 frequencies over the range of 500 to 8000 Hz, with 5 frequencies presented per octave. Intensities of the two pure-tone stimuli were 55-dB SPL for f2 (L2) and 65-dB SPL for f1 (L1). The f2/f1 ratio was 1.22. The "screen" configuration was used with the GSI 60 device. DPOAE amplitude values were calculated and analyzed with reference to published normative data available with the device (the Vanderbilt 65/65 normative region).

Approximately one-in-five (21%) of the 65 children had an abnormal finding on pure-tone audiometry, as defined by a threshold at or exceeding 20-dB HL for one or more of the test frequencies. Among this subset of children, 78.5% had average hearing thresholds meeting common criteria for hearing impairment (>20-dB HL) within the speech frequency region. Can OAEs be used to detect auditory dysfunction in children being assessed for APD, even children with normal hearing sensitivity as determined by the audiogram? Based on analysis of the data, the answer is "yes" on both counts. More than one-third of the series of children (35.5%) showed OAE abnormalities. Clearly, the proportion of children with DPOAE abnormalities exceeded the proportion with abnormal audiogram findings. Once again, DPOAEs provide information on cochlear function in children

with APD that is not available from the conventional pure-tone audiogram.

Smurzynski and Probst (1999) documented the impact of "subtle" cochlear deficits, as confirmed by OAEs, on several typical auditory measures used in the diagnostic assessment of APD. Whether spontaneous OAEs were "strong" or "weak" was related to performance on tasks of just noticeable differences in intensity for pure tones, temporal integration, and gap detection thresholds for broad-band noise bursts. The authors concluded that cochlear status, as defined by OAEs, can influence psychoacoustic task performance, especially for signals with spectral components in the vicinity of high-level spontaneous otoacoustic emissions (SOAEs) and presented at low-intensity levels. In a study of what is referred to as King Kopetsky syndrome or, mostly in the United Kingdom "obscure auditory dysfunction," Stephens and Zhao (2000) reported "notches" in distortion product OAEs and also abnormalities in transient evoked otoacoustic emissions (TEOAEs), even though pure-tone audio-metry was normal. Difficulty with speech perception in background noise was a common complaint of the subjects with obscure auditory dysfunction, a problem compatible with auditory processing disorders.

In addition to the application of OAEs for detection of peripheral auditory dysfunction in children undergoing APD assessment, there are reports of the use of OAE for electrocoustic documentation of dysfunction in the efferent (i.e., descending and inhibitory) auditory pathways. Muchnik and colleagues (2004) studied contralateral acoustic suppression of transient OAEs (TEOAEs) in 13 children ranging in age from 8 to 13 years who were diagnosed with APD. In comparison to a control group, the children with APD showed significantly less suppression of TEOAE activity. According to the authors, their results "imply that some APD children present low activity of the MOCB system, which may indicate a reduced auditory inhibitory function and affect their ability to hear in the presence of background noise" (p. 107).

Electrophysiologic Auditory Measures

Introduction

New applications of a variety of auditory evoked responses in APD, among them ABR, the amplitude modulation following response (AMFR), the auditory late response, and the MMN response are discussed in Chapter 4 (by Banai and Kraus). According to conventional thinking, APD is most likely to involve higher-level auditory central nervous system function, especially the auditory cortex. With this anatomic perspective, the ABR would be less useful in the diagnosis and description of APD than cortical auditory evoked responses. As detailed in Chapter 4, Banai and Kraus challenge the viewpoint with original data documenting the sensitivity of ABR elicited by complex (e.g., speech) stimuli to auditory, language, and learning disorders in school-aged children. The reader is referred to Chapter 4 for a full review of this exciting new application of ABR.

In addition to their usefulness in the clinical assessment of selected children suspected of APD, cortical evoked responses have considerable value as tools to uncover principles and mechanisms of auditory processing in patients across the age span, from infants to older adults, and to establish fundamental parameters of test performance for existing behav-

ioral procedures used clinically in the assessment of APD. That is, auditory evoked responses provide information essential for our understanding of the basic neuroscience of APD. Indeed, Jerger and Musiek (2002) noted "if we are ever going to have a gold standard for APD, it will probably be in the form of electrophysiologic measures" (p. 20). Although each of the major categories of cortical auditory evoked responses can contribute to our basic understanding of normal auditory processing, and disorders of auditory processing, the MMN response is especially attractive as a research tool.

There is general agreement that verification of APD must include evidence acquired with techniques that are independent of the multiple variables (listed in the introduction and in Table 12–1) that affect behavioral measures of auditory processing. In addition, auditory evoked responses elicited by nonspeech signals permit the validation of APD independent of language status, and other *pansensory* (Musiek, Bellis, & Chermak, 2005) functions that are not auditory specific. As noted by Rosen (2005), "any useful definition of CAPD must not only exclude supramodal causes of auditory deficits, but must be based on the notion of impaired brain function demonstrable for nonspeech sounds" (p. 139). The term "supramodal causes of auditory deficits" refers to problems that have a basis in language, cognition, and/or attention. All categories of auditory evoked responses (AERs) can be evoked with nonspeech stimuli, even from young children (e.g., infants), other subjects unable to yield consistent and valid behavioral responses, and subjects with a reduced state of arousal (e.g., sleep). Of course, AERs can also be recorded from animals in experimental paradigms that permit manipulations not possible in human investigations, such as creation of lesions or single-unit recordings directly from the generator of the response. Evidence is rapidly accumulating that brainstem and cortical auditory evoked responses are objective tools for verification of auditory processing deficits, and for establishing the electrophysiologic linkage between APD and other serious educational deficiencies, such as dyslexia, an auditory-based reading impairment (e.g., Sharma et al, 2006). The use of auditory evoked responses in APD is reviewed briefly below, and also by Banai and Kraus in Chapter 4.

A review of the principles underlying auditory evoked responses (AERs), and the protocols and procedures for clinical measurement of AERs, is far beyond the scope of this chapter. Each of the major AERs, ranging from short-latency responses (ECochG and the ABR) arising from peripheral auditory structures and the brainstem, to long-latency cortical responses (e.g., AMLR, ALR, P300, and the MMN response) offer advantages and disadvantages for the clinical assessment of APD. Strengths and weaknesses of each response are summarized in Table 12-3.

Table 12-3. Advantages and Disadvantages of Different Auditory Evoked Responses in the Diagnosis of Auditory Processing Disorders (APD)

Auditory Evoked Response*	Advantages	Disadvantages
ECochG	• Highly reliable in children • Anatomy/physiology known • Not influenced by drugs • Not influenced by state of arousal • Contributes to the diagnosis of auditory neuropathy	• Information limited to cochlea and VIIIth cranial nerve • Not a test of hearing • Insensitive to most APD (usually normal)
ABR	• Accepted test protocols and analysis strategies • Anatomy/physiology known • Highly reliable in young children • Age influences are well-defined • Assesses neural temporal function • Not influenced by state of arousal • Not influenced by medications	• No information on auditory function for pathways rostral to brainstem • Dependent on synchronous firing of onset neurons • Not a test of hearing • Insensitive to most APD (usually normal)
AMLR	• Accepted test protocols and procedures • Measurable in young children	• Influenced by sleep and sedatives • Analysis strategies not well defined in APD

Table 12–3. *(continued)*

Auditory Evoked Response*	Advantages	Disadvantages
AMLR *(continued)*	• Not influenced by validity of behavioral response to sound • Information on primary auditory cortex	• Interactions among age, stimulus rate, duration • Requires (minimally) two-channel evoked response (non-inverting electrodes over each hemisphere) • Few data on relationship to behavioral APD findings
ALR	• Accepted test protocols and procedures • Origin in auditory cortex (secondary) • Closer relation to behavioral findings • Elicited by complex (e.g., speech) stimuli • May provide information on effectiveness of intervention	• Marked influence of sleep and sedatives • Test protocols and analysis in APD not well defined • Some subject cooperation required
P300 response	• Accepted test protocols and procedures • Elicited with complex stimuli • High-level origin in auditory system (e.g., cortex and hippocampus) • Closer relation to behavioral findings • May provide information on effectiveness of intervention	• Requires P300 equipment option • Marked influence by sleep and sedatives • Some subject cooperation required • Validity with attention deficits may be problem • Analysis strategies not well defined in APD
MMN response	• Patient attention to stimulus is not required • Can be recorded from infants • Complex stimuli (e.g., speech) optimal • Cortical anatomic origin • Fundamental relation to behavioral findings • Information on effectiveness of intervention	• No accepted test protocols or analyses strategies • Requires special equipment options • Reliability in individual subjects is questionable • Not a proven clinical technique

*ECochG = Electrocochleography; ABR = Auditory brainstem response; AMLR = Auditory middle latency response; ALR = Auditory late response; MMN = Mismatch negativity response

The correlation of the origin of the cortical auditory evoked responses with the suspected site of dysfunction in the majority of children with APD is an obvious asset for the application of the AMLR, ALR, and P300 response clinically, and the MMN for investigations of the mechanisms underlying APD. Papers describing longer-latency AERs, therefore, dominate the literature on APD. Banai and Kraus (Chapter 4), however, provide recent and original evidence supporting the application of the ABR in the assessment of temporal processing in children with APD. Other studies of specific ABR measurement and analysis strategies in APD, such as calculation of the binaural interaction component (BIC) of the ABR, have yielded positive findings (Delb, Strauss, Hohenberg, & Plinkert, 2003). The reader is referred to the current and comprehensive *New Handbook of Auditory Evoked Responses* for detailed information on the topic (Hall, 2007). What follows herein is an overview of selected papers published in recent years reporting findings for various AERs in subject populations meeting the authors' criteria for APD.

Clinical Application of Auditory Evoked Responses in APD

Unquestionably, abnormalities in auditory evoked responses are found in some children undergoing diagnostic audiologic assessment for APD. As illustrated in Figure 12–3, acoustic reflex and auditory evoked response abnormalities are not uncommon in an unselected series of children evaluated clinically for APD (Hall & Baer, 1992; Hall & Mueller, 1997). The proportion of abnormalities is higher, as expected, for cortical auditory evoked responses (AMLR, ALR, and P300 re-

sponse) than for the ABR. With reference to the previous discussion about acoustic reflexes in APD, it is interesting to note that acoustic reflex abnormalities were more commonly observed in the contralateral (crossed) condition than in the ipsilateral (uncrossed) condition. Whether AERs are routinely included in a test battery for assessment of APD depends upon rather diverse factors, including characteristics of the patient population (e.g., age), the availability of necessary instrumentation and equipment options (e.g., multiple channels and the P300 option), the nature of the facility (e.g., purely clinical or a clinical research center), and even monetary considerations (e.g., available of coverage by third-party payors).

Each of the major auditory evoked responses has certain advantages and disadvantages as tools for clinical assessment of APD (refer to Table 12–3). Earlier latency AERs, that is, electrocochleography (ECochG) and ABR, can be recorded even under sedation and anesthesia, permitting assessment of very young children and those difficult to test with behavioral audiometry. Unfortunately, findings are normal in the majority of children undergoing APD assessment (see Figure 12–3), even for children with clear evidence of abnormality by behavioral diagnostic measures. In contrast, the later latency AERs are remarkably sensitive to APD and, when elicited by complex (e.g., speech) stimuli, may consistently document electrophysiologic deficits in auditory processing. The AMLR, ALR, and P300 certainly can be recorded with clinical instrumentation, although the availability of more user-friendly instrumentation for elicitation of these responses with sophisticated (e.g., speech) signals and statistically based analysis strategies

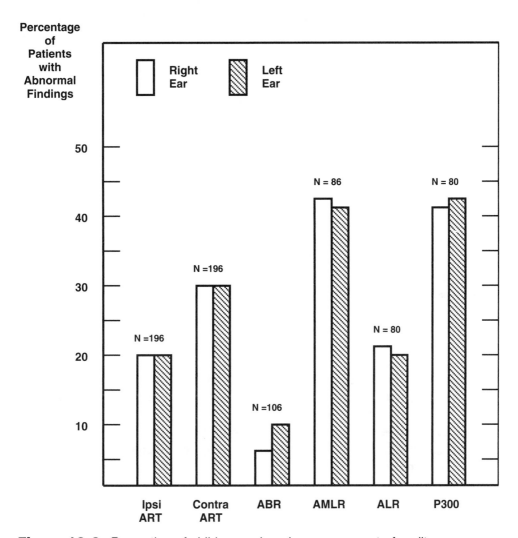

Abnormal Electroacoustic and Electrophysiologic Findings in Children with Auditory Processing Disorders (APD)

Figure 12–3. Proportion of children undergoing assessment of auditory processing disorders with abnormal findings for selected auditory evoked responses.

and software would contribute greatly to the clinical feasibility and value of the cortical AERs.

A brief review of the literature on AERs in clinical populations that include children with APD serves to highlight the potential clinical value of different responses. Mason and Mellor (1984) com-

pared AER findings for eight children with severe language disorders and six with severe motor speech disorders. Data also were collected for an age-matched normal control group. ABR latency was equivalent among groups, although amplitude was smaller in the children with speech and language disorders for all wave components. AMLR and ALR latency values also were comparable among groups. Grillon, Courchesne, and Akshoomoff (1989) recorded ABR and AMLR from eight subjects (mean age of 16 years) with "receptive developmental language disorder" (RDLD). There was no significant difference between an RDLD group and an age-matched control group for ABR or AMLR.

Since the 1980s, the AMLR has been investigated as an electrophysiologic measure of auditory dysfunction in children and adults with APD or, less specifically, children with learning disabilities (e.g., Arehole, 1995; Chermak & Musiek, 1997; Hall, 1992; Hall & Baer, 1992; Jerger & & Martin, 2004; Jerger, Martin, & McColl, 2004; Jerger et al., 1991; Jerger & Jerger 1985; Jerger, Johnson, & Loiselle, 1988; Marvel, Jerger, & Lew, 1992; Mason & Mellor, 1984; Musiek, Baran, & Pinheiro, 1994; Musiek, Baran, & Schochat, 1999; Purdy, Kelly, & Davies, 2002; Squires & Hecox, 1983; Tonnquist, 1996). With accumulated clinical experience and formal investigations, the methodology for AMLR measurement has evolved and improved with regard to the consistent and optimal detection of each component, for example, Pa and Pb. Although protocols followed in many of the earlier investigations included parameters that were not ideal for the neurodiagnostic application of the AMLR, especially in children, research has confirmed the value of AMLR for objective documentation of auditory dysfunction within the cortex. Some studies (e.g., Grillon et al., 1989; Mason & Mellor, 1984) reported no significant difference in the detection, or the latency and amplitude values, of the Pa component in children with learning disabilities (LD) or language impairment. Clearly, one possible expla-

nation for these negative findings is the absence of rigorous documentation of specific auditory processing disorder in the subjects enrolled in the studies.

A number of these investigators commented on their failure to consistently record the AMLR Pb component (e.g., Purdy, Kelly, & Davies, 2002). The most likely explanation for the apparent absence of the Pb component lies in the use of inappropriate settings for measurement parameters, as summarized at the end of this chapter (see New Directions in Research). A typical finding for AMLR in children with APD is latency prolongation and, particularly, amplitude reduction for the Na and Pa components with an electrode over one or both cerebral hemispheres. Indeed, among auditory evoked responses, the AMLR and the P300 response are abnormal most often, that is, in approximately 40% of patients referred for an APD assessment (Hall & Mueller, 1997).

Purdy, Kelly, and Davies (2002) conducted an investigation of multiple AERs (ABR, AMLR, ALR, and P300) in a small group (N = 10) of children with the rather general diagnosis of learning disabilities (LD). Age of the subjects ranged from 7 to 11 years. The AMLR was evoked with click signals (0.1-ms duration) presented monaurally and also binaurally at a rate of 8.7 per second and an intensity level of 70-dB nHL, and detected with noninverting electrodes located at midline (Cz) and hemisphere (C5 and C6) electrodes with linked earlobe inverting electrodes and bandpass filtering at 3 to 300 Hz. Longer duration (>30-ms) tonebursts are more effective in eliciting the Pb wave than clicks (0.1-ms duration) and a much slower stimulus rate (e.g., 1 per sec or slower) is required (Nelson, Hall, & Jacobson, 1997). It is not surprising, therefore, that Purdy et al. (2002) failed to record a Pb component. They did report AMLR differences for the LD versus control group, including delayed Na latency and smaller amplitude (less negativity) for the Nb component. Trends for other AMLR components, for example, Pa latency prolongation, were not statistically significant. More recent data (Schochat, Musiek, Alonso, & Ogata, 2006) have demonstrated the ability of the AMLR to differentiate children behaviorally diagnosed with APD from matched controls. The difference between the two groups was seen primarily in the amplitude of the AMLR.

Diagnostically, it has been shown that the MLR is sensitive and specific to involvement of the central auditory nervous system (Kileny, Paccioretti, & Wilson, 1987; Musiek, Charette, Kelly, Lee, & Musiek, 1999). This test efficiency is best shown by utilizing what is termed measurements of electrode and ear effects. Electrode effects are revealed by comparing amplitudes and latencies from the left and right hemispheres with electrodes positioned at C3 and T3 (left hemisphere) to electrodes at C4 and T4 (right hemisphere). Although amplitude and latency measures should both be obtained, it seems that amplitude measures are more insightful to dysfunction (Kileny, Paccioretti, & Wilson, 1987; Musiek et al., 1999; Musiek & Lee, 1997).

There are a growing number of papers on the ALR in APD and in other pediatric populations with APD as a possible coexisting disorder (Arehole, 1995; Bernal et al., 2000; Seri, Cerquiglini, Pisani, & Curatolo, 1999; Tonnquist, 1996). The ALR usually refers to the N1 and P2 wave complex. Its generators are the auditory cortex, and because of this the ALR has often been thought of as a potential that

could reflect integrity of the auditory cortex (Steinschneider, Kurtzberg, & Vaughan, 1992). Several key studies have demonstrated that lesions of the auditory cortex compromise the N1P2 more than lesions of the frontal or parietal lobe (Knight, Hillyard, Woods, & Neville, 1980; Knight, Scabini, Woods, & Clayworth, 1989) providing support for the clinical use of this potential to measure the functional status of the central auditory nervous system. In this regard, the N1 and P2 have been shown to be either reduced in amplitude and/or delayed in latency for children with APD and language disorders (Jirsa & Clontz, 1990; Tonnquist, 1996).

Longer latencies for major ALR waves (e.g., N1) in children with auditory-language impairment have been attributed to slower processing speeds (e.g., Tonnquist, 1996). Applying two sophisticated strategies (discriminant analysis [DA] and self-organizing feature maps [SOFM]) for analysis of the ALR P1, N1, P2, and N2 waves, Schonweiler et al. (2000) first correlated the evoked response findings with behavioral measures in a group of 16 children with APD versus a control group. Then, the authors validated the same ALR analysis approach against behavioral findings for a group of 37 with suspected APD. Since the mid-1990s, Nina Kraus and colleagues also have conducted dozens of studies of the ALR in children with auditory-learning problems. Their work is summarized in Chapter 4. As just noted, Purdy, Kelly, and Davies (2002) included ALR components in an investigation of cortical auditory evoked responses in children with learning disabilities, including APD, and a control group of children with no history of learning or auditory problems. The P2 component of the ALR was not consistently recorded, and was typically small in amplitude. There were also significant group differences for the ALR P1 (shorter latency in the APD group) and the N1 component (smaller amplitude in the APD group).

The auditory P300 response and the MMN response are the focus of most studies of cortical evoked responses in children with APD. Nonetheless, given the potential clinical value of the P300 response for assessment of auditory processing and cognitive function, there are surprisingly few formal published investigations in groups of children with auditory-specific processing disorders (Hall, 1992; e.g., Jirsa & Clontz, 1990). Most papers describe P300 response findings in children with other disorders that sometimes include auditory dysfunction, for example, autism, language impairment, and learning disabilities (Purdy et al., 2002; e.g., Arehole, 1995; Seri, Cerquiglini, Pisani & Curatolo, 1999). However, there are some compelling data that confirm the sensitivity of P300 to central auditory nervous system involvement. Although there are nonauditory contributors to the P300, there is evidence that lesions in the auditory regions of the cortex compromise the P300 in both latency and amplitude (see Knight, Scabini, Woods, & Clayworth, 1989 and Musiek, Baran, & Pinheiro,1992).

The application of the MMN response in auditory processing disorders (APD) is a natural outgrowth of the basic investigations of auditory processing mechanisms with the MMN. Case reports and group studies on the clinical use of MMN in the diagnosis of APD date back to the early 1990s. Among them are studies of the MMN response in dyslexia, an auditory-based reading disorder. A reconciliation of two apparently divergent explanations for dyslexia—auditory processing versus phonologic/linguistic processing —is likely to emerge from clinical data reported in the rapidly expanding literature on the MMN response in dyslexia. Difficulty perceiving speech sound differences (including vowel and consonant sounds requiring precise perception of rapid-timing changes) and in phonologic awareness (the ability to detect and manipulate speech sounds in words) are characteristic features of dyslexia. The MMN response for speech stimuli can be detected in infants before it is possible to evaluate speech perception behaviorally. The early appearance of the MMN response, and the feasibility of measurement in sleep, has led to fascinating investigations of auditory processing and speech sound perception in infants at familial risk for auditory-based reading disorders.

Banai and Kraus offer a detailed review of selected studies of the MMN in APD and dyslexia in Chapter 4. Several additional investigations are noted here. Leppänen and Lyytinen (1997) found differences in the MMN response for infants with a family history of delayed speech acquisition and dyslexia versus a control group. Studying the MMN response elicited with nonspeech (pure tones) and speech stimuli, Schulte-Körne et al. (1998) continued this line of investigation with children in adolescence finding a difference between the dyslexic and control groups in the MMN (smaller amplitude) evoked by speech stimuli, but not for tonal stimuli. Also, Baldeweg et al. (1999) reported abnormal MMN response findings in persons with dyslexia, using pure-tone standard and deviant stimuli. Smaller differences between the standard and deviant stimuli were more effective in differentiating the dyslexic subjects from the control group. One finding was particularly relevant for clinical assessment of APD. Baldeweg et al. (1999) reported a correlation between the MMN findings and behavioral performance in processing the stimuli. Kujala and colleagues (Kujala, Kallio, et al., 2001; Kujala, Karma, et al., 2001; Kujala & Näätänen, 2001) reported an abnormal MMN response when an additional sound closely followed (10 ms) a tone pattern that, when the third tone was not presented, elicited a response. The results suggest the possibility of a temporal deficit in auditory processing, and potential value of backward masking paradigms in the study of dyslexia. The very early detection with the MMN response of children at risk for such common and academically critical disorders as dyslexia raises the possibility for its use to maximize early intervention, even in infancy, and, perhaps, preventive management. Finally, there is experimental evidence that the MMN response can document effective intervention for dyslexia (Kujala, Karma, et al., 2001). Furthermore, the changes in MMN response were related to improvement in reading performance (Kujala, Karma, et al., 2001).

New Directions for Auditory Evoked Response Research in APD

Within recent years, new strategies and techniques have been reported for the investigation of auditory processing with each of the major AERs. Banai and Kraus (Chapter 4) provide a review of the application of ABR and cortical evoked responses elicited by speech stimuli in the diagnosis of APD, and the use of these responses in documenting the effectiveness of intervention. Similarly, an exciting potential strategy for assessment of APD with the AMLR will now be discussed.

As noted in the introduction to this chapter, the AMLR is appealing for assessment of APD because of the anatomic (cerebral cortex) origins of the response and simplicity of instrumentation, measurement, and analysis. The AMLR consists of two major positive components—the Pa and the Pb waves. In the clinical application of AMLR, attention has usually focused on the Pa wave, largely because of difficulties in consistently detecting the later Pb wave. In APD assessment, measurement and analysis of the AMLR Pb wave would be useful because the Pb wave represents contributions from regions of the auditory cortex not tapped by the Pa wave, presumably secondary auditory regions within the superior gyrus of the temporal lobe. It appears that the AMLR Pb wave is the same as the P1 wave of the auditory late response. Nelson, Hall, and Jacobson (1997) showed that the AMLR Pb wave is recorded consistently, even in children, with modification of the test protocol. Specifically, tone-burst stimuli (especially lower-frequency tone bursts) are more effective than click stimuli for eliciting the Pa component. Also, stimulus rate must be as slow as one or two stimuli per second, with even slower rates for children (e.g., 1 stimulus every few seconds). Among acquisition parameters, filter settings are particularly important. A high-pass filter setting as low as 1 Hz or even 0.1 Hz is necessary to capture the low-frequency energy contributing to the Pa wave. The reader is referred to the original article by Nelson, Hall, and Jacobson (1997) and to Chapter 11 in Hall (2007) for details on the optimal test protocol for measurement of the AMLR Pb wave.

With conventional test protocols, an AMLR is evoked with a series of single click or tone-burst stimuli and the resulting electrophysiologic activity is averaged periodically during the process. However, investigations of some fundamental auditory system and central nervous system processes via the AMLR also have utilized atypical stimulus paradigms, such as pairs of clicks, combinations of tone-bursts, trains of clicks, and even the oddball paradigm that is commonly associated with the P300 response (Ambrosini et al., 2001; Boutros & Belger, 1999; Boutros et al., 1995; Kisley et al., 2003).

With one test protocol, the AMLR Pb (P50) component is evoked with a pair of stimuli, a measurement approach sometimes referred to as the "double click paradigm" (e.g., Rosburg et al., 2004). The general concept is illustrated in Figure 12–4. The waveforms in the top portion of the figure depict an AMLR recorded with a conventional stimulus paradigm in which the response is averaged for a series of identical stimuli presented at a consistent rate (e.g., 1 per second) and the patient is not attending to the stimuli. Each stimulus evokes a similar response during the period of signal averaging, and similar responses are recorded for repeated averaging periods or runs. In the simplest version of the sensory-gating stimulus paradigm (middle waveform in Figure 12–4), the two identical stimuli (e.g., both of the clicks or both of the tone-bursts at the same frequency) are presented as a pair. The first stimulus (S1) is followed relatively soon after (e.g., <500 ms) by the second stimulus (S2), and then a longer interval (e.g., 8 to 10 seconds) separates the stim-

ulus pair from the subsequent signal pair. Some authors refer to the first and second stimulus as the "conditioning" and "test" stimuli, respectively (e.g., Ambrosini et al., 2001; Kisley et al., 2003). A fundamental function of the brain is to filter or "tune" out irrelevant, unimportant, or redundant information (e.g., Rosburg et al., 2004). According to investigators utilizing this stimulus paradigm, the ability of the brain to inhibit, or habituate to, irrelevant (repetitive) stimulation is reflected by the reduction in amplitude for the second stimulus in the pair. The amplitude change from the first to the second stimulus is calculated as a ratio (S2/S1) or simple mathematical difference (S1 − S2), with lower ratios and larger differences consistent with more inhibition or "gating out" of irrelevant sensory input. If the second stimulus is different from the first or "novel" stimulus, then larger ratios and smaller differences (or no difference) is consistent with "gating in," or a preattentive response of the brain indicating the ability to identify novel or potentially significant stimuli (Boutros & Belger, 1999; Rosburg et al., 2004). This novel approach for eliciting, recording, and analyzing the Pb (P50) component of the AMLR seems to be well suited for clinical application in children with APD.

With the rapidly accumulating information on the basic mechanisms of auditory processing yielded by investigations with auditory evoked responses arising from brainstem and cortical regions, and with the inclusion of paradigms and algorithms formerly found only in laboratory evoked response instrumentation within clinical evoked response devices, we appear to be on the threshold of a new era for applied auditory electrophysiology in

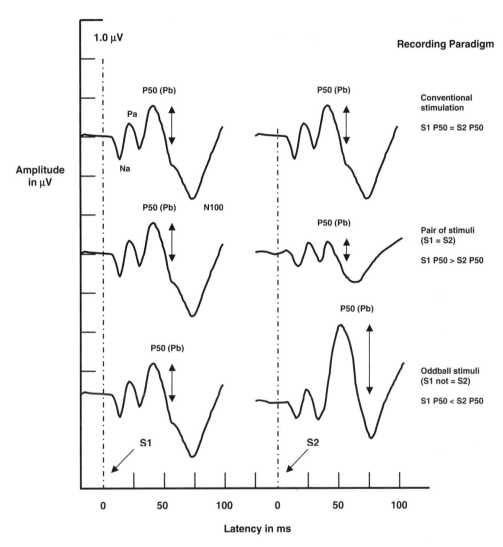

AMLR P50 (Pb) COMPONENT
An Index of Sensory Gating

Figure 12–4. Stimulus paradigm for measurement of the P50 component (the Pb wave) of the auditory middle latency response in the measurement of sensory gating, or habituation, to acoustic signals. (Used with permission from Hall, 2007).

APD. It is not hard to envision a clinically feasible diagnostic test battery for APD that includes a variety of auditory evoked responses, permitting confidence in identification and description of auditory processing even in young children. Auditory evoked responses also will be exploited in the objective documentation of the effectiveness of intervention for children, and adults, with APD.

Summary

We concur with the opinions expressed by Jerger and Musiek (2002) in response to the concerns raised by Katz and colleagues (2002) that "electrophysiological and electroacoustic measures are indispensable components of the diagnostic test battery for APD" (p. 21). We are in agreement with the participants of the Bruton Conference on APD who stressed the unique value of these techniques in the accurate and sensitive assessment of auditory function of children suspected of APD. Auditory deficits can occur anywhere within the auditory system, from the cochlea to the cortex. Although a staple in the audiologic test battery, the audiogram lacks sensitivity to some forms or degrees of cochlear dysfunction. OAEs, on the other hand, are highly sensitive to even subtle cochlear dysfunction involving the outer hair cells. Again, Jerger and Musiek (2002) articulated the point clearly: "We know that a pure tone audiogram within 'normal limits' does not guarantee normality at the auditory periphery" (p. 20). In combination, auditory evoked responses provide an objective means of documenting integrity, or dysfunction, of auditory pathways from the cochlea to the primary and secondary regions of the auditory cortex. Admittedly, for the vast majority of children undergoing APD assessment, electrocochleography (ECochG) and the ABR findings would be entirely normal. We do not recommend routinely including either ECochG or ABR in the test battery for assessing auditory processing in reasonably cooperative school-aged children. Both of these electrophysiologic techniques, however, are remarkably effective in the identification and diagnosis of certain forms of auditory dysfunction that are on occasion encountered in a large and unselected population of children suspected of APD, namely, what is commonly referred to as "auditory neuropathy." Returning once more to the collective viewpoint of the Bruton participants " . . . we know that dys-synchrony in brainstem auditory pathways (sometimes called 'auditory neuropathy') produces a distinct problem in speech understanding requiring specific intervention techniques." "The best and virtually only techniques we currently have available for excluding these two possibilities (cochlear auditory dysfunction with a normal audiogram and auditory neuropathy) are evoked OAEs and the auditory brainstem response" (p. 20). We cannot accurately evaluate higher level, central auditory processing without first ruling out auditory dysfunction in the peripheral auditory system and lower central auditory nervous system, that is, the brainstem. This is a deceptively simple, yet critically important, principle in diagnostic assessment of APD. In summary, both electroacoustic and electrophysiologic auditory measures can play a valuable and, really, indispensable role in the clinical assessment of APD in children, and as research tools to unravel the mysteries of auditory processing. (See Chapter 14 for discussion of OAEs and auditory brainstem response in the differential diagnosis of auditory neuropathy and APD.)

References

Ambrosini, A., De Pasqua, V., Afra, J., Sandor, P. S., & Schoenen, J. (2001). Reduced gating of middle-latency auditory evoked potentials (P50) in migraine patients: Another indication of abnormal sensory processing? *Neuroscience Letters, 306,* 132-134.

Arehole, S. (1995). A preliminary study of the relationship between long latency response and learning disorder. *British Journal of Audiology, 29,* 295-298.

Baldeweg, T., Williams, J. D., & Gruzelier, J. H. (1999). Differential changes in frontal and sub-temporal components of mismatch negativity. *International Journal of Psychophysiology, 33,* 143-148.

Bernal, J., Harmony, T., Rodriguez, M., Reyes, A., Yanez, G., Fernandez, T., Galan, L., Silva, J., Bouzas, A., Rodriguez, H., Guerrero, V., & Marosi, E. (2000). Auditory event-related potentials in poor readers. *International. Journal of Psychophysiology, 36,* 11-23.

Borg, E. (1971). Efferent inhibition of afferent acoustic activity in the unanesthetized rabbit. *Experimental Neurology, 31,* 301-312.

Borg, E. (1973). On the neuronal organization of the acoustic middle ear reflex. A physiological and anatomic study. *Brain Research, 49,* 101-123.

Borg, E. (1982). Time course of the human acoustic stapedius reflex. A comparison of eight different measures in normal-hearing subjects. *Scandinavian Audiology, 11,* 237-242.

Bosatra, A. (1977). Pathology of the nervous arc of the acoustic reflexes. *Audiology, 68,* 307-315.

Bosatra, A., & Russolo, M. (1976). Oscilloscopic analysis of the stapedius muscle reflex in brain stem lesions. *Archives of Otolaryngology, 102,* 284-290.

Bosatra, A., Russolo, M., & Poli, P. (1975). Modifications of the stapedius muscle reflex under spontaneous and experimental brain-stem impairment. *Acta Otolaryngologica (Stockholm), 80,* 61-66.

Boutros, N. N., & Belger, A. (1999). Midlatency evoked potentials attenuation and augmentation reflect different aspects of sensory gating. *Biological Psychiatry, 45,* 917-922.

Boutros, N. N., Torello, M. W., Barker, B. A., Tueting, P. A., Wu, S. C., & Nasrallah, H. A. (1995). The P50 evoked potential component and mismatch detection in normal volunteers: Implications for the study of sensory gating. *Psychiatry Research, 57,* 83-88.

Brodal, A. (1981). *Neurological anatomy in relation to clinical medicine*. New York: Oxford University Press.

Chermak, G. D., & Musiek, F. E. (1997). *Central auditory processing disorders: New perspectives*. San Diego, CA: Singular Publishing Group.

Delb, W., Strauss, D. J., Hohenberg, G., & Plinkert, P. K. (2003). The binaural interaction component (BIC) in children with central auditory processing disorders (CAPD). *International Journal of Audiology, 42,* 401-412.

Djupesland, G., Sundby, A., & Flottorp, G. (1973). Temporal summation in the acoustic stapedius reflex mechanism. *Acta Otolaryngologica (Stockholm), 76,* 305-312.

Djupesland, G., & Zwislocki, J. (1973). On the critical band in the acoustic stapedius reflex. *Journal of the Acoustical Society of America, 54,* 1157-1159.

Downs, D. W., & Crum, M. A. (1980). The hyperactive acoustic reflex: Four case studies. *Archives of Otolaryngology, 106,* 401-404.

Flottorp, G., Djupesland, G., & Winther, F. Ø. (1971). The acoustic stapedius reflex in relation to critical bandwidth. *Journal of the Acoustical Society of America, 49,* 457-461.

Foley, J. O., & DuBois, F. S. (1953). An experimental study of the facial nerve. *Journal of Comparative Neurology, 79,* 70-101.

Griesen, O., & Rasmussen, P. (1970). Stapedius reflexes in otoneurological examination in brain stem tumors. *Acta Otolaryngologica (Stockholm) 70,* 366-370.

Grillon, C., Courchesne, E., & Akshoomoff, N. A. (1989). Brainstem auditory evoked potentials and middle latency responses in non-retarded subjects with infantile autism and receptive developmental language disorders. *Journal of Autism and Developmental Disorders, 19,* 255-269.

Hall, J. W. III. (1981). Central auditory function in spastic dysphonia. *American Journal of Otolaryngology*, *2*, 188–198.

Hall, J. W. III. (1985a). The effects of high-dose barbiturates on the acoustic reflex and auditory evoked responses: Two case reports. *Acta Otolaryngologica (Stockholm)*, *100*, 387–398.

Hall, J. W. III. (1985b). The acoustic reflex in central auditory dysfunction. In M. L. Pinheiro & F. E. Musiek (Eds.), *Assessment of auditory dysfunction: Foundations and clinical correlates* (pp. 103–130). Baltimore: Williams & Wilkins.

Hall, J. W. III. (1992). *Handbook of auditory evoked responses*. Needham Heights, MA: Allyn & Bacon.

Hall, J. W. III. (2000). *Handbook of otoacoustic emissions*. San Diego, CA: Singular Publishing Group.

Hall, J. W. III. (2007). *New handbook of auditory evoked responses*. Boston: Allyn & Bacon.

Hall, J. W. III, & Baer, J. E. (1992). Central auditory processing disorder: Case report. *Seminars in Hearing*, *14*, 254–264.

Hall, J. W. III, Huangfu, M., & Gennarelli, T. A. (1982). Auditory function in acute head injury. *Laryngoscope 93*, 383–390.

Hall, J. W. III, & Jerger, J. F. (1976). Acoustic reflexes in spastic dysphonia. *Archives of Otolaryngology 102*, 411–415.

Hall, J. W. III , & Jerger, J. F. (1978). Central auditory function in stuttering. *Journal of Speech and Hearing Research*, *21*, 324–337.

Hall, J. W. III, & Mueller, H. G. III. (1997). *Audiologists' desk reference. Volume I*. San Diego, CA: Singular Publishing Group.

Hardie, N. A., & Shepherd, R. K. (1999). Sensorineural hearing loss during development: Morphological and physiological response of the cochlea and auditory brainstem. *Hearing Research*, *128*, 147–165.

Hayes, D., & Jerger, J. (1983). Signal averaging of the acoustic reflex: Diagnostic application of amplitude characteristics. *Scandinavian Audiology (Supplement)*, *17*, 31–36.

Jerger, J., & Jerger, S. (1974). Auditory findings in brainstem disorders. *Archives of Otolaryngology*, *99*, 342–350.

Jerger, J., & Jerger, S. (1981). *Auditory disorders: A manual for clinical evaluation*. Boston: Little, Brown & Co.

Jerger, J., Jerger, S., & Hall, J. W. III. (1979). A new acoustic reflex pattern. *Archives of Otolaryngology*, *105*, 24–28.

Jerger, J., Johnson, K., Jerger, S., Coker, N., Pirozzolo, F., & Gray, L. (1991). Central auditory processing disorder: A case study. *Journal of the American Academy of Audiology*, *2*, 36–54.

Jerger, J., & Martin, J. (2004). Hemispheric asymmetry of the right ear advantage in dichotic listening. *Hearing Research*, *198*, 125–136.

Jerger, J., Martin, J., & McColl, R. (2004) Interaural cross correlation of event-related potentials and diffusion tensor imaging in the evaluation of auditory processing disorder: A case study. *Journal of the American Academy of Audiology*, *15*, 79–87.

Jerger, J., & Musiek, F. (2000). Report of the consensus conference on the diagnosis of auditory processing disorders in school-aged children. Consensus Development Conference. *Journal of the American Academy of Audiology*, *11*, 467–474.

Jerger, J., & Musiek F. (2002). On the diagnosis of auditory processing disorder: A reply to "Clinical and research concerns regarding the 2000 APD consensus report and Recommendations." *Audiology Today*, *14*, 19–21.

Jerger, S. (1980). Diagnostic application of impedance audiometry in central auditory disorders. In J. Jerger & J. Northern (Eds.), *Clinical impedance audiometry* (2nd ed., pp. 128–140). Acton, MA: American Electromedics,.

Jerger, S., & Jerger, J. (1977). Diagnostic value of crossed versus uncrossed acoustic reflexes. Eighth nerve and brainstem disorders. *Archives of Otolaryngology*, *103*, 445–453.

Jerger S, & Jerger J. (1985). Audiologic applications of early, middle, and late auditory evoked potentials. *The Hearing Journal, 38,* 31-36.

Jerger, S., Johnson, K., & Loiselle, L. (1988). Pediatric central auditory dysfunction. Comparison of children with confirmed lesions versus suspected processing disorders. *American Journal of Otology* (Suppl. 9), 63-71.

Jirsa, R. E., & Clontz, K. B. (1990). Long latency auditory event-related potentials from children with auditory processing disorders. *Ear and Hearing, 11,* 222-232.

Katz, J., Johnson, C.D., Brandner, S., Delagrange, T., Ferre, J., King, J., Kossover-Wechter, D., Lucker, J., Medwetsky, L., Saul, R., Rosenberg, G. G., Stecker, N., & Tillery, K. (2002). Clinical and research concerns regarding the 2000 APD consensus report and recommendations. *Audiology Today, 14,* 14-17.

Keith, R. W., Murphy, K. T., & Martin, F. (1977). Acoustic reflex measurement in children with cerebral palsy. *Folia Phoniatrica (Basel), 29,* 311-314.

Kileny, P., Paccioretti, D., & Wilson, A. (1987). Effects of cortical lesions on middle latency evoked responses (MLR). *Electrocephalography and Clinical Neurophysiology, 66,* 108-120.

Kisley, M. A., Polk, S. D., Ross, R. G., Levisohn, P. M., & Freedman, R. (2003). Early postnatal development of sensory gating. *NeuroReport, 14,* 693-697.

Kitzes, L. (1996). Anatomical and physiological changes in the brainstem induced by neonatal ablation of the cochlea In R. Salvi, D. Henderson, F. Fiorino, & V. Colletti (Eds.), *Auditory system plasticity and regeneration* (pp. 256-274). New York: Thieme.

Knight, R., Hillyard, S., Woods, D., & Neville, H. (1980) The effects of frontal and temporal-parietal lesions on the auditory evoked potential in man. *Electrocephalography and Clinical Neurophysiology, 50,* 112-124.

Knight, R., Scabini, D., Woods, D., & Clayworth, C. (1989). Contributions of the temporal-parietal junction to human auditory P3. *Brain Research, 502,* 109-116.

Kujala, T., Kallio, J., Tervaniemi, M., & Naatanen R. (2001) The mismatch negativity as an index of temporal processing in audition. *Clinical Neurophysiology, 112,* 1712-1719.

Kujala, T., Karma, K., Ceponiene, R., Belitz, S., Turkkila, P., Tervaniemi, M., & Näätänen, R. (2001). Plastic neural changes and reading improvement caused by audiovisual training in reading-impaired children. *Proceedings of the National Academy of Sciences, USA, 98,* 10509-10514.

Kujala, T. & Näätänen, R. (2001) The mismatch negativity in evaluating central auditory dysfunction in dyslexia. *Neuroscience Biobehavioral Review, 25,* 535-543.

Leppänen, P.H., & Lyytinen, H. (1997). Auditory event-related potentials in the study of developmental language-related disorders. *Audiology and Neuro-Otology, 2,* 308-340

Lorente de Nó, R (1933). The reflex contractions of the muscles of the middle ear as a hearing test in experimental animals. *Transactions of the American Laryngology Rhinology Otology Society, 39,* 26-42.

Marvel, J. B., Jerger, J. F., & Lew, H. L. (1992). Asymmetries in topographic brain maps of auditory evoked potentials in the elderly. *Journal of the American Academy of Audiology, 3,* 361-368.

Mason, S.M., & Mellor, D.H. (1984). Brainstem, middle latency and late cortical evoked potentials in children with speech and language disorders. *Electroencephalography and Clinical Neurophysiology, 59,* 297-309.

Muchnik, C., Ari-Even Roth, D., Othman-Jebara, R., Putter-Katz, H., Shabtai, E. L. & Hildesheimer, M. (2004) Reduced medial olivocochlear bundle system function in children with auditory processing disorders. *Audiology Neuro-Otology, 9,* 107-114.

Musiek, F. E, Baran, J. A, & Pinheiro, M. (1992). P300 results in patients with lesions of the auditory areas of the cerebrum. *Journal of the American Academy of Audiology, 3,* 5-15.

Musiek, F. E., Baran, J. A, & Pinheiro, M. (1994). *Neuroaudiology: Case studies.* San Diego, CA: Singular Publishing Group.

Musiek, F. E., Bellis, T. J., & Chermak, G. D. (2005). Nonmodularity of the central auditory nervous system: Implications for (central) auditory processing disorder. *American Journal of Audiology, 14,* 128–138.

Musiek, F., Charette, L., Kelly, T., Lee, W., & Musiek, E. (1999b). Hit and false positive rates for the middle latency response in patients with central nervous system involvement. *Journal of the American Academy of Audiology, 10,* 124–132.

Musiek, F., & Lee, W. W. (1997). Conventional and maximum length sequences middle latency response in patients with central nervous system lesions. *Journal of the American Academy of Audiology, 8,* 173–180.

Neijenhuis, K., Tschur, H., & Snik, A. (2004). The effect of mild hearing impairment on auditory processing tests. *Journal of the American Academy of Audiology, 15,* 6–16.

Nelson, M. D., Hall, J. W. III, & Jacobson, G. P. (1997). Factors influencing the auditory middle latency response Pb component (P1). *Journal of the American Academy of Audiology, 8,* 89–99.

Purdy, S. C, Kelly, A. S., & Davies, M. G. (2002). Auditory brainstem response, middle latency response, and late cortical evoked potentials in children with learning disabilities. *Journal of the American Academy of Audiology, 13,* 367–382.

Recanzone, G., Schreiner, C., & Merzenich, M. (1993). Plasticity in the frequency representation of primary auditory cortex following discrimination training in adult owl monkeys. *Journal of Neuroscience, 13,* 97–103.

Rosburg, T., Marinou, V., Haueisen, J., Smesny, S., & Sauer, H. (2004). Effects of lorazepam on the neuromagnetic mismatch negativity (MMNm) and auditory evoked field component N100m. *Neuropsychopharmacology, 29,* 1723–1733.

Rosen, S. (2005). "A riddle wrapped in a mystery inside an enigma": Defining central auditory processing disorder. *American Journal of Audiology, 14,* 139–142.

Schochat, E., Musiek, F. E., Alonso, R., & Ogata, J. (2006). *The effects of auditory training on the middle latency response (MLR) in children with APD.* Manuscript submitted for publication.

Schonweiler, R., Wubbelt, P., Tolloczko, R., Rose, C., & Ptok, M. (2000). Classification of passive auditory event-related potentials using discriminant analysis and self-organizing feature maps. *Audiology and Neuro-Otology, 5,* 69–82.

Schulte-Körne, G., Deimel, W., Bartling, J., & Remschmidt, H. (1998). Auditory processing and dyslexia: Evidence for a specific speech processing deficit. *NeuroReport, 9,* 337–340.

Schwaber, M., Garraghty, P., & Kaas, J. (1993). Neuroplasticity of the adult primate auditory cortex following cochlear hearing loss. *American Journal of Otology, 14,* 252–258.

Seri, S., Cerquiglini, A., Pisani, F., & Curatolo, P. (1999) Autism in tuberous sclerosis: Evoked potential evidence for a deficit in auditory sensory processing. *Clinical Neurophysiology, 110,* 1825–1830.

Sharma, M., Purdy, S. C., Newall, K., Wheldall, P., Beaman, R., & Dillon, H. (2006). Electrophysiological and behavioral evidence of auditory processing deficits in children with reading disorder. *Clinical Neurophysiology, 117,* 1130–1144.

Smurzynski, J., & Probst, R. (1999). Intensity discrimination, temporal integration and gap detection by normally hearing subjects with weak and strong otoacoustic emissions. *Audiology, 38,* 251–256.

Spitzer, J. B., & Ventry, I. M. (1980). Central auditory dysfunction among chronic alcoholics. *Archives of Otolaryngology, 106,* 224–229.

Squires, K. C., & Hecox, K. E. (1983). Electrophysiological evaluation of higher level auditory processing. *Seminars in Hearing, 4,* 415–433.

Steinschneider, M., Kurtzberg, D., & Vaughan, H. (1992). Event-related potentials in developmental neural psychology. In I. Lapin & S. Segalowitz (Eds.), *Handbook of neural psychology*, *Vol. 6, Child neuropsychology* (pp. 239–299). Amsterdam: Elsevier.

Stephens, D., & Zhao, F. (2000). The role of a family history in King Kopetzky Syndrome (obscure auditory dysfunction). *Acta Otolaryngologica, 120,* 197–200.

Thomas, W. G., McMurry, G., & Pillsbury, H. C. (1985). Acoustic reflex abnormalities in behaviorally disturbed and language delayed children. *Laryngoscope, 95,* 811–817.

Tonnquist, U. (1996). Topography of auditory evoked long-latency potentials in children with severe language impairment: The P2 and N2 components. *Ear and Hearing, 17,* 314–326.

Webster, D., & Webster, M. (1977). Neonatal sound deprivation affects brainstem auditory nuclei. *Archives of Otolaryngology, 103,* 392–396.

SECTION III

Differential Diagnosis

CHAPTER 13

DIFFERENTIAL DIAGNOSIS OF (CENTRAL) AUDITORY PROCESSING DISORDER IN OLDER LISTENERS

TERI JAMES BELLIS

Much of the focus in (central) auditory processing disorders ([C]APD) has been on the relationship between central auditory dysfunction and learning, language, listening, communication, and related function in school-aged children. However, in recent years, attention has turned to the relative contribution of central auditory nervous system (CANS) function to the listening and speech understanding abilities of older adults. It is generally accepted that elderly individuals have difficulty with understanding spoken language, particularly in situations of competing background messages. What is less clear, however, is the underlying cause(s) of the speech perceptual difficulties of aging listeners.

Historically, many investigators have attributed the majority of the decreased auditory processing and speech percep-

tual abilities of the elderly to age-related changes in peripheral hearing sensitivity (e.g., Cooper & Gates, 1991, 1992; Divenyi & Haupt, 1997; Humes, 1996; Humes & Christopherson, 1991; Humes & Roberts, 1991; van Rooij & Plomp, 1991; Wiley, Cruickshanks, Nondahl, Tweed, Klein, & Klein, 1998). However, others have emphasized central (e.g., Bellis & Wilber, 2001; Golding, Mitchell, & Cupples, 2005; Jerger, 1992; Jerger & Chmiel, 1997; Jerger, Jerger, Oliver, & Pirrozzolo, 1989; Stach, Spretnjak, & Jerger, 1990; Strouse, Hall, & Burger, 1995) and/or cognitive (Gates, Cobb, Linn, Rees, Wolf, & D'Agostino, 1996; Gordon-Salant & Fitzgibbons, 1997; e.g., Hallgren, Larsby, Lyxell, & Arlinger, 2001; Sommers, 1996, 1997) factors. Although studies of the effects of biological aging and peripheral auditory dysfunction on neural encoding in the animal model may be found in the literature (e.g., Malmo & Malmo, 1982; Willott, 1986; Willott, Parkham, & Hunter, 1988a, 1988b, 1988c), the majority of earlier human studies failed to control for peripheral auditory dysfunction, including very subtle dysfunction that may not readily be apparent on behavioral audiometric testing. Nonetheless, more recent research has begun to investigate in a systematic manner the relative contribution of peripheral auditory, central auditory, and cognitive factors to listening and speech recognition in aging adults.

In this chapter, the factors contributing to listening and auditory processing difficulties in older listeners are explored. Particular attention is paid to methods of disentangling peripheral auditory and cognitive deficits from central auditory dysfunction for purposes of differential diagnosis of (C)APD in older listeners. Finally, key intervention strategies for older listeners who exhibit central auditory dysfunction with and without concomitant peripheral hearing is discussed.

Prevalence of and Risk Factors for (C)APD in Older Listeners

Various figures have been offered for the prevalence of (C)APD in older listeners. Stach et al. (1990) were perhaps the first to investigate what they termed "central presbycusis" in the older population while, at the same time, attempting to control for confounding effects of peripheral hearing loss and general cognitive decline. Their results indicated that 70% of adults older than 60 years in their clinical population exhibited some degree of central auditory dysfunction. (C)APD

prevalence increased with increasing age, with 17% prevalence in the 50 to 54-year-old age group but a remarkable 95% prevalence in the clinical population aged 80 years and older. In their nonclinical sample, they found a lower, yet still significant, prevalence, with 61% of those aged 75 to 79 years and 72% of those aged 80 years and older demonstrating some degree of (C)APD.

In contrast to the Stach et al. (1990) study, Cooper and Gates (1991) found a much lower prevalence of central auditory disorder in older listeners. Using the Framingham cohort, the authors found a 22.6% overall prevalence in their subjects aged 65 to 93 years, with no significant effect of gender on (C)APD prevalence. As with the previous study, Cooper and Gates (1991) found that the prevalence of (C)APD increased with increasing age but that age alone accounted for only 15% of the total variability in their study. Other estimates of the prevalence of (C)APD in the aging population have been offered (e.g., Jerger et al., 1989; Rodriguez, DiSarno, & Hardiman, 1990). Differences in prevalence estimates likely are due to widely differing methods of defining and diagnosing (C)APD, degrees to which peripheral auditory and cognitive factors were controlled for, whether a clinical or population-based sample was used, and a host of other factors.

In a more recent, population-based study of the prevalence of (C)APD in 2,015 Australian adults aged 55 years and older, Golding, Carter, Mitchell, and Hood (2004) found, as with previous studies, that the prevalence of central auditory disorder increased with increasing age, with older listeners more likely to perform poorly on a greater number of tests of auditory function. Depending upon how the disorder was defined, prevalence figures ranged from 2% (strict criterion of failure on all seven measures of auditory function employed in the study) to 76.4% (lax criterion of failure on one or more measure). Neither peripheral hearing loss nor cognitive factors could account for their findings. The authors also found that the prevalence of central auditory disorder was higher in men than in women, a finding that had been reported previously (e.g., Dubno, Lee, Matthews, & Mills, 1997; Jerger, Chmiel, Allen, & Wilson, 1994; Wiley et al., 1998). The authors concluded, as did most authors before them, that the prevalence of (C)APD in the aging population is of sufficient significance that its impact cannot be ignored.

Golding et al. (2005) further examined the above-mentioned Australian cohort to delineate risk factors associated with central auditory dysfunction in older listeners. They found that moderate or severe (C)APD was more prevalent with increasing age and resulted in increased self-perceived hearing handicap. Severe (C)APD was more common in men than in women; however, gender did not appear to be a predictive factor for more mild or moderate (C)APD. Decreased cognitive function was a significant predictor for central auditory dysfunction of all severities. Finally, general physiologic and life-related factors such as cardiovascular health, diabetes, alcohol consumption, presence of a social network, living alone, and other factors were not associated with increased (C)APD prevalence.

When taken together, results of these studies indicate that central auditory dysfunction is of sufficient prevalence in the aging population to be of clinical concern. Potential impact of the disorder in aging includes increased self-assessment of hearing handicap (e.g., Chmiel & Jerger, 1996; Golding et al., 2005; Jerger, Oliver, & Pirozzolo, 1990) and, when occurring comorbidly with peripheral hearing loss, may have an adverse impact on an individual's ability to realize benefit from the use of amplification (e.g., Chmiel & Jerger, 1996; Chmiel, Jerger, Murphy, Pirozzolo, & Tooley-Young, 1997; Jerger et al., 1990). Although men appear to be more at risk for age-related central auditory dysfunction than women, the relationship between gender and (C)APD in aging is less than clear, and may differ by gender depending upon the nature of the (C)APD and the point of time in the life span (Bellis & Wilber, 2001), with some forms of central auditory dysfunction occurring during the middle-aged years (e.g., Bellis, Nicol, & Kraus, 2000; Bellis & Wilber, 2001; Jaaskelainen, Varonen, Näätänen, & Pekkonen, 1999). Finally, both peripheral hearing loss and cognitive decline interact in a complex manner with central auditory dysfunction, and the presence of (C)APD may influence results of psychiatric assessment of older patients and may be an early marker for the onset of dementia in some cases (e.g., Gates et al., 1996; Strouse et al., 1995).

Factors Affecting Auditory Processing and Speech Recognition in Older Listeners

It is well accepted that difficulties with spoken message recognition, especially in the presence of competing backgrounds of noise, commonly accompany aging. Three primary hypotheses have been offered for the decreased speech perceptual abilities of older listeners (CHABA, 1988; Humes, 1996): The peripheral hypothesis attributes the speech perceptual difficulties experienced by aging individuals to age-related dysfunction in the cochlea and VIIIth nerve. The central hypothesis suggests that age-related changes in the CANS, independent of peripheral auditory dysfunction, lead to decreased speech perceptual abilities in the elderly. Finally, the cognitive hypothesis suggests that general age-related cognitive deterioration leads to processing difficulties in a variety of modalities, including those that are specific to listening and speech perception. Recent evidence suggests, however, that all three factors interact in a complex and multiplicative manner, and the relative contribution of each to listening and communicative function is highly individualized.

Peripheral Auditory Factors

Studies of the effects of peripheral auditory dysfunction and biological aging in the animal model have demonstrated that the presence of high-frequency hearing loss not only results in decreased audibility of certain spectral components of the acoustic signal, but also leads to a disruption in the tonotopic organization of the CANS (Willott, 1986; Willott & Lu, 1982; Willott et al., 1988a, 1988b, 1988c). Specifically, it has been found that neurons at the level of the inferior colliculus that may have responded previously to high-frequency acoustic signals exhibit lower characteristic frequencies (CFs) following the advent of cochlear hearing loss, resulting in a disproportionately greater representation of low-frequency information in the CANS. It may be pre-

dicted that this would lead to degraded encoding of high-frequency spectral components of the speech signal. Furthermore, because low-frequency auditory channels exhibit inherently poorer temporal resolving abilities (Phillips, Rappaport, & Gulliver, 1994; Stuart & Phillips, 1996; Stuart, Phillips, & Green, 1995), it is likely that such tonotopic reorganization secondary to peripheral auditory dysfunction may result in degradation of temporal encoding of the acoustic signal. These factors, combined with reduced audibility of certain spectral components of the acoustic signal, may be predicted to lead to significant disruptions in auditory processes that rely on precise temporal and frequency encoding, including speech perception.

A number of investigators have concluded that the single most important factor affecting speech perceptual abilities in the elderly is peripheral hearing sensitivity and signal audibility (Bess & Townsend, 1977; Humes & Christopherson, 1991; Humes & Roberts, 1990; Marshall & Bacon, 1981; van Rooij & Plomp, 1991). Cooper and Gates (1991), in their study of 1,026 older adults, demonstrated that pure-tone average (PTA) accounted for 30% of the variability in performance on a test of central auditory function and that it was the PTA, rather than aging alone, that correlated most significantly with central auditory performance. Similarly, Divenyi and Haupt (1997) emphasized that peripheral hearing loss was a primary factor affecting auditory performance in both elderly and young listeners. As a result, they cautioned that even very mild pure-tone threshold elevations may influence performance on any auditory test. Neijenhus, Tschur, and Snik (2004) also found that mild hearing loss can impact even those central auditory measures previously thought to be resistant to peripheral hearing impairment, underscoring the need to consider carefully the relative influence of peripheral factors on "central" auditory function. Jerger and Chmiel (1997) reported that both low-frequency and high-frequency hearing sensitivity were significant factors contributing to overall auditory impairment in elderly individuals. It is clear from these and other studies that the integrity of the auditory periphery is a key factor contributing to listening and related auditory function in aging adults, particularly given the high prevalence of peripheral hearing loss in this population.

Central Auditory Factors

Notwithstanding the importance of the auditory periphery to listening and speech recognition in aging, the vast majority of studies have concluded that peripheral hearing loss alone cannot account for the auditory performance decrements seen in older listeners. Instead, even when peripheral hearing loss is taken into account and/or corrected for, or when participants are free of peripheral auditory dysfunction, older listeners tend to perform more poorly on a variety of auditory measures. Moreover, these performance decrements are accompanied by age-related changes in the neurophysiologic representation of acoustic stimuli that cannot be attributed to changes in the auditory periphery alone.

Age-Related Changes in Neurophysiologic Representation of Acoustic Signals

Animal studies of the effects of biological aging in the absence of peripheral audi-

tory dysfunction have suggested that the effects of aging, per se, on the neural encoding of acoustic input may be relatively subtle. However, studies have demonstrated that an increase in spontaneous neural activity, possibly resulting from a decrease in inhibitory GABA, accompanies advancing age and may be indicative of increased "neural noise" in the aging CANS (Caspary, Raza, Lawhorn Armour, Pippin, & Arneric, 1990). It has been postulated that this increase in neural noise may underlie the speech perceptual difficulties of elderly listeners in competing acoustic backgrounds (Gregory, 1974; Novak & Anderson, 1982; Salthouse & Lichty, 1985). Furthermore, it has been shown that the number of neurons that exhibit precise temporal encoding is reduced in the inferior colliculus of aging mice, accompanied by a higher proportion of neurons that display sluggish temporal response properties (Willott et al., 1988a).

Human studies of the effects of aging on neurophysiologic encoding of auditory stimuli have revealed differences between young and elderly subjects. For example, studies have shown that the absolute latencies of auditory brainstem response (ABR) waves demonstrate a slight increase and that wave amplitudes diminish with advancing age (Harkins, 1981; Jerger & Hall, 1980; Patterson, Michalewski, Thompson, Bowman, & Litzelman, 1981; Rosenhamer, Lindstron, & Lundborg, 1980; Soucek, & Mason, 1990). Likewise, an increase in latency of peak components of the middle latency response (MLR) (Lenzi, Chiarelli, & Sambataro, 1989; Ryan, 1989; Woods & Clayworth, 1986) as well as in late components of the auditory evoked response (Goodin, Squires, Henderson, & Starr, 1978; Pfefferbaum, Ford, Roth, Hopkins, &

Kopell, 1979; Pfefferbaum, Ford, Roth, & Kopell, 1980; Picton, Stuss, Champagne, & Nelson, 1984) have been documented in elderly subjects. However, the underlying cause(s) of these changes in neurophysiologic measures are difficult to interpret, as such changes may be due to peripheral (e.g., decrease in the short-latency response from the basal end of the cochlea secondary to high-frequency hearing loss) or central (e.g., decreased neural synchrony/increased neural noise) factors. Finally, the finding that peak Pa of the MLR demonstrates an increase in amplitude with advancing age (e.g., Chambers & Griffiths, 1991; Jerger, Oliver, & Chmiel, 1988; Woods & Clayworth, 1986) suggests a possible impairment in inhibition in the aging organism, which is consistent with the findings of decreased GABA levels in animals discussed previously. Bellis et al. (2000) also postulated that a decrease in inhibition of right-hemisphere neural activity may underlie the lack of typical hemispheric asymmetry in the neural representation of speech sounds in older, normally hearing women.

More recent studies of the neurophysiologic representation of acoustic signals in aging populations have suggested that age effects may be more pronounced when complex speech signals and/or challenging tasks paradigms are employed than when simple, nonverbal acoustic stimuli are utilized to elicit neural responses (e.g., Fisher, Hymel, Cranford, & DeChicchis, 2000; Jerger & Lew, 2004; Tremblay, Billings, & Rohila, 2004). Tremblay, Piskosz, and Souza (2002, 2003) reported that the cortical event-related potentials elicited by speech signals differing in voice-onset time (VOT) were different in older listeners when compared to younger controls. These neuro-physiologic differences were accompanied by concomitant difficulty in psychophysical discrimination of the same VOT contrasts in the older adults, with performance decrements more pronounced in older adults who also exhibited peripheral hearing loss. The authors concluded that at least some of the speech perceptual difficulties exhibited by aging adults may be due to age-related changes in excitatory and inhibitory neural factors affecting neural synchrony, leading to poorer temporal precision in the central auditory pathways of older listeners. The fact that these difficulties were compounded in listeners with peripheral hearing loss may hold implications for hearing aid success in older adults with comorbid central and peripheral auditory dysfunction. In a subsequent study, Tremblay et al. (2004) demonstrated that the abnormalities seen in the neural responses of aging adults were not attributable merely to presentation rate of the stimuli alone, but were due to signal complexity as well. That is, both the speed of presentation/interstimulus intervals of consecutive stimulus onsets as well as stimulus complexity (i.e., speech versus nonspeech signals) affected various components of the cortical responses in older listeners, providing additional evidence for age-related temporal processing deficits, especially for complex signals such as speech.

Bertoli, Smurzynski, and Probst (2005) also found that the presence of peripheral hearing loss affected frequency discrimination abilities in older listeners, especially in backgrounds of competing noise, and that the psychophysical findings were accompanied by age-related differences in cortical auditory event-related potentials. Although they found that normally hearing older adults exhibited preserved discrimination abilities for simple frequency contrasts, the age-related differences in neural representation of the stimuli suggested that the aging adults used different processing strategies than the younger controls and that behavioral maintenance of discrimination abilities in older listeners was more effortful even in the absence of peripheral hearing loss.

Other studies have focused on age-related changes in interhemispheric asymmetries in the neural representation of auditory signals. These studies, in combination, have demonstrated that the pattern of hemispheric asymmetry in the neural representation of auditory signals is different in older adults when compared to younger listeners. In a study of whole-head auditory evoked magnetic fields in young versus elderly subjects, Pekkonen and colleagues (Pekkonen, Huotilainen, Virtanen, Sinkkonen, Rinne, Ilmoniemi, & Näätänen, 1995) found that the interhemispheric latency difference of the N100m component to simple tone pips was significantly increased in older adults, suggesting that age affects signal processing in the ipsilateral auditory cortex. Bellis et al. (2000) demonstrated that the obligatory P1-N1 complex elicited by synthetic speech syllables did not exhibit the expected left-hemisphere dominance in older, normally hearing women and that this decrease in typical interhemispheric asymmetry was accompanied by deficits in the behavioral discrimination of the same speech syllables. These findings provided evidence for a biological, age-related change in the basic sensory representation of elemental speech stimuli.

Jerger and colleagues (e.g., Greenwald & Jerger, 2001; Jerger, Alford, Lew, Rivera & Chmiel, 1995; Jerger, Moncrieff, Green-wald, Wambacq, & Seipel, 2000), in a series of studies combining behavioral and electrophysiologic measures of dichotic listening, demonstrated that aging adults exhibit increased interaural asymmetry (i.e., left-ear deficit) for dichotic speech stimuli and that this pattern is reflected in the electrophysiologic representation of the same stimuli. Moreover, a reversed pattern is seen when nonverbal signals are used. The patterns observed both behaviorally and electrophysiologically were strikingly similar to those seen in individuals with corpus callosum dysfunction, leading to a hypothesis of decreased interhemispheric transfer of auditory information in aging adults. Further supporting this hypothesis is the finding of decreased interhemispheric coherence of electroencephalographic (EEG) activity with advanced age (Duffy, Mcanulty, & Albert, 1996).

Finally, in an attempt to disentangle possible age-related difficulties in processing speech in competing backgrounds from higher level selective attention deficits, Hymel and colleagues (DeChicchis, Carpenter, Cranford, & Hymel, 2002; Fisher et al., 2000; Hymel, Cranford, & Stuart, 1998) demonstrated that aging affects the electrophysiologic correlate of stimulus competition. In contrast, the biologic mechanisms underlying the ability to attend selectively to target stimuli appear to be more resistant to the aging process. These findings provide further evidence of a fundamental signal-in-competition deficit in older listeners that cannot be attributed to higher level attention or other cognitive factors.

When taken together, studies of the neurophysiologic representation of auditory signals in older adults demonstrate decreased temporal precision and neural synchrony, atypical interhemispheric asymmetry, poorer interhemispheric communication and transfer of auditory information, and changes in the neural representation of stimulus competition with aging. These findings are most pronounced for speech signals, especially those involving rapid spectrotemporal acoustic changes. Although these effects are compounded by the presence of peripheral hearing loss, they cannot be accounted for by peripheral factors or by higher level attention or cognitive factors. Therefore, these studies provide compelling evidence of age-related changes in the central auditory mechanisms underlying binaural listening and speech perception, especially in backgrounds of competition.

On a final note, the auditory P300 event-related potential has been demonstrated to be instrumental in evaluating cognitive effects of aging and in the clinical assessment of dementia (e.g., Katado, Sato, Ojika, & Ueda, 2004; Knott et al., 2003). Thus, the combined use of brainstem, cortical, and cognitive auditory electrophysiologic responses may provide useful information regarding sensory encoding and cognitive processing of auditory stimuli in aging adults (see Olichney & Hillert, 2004, for review).

Age-Related Changes in Psychophysical Measures of Central Auditory Function

Several studies have examined the effects of aging on a variety of psychophysical measures of fundamental auditory skills. Age-related declines in frequency resolution have been documented (Glasberg, Moore, Patterson, & Nimmo-Smith, 1984; Lutman, Gatehouse, & Worthington, 1991; Matschke, 1991; Patterson, Nimmo-Smith, Weber, & Milroy, 1982), as have decreased

temporal processing abilities in elderly listeners on tasks including frequency and duration discrimination (Abel, Krever, & Alberti, 1990; Fitzgibbons & Gordon-Salant, 1994, 1998; Konig, 1957; Marshall, 1981; Meurman, 1954; Phillips, Gordon-Salant, Fitzgibbons, & Yeni-Komishian, 1994), gap detection (Ludlow, Cudahy, & Bassich, 1982; Lutman, 1991; Moore, Peters, & Glasberg, 1992; Schneider, Speranza, & Pichora-Fuller, 1998; Snell & Frisina, 2000; Strouse, Ashmead, Ohde, & Grantham, 1998; Walton, Frisina, & O'Neill, 1998), precedence effect (Cranford, Boose, & Moore, 1990), and backward masking (Cobb, Jacobson, Newman, Kretschmer, & Donnelly, 1993). It should be noted that the effects of aging on gap detection, in particular, may be complex, with evidence suggesting that it is influenced by condition (e.g., across-channel versus within-channel gap detection; Roberts & Lister, 2004), distance between the gap and the onset or offset of the signal (He, Horwitz, Dubno, & Mills, 1999), marker duration (Schneider & Hamstra, 1999), and other factors, including the presence of competing noise (Snell, 1997). Furthermore, age effects on gap detection performance may not be apparent with some gap detection paradigms when attention is directed toward the task, despite being evident during electrophysiologic measures of preattentive temporal processing (e.g., Bertoli, Smurzynski, & Probst, 2002). In addition, animal studies suggest that stimulus level also may play a role in aging effects on gap detection performance (Allen, Burkard, Ison, & Walton, 2003).

A plethora of studies have investigated the ability of elderly subjects to process speech stimuli, both in quiet and under conditions of background noise and/or various forms of signal distortion. Results of these investigations have suggested that older individuals have more difficulty than younger listeners in noisy or reverberant conditions (e.g., Dubno, Dirks, & Morgan, 1984; Harris, & Reitz, 1985; Nabalek, 1988; Nabalek, & Robinson, 1982; Wiley et al., 1998), and with temporally distorted speech (Gordon-Salant & Fitzgibbons, 1993a, 1993b, 2001; Rastatter, Watson, & Strauss-Simmons, 1989). In the absence of significant hearing loss, the speech perceptual abilities of elderly listeners do not appear to be greatly affected in quiet listening conditions (Dubno et al., 1984; Holmes, Kricos, & Kessler, 1988; Surr, 1977; Townsend & Bess, 1980). However, when the listening condition is made difficult either through the addition of competing noise or via introduction of some form of distortion in the speech signal, even normally hearing elderly listeners exhibit reduced speech perceptual abilities as compared to younger listeners (e.g., Helfer & Wilber, 1990; Rodriguez et al., 1990).

Many investigations of speech perception and aging have used either presbycusic listeners or listeners with "normal hearing for age/minimal hearing loss." Because a decline in peripheral hearing sensitivity typically accompanies aging, it is difficult to determine what proportion of the difficulties exhibited by elderly subjects in these studies may be due to central effects of biological aging alone versus central effects of subtle peripheral dysfunction. Because even minimal peripheral auditory dysfunction may degrade the neural input to the CANS, resulting in frequency, intensity, and temporal distortions of the acoustic signal, one cannot underestimate the possible detrimental effect of even very subtle peripheral dysfunction on those "central" processes presumed to be impor-

tant for speech perception (Willott, 1991). In fact, findings by Wilson and Weakley (2005) suggested that, in their study, word recognition performance in a background of multitalker babble was influenced more by the degree of peripheral hearing loss than by the age of the subjects, per se. Nonetheless, and as discussed previously in this chapter, other authors have demonstrated that the speech perceptual difficulties exhibited by aging listeners are independent of and/or cannot be accounted for entirely by peripheral hearing loss (e.g., Golding et al., 2005; Gordon-Salant & Fitzgibbons, 1993a, 1993b; Jerger & Chmiel, 1997; Wiley et al., 1998).

One way to separate the effects of peripheral hearing loss from central auditory deficits is to examine ear differences in performance on central auditory tests. That is, the presence of a significant ear effect despite symmetric hearing sensitivity or, alternatively, the presence of an ear deficit in the ear with *better* peripheral hearing sensitivity in cases of asymmetric hearing loss, can be taken as evidence in favor of a central auditory deficit rather than a peripheral explanation. Studies of dichotic listening performance in elderly listeners have been particularly useful in this regard. The presence of a significant left-ear deficit (or greater than normal right ear advantage, REA) on dichotic speech tests in aging adults has been reported in numerous studies (e.g., Bellis & Wilber, 2001; Chmiel & Jerger, 1996; Cowell & Hugdahl, 2000; Hallgren et al, 2001; Jerger & Chmiel, 1997; Jerger et al., 1994, 1995).

Bellis and Wilber (2001) demonstrated that the effects of aging on auditory and visual-motor indices of interhemispheric function, including dichotic listening and temporal patterning as well as visual-motor interhemispheric transfer time (IHTT), differed depending upon gender and point of time in the adult life span. In their study of 120 adults with 15 females and 15 males in each of four discrete age groups from 20 to 75 years of age, they demonstrated that males exhibited maximum interhemispheric auditory function in the early adult years, followed by a gradual and linear decline in interhemispheric abilities with increased age. Women, on the other hand, demonstrated preserved function throughout the child-rearing years up to approximately age 55, at which point a rapid decline in function occurred. No gender differences were observed in the oldest or youngest age groups. These findings mirrored previously reported anatomic changes in corpus callosum structure as a function of gender and point of time in the life span (Cowell, Allen, Zaltimo, & Dennenberg, 1992). This complex interaction between gender and point of time in the life span may explain, at least in part, previous contradictory findings regarding gender, aging, and dichotic listening performance. An additional, rather serendipitous, finding of Bellis and Wilber's (2001) study was that women tended also to exhibit a deficit in right-hemisphere-based central auditory function presumed to underlie perception of rhythm, stress, and intonational prosodic cues of speech during the immediate postmenopausal years which subsequently improved in later years. It was hypothesized that this latter finding may provide insight into a biological mechanism underlying, at least in part, the oft-reported difficulty in interpreting tone-of-voice cues in postmenopausal women.

In summary, studies of aging and central auditory function indicate that older adults exhibit difficulties in a variety of fundamental auditory processes as well as in speech recognition in backgrounds of competition and binaural listening abilities. Although peripheral auditory dysfunction compounds these difficulties, it cannot account for all the auditory effects observed.

Cognitive Factors

Age-related changes in cognitive functions such as working memory and information processing speed have been hypothesized to be responsible for some of the speech perception difficulties of older adults (e.g., Birren & Fisher, 1995; CHABA, 1988). Relationships between cognitive function and performance on central auditory tests have been reported in the literature (e.g., Gates et al., 1996; Golding et al., 2005, Gordon-Salant & Fitzgibbons, 1997; Strouse et al., 1995). Hallgren et al. (2001) found that dichotic listening performance correlated with measures of general cognitive ability, including working memory and processing speed, particularly when the listener is forced to attend to and report stimuli presented to the left ear. They attributed these findings to a decrease in working memory in the older adults and argued that such findings support the cognitive explanation of auditory deficits in aging. Others also have found a significant relationship between cognitive performance and directed report of stimuli to the left ear during dichotic listening performance (e.g., Cowell & Hugdahl, 2000), and suggest that the forced-left report condition may reflect additional attentional and cognitive mechanisms rather than true perceptual asymmetries. These findings hold implications for the use of directed-report versus free-report conditions during dichotic listening testing, which is discussed in a subsequent section of this chapter.

In these and similar studies, it might be assumed that cognitive decline affects older adults' performance on central auditory tests. However, an alternative explanation is equally, perhaps even more, likely. There is a great deal of evidence to suggest that the presence of perceptual deficits results in the need for greater resources to be allocated to auditory processing, thus leaving fewer resources available "upstream" for central cognitive processes required for storage and retrieval of auditory information (e.g., McCoy, Tun, Cox, Colangelo, Stewart, & Wingfield, 2005; Pichora-Fuller, Schneider, & Daneman, 1995;). In this resource allocation model, apparent "cognitive" changes are actually a consequence of a decline in auditory abilities and are exacerbated by both perceptual and cognitive stressors (McCoy et al., 2005; Murphy, Craik, Li, & Schneider, 2000; Pichora-Fuller, 2003; Pichora-Fuller et al., 1995; Rabbitt, 1991; Schneider, Daneman, & Murphy, 2005; Schneider, Daneman, & Pichora-Fuller, 2002).

That the central auditory and speech recognition difficulties of aging adults cannot be explained entirely or even primarily by cognitive decline is bolstered further by the finding that degree of cognitive deficit, unlike presence of central auditory dysfunction, does not correlate with perceived self-assessment of hearing handicap in older listeners (Jerger et al., 1990), and that measures of working memory and sequence-learning ability do not demonstrate a significant association with various measures of speech recognition in elderly listeners (e.g., Humes & Floyd, 2005). Indeed, Strouse et al. (1995) cautioned that the presence of auditory processing deficits may lead to poorer performance on cognitive tests and, thus, may influence results of psychiatric assessment in older adults. Finally,

although it has been demonstrated that older adults exhibit poorer performance than younger listeners on speech recognition tasks in the presence of meaningful competition, which has been taken as evidence that elderly listeners exhibited reduced attentional control (e.g., Tun, O'Kane, & Wingfield, 2002), neurophysiologic studies discussed previously suggest that it appears to be the processing of the signal in competition itself, rather than the ability to selectively attend, that is impaired in older adults (DeChicchis et al., 2002; Fisher et al., 2000; Hymel et al., 1998).

In contrast, research indicates that the linguistic experience of older adults actually facilitates their ability to compensate for deficits in sensory and perceptual processing. This is evident from studies demonstrating that older adults are better than younger listeners at using context to recognize words (Cohen & Faulkner, 1983; Jerger & Martin, 2005), and are better able to rely on previous linguistic knowledge and short-term conceptual memory when recognizing accelerated speech (e.g., Gordon-Salant & Fitzgibbons, 2001; Wingfield, Tun, Koh, & Rosen, 1999). Furthermore, the ability to make use of prosodic information, including clausal structure, to facilitate spoken word recognition is preserved in normal aging (Fallon, Kuchinsky, & Wingfield, 2004; Wingfield, Lindfield, & Goodglass, 2000).

In conclusion, a review of the literature on aging and speech perception suggests that many of the speech perception difficulties experienced by the elderly may be attributed to peripheral auditory dysfunction. On the other hand, age-related changes in neural synchrony and neural signal-to-noise ratios, along with declines in temporal processing and inefficient interhemispheric transfer of auditory information, also may give rise to degradation in the neural encoding of acoustic stimuli, leading to speech perceptual difficulties in the absence of peripheral auditory dysfunction, especially in backgrounds of competing noise. These central effects of biological aging may differ by gender and by point of time in the life span. Furthermore, it seems clear that the combination of peripheral auditory dysfunction and subtle age-related changes in auditory encoding results in a multiplicative effect, leading to significant speech perceptual difficulties in presbycusic listeners that cannot be predicted from the effects of biological aging or peripheral auditory dysfunction alone. Finally, the presence of peripheral and/or central auditory deficits may result in decreased resources available for storage and retrieval of auditory information. However, the ability to use linguistic, contextual, and prosodic knowledge to facilitate spoken language recognition may assist in offsetting the negative impact of peripheral and central auditory decline in older listeners.

Implications of Research for Auditory Assessment and Intervention in Older Adults

Several clinical implications can be drawn from the research regarding speech recognition, auditory processing, and aging. First, because the presence of peripheral auditory dysfunction has a deleterious effect on speech recognition and related abilities, particularly in backgrounds of noise, it is clear that a complete evaluation of peripheral auditory function is indicated in any case of reported listening or related difficulty, including physiologic measures to rule out subtle cochlear dysfunction that may not be apparent from the pure-tone audiogram. Furthermore, even when results of peripheral auditory evaluation suggest normal hearing, one should not assume that the entire auditory system is, therefore, normal. Evaluation of peripheral auditory function is merely the first step in the assessment process. Finally, clinicians should be cautious in interpreting traditional tests of speech recognition in quiet as it has been demonstrated clearly, first, that the speech perceptual difficulties of older adults often are apparent only in conditions of competition and/or signal distortion and, second, that auditory processing abilities cannot be predicted from traditional word-recognition-in-quiet scores. Therefore, more thorough evaluation of auditory function is indicated, particularly for those cases in which reported listening and related difficulties are greater than would be expected on the basis of the audiogram alone.

Second, based on findings related to prevalence of (C)APD in the aging population, beginning as early as the middle-age years, as well as the potential impact of central auditory dysfunction on self-perceived hearing handicap, benefit from amplification, and other factors, it may not be unreasonable to suggest that some type of central auditory assessment or screening be included as part of every audiologic evaluation involving older adults whenever possible. The role of the audiologist is to evaluate hearing, and the act of hearing involves mechanisms beyond just the peripheral auditory system. Given the significant adverse effects of central auditory dysfunction on listening and communication function, it behooves clinicians to obtain as much information as possible regarding auditory function so that intervention efforts can be directed appropriately. Issues related to diagnosing (C)APD and principles of intervention are discussed later in this chapter. Furthermore, because both gender and point of time in the life span may affect central auditory function differentially, intervention likely should include cross-gender counseling of spouses, family members, and other communicative partners.

Finally, there is some evidence to suggest that evaluation of peripheral and central auditory function may be important in cases of suspected dementia or other cognitive disorder in older adults (e.g., Gates et al., 1996; Strouse et al., 1995). Because the presence of sensory or perceptual deficit can result in "upstream" effects on memory and related cognitive abilities due to insufficient processing resources, it is critical that audiologists work as team members with psychiatrists, speech-language pathologists, and other professionals in the evaluation of older adults in an effort to disentangle the relative effects of peripheral and central auditory dysfunction from higher level cognitive, language, and other deficits. Thus, as with children, a multidisciplinary team approach is critical to the accurate and effective diagnosis of and intervention for (C)APD in the older population.

Differential Diagnosis of (C)APD in Older Listeners

Because many older adults exhibit peripheral hearing loss, and because even mild peripheral auditory dysfunction may affect performance on many tests of central auditory function, behavioral central auditory assessment in this population must be undertaken with caution. Nonetheless, it is possible to separate the relative effects of peripheral and central auditory dysfunction in many cases. However, clinicians must be familiar with the research underlying the available test procedures and select those that have been shown to be relatively resistant to peripheral hearing impairment. Furthermore, clinicians should be cautious in interpreting any test of central auditory function when peripheral hearing loss is present, even if previous research indicates that the test is relatively unaffected by peripheral disorder (Neijenhus et al., 2004).

Based on research discussed previously in this chapter, dichotic speech tests may provide the most useful information regarding central auditory function in older listeners. However, not all dichotic speech tests are equal in terms of resistance to peripheral hearing loss. As a general rule, dichotic speech tests that also require fine-grained discrimination of minimal-pair speech-sound contrasts, such as Dichotic Consonant-Vowel (CV) tests, also are most likely to be influenced adversely by peripheral hearing loss (e.g., Speaks, Niccum, & Van Tassell, 1985). In contrast, dichotic speech stimuli that carry a light linguistic load and do not require fine-grained auditory discrimination, such as the Dichotic Digits test (Musiek, 1983), appear to be most resistant to cochlear dysfunction (Musiek, Gollegly, Kibbe, & Verkest-Lenz, 1991). An additional advantage of the Dichotic Digits test is its ease and rapidity of administration (Musiek, 1983; Musiek et al., 1991), rendering it particularly appropriate as a screening tool for inclusion in standard audiologic test batteries. Moreover, the Dichotic Digits test has been shown to have good test-retest reliability even in elderly listeners with Alzheimer's disease, as well as in elderly listeners with no evidence of dementia (Strouse & Hall, 1995). Other dichotic speech tests that have been demonstrated to be relatively resistant to peripheral hearing loss include the Dichotic Sentence Identification (DSI) test (Fifer, Jerger, Berlin, Tobey, & Campbell, 1983) and the Staggered Spondaic Word Test (SSW; Arnst, 1982; Katz, 1962).

When administering any dichotic speech test, clinicians first should ensure that the test does not exceed the patient's working memory capacity. Thus, for example, if a test requires a patient to repeat four digits, as is the case with the Dichotic Digits test, clinicians first should ensure that the patient's digit span well exceeds the threshold level of four in a noncompeting condition prior to presenting the stimuli in the dichotic, competing condition. This provides at least one within-patient control for possible confounding effects of cognition and memory on central auditory test performance and assists in ensuring that dichotic speech deficits are due more likely to the introduction of the stimulus competition rather than to generalized memory problems.

Additional consideration should be given to the report condition required by tests of dichotic listening. When testing dichotically, two report conditions are possible. In the free report (FR) condition, listeners are instructed to repeat stimuli directed to both ears, usually in any order. This assesses the process of binaural integration (e.g., Bellis & Ferre, 1999; Bellis, 2003a; Chermak & Musiek, 1997). In the directed report (DR) condition, listeners typically are instructed to attend to and report the stimuli delivered

to the target ear only, thus assessing the process of binaural separation (Bellis & Ferre, 1999; Bellis, 2003a; Chermak & Musiek, 1997). Although it may appear at the outset that the FR condition is more susceptible to cognitive and/or memory confounds as it requires the listener to report a greater number of stimuli, previous research indicates that it is the DR condition that correlates most closely with cognitive function (e.g., Cowell & Hugdahl, 2000; Hallgren et al., 2001), particularly when the listener is directed to attend to the left ear, as this condition requires the listener to recruit additional cognitive and attentional mechanisms. These studies, therefore, concluded that performance decrements in the FR condition are more likely to be a consequence of true auditory perceptual asymmetries than are performance decrements in the DR (left) condition. Therefore, clinicians should be very careful in assigning central auditory versus cognitive explanations to differences in performance on dichotic speech tests based upon report condition. Instead, because the two report conditions tap into different underlying auditory processes, the use of both FR and DR conditions may, when administered and interpreted appropriately, provide useful insight into the specific auditory processes that are impacted by a given central auditory disorder. This information then may be used in designing a deficit-specific intervention plan to address the presenting auditory deficit profile.

An additional control that assists in disentangling the effects of peripheral and/or cognitive confounds from true central auditory dysfunction is the use of within-test comparisons of ear performance. Thus, and as previously discussed, the presence of a significant ear-specific deficit on dichotic speech tasks in the presence of normal or symmetric hearing sensitivity or, alternatively, the presence of a deficit in the ear with the better hearing thresholds in the case of asymmetric hearing sensitivity, may be taken as evidence of central auditory involvement.

Other behavioral tests of central auditory function also have been shown to be resistant to peripheral hearing loss as long as the signals are audible to the listener, including temporal patterning tests such as Frequency Patterns and Duration Patterns (Musiek, Baran, & Pinheiro, 1990; Musiek & Pinheiro, 1987). Again, ensuring that listeners can perform the task using live-voice modeling and employing within-test comparisons of contrasting report conditions (i.e., linguistic labeling of the stimuli versus nonverbal or humming report) can assist in controlling for potential cognitive and/or memory confounds and ensure that performance decrements observed are due to central auditory disorder.

A final control that assists in differentiating true central auditory dysfunction from more generalized cognitive, motivational, hearing, or other confounds is the use of intertest and multidisciplinary test analysis. Specifically, measures are examined for *patterns* of performance across tests that conform to well-established neuroscience tenets drawn from cases of known central auditory dysfunction. For example, the finding of left-ear deficits on dichotic speech tasks combined with a deficit on temporal patterning tests in the linguistic labeling condition only has been demonstrated in cases of known interhemispheric dysfunction involving the corpus callosum (e.g., Baran, Musiek, & Reeves, 1986; Musiek, Kibbe, & Baran, 1984). The emergence of this same pattern has been observed in aging adults

and correlates with anatomic changes in corpus callosum structure with aging (Bellis & Wilber, 2001; Cowell et al., 1992). Additional decrements in visual-motor interhemispheric transfer time, bimanual and/or bipedal difficulties, and other multidisciplinary findings indicative of inefficient interhemispheric function also may be seen on multidisciplinary tests (Bellis & Wilber, 2001).

In contrast, absence of a clear pattern of performance across tests, inconsistency in test performance, poor performance on all measures in all report conditions, or contradictory test findings (e.g., a left-ear deficit on one dichotic speech task accompanied by a right-ear deficit on another) argues for a nonauditory explanation and may be due to a host of factors, including generalized cognitive difficulty, motivational issues, lack of understanding of the test procedures, or other confounding factors. In these cases, diagnosis of a (C)APD would not be supported.

Although several other behavioral tests of central auditory function are available, the majority of them are affected adversely by cochlear pathology. Therefore, unless the listener presents with normal peripheral hearing status, these tests may not be appropriate for use in differential diagnosis of (C)APD in older listeners. For a detailed discussion of effects of cochlear, brainstem, and cortical (including corpus callosum) pathology on behavioral tests of central auditory function, as well as for information regarding administration and interpretation of these tests, readers are referred to Bellis (2003a).

As has been seen earlier in this chapter, electrophysiologic measures of central auditory function also hold great promise for differential diagnosis of (C)APD in older listeners, particularly when complex (e.g., speech) stimuli are used. Although many of the electrophysiologic paradigms discussed previously are not in general clinical use at this time, there is no doubt that they can be a useful addition to the clinician's differential diagnostic armamentarium (e.g., Jerger & Lew, 2004).

Finally, the use of speech-in-noise testing for (C)APD diagnosis should be mentioned. Although tests of speech in noise may provide a great deal of information about how an individual functions in backgrounds of competition, they may be affected by peripheral and central auditory disorders as well as other factors, and normative values will necessarily be different depending upon the stimuli, type and signal-to-noise levels of the competing signal, degree and configuration of hearing loss, and a number of other factors. Therefore, this author does not recommend their use for the diagnosis of (C)APD, per se. Nonetheless, they can assist clinicians both in determination of functional impact of auditory disorders as well as in investigating post-treatment outcomes. Several speech-in-noise tests have been developed for use with hearing-impaired populations, including the Quick-SIN (Etymotic Research, 2001) and the Hearing in Noise Test (HINT, Nillson, Soli, & Sullivan, 1994). Similarly, the use of self-assessments of hearing handicap such as the Hearing Handicap Inventory for the Elderly (HHIE; Ventry & Weinstein, 1982), Hearing Handicap Inventory for Adults (HHIA; Newman, Weinstein, Jacobson, & Hug, 1990), or the Communication Scale for Older Adults (CSOA; Kaplan, Bally, Brandt, Busacco, & Pray, 1997) may provide invaluable information regarding impact of the individual's auditory disorder on daily life and also may be useful in assessing post-treatment outcomes.

To obtain information regarding cognitive function, processing speed, working memory, and other factors that might affect performance on central auditory tests, clinicians also may wish to include general measures of these abilities. Some useful tools include the Mini-Mental State Examination (MMSE; Folstein, Folstein, & McHugh, 1975), a test of processing speed and interference such as the Stroop Color-Word Test (Uttl & Graf, 1997), and formal or informal listening span tests (e.g., Pichora-Fuller et al., 1995). Although none of these tests should be considered diagnostic for central auditory or cognitive disorder, they may provide important insight into the listener's overall levels of functioning across a variety of domains. Nonetheless, it should be emphasized that, as with any case of suspected (C)APD, a multidisciplinary approach is important to understanding fully the overall capabilities of the individual, and all efforts should be made to include physicians, psychologists, speech-language pathologists, and other professionals in the overall assessment process when indicated.

General Principles of Intervention for (C)APD in Older Adults

As with any (C)APD, it is important that intervention for older adults incorporate both bottom-up and top-down approaches. That is, intervention should focus both on the acoustic signal itself (bottom-up) and on the deployment of higher level language, cognitive, and related strategies to buttress deficient auditory skills (top-down). Furthermore, the precise nature of the intervention approaches will be dependent upon the individual's presenting deficit profile, lifestyle demands and communicative needs, and the presence of comorbid conditions, if applicable. As such, a multidisciplinary approach to intervention for (C)APD in older adults is just as critical as it is when considering the pediatric population. Although it is not within the scope of this chapter to provide detailed information regarding intervention approaches for adults with (C)APD, readers are referred to Volume II of this Handbook, as well as to Bellis (2002, 2003a, 2003b, in press), for a more in-depth discussion of treatment and management activities applicable to adults with (C)APD.

Research indicates that older listeners are able to use their linguistic knowledge and other top-down skills to assist in mitigating the effects of auditory deficits. To this end, compensatory strategies, or central resources, training is critical to assist patients in making optimum use of language, metalanguage, and cognitive, metacognitive, and related skills during listening. Specific details regarding central resources training are provided in Volume II of this Handbook.

In addition, particular attention should be paid to the listening and communicative environment of older adults. For those adults who are still in the workplace, or who regularly attend functions that require the ability to hear a speaker well (e.g., church, Bingo, the theater), consideration may be given to assistive-listening technology (ALDs) to improve the signal-to-noise ratio in these environments. Even older adults who spend a great deal of time at home may benefit from ALDs to assist in hearing the television or radio. Communication repair strategies and auditory-visual speech perception training also is an integral part of intervention for older adults with auditory disorders, including (C)APD and peripheral hearing loss. It is critical that family members, spouses, and other communicative partners be involved in the intervention and counseling process, and that mutually agreed-upon solutions to communicative dilemmas be developed.

The use of clear speech to enhance acoustic cues has been demonstrated to improve signal clarity and speech recognition for listeners with auditory disorders. Clear speech consists of several acoustic modifications, including a reduction in speaking rate, increase in duration of consonants and vowels, complete release of stop-consonants, increased consonant-to-vowel intensity ratio, and other parameters (e.g., Bradlow, Kraus, & Hayes, 2003; Ferguson & Kewley-Port, 2002; Pichenyi, Durlach, & Braida, 1986). Although research has shown that simply asking communicative partners to speak clearly is effective in achieving these acoustic modifications, resulting in improved speech recognition on the part of the listener, there is recent evidence to indicate that overtly *training* communicative partners in clear speech production results in greater speech recognition benefits (Caissie, Campbell, Frenette, Scott, Howell, & Roy, 2005). Furthermore, as discussed previously in this chapter, cross-gender counseling also may be of benefit for life partners to assist in understanding the opposite gender's listening and related difficulties (Bellis & Wilber, 2001).

Because so many older adults also present with peripheral hearing loss, it is important to remember that there is some evidence to suggest that the presence of (C)APD may affect the ability to receive optimum benefit and/or satisfaction from binaural amplification (e.g., Chmiel & Jerger, 1996; Chmiel et al., 1997). Although this does not by any means indicate that binaural amplification should not be considered for patients with peripheral hearing loss and comorbid (C)APD, it does indicate that special care may need to be taken to ensure optimum adjustment to binaural amplification in these cases. Indeed, recent evidence is emerging that individualized, intensive auditory training may improve hearing aid outcomes in general (e.g., Sweetow, 2005; Sweetow & Henderson-Sabes, 2004, in press; Sweetow & Palmer, 2005). This is consistent with research indicating that auditory plasticity extends throughout the life span and that adults demonstrate both stimulation- and deprivation-induced plasticity in the central auditory pathways (e.g., Blake, Strata, Churchland, & Merzenich, 2002; Silman & Silverman, 1993; Tremblay, Kraus, Carrell, & McGee, 1997; Tremblay, Kraus, & McGee, 1998; Tremblay, Kraus, McGee, Ponton, & Otis, 2001). Thus, although greater attention has been given historically to methods of assisting older adults in compensating for auditory deficits through acoustic signal enhancement and communication strategy training approaches, the role of deficit-specific, intensive auditory training for adults should not be overlooked.

In conclusion, intervention for (C)APD in older adults, as with children, should focus on three primary areas: environmental modifications (bottom-up and top-down approaches) to improve acoustic signal clarity and enhance access to the auditory signal, compensatory strategies (top-down) to strengthen and recruit central resources to assist in buttressing deficient auditory skills, and direct auditory training (bottom-up) to address specifically the specific auditory deficits present.

Summary

This chapter focused on the various factors that contribute to the well-recognized speech recognition difficulties of older adults. Specifically, peripheral hearing loss, changes in central auditory function, and cognitive factors often interact multiplicatively to impact adversely an adult's ability to listen and communicate effectively. Methods of differentially diagnosing (C)APD in older adults must take into account all three of these factors, as well as the lifestyle and communicative needs of the individual patient. Intervention for (C)APD in older adults should focus on improving the acoustic and communicative environment and utilizing central resources to compensate for auditory deficits. Finally, the potential importance of deficit-specific auditory training for maximizing listening and communication success in older listeners should not be discounted.

References

Abel, S. M., Krever, E. M., & Alberti, P. W. (1990). Auditory detection, discrimination and speech processing in ageing, noise-sensitive and hearing-impaired listeners. *Scandinavian Audiology, 19,* 43–54.

Allen, P. D., Burkard, R. F., Ison, J. R., & Walton, J. P. (2003). Impaired gap encoding in aged mouse inferior colliculus at moderate but not high stimulus levels. *Hearing Research, 186,* 17-29.

Arnst, D. J. (1982). SSW test results with peripheral hearing loss. In D. Arnst & J. Katz (Eds.), *The SSW test: Development and clinical use* (pp. 287-293). San Diego, CA: College-Hill Press.

Baran, J. A., Musiek, F. E., & Reeves, A. G. (1986). Central auditory function following anterior sectioning of the corpus callosum. *Ear and Hearing, 7,* 359-362.

Bellis, T. J. (2002). *When the brain can't hear: Unraveling the mystery of auditory processing disorder.* New York: Simon & Schuster.

Bellis, T. J. (2003a). *Assessment and management of central auditory processing disorders in the educational setting: From science to practice* (2nd ed.). Clifton Park, NY: Thomson-Delmar Learning.

Bellis, T. J. (2003b). Auditory processing disorders: It's not just kids who have them. *The Hearing Journal, 56,* 10-20.

Bellis, T. J. (in press). Treatment options for patients with (central) auditory processing disorders. In R. Roeser, M. Valente, & H. Hosford-Dunn (Eds.), *Audiology: Treatment* (2nd ed.). New York: Thieme.

Bellis, T. J., & Ferre, J. M. (1999). Multidimensional approach to the differential diagnosis of central auditory processing disorders in children. *Journal of the American Academy of Audiology, 10,* 319-328.

Bellis, T. J., Nicol, T., & Kraus, N. (2000). Aging affects hemispheric asymmetry in the neural representation of speech sounds. *Journal of Neuroscience, 20,* 791-797.

Bellis, T. J., & Wilber, L. A. (2001). Effects of aging and gender on interhemispheric function. *Journal of Speech, Language, and Hearing Research, 44,* 246-263.

Bertoli, S., Smurzynski, J., & Probst, R. (2002). Temporal resolution in young and elderly subjects as measured by mismatch negativity and a psychoacoustic gap detection task. *Clinical Neurophysiology, 113,* 396-406.

Bertoli, S., Smurzynski, J., & Probst, R. (2005). Effects of age, age-related hearing loss, and contralateral cafeteria noise on the discrimination of small frequency changes: Psychoacoustic and electrophysiologic measures. *Journal of the Association of Research in Otolaryngology, 6,* 207-222.

Bess, F. H, & Townsend, T. H. (1977). Word discrimination for listeners with flat sensorineural hearing losses. *Journal of Speech and Hearing Disorders, 42,* 232-237.

Birrin, J. E., & Fisher, L. M. (1995). Speed of behavior: Possible consequences for psychological functioning. *Annual Review of Psychology, 46,* 329-353.

Blake, D. T., Strata, F., Churchland, A. K., & Merzenich, M. M. (2002). Neural correlates of instrumental learning in primary auditory cortex. *Proceedings of the National Academy of Sciences, USA, 99,* 10114-10119.

Bradlow, A. R., Kraus, N., & Hayes, E. (2003). Speaking clearly for children with learning disabilities: Sentence perception in noise. *Journal of Speech, Language, and Hearing Research, 46,* 80-97.

Caissie, R., Campbell, M. M., Frenette, W. L., Scott, L., Howell, I., & Roy, A. (2005). Clear speech for adults with a hearing loss: Does intervention with communication partners make a difference? *Journal of the American Academy of Audiology, 16,* 157-171.

Caspary, D. M, Raza, A., Lawhorn Armour, B. A., Pippin, J., & Arneric, S. P. (1990). Immunocytochemical and neurochemical evidence for age-related loss of GABA in the inferior colliculus: Implications for neural presbycusis. *Journal of Neuroscience, 10,* 2363-2372.

CHABA. (1988). Speech understanding and aging. *Journal of the Acoustical Society of America, 83,* 859-894.

Chambers, R. D., & Griffiths, S. K. (1991). Effects of age on the adult auditory middle latency response. *Hearing Research, 51,* 1-10.

Chermak, G. D., & Musiek, F. E. (1997). *Central auditory processing disorders: New perspectives.* San Diego, CA: Singular Publishing Group.

Chmiel, R., & Jerger, J. (1996). Hearing aid use, central auditory disorder, and hearing handicap in elderly persons. *Journal of the American Academy of Audiology, 7*, 190–202.

Chmiel, R., Jerger, J., Murphy, E., Pirozzolo, F., & Tooley-Young, C. (1997). Unsuccessful use of binaural amplification by an elderly person. *Journal of the American Academy of Audiology, 8*, 1–10.

Cobb, F. E., Jacobson, G. P., Newman, C. W., Kretschmer, L. W., & Donnelly, K. A. (1993). Age-associated degeneration of backward masking task performance: Evidence of declining temporal resolution abilities in normal listeners. *Audiology, 32*, 260–271.

Cohen, G., & Faulkner, D. (1983). Word recognition: Age differences in contextual facilitation effects. *British Journal of Psychology, 74*, 239–251.

Cooper, J. C., & Gates, G. A. (1991). Hearing in the elderly—the Framingham cohort, 1983–1985. Part II. Prevalence of central auditory processing disorders. *Ear and Hearing, 12*, 304–311.

Cooper, J. C., & Gates, G. A. (1992). Central auditory processing disorders in the elderly: The effects of pure tone average and maximum word recognition. *Ear and Hearing, 13*, 278–280.

Cowell, P. E., Allen, L. S., Zaltimo, N. S., & Dennenberg, V. H. (1992). A developmental study of sex and age interactions in the human corpus callosum. *Developmental Brain Research, 66*, 187–192.

Cowell, P., & Hugdahl, K. (2000). Individual differences in neurobehavioral measures of laterality and interhemispheric function as measured by dichotic listening. *Developmental Neuropsychology, 18*, 95–112.

Cranford, J. L., Boose, M., & Moore, C. A. (1990). Effects of aging on the precedence effect in sound localization. *Journal of Speech and Hearing Research, 33*, 654–659.

DeChicchis, A. R., Carpenter, M., Cranford, J. L., & Hymel, M. (2002). Electrophysiologic correlates of attention versus distraction in young and elderly listeners. *Journal of the American Academy of Audiology, 13*, 383–391.

Divenyi, P. L., & Haupt, K. M. (1997). Audiological correlates of speech understanding deficits in elderly listeners with mild-to-moderate hearing loss. I. Age and lateral asymmetry effects. *Ear and Hearing, 18*, 42–61.

Dubno, J. R., Dirks, D. D., & Morgan, D. E. (1984). Effects of age and mild hearing loss on speech recognition in noise. *Journal of the Acoustical Society of America, 76*, 87–96.

Dubno, J. R., Lee, F-S., Matthews, L. J., & Mills, J. H. (1997). Age-related and gender-related changes in monaural speech recognition. *Journal of Speech, Language, and Hearing Research, 40*, 444–452.

Duffy, F. H., Mcanulty, G. B., & Albert, M. S. (1996). Effects of age upon interhemispheric EEG coherence in normal adults. *Neurobiology of Aging, 17*, 587–599.

Etymotic Research. (2001). *QuickSIN Speech in Noise Test.* Elk Grove Village, IL: Author.

Fallon, M., Kuchinsky, S., & Wingfield, A. (2004). The salience of linguistic clauses in young and older adults' running memory for speech. *Experimental Aging Research, 30*, 359–371.

Ferguson, S. H., & Kewley-Port, D. (2002). Vowels intelligibility in clear and conversational speech for normal-hearing and hearing-impaired listeners. *Journal of the Acoustical Society of America, 112*, 259–271.

Fifer, R., Jerger, J., Berlin, C., Tobey, E., & Campbell, J. (1983). Development of a dichotic sentence identification test for hearing impaired adults. *Ear and Hearing, 4*, 300–305.

Fisher, A. L., Hymel, M. R., Cranford, J. L., & DeChicchis, A. R. (2000). Electrophysiologic signs of auditory distraction in elderly listeners. *Journal of the American Academy of Audiology, 11*, 36–45.

Fitzgibbons, P. J., & Gordon-Salant, S. (1994). Age effects on measures of auditory duration discrimination. *Journal of Speech and Hearing Research, 37,* 662–670.

Fitzgibbons, P. J., & Gordon-Salant, S. (1998). Auditory temporal order perception in younger and older adults. *Journal of Speech and Hearing Research, 41,* 1052–1060.

Folstein, M. F., Folsein, S. E., & McHugh, P. R. (1975). Mini mental state: A practical guide for grading the mental state of patients for the clinician. *Journal of Psychiatric Research, 12,* 189–198.

Gates, G. A., Cobb, J. L., Linn, R. T., Rees, T., Wolf, P. A., & D'Agostino, R. B. (1996). Central auditory dysfunction, cognitive dysfunction, and dementia in older people. *Archives of Otolaryngology, 119,* 156–161.

Glasberg, B. R., Moore, B. J., Patterson, R. D., & Nimmo-Smith, I. (1984). Dynamic range and asymmetry of the auditory filter. *Journal of the Acoustical Society of America, 76,* 419–427.

Golding, M., Carter, N., Mitchell, P., & Hood, L. J. (2004). Prevalence of central auditory processing (CAP) abnormality in an older Australian population: The Blue Mountains hearing study. *Journal of the American Academy of Audiology, 15,* 633–642.

Golding, M., Mitchell, P., & Cupples, L. (2005). Risk markers for the graded severity of auditory processing abnormality in an older Australian population: The Blue Mountains hearing study. *Journal of the American Academy of Audiology, 16,* 348–356.

Goodin, D. S., Squires, K. C., Henderson, B. H., & Starr, A. (1978). Age-related variations in evoked potentials to auditory stimuli in normal human subjects. *Electroencephalography and Clinical Neurophysiology, 44,* 447–458.

Gordon-Salant, S., & Fitzgibbons, P. J. (1993a). Recognition of multiply degraded speech by young and elderly listeners. *Journal of Speech and Hearing Research, 38,* 1150–1156.

Gordon-Salant, S., & Fitzgibbons, P. J. (1993b). Temporal factors and speech recognition performance in young and elderly listen-ers. *Journal of Speech and Hearing Research, 36,* 1276–1285.

Gordon-Salant, S, & Fitzgibbons, P. J. (1997). Selected cognitive factors and speech recognition performance among young and elderly listeners. *Journal of Speech, Language, and Hearing Research, 40,* 423–431.

Gordon-Salant, S., & Fitzgibbons, P. J. (2001). Sources of age-related recognition difficulty for time-compressed speech. *Journal of Speech, Language, and Hearing Research, 44,* 709–719.

Gregory, R. L. (1974). Increase in neurological noise as a factor in aging. In R. L. Gregory (Ed.), *Concepts and mechanisms of perception.* London: Duckworthy & Co.

Greenwald, R. R., & Jerger, J. (2001). Aging affects hemispheric asymmetry on a competing speech task. *Journal of the American Academy of Audiology, 12,* 167–173.

Hallgren, M., Larsby, B., Lyxell, B., & Arlinger, S. (2001). Cognitive effects in dichotic speech testing in elderly persons. *Ear and Hearing, 22,* 120–129.

Harkins, S. W. (1981) Effects of age and interstimulus interval on the brainstem auditory evoked potential. *International Journal of Neuroscience, 15,* 107–118.

Harris, R. W., & Reitz, M. L. (1985). Effects of room reverberation and noise on speech discrimination by the elderly. *Audiology, 24,* 319–324.

He, N. J., Horwitz, A. R., Dubno, J. R., & Mills, J. H. (1999). Psychometric functions for gap detection in noise measured from young and aged subjects. *Journal of the Acoustical Society of America, 106,* 966–978.

Helfer, K. S., & Wilber, L. A. (1990). Hearing loss, aging, and speech perception in reverberation and noise. *Journal of Speech and Hearing Research, 33,* 149–155.

Holmes, A. E., Kricos, P. B., & Kessler, R. A. (1988). A closed-versue open-set measure of speech discrimination in normally hearing young and elderly adults. *British Journal of Audiology, 22,* 29–33.

Humes, L. E. (1996). Speech understanding in the elderly. *Journal of the American Academy of Audiology, 7*, 161–167.

Humes, L. E., & Christopherson, L. (1991). Speech identification difficulties of hearing-impaired elderly persons: The contributions of auditory-processing deficits. *Journal of Speech and Hearing Research, 34*, 686–693.

Humes, L. E., & Floyd, S. S. (2005). Measures of working memory, sequence learning, and speech recognition in the elderly. *Journal of Speech, Language, and Hearing Research, 48*, 224–235.

Humes, L., & Roberts, L. (1990). Speech-recognition difficulties of the hearing-impaired elderly: The contributions of audibility. *Journal of Speech and Hearing Research, 33*, 726–735.

Humes, L. E., & Roberts, L. (1991). Speech-recognition difficulties of the hearing-impaired elderly: the contributions of audibility. *Journal of Speech and Hearing Research, 33*, 726–735.

Hymel, M. R., Cranford, J. L., & Stuart, A. (1998). Effects of contralateral speech competition on auditory event-related potentials recorded from elderly listeners: Brain map study. *Journal of the American Academy of Audiology, 9*, 1–13.

Jaaskelainen, I. P., Varonen, R., Näätänen, R., & Pekkonen, E. (1999). Decay of cortical pre-attentive sound discrimination in middle-age. *NeuroReport, 10*, 123–126.

Jerger, J. (1992). Can age-related decline in speech understanding be explained by peripheral hearing loss? *Journal of the American Academy of Audiology, 3*, 33–38.

Jerger, J., Alford, B., Lew, H., Rivera, V., & Chmiel, R. (1995). Dichotic listening, event-related potentials, and interhemispheric transfer in the elderly. *Ear and Hearing, 16*, 482–498.

Jerger, J., & Chmiel, R. (1997) Factor analytic structure of auditory impairment in elderly persons. *Journal of the American Academy of Audiology, 8*, 269–276.

Jerger, J., Chmiel, R., Allen, J., & Wilson, A. (1994). Effects of age and gender on dichotic sentence identification. *Ear and Hearing, 15*, 274–286.

Jerger, J, & Hall, J. (1980) Effects of age and sex on auditory brainstem response. *Archives of Otolaryngology, 106*, 387–391.

Jerger, J., Jerger, S, Oliver, T, & Pirozzolo, F. (1989) Speech understanding in the elderly. *Ear and Hearing, 10*, 79–89.

Jerger, J., & Lew, H. L. (2004). Principles and clinical applications of auditory evoked potentials in the geriatric population. *Physical Medicine and Rehabilitation Clinics of North America, 15*, 235–250.

Jerger, J., & Martin, J. (2005). Some effects of aging on event-related potentials during a linguistic monitoring task. *International Journal of Audiology, 44*, 321–330.

Jerger, J., Moncrieff, D., Greenwald, R., Wambacq, I., & Seipel, A. (2000). Effect of age on interaural asymmetry of event-related potentials in a dichotic listening task. *Journal of the American Academy of Audiology, 11*, 383–389.

Jerger, J., Oliver, T., & Chmiel, R. (1988). Auditory middle latency response: A perspective. *Seminars in Hearing, 9*, 75–85.

Jerger, J., Oliver, T. A., & Pirozzolo, F. (1990). Impact of central auditory processing disorder and cognitive deficit on the self-assessment of hearing handicap in the elderly. *Journal of the American Academy of Audiology, 1*, 75–80.

Kaplan, H., Bally, S., Brandt, F., Busacco, D., & Pray, J. (1997). Communication scale for older adults (CSOA). *Journal of the American Academy of Audiology, 8*, 203–217.

Katada, E., Sato, K., Ojika, K., & Ueda, R. (2004). Cognitive event-related potentials: Useful clinical information in Alzheimer's disease. *Current Alzheimer Research, 1*, 63–69.

Katz, J. (1962). The use of staggered spondaic words for assessing the integrity of the central auditory nervous system. *Journal of Auditory Research, 2*, 327–337.

Knott, V., Bradford, L., Dulude, L., Millar, A., Alwahabi, F., Lau, T., Shea, C., & Wiens, A. (2003). Effects of stimulus modality and response mode on the P300 event-related potential differentiation of young and elderly adults. *Clinical Electroencephalography, 34,* 182-190.

Konig, E. (1957) Pitch discrimination and age. *Acta Oto-laryngologica, 48,* 475-489.

Lenzi, A., Chiarelli, G., & Sambataro, G. (1989). Comparative study of middle-latency responses and auditory brainstem responses in elderly subjects. *Audiology, 28,* 144-151.

Ludlow, C. L., Cudahy, E. A., & Bassich, C. J. (1982). Developmental, age, and sex effects on gap detection and temporal order. *Journal of the Acoustical Society of America,* 71, S47.

Lutman, M. E. (1991) Degradations in frequency and temporal resolution with age and their impact on auditory function. *Acta Oto-laryngologica Supplement, 476,* 120-126.

Lutman, M. E., Gatehouse, S., & Worthington, A. G. (1991). Frequency resolution as a function of hearing threshold level and age. *Journal of the Acoustical Society of America, 89,* 320-328.

Malmo, H. P., & Malmo, R. B. (1982). Multiple unit activty recorded longitudinally in rats from pubescence to old age. *Neurobiology of Aging, 3,* 43-53.

Marshall, L. (1981). Auditory processing in aging listeners. *Journal of Speech and Hearing Disorders, 46,* 226-240.

Marshall, L., & Bacon, S. P. (1981) Prediction of speech discrimination scores from audiometric data. *Ear and Hearing, 2,* 148-155.

Matschke, R. G. (1991). Frequency selectivity and psychoacoustic tuning curves in old age. *Acta Oto-laryngologica Supplement, 476,* 114-119.

McCoy, S. L., Tun, P. A., Cox, L. C., Colangelo, M., Stewart, R. A., & Wingfield, A. (2005). Hearing loss and perceptual effort: Downstream effects on older adults' memory for speech. *Journal of Experimental Psychology, 58*(1), 22-33.

Meurman, O. H. (1954). The difference limen of frequency in tests of auditory function. *Acta Oto-laryngologica Supplement, 118,* 144-155.

Moore, B. C. J., Peters, R. W., & Glasberg, B. R. (1992). Detection of temporal gaps in sinusoids by elderly subjects with and without hearing loss. *Journal of the Acoustical Society of America, 92,* 1923-1932.

Murphy, D. R., Craik, F. I., Li, K. Z., & Schneider, B. A. (2000). Comparing the effects of aging and background noise on short-term memory performance. *Psychological Aging, 15,* 323-334.

Musiek, F. E. (1983). Assessment of central auditory dysfunction: The Dichotic Digits Test revisited. *Ear and Hearing, 4,* 79-83.

Musiek, F. E., Baran, J. A., & Pinheiro, M. L. (1990). Duration pattern recognition in normal subjects and patients with cerebral and cochlear lesions. *Audiology, 29,* 304-313.

Musiek, F. E., Gollegly, K. M., Kibbe, K. S., & Verkest-Lenz, S. B. (1991). Proposed screening test for central auditory disorders: Follow-up on the Dichotic Digits Test. *American Journal of Otology, 12,* 109-113.

Musiek, F. E., Kibbe, K., & Baran, J. A. (1984). Neuroaudiological results from split-brain patients. *Seminars in Hearing, 5,* 219-229.

Musiek, F. E., & Pinheiro, M. L. (1987). Frequency patterns in cochlear, brainstem, and cerebral lesions. *Audiology, 26,* 79-88.

Nabalek, A. K. (1988). Identification of vowels in quiet, noise, and reverberation: Relationships with age and hearing loss. *Journal of the Acoustical Society of America, 84,* 476-484.

Nabalek, A. K., & Robinson, P. K. (1982). Monaural and binaural speech perception in reverberation for listeners of various ages. *Journal of the Acoustical Society of America, 71,* 1242-1248.

Neijenhuis, K., Tschur, H., & Snik, A. (2004). The effect of mild hearing impairment on auditory processing tests. *Journal of the American Academy of Audiology, 15,* 6-16.

Newman, C. W., Weinstein, B. E., Jacobson, G. P., & Hug, G. A. (1990). The Hearing Handicap Inventory for Adults: Psychometric adequacy and audiometric correlates. *Ear and Hearing, 11,* 430-433.

Nillson, M., Soli, S. D., & Sullivan, J. A. (1994). Development of the Hearing in Noise Test for the measurement of speech reception thresholds in quiet and in noise. *Journal of the Acoustical Society of America, 95,* 1085-1099.

Novak, R. E, & Anderson, C. V. (1982). Differentiation of types of presbycusis using the masking-level difference. *Journal of Speech and Hearing Research, 25,* 504-508.

Olichney, J. M., & Hillert, D. G. (2004). Clinical applications of cognitive event-related potentials in Alzheimer's disease. *Physical Medicine and Rehabilitation Clinics of North America, 15,* 205-233.

Patterson, J. V., Michalewski, H. J., Thompson, L. W., Bowman, T. E., & Litzelman, D. K. (1981). Age and sex differences in the human auditory brainstem response. *Journal of Gerontology, 36,* 455-462.

Patterson, R. D., Nimmo-Smith, I., Weber, D. I., & Milroy, R. (1982). The deterioration of hearing with age: Frequency selectivity, the critical ratio, the audiogram, and speech threshold. *Journal of the Acoustical Society of America, 72,* 1788-1804.

Pekkonen, E., Huotilainen, M., Virtanen, J., Sinkkonen, J., Rinne, T., Ilmoniemi, R. J., & Näätänen, R. (1995). Age-related functional differences between auditory cortices: A whole-head MEG study. *NeuroReport, 6,* 1803-1806.

Pfefferbaum, A., Ford, J. M., Roth, W. T., Hopkins, W. F., & Kopell, B. (1979). Event-related potential changes in healthy aged females. *Electroencephalography and Clinical Neurophysiology, 46,* 81-86.

Pfefferbaum, A., Ford, J. M., Roth, W. T., & Kopell, B. (1980). Age related changes in auditory event-related potentials. *Electroencephalography and Clinical Neurophysiology, 49,* 266-276.

Phillips, D. P., Rappaport, J. M., & Gulliver J. M. (1994). Impaired word recognition in noise by patients with noise-induced cochlear hearing loss: Contribution of a temporal resolution deficit. *American Journal of Otology, 15,* 679-686.

Phillips, S. L., Gordon-Salant, S., Fitzgibbons, P. J., & Yeni-Komishian, G. H. (1994). Auditory duration discrimination in young and elderly listeners with normal hearing. *Journal of the American Academy of Audiology, 5,* 210-215.

Pichenyi, M. A., Durlach, N. I., & Braida, L. D. (1986). Speaking clearly for the hard of hearing II: Acoustic characteristics of clear and conversational speech. *Journal of Speech and Hearing Research, 29,* 434-446.

Pichora-Fuller, M. K. (2003). Cognitive aging and auditory information processing. *International Journal of Audiology, 42* (Suppl. 2), 26-32.

Pichora-Fuller, M. K., Schneider, B. A., & Daneman, M. (1995). How young and old adults listen to and remember speech in noise. *Journal of the Acoustical Society of America, 97,* 593-608.

Picton, T. W., Stuss, D. T., Champagne, S. C., & Nelson, R. F. (1984). The effects of age on human event-related potentials. *Psychophysiology, 21,* 312-326.

Rabbitt, P. (1991) Mild hearing loss can cause apparent memory failures which increase with age and reduce with IQ. *Acta Otolaryngologica Supplement, 476,* 167-176.

Rastatter, M., Watson, M., & Strauss-Simmons, D. (1989). Effects of time-compression on feature and frequency discrimination in aged listeners. *Perceptual and Motor Skills, 68,* 367-372.

Roberts, R. A., & Lister, J. J. (2004). Effects of age and hearing loss on gap detection and the precedence effect: Broadband stimuli.

Journal of Speech, Language, and Hearing Research, *47*, 965-978.

Rodriguez, G. P,. DiSarno, N. J., & Hardiman, C. J. (1990). Central auditory processing in normal-hearing elderly adults. *Audiology*, *18*, 320-324.

Rosenhamer, H. J., Lindstron, B., & Lundborg, T. (1980). On the use of click-evoked electric brainstem responses in audiological diagnosis. II. The influence of sex and age upon the normal response. *Scandinavian Audiology*, *9*, 93-100.

Ryan, J. N. (1989). *Middle latency auditory evoked potentials as a function of age.* Unpublished doctoral dissertation, Dallas: University of Texas.

Salthouse, T. A., & Lichty, W. (1985). Tests of the neural noise hypothesis of age-related cognitive change. *Journal of Gerontology*, *40*, 443-450.

Schneider, B. A., Daneman, M., & Murphy, D. R. (2005). Speech comprehension difficulties in older adults: Cognitive slowing or age-related changes in hearing? *Psychological Aging*, *20*, 261-271.

Schneider, B. A., Daneman, M., & Pichora-Fuller, M. K. (2002). Listening in aging adults: From discourse comprehension to psychoacoustics. *Canadian Journal of Experimental Psychology*, *56*, 139-152.

Schneider, B. A., & Hamstra, S. J. (1999). Gap detection thresholds as a function of tonal duration for younger and older listeners. *Journal of the Acoustical Society of America*, *106*, 371-380.

Schneider, B., Speranza, F., & Pichora-Fuller, M. K. (1998). Age-related changes in temporal resolution: Envelope and intensity effects. *Canadian Journal of Experimental Psychology*, *52*, 184-191.

Silman, S., & Silverman, C. A. (1993). Effects of prolonged lack of amplification on speech-recognition performance: Preliminary findings. *Journal of Rehabilitation Research and Development*, *30*, 326-332.

Snell, K. B. (1997). Age-related changes in temporal gap detection. *Journal of the Acoustical Society of America*, *101*, 2214-2220.

Snell, K. B., & Frisina, D. R. (2000). Relationships among age-related differences in gap detection and word recognition. *Journal of the Acoustical Society of America*, *107*, 1615-1626.

Sommers, M. S. (1996). The structural organization of the mental lexicon and its contribution to age-related declines in spoken-word recognition. *Psychology and Aging*, *11*, 333-341.

Sommers, M. S. (1997). Stimulus variability and spoken word recognition. II. The effects of age and hearing impairment. *Journal of the Acoustical Society of America*, *101*, 2278-2288.

Soucek, S., & Mason, S. M. (1990). Investigation of stimulus rate effects in the elderly using non-invasive electrocochleography and auditory brainstem response. *Association for Research in Otolaryngology Abstracts*, *13*, 218.

Speaks, C., Niccum, N., & Van Tassell, D. (1985). Effects of stimulus material on the dichotic listening performance of patients with sensorineural hearing loss. *Journal of Speech and Hearing Research*, *28*, 16-25.

Stach, B. A., Spretnjak, M. L., & Jerger, J. (1990). The prevalence of central presbycusis in a clinical population. *Journal of the American Academy of Audiology*, *1*, 109-115.

Strouse, A., Ashmead, D. H., Ohde, R. N., & Grantham, D. W. (1998). Temporal processing in the aging auditory system. *Journal of the Acoustical Society of America*, *104*, 2385-2399.

Strouse, A. L., & Hall, J. W. (1995). Test-retest reliability of a dichotic digits test for assessing central auditory function in Alzheimer's disease. *Audiology*, *34*, 85-90.

Strouse, A. L., Hall, J. W., & Burger, M. C. (1995). Central auditory processing disorder in Alzheimer's disease. *Ear and Hearing*, *16*, 230-238.

Stuart, A., & Phillips, D. P. (1996). Word recognition in continuous and interrupted broadband noise by young normal-hearing, older normal-hearing, and presbyacusic listeners. *Ear and Hearing, 17,* 478–489.

Stuart, A., Phillips, D. P., & Green W. B. (1995). Word recognition performance in continuous and interrupted noise by normal-hearing and hearing-impaired listeners. *American Journal of Otology, 16,* 658–663.

Surr, R. K. (1977). Effect of age on clinical hearing aid evaluation results. *Journal of the American Audiological Society, 3,* 1–5.

Sweetow, R. W. (2005). Training the adult brain to listen. *The Hearing Journal, 58,* 10–16.

Sweetow, R. H., & Henderson-Sabes, J. (2004). The case for LACE: Listening and auditory communication enhancement training. *The Hearing Journal, 57,* 32–38.

Sweetow, R. H., & Henderson-Sabes, J. (in press). The need for and development of an adaptive listening and communication enhancement (LACE™) program. *Journal of the American Academy of Audiology.*

Sweetow, R., & Palmer, C. V. (2005). Efficacy of individual auditory training in adults: A systematic review of the evidence. *Journal of the American Academy of Audiology, 16,* 494–504.

Townsend, T. H., & Bess, F. H. (1980). Effects of age and sensorineural hearing loss on word recognition. *Scandinavian Audiology, 9,* 245–248.

Tremblay, K. L., Billings, C., & Rohila, N. (2004). Speech evoked cortical potentials: Effects of age and stimulus presentation rate. *Journal of the American Academy of Audiology, 15,* 226–237.

Tremblay, K., Kraus, N., Carrell, T., & McGee, T. (1997). Central auditory system plasticity: Generalization to novel stimuli following listening training. *Journal of the Acoustical Society of America, 102,* 3762–3773.

Tremblay, K., Kraus, N., & McGee, T. (1998). The time course of auditory perceptual learning: Neurophysiologic changes during speech-sound training. *NeuroReport, 9,* 3557–3560.

Tremblay, K., Kraus, N., McGee, T., Ponton, C., & Otis, B. (2001). Central auditory plasticity: Changes in the N1-P2 complex after speech-sound training. *Ear and Hearing, 22,* 1–11.

Tremblay, K. L., Piskosz, M., & Souza, P. (2002). Aging alters the neural representation of speech cues. *NeuroReport, 13,* 1865–1870.

Tremblay, K. L., Piskosz, M., & Souza, P. (2003). Effects of age and age-related hearing loss on the neural representation of speech cues. *Clinical Neurophysiology, 114,* 1332–1343.

Tun, P. A., O'Kane, G., & Wingfield, A. (2002). Distraction by competing speech in young and older adult listeners. *Psychological Aging, 17,* 453–467.

Uttl, B., & Graf, P. (1997). Color-Word Stroop test performance across the adult life span. *Journal of Clinical and Experimental Neuropsychology, 19,* 405–420.

van Rooij, J. C. G. M. & Plomp, R. (1991) Auditive and cognitive factors in speech perception by elderly listeners. *Acta Otolaryngologica Supplement, 476,* 177–181.

Ventry, I. M., & Weinstein, B. E. (1982). The hearing handicap inventory for the elderly: A new tool. *Ear and Hearing, 3,* 128–134.

Walton, J. P., Frisina, R. D., & O'Neill, W. E. (1998). Age-related alteration in processing of temporal sound features in the auditory midbrain of the CBA mouse. *Journal of Neuroscience, 18,* 2764–2776.

Wiley, R., Cruikshanks, K., Nondahl, D., Tweed, T., Klein, R., & Klein, B. (1998). Aging and word recognition in competing message. *Journal of the American Academy of Audiology, 9,* 191–198.

Willott, J. F. (1986). Effects of aging, hearing loss, and anatomical location on thresholds of inferior colliculus neurons in C57BL/6 and CBA mice. *Journal of Neurophysiology, 56,* 391–408.

Willott, J. F. (1991). *Aging and the auditory system: Anatomy, physiology, and psychophysics.* San Diego, CA: Singular Publishing Group.

Willott, J. F., Lu, S-M. (1982). Noise-induced hearing loss can alter neural coding and increase excitability in the central nervous system. *Science, 216*, 1331–1332.

Willott, J. F., Parkham, I., & Hunter, K. P. (1988a). Response properties of inferior colliculus neurons in young and very old CBA/J mice. *Hearing Research, 37*, 1–14.

Willott, J. F., Parkham, I., & Hunter, K. P. (1988b). Response properties of inferior colliculus neurons in middle-aged C57BL/6J mice with presbycusis. *Hearing Research, 37*, 15–28.

Willott, J. F., Parkham, I., & Hunter, K. P. (1988c). Response properties of cochlear nucleus neurons in young and middle aged C57BL/6J mice with presbycusis. *Society for Neuroscience Abstracts, 14*, 646.

Wilson, R. H., & Weakley, D. G. (2005). The 500 Hz masking-level difference and word recognition in multitalker babble for 40- to 89-year-old listeners with symmetrical sensorineural hearing loss. *Journal of the American Academy of Audiology, 16*, 367–382.

Wingfield, A., Lindfield, K. C., & Goodglass, H. (2000). Effects of age and hearing sensitivity on the use of prosodic information in spoken word recognition. *Journal of Speech, Language, and Hearing Research, 43*, 915–925.

Wingfield, A., Tun, P. A., Koh, C. K., & Rosen, M. J. (1999). Regaining lost time: Adult aging and the effect of time restoration on recall of time-compressed speech. *Psychological Aging, 14*, 380–389.

Woods, D. L., & Clayworth, C. C. (1986). Age-related changes in human middle latency auditory evoked potentials. *Electroencephalography and Clinical Neurophysiology, 65*, 297–303.

CHAPTER 14

DIFFERENTIAL DIAGNOSIS OF (CENTRAL) AUDITORY PROCESSING DISORDER AND NEUROPATHY

ANNETTE HURLEY and RAYMOND M. HURLEY

Auditory neuropathy (AN) is characterized by normal otoacoustic emissions (OAEs), a recordable cochlear microphonic (CM), and an absent auditory brainstem response (ABR) (Sininger & Oba, 2001). The primary complaint of a person diagnosed with AN is difficulty understanding speech, especially in background noise. Similarly, difficulty understanding speech in background noise is a hallmark symptom of individuals with (central) auditory processing disorder ([C]APD) (Chermak & Musiek, 1997). (C)APD refers to deficits in the neural processing of auditory stimuli (not the result of cognitive, language, or related factors) and is characterized by poor performance in one or more of the following auditory areas: sound localization and lateralization; auditory discrimination; auditory pattern recognition; temporal discrimination (e.g.,

temporal gap detection), temporal ordering, and temporal masking. In addition, listeners with (C)APD have reduced performance with certain speech perception paradigms such as dichotic listening and compressed/filtered speech (ASHA, 2005). Although both AN and (C)APD can present with some of the same auditory problems and overlapping symptomatology, AN can be distinguished from (C)APD through careful assessment with an appropriate test battery.

There is little question that a comprehensive test battery is the best approach to confirm a (C)APD diagnosis (ASHA, 2005; Jerger & Musiek, 2000). In addition, interpretation of the (C)APD test battery may provide insight into the anatomic site of the auditory dysfunction (Bellis, 2003). Recent advances in diagnostic testing have also enabled clinicians to gain a better understanding of the dysfunctional site(s) responsible for AN. An investigation by Rapin and Gravel (2003) suggested that complete, comprehensive testing may lead to an anatomically based diagnosis of auditory neuropathy (AN). Furthermore, these investigators contend that the term AN has been overused to describe a heterogeneous group of disorders without regard to the anatomic site of neuropathy. These authors suggested that the term AN should only be used when the spiral ganglion cells, their processes, and the VIIIth nerve fibers are affected. Thus, the term AN is only appropriate when the peripheral auditory system is affected. Berlin and colleagues (2002) recognized that the term AN lacks a precise anatomic basis and suggested that the term auditory dys-synchrony (AD) be used to avoid the implication of an anatomic diagnosis. To avoid the anatomic implications, the term auditory neuropathy/auditory dys-synchrony (AN/AD) will be used in this chapter.

AN/AD is not a new disorder, as reports which predate the use of the AN/AD term have described patients who have abnormal or absent ABR recordings, but have normal pure tone audiograms (Davis & Hirsh, 1979; Worthington & Peters, 1980). For many years, these patients have been poorly understood, misdiagnosed, improperly managed, and sometimes dismissed as not having an organically based hearing loss (Kraus, 2001). Some patients, diagnosed with a sensorineural hearing loss at a time before OAE testing became routine, may have rejected hearing aids (Berlin, Hood, Hurley, & Wen, 1996) or had a history of responding inconsistently to sound (Kraus, 2001).

Kraus, Ozdamar, Stein, and Reed (1984) first reported what is now known and described as AN/AD. In their retrospective study, these investigators reported that 49 of 543 children who were evaluated for hearing loss had absent ABRs. Of these 49 patients, 42 had severe to profound hearing loss that was later confirmed by behavioral thresholds. Seven of the 49 patients with absent ABRs had behavioral thresholds that were no greater than a moderate hearing loss and would most likely, with OAE data, be diagnosed with AN/AD. Thus, the AN/AD incidence which is the number of newly diagnosed cases in a given year would be 1.3% (Kraus et al., 1984). Others have reported the incidence of auditory neuropathy to range from 5% (Davis & Hirsh, 1979) to 12 to 14% (Berlin et al., 1998). Chermak and Musiek (1997) estimated that (C)APD affects approximately 2 to 3% of the school-age population, whereas Goldberg (1998) maintained that auditory processing deficits impacted 5% of children. AN/AD prevalence (i.e., the total number of individuals with the disorder) is generally higher than the prevalence of (C)APD in the general population; however, the reported prevalence of AN/AD may be inflated due to the use of an inappropriate diagnostic criterion that requires only an abnormal ABR for diagnosis versus the more stringent requirement of an absent ABR.

Risk Factors for AN/AD and APD

Just as there is no single cause for hearing loss, there is no single cause for AN/AD or (C)APD. Sininger and Oba (2001) reported that 80% of 25 patients with AN/AD who had symptoms before age 2 had neonatal risk factors for hearing impairment. The predisposing risk factors associated with hearing loss, AN/AD and (C)APD are listed in Table 14-1.

Interestingly, several risk factors, such as hyperbilirubinemia and a positive family history, are associated with hearing loss, AN/AD, and (C)APD. The central auditory system is highly sensitive to bilirubin toxicity. Damage occurs in the auditory nuclei of the brainstem, with the neurons in the cochlear nuclei being severely affected or completely destroyed resulting in a central pathology (Dublin, 1985). In contrast, bilirubin does not appear toxic to the peripheral auditory structures, including the VIIIth nerve or

Table 14-1. Associated Risk Factors for Hearing Loss, AN/AD, and (C)APD

Hearing Loss	AN/AD	(C)APD
Family history	Family history	Family history
Infections: (Toxoplasmosis, Rubella, Cytomegalovirus [CMV], Herpes virus, Syphilis)	Infections: (Toxoplasmosis, Rubella, Cytomegalovirus [CMV], Herpes virus, Syphilis)	Infections: (Toxoplasmosis, Rubella, Cytomegalovirus [CMV], Herpes virus, Syphilis)
Hyperbilirubinemia	Hyperbilirubinemia	Hyperbilirubinemia
Craniofacial anomalies	Immune disorders (Type 1 Diabetes) Uremia	Rh incompatibility
Low birth weight		Difficulty during birth
Other syndromes	Genetic/Syndrome	Toxic exposures
Ototoxic medications		Ototoxic medications
Prematurity		Prematurity
Anoxia		Anoxia
Infections after birth		Infections after birth
Mechanical ventilation		Head trauma
Bacterial meningitis		Cerebrovascular disorders
		Metabolic disorders
		Epilepsy
		Recurrent otitis media
		Meningitis/Encephalitis
		Developmental disorders (e.g., Dyslexia, Learning disability, Language impairment, Attention deficit hyperactivity disorder)

hair cells (Dublin, 1985). As noted above, Rapin and Gravel (2003) suggested that AN/AD should not be diagnosed in the absence of involvement of the spiral ganglion cells, their processes, and the VIIIth nerve. Just as many siblings are diagnosed with (C)APD, investigators have reported positive sibling histories of AN/AD (Starr et al., 1998). For example, Sininger and Oba (2001) reported 46% of 59 subjects had a positive family history of AN/AD. In the case of (C)APD, there are postnatal factors that may contribute to (C)APD such as frequent bouts of otitis media, meningitis, high fever, lead or other toxic substance exposure. In addition, any type of neurologic disorder or head injury which also may be associated with AN/AD also can cause (C)APD (Barr, 1976; Brown, 1994; Chedru, Bastard, & Efron, 1978; Gravel & Wallace, 1992; Hall & Grose, 1993; Musiek, Baran, & Shinn, 2004; Willeford & Burleigh, 1985). Some patients with AN/AD will have other neurologic abnormalities or other peripheral neuropathies that may only be recognized during a neurologic examination. AN/AD can be part of a syndrome, occur with other medical conditions, or occur with nonauditory neuropathies such as Freidrech's ataxia (Taylor, McMenamin, Andermann & Watters, 1982), Stevens-Johnson syndrome, Ehrlers-Danlos syndrome, and Charcot-Marie Tooth syndrome (Berlin, Hood, Cecola, Jackson, & Szabo, 1993; Deltenre, Mansbach, Bozet, Clercx, & Hecox, 1997).

Site of AN/AD Dysfunction

The underlying physiologic site of auditory dysfunction that results in AN/AD may be determined using an extensive behavioral and electrophysiologic test battery (Rapin & Gravel, 2003). There are several hypothesized anatomic sites for this disorder and there may be more than one site of physiologic dysfunction which results in AN/AD. Investigators have reported the underlying physiologic site of AN/AD could possibly be a mechanical dysfunction of the outer and inner hair cells (Harrison, 1988), or a dysfunction of the VIIIth nerve axons, cell bodies, and/or myelin sheath (Starr, Picton, Sininger, Hood, & Berlin, 1996). Rapin and Gravel (2003) report site-specific test results for AN/AD. For example, an inner hair cell etiology would result in recordable otoacoustic emissions (OAEs) and CM, but an absent ABR, and abnormal psychoacoustic tests, would classify this as an isolated site-specific AN/AD. This is in contrast to an isolated brainstem lesion, which would result in absent acoustic reflexes (either ipsilaterally, contralaterally or both (depending on the size and site of the lesion), recordable OAEs and CM, recordable waves I, and II of the ABR, but absent (or delayed) waves III and V, and abnormal psychoacoustic tests. Rapin and Gravel (2003) would classify these results as representing a central auditory disorder, not an AN/AD.

Profiles or subtypes have been proposed to better understand the anatomic site(s) of auditory dysfunction and its behavioral manifestations for both AN/AD and (C)APD (Bellis & Ferre, 1999; Katz, 1992; Musiek & Gollegly, 1988; Rapin & Gravel, 2003; Starr, Picton, & Kim, 2001). Four types of AN/AD have been proposed. In the first type, demyelinating neuropathies affect the Schwann cells that compose the myelin sheaths and affect the rapid transmission of information exchange from one neuron to another (Starr, Picton, & Kim, 2001). In the second type, axonal neuropathies result in muscular weakness and muscular atrophy (Starr et al., 2001). In the third type, sensory axonal neuropathies cause impaired sensation (Starr et al., 2001). Mixed neuropathies affect both the myelin sheath and neuron axon in the fourth type (Starr et al., 2001) and may occur as a progressive degeneration from axonal to demyelinating neuropathy or vice versa (Rapin & Gravel, 2003). If the pathology extends to the brainstem, however, this lesion should be characterized as a central lesion, not AN/AD (Rapin & Gravel, 2003).

Although no (C)APD subtypes have been universally accepted, investigators have attempted to document the heterogeneous nature of (C)APD by describing the characteristics in terms of commonalities (Bellis & Ferre, 1999; Katz, 1992; Musiek & Gollegly, 1988). For example, Musiek and Gollegly (1988) reported three causes of (C)APD in children with learning disabilities: one based on neuromaturational delay, a second resulting from a neuromorphologic disorder, and a third arising from neurologic disease or insult. More recently, research has documented the neurobiological underpinnings of (C)APD in children pointing out the neurologic bases of inefficient interhemispheric transfer of auditory information and/or lack of appropriate hemispheric lateralization, and atypical hemispheric asymmetries experienced by patients with (C)APD. A much less frequent etiology of (C)APD, is a neurologic disorder, insult, or abnormality in children (Jerger & Musiek, 2000; Kraus et al., 1996; Musiek, Baran, & Pinheiro, 1994). In adults, (C)APD may result from accumulated damage or deterioration to the central auditory nervous system (CANS)

due to neurologic/neurodegenerative diseases, disorders or insults, and the aging process itself, which leads to poorer neural synchrony, slower refractory periods, decreased central inhibition, and interhemispheric transfer asymmetry/deficits (Bellis, Nicol, & Kraus, 2000; Bellis & Wilber, 2001; Jerger, Greenwald, Wambacq, Seipel, & Moncrieff, 2000; Pichora-Fuller & Souza, 2003; Tremblay, Piskosz, & Souza, 2003; Willott, 1996; Woods & Clayworth, 1986). Nonetheless, it is not yet possible to definitively determine the etiology, or subtypes of (C)APD using today's clinical tools.

Differential Diagnosis

Given the overlapping symptomatology, etiology, and similar anatomic sites that may contribute to both (C)APD and AN/AD, it is necessary to administer a complete test battery to differentially diagnose these two disorders. Rapin and Gravel (2003) commented that it is unfortunate that few patients have received the thorough test battery required, which has resulted in the current confusion in the audiology literature regarding physiologic and behavioral test results in patients with presumed AN/AD. Performance differences across a number of behavioral tests, and electrophysiologic and electroacoustic procedures are reviewed in the following sections.

Pure Tone Audiometry

Patients with AN/AD may present with normal hearing or any degree of hearing loss from mild to profound and with various configurations such as flat, reverse slope, or high frequency (Sininger & Oba, 2001). Most importantly, hearing thresholds for patients with AN/AD may also fluctuate as reported by some investigators (Sininger & Oba, 2001). Specifically, hearing thresholds for some patients with AN/AD may deteriorate over time, but remain stable in other patients (Sininger & Oba, 2001). Investigators have also reported a "temperature-sensitive" AN/AD in which pure tone thresholds change from normal to profound hearing loss as a function of internal temperature (Gorga, Stelmachowitz, Barlow, & Brookhouser, 1995; Starr et al., 1998). In short, there is a great deal of variance in the audiometric threshold results for AN/AD patients. Unlike AN/AD, pure-tone audiometric thresholds for patients with (C)APD are, by definition, normal, although individuals with (C)APD can also present comorbid hearing impairment, particularly among older adults (Stach, Spretnjak, & Jerger, 1990). However, on the average, pure tone thresholds are normal and do not fluctuate.

Immittance Testing

Generally, tympanometry is normal for patients with AN/AD, thus indicating normal middle ear pressure and compliance. These measures are also generally normal in patients with (C)APD, although children with (C)APD may experience otitis media and resulting abnormal tympanometry (Willeford & Burleigh, 1985). Acoustic reflexes can provide valuable information about the integrity of the middle ear, cochlea, VIIIth nerve, and lower brainstem. Acoustic reflexes are generally abnormal or elevated in patients with AN/AD (Berlin et al., 1993; Hood, 1998a; Sininger & Oba, 2001) whereas, generally, acoustic reflexes are present at

normal levels in patients with (C)APD, unless there is a lower brainstem lesion. In some patients with (C)APD who had a positive history of otitis media, however, acoustic reflexes may be slightly elevated or absent due to the middle ear effect of the otitis media (Willeford & Burleigh, 1985).

Otoacoustic Emissions (OAEs)

Otoacoustic emissions (OAEs) are expected to be present in patients with normal middle and inner ear function; however, a diagnosis of AN/AD should be suspected if a person has recordable (normal) OAEs with an audiogram that shows a sensorineural hearing loss (SNHL) greater than 35-dB HL (Starr, 2001). Present OAEs and an SNHL may, however, be a confounding factor in some patients with AN/AD due to the fact that OAEs may deteriorate over time (Deltenere et al., 1997). Generally, patients with AN/AD have present OAEs that may not be in agreement with their pure tone thresholds. Similar to AN/AD patients, individuals with (C)APD are expected to have normal OAEs. The obvious exceptions in either group are the patients who have histories of protracted otitis media, resulting in absent or abnormal OAEs, which reflects a mild impairment of sound transmission through the middle ear (Rappaport & Provencal, 2002).

Speech Audiometry

One of the most common complaints of individuals with AN/AD is difficulty understanding speech especially in background noise (Sininger & Oba, 2001). Word recognition ability in quiet in suspected AN/AD patients is usually poorer than expected based on their behavioral pure tone thresholds (Sininger & Oba, 2001). Furthermore, patients with AN/AD may often have histories of reporting that speech is not clear, often sounding distorted (Berlin, Hood, & Rose, 2002). Likewise, many patients (C)APD present this auditory complaint of difficulty hearing in background noise (Bellis, 2003).

Electrophysiologic Assessment

Cochlear Microphonic

It is believed that the cochlear microphonic (CM) response is generated primarily by the outer hair cells (Dallos, 1973); however, the inner hair cells may likewise contribute to this response (Dallos, 1997). The CM is expected to be present in AN/AD patients, albeit at an amplitude that may be larger than expected (Sininger & Oba, 2001). Conversely, in (C)APD, the CM is expected to be of normal amplitude. To ensure accurate interpretation, clinicians are encouraged to obtain CM recordings using both rarefaction and condensation clicks, which allows ABR waves to be separated from the CM response (Berlin et al., 1998).

Auditory Brainstem Response (ABR)

The auditory brainstem response (ABR) is a short latency response, less than 10 msec poststimulus onset, which provides objective evidence of the integrity of the auditory brainstem. The ABR consists of a waveform complex that reflects synchronous firing of the auditory nerve through the brainstem; it is a test of neurosynchrony (Hood, 1998b). Historically,

the ABR has also been used in the diagnosis of central nervous system disorders such as demyelinating diseases (Jerger, Oliver, Chmiel, & Rivera, 1986), degenerative diseases (Harkins 1981), and asynchronous disorders such as AN/AD (Hood, 1998a; Starr et al., 1996). Unlike imaging techniques, which have superior spatial resolution and are useful in identifying structural defects, the ABR has excellent temporal resolution and is useful in detecting central auditory brainstem disorders (Hall, 1992). In short, the ABR is a test of physiology whereas most imaging techniques examine anatomic structure.

One of the primary criteria for the diagnosis of AN/AD is an absent ABR (Hood & Berlin, 2001; Sininger & Oba, 2001; Zeng, Oba, Garde, Sininger, & Starr 2001). Other investigators have broadened the diagnosis of AN/AD to include abnormal ABRs (Starr, 2001). This may possibly lead to a diagnosis of AN/AD when there is a central auditory deficit (Rapin & Gravel, 2003). The ABR abnormality begins with an absent wave I, which implies asynchronous firing at the synapse between the hair cells and auditory nerve (see Figure 14-1). Sininger and Oba (2001) reported absent ABRs in 70% of their 59 subjects with confirmed AN/AD, abnormal ABRs in 6% of these subjects, whereas 19% of these subjects had only wave V in the ABR recording, implying asynchrony in the lower brainstem. Thus, an absent ABR is most indicative of AN/AD. In contrast, most investigations report normal ABRs in children with (C)APD (Hurley, 2004; Mason & Mellor, 1984; Roush & Tait, 1984). However, reports of compromised ABR in patients with CANS dysfunction demonstrate the importance of this potential in the central auditory processing battery (Musiek, Charette, Morse, & Baran, 2004).

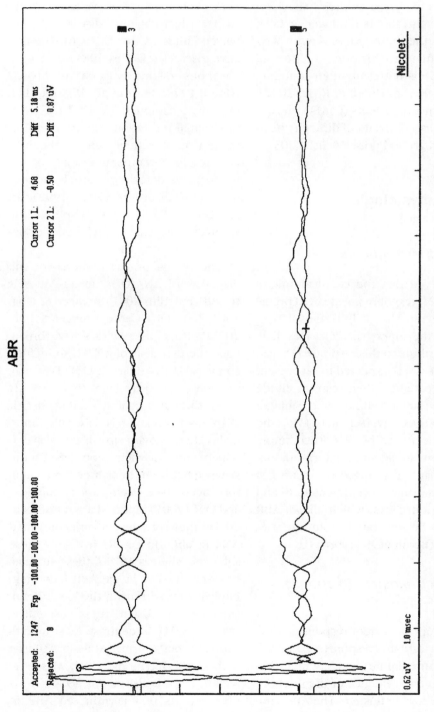

Figure 14–1. The auditory brainstem response (ABR) recording from a 15-year-old female which illustrates the common finding of a biphasic response in AN/AD cases. Also note a complete inversion of elements even beyond 2 msec. This patient presented a flat, bilateral sensorineural hearing loss of moderate degree; however, distortion product otoacoustic emissions for most of the 1000 to 8000 Hz test range were within normal limits.

Also, ABR is a very valuable tool in (C)APD assessment as it will provide objective evidence of any CANS involvement, especially in patients with protracted histories of otitis media or hyperbilirubinemia (Dublin, 1985).

Auditory Middle Latency Response (AMLR)

The underlying auditory generators of the auditory middle latency response (AMLR) include the thalamocortical pathway (Kileny, Paccioretti, & Wilson, 1987; Kraus, Ozdamar, Hier, & Stein, 1982; Ozdamar, & Kraus, 1983), the reticular formation (Kraus, Kileny, & McGee, 1994), and the inferior colliculus (McGee, Kraus, Comperatore, & Nicole, 1991). Specifically, the early AMLR components, waves Na and Pa might arise from the medial geniculate and thalamus, whereas the association areas of the cortex might be responsible for waves Nb and Pb (Geisler, Frishkopt, & Rosenblith, 1958).

There is no consistent pattern for the AMLR in patients with AN/AD. Starr et al. (1998) reported absent AMLRs in four patients, two patients had abnormal AMLR recordings, and one patient had a normal AMLR recording. Absent AMLR recordings have also been reported in other published case reports (Hood & Berlin, 2001). The presence or absence of the AMLR is dependent on where the site of auditory dysfunction lies along the central auditory pathway. Thus, the inclusion of the AMLR response may provide valuable information to the site of the auditory dysfunction.

The AMLR recording is also a valuable tool in assessing maturity of the central auditory pathway with a multiple electrode montage being recommended in (C)APD assessment (Chermak & Musiek,

1997). Unlike the standard ABR, amplitude measures may be a more sensitive measure than latency in (C)APD assessment using the AMLR (Kraus et al., 1982; Scherg & von Cramon, 1986). The multisite amplitude measures are compared over hemispheres to determine if there is an electrode effect (Musiek, Baran & Pinheiro, 1994) or ear effect (Musiek, et al., 1999). Pre- and post-AMLR recordings may also be useful to assess the efficacy of AN/AD and (C)APD training programs, and to study auditory maturation in young children (Musiek et al., 2004).

Auditory Long-Latency Response (ALLR)

The auditory long-latency response (ALLR) is a set of cortical responses that can be divided into sensory potentials (auditory late response [ALR]) and processing contingent potentials (P300) (Davis, 1976; Steinschneider, Kurtzberg & Vaughan, 1992). These potentials have generators that are located in the auditory cortex and are believed to reflect higher order processing in individuals (Steinschneider et al., 1992). Waves N1 and P2 of the ALR, also referred to as N100 and P200 as they occur at approximately 100 and 200 msec poststimulus, occur in response to clicks, tones, or speech. These sensory potentials are sometimes referred to as exogenous potentials (stimulus related). Specifically, the generator of the N1 and P2 components is believed to be the auditory cortex (Näätänen & Picton, 1987), whereas the P2 component may also reflect activity in the reticular formation (Näätänen & Picton, 1987).

The P300 response is a processing-contingent potential and is also referred to as an endogenous response (subject-related) (Squires & Hecox, 1983). This potential is usually elicited by an oddball paradigm in which the subject actively attends to an occasional rare stimulus as opposed to the standard stimuli (Sutton, Braren, Zubin, & John, 1965). Thus, attention, discrimination, and memory are reflected in the P300 recording (Picton & Hillyard, 1988). The underlying generators are not completely defined, but evidence shows that the hippocampus, auditory cortex, and temporal lobe contribute to this response (Buchwald, 1990; McPherson, 1996).

Similar to the AMLR, a multiple-electrode montage is recommended when recording ALLRs (Chermak & Musiek, 1997; Peronnet & Mickel, 1977) as this will provide amplitude and latency measures to objectively determine hemispheric involvement for ear or electrode effects. Chermak and Musiek (1997) recommended recording N1 and P2 from electrode sites C3, C4, and Cz and the P300 from Fz, Pz, and Cz, and additionally C3 and C4. As with AMLR recordings, the ALR and P300 studies may be useful in longitudinal studies to monitor or assess the effectiveness of an auditory training program.

Neural synchrony is represented differently in the ALLR than in the early ABR as disrupted neural synchrony in the earlier auditory evoked potentials does not lead to asynchronous ALLRs. Starr et al., (1996) reported differing results in a group of patients with AN/AD. All patients had abnormal ABRs, yet two patients had normal ALRs, two had abnormal ALRs, and two had absent ALR recordings. Hood and Berlin (2001) also reported absent ALRs in one patient with AN/AD. Again, the presence or absence of these potentials appears to be dependent upon the site of disorder in the central auditory pathway.

Jirsa and Clontz (1990) reported prolonged P300 latencies in a group of children with APD. Similar, prolonged P300 latencies have also been reported in a group of patients with cerebral lesions (Musiek, Baran, & Pinhero, 1994. It is important to note that nonauditory factors may affect the P300 recording (Knight, 1990); thus, an absent or abnormal ALR and P300 recording does not warrant a diagnosis for (C)APD. However, inclusion of the ALR and P300 recordings in the (C)APD battery may provide objective evidence to support the diagnosis of an (C)APD (Jerger, Chmiel, Tonini, Murphy, & Kent, 1999; Purdy, Kelly & Davies, 2002; Wible, Nicol, & Kraus, 2005). (See Chapter 12 for discussion of auditory evoked potentials in (C)APD diagnosis.)

Behavioral Tests of Temporal Processing

Temporal processing requires synchronous discharge of neurons of the peripheral and central auditory pathway (Phillips, 1995). Sound undergoes complex processing by intricate neural mechanisms and neural networks, which are composed of structures located in the brainstem, subcortex, primary and association areas of the auditory cortex, and the corpus callosum (Phillips, 1995). In addition, these mechanisms are responsible for transmitting, enhancing/inhibiting, reshaping, refining, and assigning recognition and meaning to sound. (See Chapter 3 for review of neurorepresentation of time in the CANS.)

Temporal processing is critical in speech perception as all acoustic signals such as speech vary over time (Tallal, 1985). In order to extract meaning from these varying acoustic signals, the listener must be able to detect very small and rapid time variations. Physiologic changes such as axonal loss and demyelination can easily disrupt temporal pattern coding in the auditory system. Although temporal processes are critical in a number of auditory behaviors, there are a limited number of clinical tests available to assess temporal processing abilities (e.g., pitch and duration pattern tests, gap detection tests, and masking level differences). (See Chapter 10 for discussion of behavioral tests of temporal processing.)

There are limited data reporting the results of temporal processing tasks by listeners with AN/AD. Zeng et al. (2001) showed that gap detection ability was impaired in all subjects with AN/AD as was the temporal modulation transfer function performance. Zeng et al. (2001) also assessed the performance of AN/AD patients on other psychoacoustic tasks and reported abnormal loudness growth measures in one patient with AN/AD, normal intensity discrimination in four subjects with AN/AD, and poorer frequency discrimination for frequencies less than 2000 Hz for all patients with AN/AD. Interestingly, as the test frequency increased, the AN/AD patient's frequency discrimination for higher frequencies improved.

Audiologic Summary

Table 14–2 lists many of the expected outcomes for the tests that may be used in AN/AD assessment. One of the most important distinguishable differences in AN/AD and (C)APD is hearing loss. Although there is no distinct audiometric configuration and pure tone thresholds may fluctuate, there is documented SNHL

in most patients with AN/AD; however, patients with (C)APD generally have normal hearing. Acoustic reflexes are generally absent or elevated in patients with AN/AD; whereas, the acoustic reflexes are generally normal in patients with (C)APD. Also important is the finding that the standard ABR is expected to be absent in patients with AN/AD, but typically is normal in most patients with (C)APD (Hurley, 2004; Mason & Mellor, 1984; Roush & Tait, 1984).

Intervention

Accurate differential diagnosis should lead to more targeted, efficient, and effective intervention. Clearly, there are challenges in managing patients with AN/AD and (C)APD. As with (C)APD, children with AN/AD should have an appropriate individual intervention and educational plan. Each case of AN/AD is unique and may require modifications to the habilitation plan over time. The habilitation plan should include therapy that is directed toward the improvement of cognitive, language and auditory skills (Bellis, 2003; Chermak & Musiek, 1997). The use of amplification, however, with AN/AD patients remains controversial. Starr et al. (1996) reported no benefit for patients with AN/AD with the use of wearable amplification. Conversely, Rance et al. (1999) reported benefit from wearable amplification in half of their patients with AN/AD. Other patients have reported benefit using FM systems (Hood, 1998a). The differing results with amplification may reflect the heterogeneous makeup of the AN/AD patient group.

Two other management strategies for AN/AD have been suggested. Cued

Table 14–2. Expected Test Results For Patients With AN/AD and (C)APD

Audiometric Test/Procedure	Auditory Neuropathy	(C)APD
Pure tone thresholds	Various degrees of hearing loss and configurations	Usually within normal limits
Tympanometry	Normal	Normal
Acoustic reflexes	Elevated or absent	Usually within normal limits depending on site(s) of central auditory nervous system (CANS) dysfunction
Speech recognition in noise	Poor	Variable, depending on site(s) of CANS dysfunction
Otoacoustic emissions	Present	Present
Gap detection	Abnormal	Often abnormal, depending on site(s) of CANS dysfunction
ABR	Absent	Usually normal
MLR	Questionable	Variable, depending on site(s) of CANS dysfunction
ALLR/P300	Questionable	Variable, depending on site(s) of CANS dysfunction

speech, a visual aide to communication, has been recommended (Berlin et al., 1998; Hood, 1998a). Cochlear implants have also been recommended for patients with AN/AD (Shallop et al., 2001; Trautwein, Sininger, & Nelson, 2000). Investigators have suggested that although a cochlear implant may appear counterintuitive given possible peripheral anatomic sites of AN/AD (i.e., inner hair cells) (Harrison, 1988), patients have shown benefit (Hood, 1998a; Shallop et al., 2001; Trautwein et al., 2000). The present situation suggests that there does not appear to be one and only one correct or successful management plan for AN/AD treatment, which gives further support to the contention that the AN/AD group is heterogeneous; it is not one disorder, but rather a family of disorders.

Similarly, management for (C)APD must be appropriate for the specific auditory deficits. A comprehensive management plan includes three approaches: (1) environmental modifications to improve access to the auditory signal (e.g., FM system); (2) direct therapy to enhance perceptual auditory skills (i.e., auditory training);

and (3) central resources training to develop compensatory language, cognitive, and metacognitive skills and strategies (Bellis, 2003; Chermak & Musiek, 1997). The particular emphasis within and across these three approaches depend upon the specific clinical deficit profile (ASHA, 2005; Bellis, 2003). It is important to note that although some of these management approaches may be considered for both patients with (C)APD and AN/AD (i.e., FM systems and auditory training), (C)APD and AN/AD are distinct disorders and management must be tailored to the behavioral deficits with recognition of the underlying physiologic differences that characterize these two disorders.

Summary

Although differential diagnosis of AN/AD and (C)APD is possible using current behavioral and electrophysiologic techniques, additional research is needed to distinguish more clearly the underlying physiologic deficit(s), perceptual correlates, and functional capabilities of AN/AD. Although patients with AN/AD and (C)APD present some similar complaints, these are distinct auditory disorders that can be distinguished by a comprehensive behavioral, electrophysiologic, and psychoacoustic test battery. The results of Zeng's (2001) work indicate the value of including psychoacoustic tests in the test battery which might enable the clinician to better understand a patient's communication difficulties. Furthermore, interpretation of a comprehensive battery can lead to inferences regarding the gross anatomic site of auditory dysfunction. Careful interpretation will allow clinicians to better understand the underlying physiologic site of disorder and the consequent communication difficulties that many patients face and may be valuable in tailoring an auditory training program. The effectiveness of treatment and management for these complex disorders depends on accurate and thorough diagnosis and assessment.

References

American Speech-Language-Hearing Association. (2005). *Central auditory processing disorders.* Technical Report. Rockville, MD.

Barr, D. F. (1976). *Auditory perceptual disorders* (2nd ed.). Springfield, MA; Charles C. Thomas.

Bellis, T. (2003). *Assessment and management of central auditory processing disorders in the educational setting: From science to practice.* Clifton Park, NY: Thomson-Delmar Learning.

Bellis, T. J., & Ferre, J. M. (1999) Multidimensional approach to the differential diagnosis of central auditory processing disorders in children. *Journal of the American Academy of Audiology, 10,* 319–328.

Bellis, T. J., Nicol, T., & Kraus, N. (2000). Aging affects hemispheric asymmetry in the neural representation of speech sounds. *Journal of Neuroscience, 20,* 791–797.

Bellis, T. J., & Wilber, L. A. (2001). Effects of aging and gender on interhemispheric function. *Journal of Speech, Language, and Hearing Research, 44,* 246–263.

Berlin, C., Bordelon, J., St. John, P., Wilensky, D., Hurley, A., Kluka, E., & Hood, L. (1998). Reversing click polarity may uncover auditory neuropathy in infants. *Ear and Hearing, 19,* 37–47.

Berlin, C. I., Hood, L. J., Cecola, R. P., Jackson, D., & Szabo, P. (1993). Afferent-efferent disconnection in humans. *Hearing Research, 65,* 40–50.

Berlin, C. E., Hood, L. J., Hurley, A., & Wen, H. (1996). Hearing aids: Only for hearing-impaired patients with abnormal oto-acoustic emissions (pp. 99–112). In C. I. Berlin (Ed.), *Hair cells and hearing aids.* San Diego, CA: Singular Publishing Group.

Berlin, C., Hood, L., & Rose, K. (2002). On renaming auditory neuropathy as auditory dys-synchrony. *Audiology Today, 13,* 15–17.

Brown, D. P. (1994). Speech recognition in recurrent otitis media: Results in a set of identical twins. *Journal of the American Academy of Audiology, 5,* 1–6.

Buchwald, J. (1990). Animal models of event-related potentials. In J. Rohrbaugh, R. Para-suraman, & R. Johnson (Eds.), *Event related potentials of the brain* (pp. 57–75). New York: Oxford Press.

Chedru, F., Bastard, V., & Efron, R. (1978). Auditory micropattern discrimination in brain damaged subjects. *Neuropsychologia, 16,* 141–149.

Chermak, G. D., & Musiek, F. E. (1997). *Central auditory processing disorders: New perspectives.* San Diego, CA: Singular Publishing Group.

Dallos, P. (1973). *The auditory periphery.* New York: Academic Press.

Dallos, P. (1997). Outer hair cells: The inside story. *American Academy of Audiology 9th Annual Convention Program,* 70 (A).

Davis, H. (1976). Principles of electric response audiometry. *Annals of Otology, Rhinology, and Laryngology, 85,* 1–96.

Davis, H., & Hirsh, S. (1979). A slow brainstem response for low-frequency audiometry. *Audiology, 18,* 445–461.

Deltenre, P., Mansbach, A. L., Bozet, C., Clercx, A., & Hecox, K. E. (1997). Auditory neuropathy: A report on three cases with early onsets and major neonatal illnesses. *Electroencephalography and Clinical Neurophysiology, 104,* 17–22.

Dublin, W. (1985). The cochlear nuclei—pathology. *Otolaryngology-Head and Neck Surgery, 93,* 448–463.

Geisler, C. D., Frishkopf, L. S., & Rosenblith, W. A. (1958). Extracranial responses to acoustic clicks in man. *Science, 128,* 1210–1211.

Goldberg, J. (1998). Out of control. *Parents, 73,* 108–109.

Gorga, M. P., Stelmachowicz, P. G., Barlow, S. M., & Brookhouser, P. E., (1995). Cases of recurrent, reversible, sudden sensorineural hearing loss in a child. *Journal of the American Academy of Audiology, 6,* 163–172.

Gravel, J. S., & Wallace, I. F. (1992). Listening and language at four years of age: Effects of early otitis media. *Journal of Speech and Hearing Research, 35,* 588–595.

Hall, J. W. III. (1992). *Handbook of auditory evoked responses.* Needham Heights, MA: Allyn & Bacon.

Hall, J. W., & Grose, J. H. (1993). The effect of otitis media with effusion on the masking level difference and the auditory brainstem response. *Journal of Speech and Hearing Research, 36,* 210–217.

Harkins, S. W. (1981). Effects of presenile dementia of the Alzheimer's type on brainstem transmission time. *International Journal of Neuroscience, 15,* 165–170.

Harrison, R. (1988). An animal model of auditory neuropathy. *Ear and Hearing, 19,* 355–361.

Hood, L. J. (1998a). *Clinical applications of the auditory brainstem response.* San Diego, CA: Singular Publishing Group.

Hood, L. J. (1998b). Auditory neuropathy: What is it and what can we do about it? *Hearing Journal, 51,* 10–18.

Hood, L. J., & Berlin, C. I. (2001). Auditory neuropathy (auditory dys-synchrony) disables efferent suppression of otoacoustic emissions. In Y. Sininger & A. Starr (Eds.), *Auditory neuropathy: A new perspective on hearing disorders* (pp. 183–202). San Diego, CA: Singular Publishing Group.

Hurley, A. (2004). *Behavioral and electrophysiological assessment of children with a specific temporal processing disorder.* Doctoral dissertation. Louisiana State University and Agricultural and Mechanical College, Baton Rouge.

Jerger, J., Chmiel, R., Ronini, R., Murphy, E., & Kent, M. (1999). Twin study of auditory processing disorder. *Journal of the*

American Academy of Audiology, *10*, 521-528.

Jerger, J., Greenwald, R., Wambacq, I., Seipel, A., & Moncrieff, D., (2000). Effect of age on interaural asymmetry of event-related potentials in a dichotic listening task. *Journal of the American Academy of Audiology*, *11*, 383-389.

Jerger, J., & Musiek, F. (2000). Report of the consensus conference o the diagnosis of auditory processing disorders in school-aged children. *Journal of the American Academy of Audiology*, *11*, 467-474.

Jerger, J., Oliver, T., Chmiel, R., & Rivera, V. (1986). Patterns of auditory abnormality in multiple sclerosis. *Audiology*, *25*, 193-209.

Jerger, J., Thibodeau, L, Martin, J., et al. (2002). Behavioral and electrophsyiological evidence of auditory processing disorder: A twin study. *Journal of the American Academy of Audiology*, *13*, 438-460.

Jirsa, R. E., & Clontz, K. B. (1990). Long latency auditory event-related potentials from children with auditory processing disorders. *Ear and Hearing*, *11*, 222-232.

Katz, J. (1992). Classification of auditory processing disorders. In J. Katz, N. A. Stecker, & D. Henderson (Eds.), *Central auditory processing disorders: Problems of speech, language and learning* (pp. 269-296). Baltimore: University Park Press.

Kileny, P. R., Paccioretti, D., & Wilson, A. F. (1987). Effects of cortical lesions on middle-latency auditory evoked responses (MLR). *Electroencephalography and Clinical Neurophysiology*, *66*, 108-120.

Knight, R. (1990). Neuromechanisms of event-related potentials: Evidence from human lesion studies. In J. Roharaboaugh, R. Parassurman, & R. Johnson (Eds.), *Event-related potentials: Basic issues in applications* (pp. 3-18). New York: Oxford University Press.

Kraus, N. (2001). Auditory neuropahy; An historical and current perspective. In Y. Sininger & A. Starr (Eds.), *Auditory neuropathy: A new perspective on hearing disorders* (pp. 1-14). San Diego, CA: Singular Publishing Group.

Kraus, N., Kileny, P., & McGee, T. (1994). The MLR: Clinical and theoretical principles. In J. Katz (Ed.), *Handbook of Clinical Audiology* (3rd ed., pp. 387-402). Baltimore: Williams and Wilkins.

Kraus, N., McGee, T., Carrell, T., Zecker, S., Nicol, T., & Koch, D. (1996). Auditory neurophysiologic responses and discrimination deficits in children with learning problems. *Science*, *273*, 971-973.

Kraus, N., Ozdamar, O, Hier, D. & Stein, L, (1982). Auditory middle latency response (MLRs) in patients with cortical lesions. *Electroencephalogry and Clinical Neurophysiology*, *54*, 275-287.

Kraus, N., Ozdamar, O., Stein, L., & Reed, N. (1984). Absent auditory brain stem response: Peripheral hearing loss or brain stem dysfunction? *Laryngoscope*, *94*, 400-406.

Mason, S., & Mellor, D. (1984). Brainstem, middle latency and late cortical potentials in children with speech and language disorders. *Electroencephalography and Clinical Neurophysiology*, *59*, 297-309.

McGee, T., Kraus, N., Comperatore, C., & Nicole, T. (1991). Subcortical and cortical components of the MLR generating system. *Brain Research*, *54*, 211-220.

McPherson, D. (1996). *Late potentials of the auditory system*. San Diego, CA: Singular Publishing Group.

Musiek, F. E., Baran, J. A., & Pinheiro, M. L. (1994). *Neuroaudiology case studies*. San Diego, CA: Singular Publishing Group.

Musiek, F. E., Baran, J. A., & Shinn, J. (2004). Assessment and remediation of an auditory processing disorder associated with head trauma. *Journal of the American Academy of Audiology*, *15*, 117-132.

Musiek, F. E., Charette, L., Kelly, T., Lee, W. W., & Musiek, E. (1999). Hit and false positive rates for the middle latency response in patients with central nervous system involvement. *Journal of the American Academy of Audiology*, *10*, 124-132.

Musiek, F. E., Charette, L., Morse, D., & Baran, J. A. (2004). Central deafness associated with a midbrain lesion. *Journal of the*

American Academy of Audiology, 15, 133-151.

Musiek, F. E., & Gollegly, K. (1988). Maturational considerations in the neuroauditory evaluation of children (pp. 231-252). In F. Bess (Ed.), *Hearing impairment in children.* Parkton, MD: York Press.

Näätänen, R., & Picton, T. W. (1987). The N1 wave of the human electric and magnetic response to sound: A review and analysis of the component structure. *Psychophysiology, 24,* 375-425.

Ozdamar, O. & Kraus, N. (1983). Auditory middle latency responses in humans. *Audiology, 22,* 34-49.

Peronnet, F., & Mickel, F. (1977). The asymmetry of auditory evoked potentials in normal man and patients with brain lesions. In J. Desmedt (Ed.), *Auditory evoked potentials in man: Psychopharmacology correlates of EPS* (pp. 130-141). Basel, Switzerland: Karger.

Phillips, D. P. (1995). Central auditory processing: A view from auditory neuroscience. *The American Journal of Otology, 16,* 338-352.

Pichora-Fuller, M. K., & Souza, P. E. (2003). Effects of aging on auditory processing of speech. *International Journal of Audiology, 42,* 2S11-2S16.

Picton, T. W., & Hillyard, S. A. (1988). Endogenous event-related potentials. In T. W. Picton (Ed.), *Handbook of electroencephalography and clinical neurophysiology Vol. 3: Human event-related potentials* (pp. 361-426). Amsterdam: Elsevier.

Purdy, S., Kelly, A., & Davies, M. (2002). Auditory brainstem response, middle latency response, and late cortical evoked potentials in children with learning disabilities. *Journal of the American Academy of Audiology, 13,* 367-382.

Rance, G., Beer, D. E., Cone-Wesson, B., Shepherd, R. K., Dowell, R. C., King, A. M., Richards, F. W., & Clark, G. M. (1999). Clinical findings for a group of infants and young children with auditory neuropathy. *Ear and Hearing, 20,* 238-252.

Rapin, I., & Gravel, J. (2003). "Auditory neuropathy": Physiologic and pathologic evidence calls for more diagnostic specificity. *International Journal of Pediatric Otorhinolaryngology, 67,* 707-728.

Rappaport, J. M. & Provencal, C. (2002). Neuro-otology for audiologists. In J. Katz (Ed.), *Handbook of clinical audiology* (5th ed.). Philadelphia: Lippincott Williams & Wilkins.

Roush, J., & Tait, C. A. (1984). Binaural fusion, masking level differences, and auditory brain-stem responses in children with language-learning disabilities. *Ear and Hearing, 5,* 37-41.

Scherg, M., & von Cramon, D. (1986). Evoked dipole source potentials of the human auditory cortex. *Electroencephalography and Clinical Neurophysiology, 65,* 344-360.

Shallop, J. K., Peterson, A., Facer, G. W., Fabry, L. B., & Driscoll, C. L. W. (2001). Cochlear implants in five cases of auditory neuropathy: Postoperative findings and progress. *Laryngoscope, 111,* 555-562.

Sininger, Y. & Oba, S. (2001). Patients with auditory neuropathy: Who are they and what can they hear? In Y. Sininger & A. Starr (Eds.), *Auditory neuropathy: A new perspective on hearing disorders* (pp. 15-35). San Diego, CA: Singular Publishing Group.

Squires, K., & Hecox, K. (1983). Electrophysiological evaluation of higher level auditory processing. *Seminars in Hearing, 4,* 415-432.

Stach, B. A., Spretnjak, M., & Jerger, J. (1990). The prevalence of central presbycusis in a clinical population. *Journal of the American Academy of Audiology, 1,* 109-115.

Starr, A. (2001). The neurology of auditory neuropathy: In Y. Sininger & A. Starr (Eds.), *Auditory neuropathy: A new perspective on hearing disorders* (pp. 37-49). San Diego, CA: Singular Publishing Group.

Starr, A., Picton, T. W., & Kim, R. (2001). Pathophysiology of auditory neuropathy: In Y. Sininger & A. Starr (Eds.), *Auditory neuropathy: A new perspective on hear-*

ing disorders (pp. 67–82). San Diego, CA: Singular Publishing Group.

Starr, A., Picton, T. W., Sininger, Y., Hood, L. J., & Berlin, C. I. (1996). Auditory neuropathy. *Brain, 119*, 741–753.

Starr, A., Sininger, Y., Winter, M., Derebery, M. J., Oba, S., & Michalewski, H. J. (1998). Transient deafness due to temperature sensitive auditory neuropathy. *Ear and Hearing, 19*, 169–179.

Steinschneider, M., Kurtzberg, D., Vaughan, H. G. Jr. (1992). Event-related potentials in developmental psychology. In I. Rapin & S. J. Segalowitz (Eds.), *Child Neuropsychology, Vol. 6.* (pp. 239–299) Amsterdam: Elsevier.

Sutton, S., Braren, M., Zubin, J., & John, E. (1965). Evoked potential correlates of stimulus uncertainty. *Science, 150*, 1187–1188.

Tallal, P. (1985). Neuropsychological research approaches to the study of central auditory processing. *Human Communications, 9*, 17–22.

Taylor, M. J., McMenamin, J. B., Andermann, E., & Watters, G. V. (1982). Electrophysiological investigation of the auditory system in Friedreich's ataxia. *Canadian Journal of Neurological Science, 9*, 131–135.

Trautwein, P., Sininger, Y., & Nelson, R. (2000). Cochlear implantation of auditory neuropathy. *Journal of the American Academy of Audiology, 11*, 309–315.

Tremblay, K. L. Piskosz, M., & Souza, A. (2003). Effects of age and age-related hearing loss on the neural representation of speech-cues. *Clinical Neurophysiology, 114*, 1332–1343.

Wible, B., Nicol., T. G., & Kraus, N. (2005). Correlation between brainstem and cortical auditory processes in normal and language-impaired children. *Brain, 128*, 417–423.

Willeford, J. A., & Burleigh, J. M. (1985) *Handbook of central auditory processing disorders in children*. Orlando, FL: Grune & Stratton.

Willott, J. F. (1996). Anatomic and physiologic aging: A behavioral neuroscience perspective. *Journal of the American Academy of Audiology, 7*, 141–151.

Woods, D. L., & Clayworth, C. C. (1986). Age-related changes in human middle latency auditory evoked potentials. *Electroencephalography and Clinical Neurophysiology, 65*, 297–303.

Worthington, D., & Peters, J. (1980). Quantifiable hearing and no ABR: Paradox or error? *Ear and Hearing, 5*, 281–285.

Zeng, F. G., Oba, S., Garde, S., Sininger, Y., & Starr, A. (2001). Psychoacoustics and speech perception in auditory neuropathy. In Y. Sininger & A. Starr (Eds.), *Auditory neuropathy: A new perspective on hearing disorders* (pp. 141–164). San Diego, CA: Singular Publishing Group.

CHAPTER 15

DIFFERENTIAL DIAGNOSIS OF (CENTRAL) AUDITORY PROCESSING DISORDER AND ATTENTION DEFICIT HYPERACTIVITY DISORDER

GAIL D. CHERMAK

Individuals diagnosed with attention deficit hyperactivity disorder (ADHD) frequently present difficulties performing tasks that challenge the central auditory nervous system (CANS). Individuals diagnosed with (central) auditory processing disorder ([C]APD) often demonstrate central auditory dysfunction that presents comorbidly with other valid diagnoses. In children, (C)APD frequently co-occurs with ADHD, language impairment, and learning disability (Chermak, Hall, & Musiek, 1999). Tests with documented sensitivity and specificity for CANS dysfunction are *necessary* for a diagnosis of (C)APD. Likewise, accurate diagnosis of ADHD depends on the sensitivity and specificity of the rating scales commonly used to infer the presence of ADHD. Multidisciplinary assessment, evaluating the role of higher order global, supramodal, or pansensory, cognitive, attention, language, and related disorders, is essential for *differential* diagnosis (Bellis, 2003; Chermak & Musiek, 1997; Musiek, Bellis, & Chermak, 2005). Accurate knowledge of an individual's problems derived from multidisciplinary evaluations leads to the most effective intervention programs. In cases of comorbidity, (C)APD and ADHD must be diagnosed fully and accurately and a treatment program must be developed and implemented by a team of professionals to address all significant functional deficits.

Spectrum of Comorbid Disorders

The association observed between attention deficits and performance on central auditory tests (Campbell & McNeil, 1985;

Cook et al., [1993]; Gascon, Johnson, & Burd, 1986; Pillsbury, Grose, Coleman, Conners, & Hall, 1995) has elicited suggestions of linkage between ADHD and (C)APD. Some have questioned whether (C)APD is a manifestation of impaired attention (Burd & Fisher, 1986; DeMarco, Harbour, Hume, & Givens, 1989; Robin, Tomblin, Kearney, & Hug, 1989) and whether (C)APD and ADHD reflect a single developmental disorder (Cook et al., 1993; Gascon et al., 1986). Others have interpreted central auditory performance deficits among children with ADHD as a reflection of the co-occurrence or co-morbidity of (C)APD and ADHD (Keith & Engineer, 199; Riccio, Cohen, Garrison, & Smith, 2005; Riccio, Hynd, Cohen, & Gonzales, 1993; Riccio, Hynd, Cohen, & Molt, 1996). For example, finding low correlations between performance on the *Staggered Spondaic Word* (SSW) *Test* and behaviors characteristic of ADHD (i.e., inattention, hyperactivity, and impulsivity), Riccio et al. (1996) concluded that ADHD and (C)APD are distinct entities that may nonetheless both involve deficits in auditory processing. Extending their earlier findings, Riccio et al. (2005) found no significant correlations between measures of attention (i.e., continuous performance test and rating scales for attention problems and hyperactivity) and measures of central auditory processing (i.e., the SSW and the Screening Test for Auditory Processing Disorders [SCAN]). Riccio and colleagues concluded that deficits in auditory processing may not necessarily be associated with ADHD or attention deficits. Despite overlapping clinical profiles and co-morbidity, converging lines of evidence indicate that (C)APD and ADHD are clinically distinctive entities (Chermak, Hall, & Musiek,

1999). The two disorders can be differentially diagnosed, leading to distinctive treatment and management strategies.

That central auditory performance deficits among children with ADHD may reflect the presence of (C)APD rather than the ADHD per se is supported further by the frequently reported history of chronic otitis media in children with ADHD (Adesman, Altshuler, Lipkin, & Walco, 1990; Feagans, Sanyal, Henderson, Collier, & Appelbaum, 1987; Pillsbury et al., 1995; Roberts, Burchinal, Collier, Ramey, Koch, & Henderson, 1989; Silva, Kirkland, Simpson, Stewart, & Williams, 1982). The association between chronic otitis media and (C)APD, with persistence of central auditory processing deficits even after resolution of the otitis media and return to normal hearing levels (Adesman et al., 1990; Brown, 1994; Ferguson, Cook, Hall, Grose, & Pillsbury, 1998; Gravel & Wallace, 1992; Hall & Grose, 1993, 1994; Hall, Grose, & Pillsbury, 1994, 1995; Hutchings, Meyer, & Moore, 1992; Jerger, Jerger, Alford, & Abrams, 1983; Moore, Hutchings, & Meyer, 1991; Pillsbury, Grose, & Hall, 1991; Silva, Chalmers, & Stewart, 1986) suggests that children with ADHD may experience central auditory performance deficits subsequent to chronic otitis media. Indeed, the frequently observed co-occurrence of (C)APD and learning disability (Breedin, Martin, & Jerger, 1989; Chermak, Vonhof, & Bendel, 1989; Elliott & Hammer, 1988; Ferre & Wilber, 1986; Jerger, Martin, & Jerger, 1987; King, Warrier, Hayes, & Kraus, 2002; Kraus, McGee, Carrell, Zecker, Nicol, & Koch, 1996; Purdy, Kelly, & Davies, 2002; Warrier, Johnson, Hayes, Nicol, & Kraus, 2004) and (C)APD and language impairment (Lubert, 1981; Marler, Champlin, Gillam, 2002; Sloan, 1980; Tallal, 1980a,

1980b; Tallal & Piercy, 1973a; Tallal, Stark, & Mellits, 1985; Tallal et al., 1996) have led to speculation that these deficits also may be causally related (Katz & Illmer, 1972; Keith, 1981; Knox & Roeser, 1980; Lubert, 1981; Merzenich et al., 1996; Miller, Kail, Leonard, & Tomblin, 2001; Rey, De Martino, Espesser, & Habib, 2002; Sloan, 1980; Tallal, 1980; Tallal & Piercy, 1973a; Tallal, Stark, & Mellits, 1985; Tallal et al., 1996). Temporal processing deficits have been linked to language and learning problems; however, this purported linkage is controversial (see for example, Studdert-Kennedy & Mody, 1995; Bishop et al., 1999; Nittrouer, 1999). Finding perceptual deficits cutting across diagnostic categories, including children with diagnoses of learning disability, ADHD, and dyslexia, Kraus (2001) concluded that there is a common perceptual deficit in a subset of children with various clinical diagnoses.

Brain Organization Underlies Comorbidity

The literature is replete with reports of individuals with concurrent diagnoses of (C)APD, attention deficits, and learning disabilities (Cunningham, Nicol, Zecker, Bradlow, & Kraus, 2001; Katz, 1992; Keith, 1986; Keller, 1992; King, Warrier, Hayes, & Kraus, 2002; Kraus, 2001; Kraus, McGee, Carrell, Zecker, Nicol, & Koch, 1996; Musiek, Charette, Kelly, Lee, & Musiek, 1999; Newhoff, Cohen, Hynd, Gonzalez, & Riccio, 1992; Pillsbury et al., 1995; Purdy et al 2002; Riccio et al., 1993, 1996; Warrier, Johnson, Hayes, Nicol, & Kraus, 2004; Wible, Nicol, & Kraus, 2002). The relationships among these comorbid con-

ditions are complex and not completely understood. Tremendous gains in our understanding of brain organization and function, however, have provided insights regarding linkages and distinctions.

Comorbidity is the result of the complex organization of the brain that is temporally coupled across the cortex, modalities, and hemispheres (Merzenich, Shreiner, Jenkins, & Wang 1993). Although there may be some brain regions that are auditory-specific, the brain's organization is predominantly nonmodular and non-exclusively segregated (Streitfeld, 1980). Neurons in so-called *auditory areas* may respond *primarily*, although not exclusively to auditory stimuli (Musiek, Bellis, & Chermak, 2005). Moreover, auditory neurons in the cerebrum exhibit inter-connectedness with a variety of neurons in other nonauditory areas of the brain, including the limbic system, cingulate gyrus, hippocampus, and the frontal lobe (Streitfeld, 1980). Additional areas of the brain that have been identified as auditory responsive include the amygdala, striatum, and frontal lobe (Poremba, Saunders, Crane, Cook, Sokoloff, & Mishkin, 2003; Salvi, Lockwood, Frisina, Coad, Wack, & Frisina, 2002). Many of the auditory responsive and interconnected areas support attention, executive control, and motor regulation and are implicated in the underlying pathophysiology of ADHD (Castellanos, 1997; Sowell, Thompson, Welcome, Henkenius, Toga, & Peterson, 2003). In addition, central auditory lesions often extend beyond artificial boundaries that are increasingly recognized as inaccurate reflections of true brain organization (Musiek, Bellis, & Chermak, 2005). Even if auditory lesions were relatively circumscribed, the fact that most brain regions are not modality-specific likely results in comorbid dysfunction in other systems due to shared neurophysiological substrates. Hence, the often reported comorbidity of (C)APD and ADHD may be explained by shared physiologic and neurologic networks.

Neurobiologic Correlates

Brain imaging studies and postmorten examinations of individuals with dyslexia, learning disabilities, ADHD, and normal controls have revealed morphologic and structural differences in auditory areas of the brain which are activated when listening to simple tonal complexes, language, and music (i.e., superior temporal gyrus, Heschl's gyrus, planum temporale, posterior portion of the insula, sulcus of the corpus callosum) (Galaburda & Kemper, 1978; Hynd, Semrud-Clikeman, Lorys, Novey, & Eliopulos, 1990; Hynd, Semrud-Clikeman, Lorys, Novey, Eliopulos, & Lyytinen 1991). The accumulating data suggests a neurobiologic basis for the often observed co-occurrence of (C)APD, auditory attention deficits, dyslexia, and learning disabilities. At the same time, a number of studies also reveal activation patterns that may help distinguish (C)APD from ADHD (e.g., see Tannock, 1998 for a review).

Postmortem studies have documented brain abnormalities (e.g., nests of ectopic [misplaced] and underdeveloped cells) involving auditory regions of the brain in children with learning disabilities and dyslexia (Galaburda & Eidelberg, 1982; Galaburda & Kemper, 1978; Galaburda, Sherman, Rosen, Aboitiz, & Geschwind, 1985). Brain imaging studies have revealed morphologic and structural differences in auditory areas, as well as motor regulation/behavioral inhibition areas (pre-

frontal lobes and striatum) of the brains of children with ADHD, as compared with the brains of normal children, implicating some deviation in normal brain development (Hynd & Semrud-Clikeman, 1989; Hynd et al., 1990; Lou, Henriksen, Bruhn, Borner, & Nielsen, 1989; Mann, Lubar, Zimmerman, Miller, & Muenchen, 1992; Tannock, 1998; Voeller, 1991; Zametkin et al., 1990).

The corpus callosum was reported smaller in children with ADHD relative to normal controls and the morphology of Heschl's gyrus may also differ in children with ADHD, as compared with normal controls (Baumgardner et al., 1996; Castellanos et al., 1996; Giedd et al., 1994; Hynd et al., 1991; Semrud-Clikeman et al., 1994). The planum temporale was reported shorter in the left hemisphere, and of reversed asymmetry (R>L), in subjects with dyslexia relative to normal controls (Hynd et al., 1990). Similarly, the insular region of the brains of children with dyslexia are smaller bilaterally than normal controls (Hynd et al., 1990). Using high-resolution magnetic resonance imaging, Sowell et al. (2003) reported abnormal morphology and reduced size of the frontal cortices of children and adolescents with ADHD relative to normal controls. Prominent increases in gray matter in large portions of the posterior temporal and inferior parietal cortices of subjects with ADHD also were reported.

Morphologic differences and possible dysfunction in areas of the brain associated with motor regulation and self-control (e.g., frontal region, caudate nucleus) suggest a neurobiological basis for co-occurring central auditory deficits and behavioral regulation problems in ADHD (Gallagher & Schoenbaum, 1999; Paus, 2000). Lou et al. (1989) reported decreased metabolism in the caudate nucleus associated with ADHD. Mann et al. (1992) found increased slow wave activity in the frontal regions and decreased beta activity in the temporal regions in boys with ADHD, compared to normal control subjects. Hynd et al. (1990) reported bilaterally smaller anterior cortexes in children with ADHD and dyslexia relative to a control group of children, reflecting significantly decreased right frontal lobe width. Positron emission tomography (PET) studies revealed widespread and bilateral reduction in glucose metabolism, in the premotor and superior frontal cortices, as well as in the striatum and the thalamus (Zametkin et al., 1990). In addition, the children with dyslexia showed hemispheric symmetry in this region in contrast to the typical pattern of the right frontal lobe being larger than the left (Hynd et al., 1990). Giedd et al. (1994) concluded that anatomic differences in several regions of the corpus callosum support theories of abnormal frontal lobe development and function in ADHD. Sowell et al. (2003) suggested that abnormal morphology of the frontal cortices in children and adolescents with ADHD may underlie attention and behavioral inhibition problems.

Finally, event-related potential (ERP) studies document the neurobiologic basis for the often observed comorbidity between (C)APD and ADHD. Compared to normal controls, individuals with ADHD exhibit smaller amplitude and longer latency auditory P300, possibly reflecting the longer time and difficulty required to complete stimulus evaluation (Klorman, 1991). Also suggesting impairment in processing of auditory stimuli in ADHD are findings of abnormal auditory brainstem evoked responses (ABR) and abnormalities in the N1, N2 of the auditory late response (ALR), and the auditory P300

(Jonkman et al., 1997; Lahat et al., 1995). Similarly, children and adults diagnosed with (C)APD and/or lesions of the CANS present longer latency and decreased amplitude auditory P300 (Jirsa & Clontz, 1990; Krishnamurti, 2001; Musiek, Baran, & Pinheiro, 1992), increased ABR latencies (Musiek & Lee, 1995), and other evoked potential abnormalities (e.g., middle-latency response (MLR) (Musiek, Baran, & Pinheiro, 1994). (See Chapter 17 by Maerlender for additional review of the neurobiology of ADHD.)

(Central) Auditory Processing Disorder: An Overview

(C)APD results from difficulties in the perceptual processing of auditory information in the central nervous system and the associated changes in the neurobiologic activity that underlies those processes and gives rise to the electrophysiologic auditory potentials (ASHA, 2005). In some cases, neurobiologic dysfunction may involve interhemispheric transfer deficits, lack of appropriate hemispheric lateralization, reversed hemispheric asymmetries, or imprecise synchrony of neural firing (Jerger et al., 2002; Kraus, McGee, Carrell, Zecker, Nicol, & Koch, 1996; Moncrieff, Jerger, Wambacq, Greenwald, & Black, 2004). (C)APD also may coexist with more global dysfunction that affects performance across modalities (e.g., attention deficit, neural timing deficit, language representation deficit) (ASHA, 2005; Chermak & Musiek, 1997). (C)APD has been observed in diverse clinical populations, including those where central nervous system (CNS) pathology or neurodevelopmental disorder is suspected (e.g., developmental language disorder, dyslexia, learning disability, attention deficit disorder) and those where evidence of CNS pathology is clear (e.g., aphasia, multiple sclerosis, epilepsy, traumatic brain injury, tumor, and Alzheimer's disease) (ASHA, 1996). (C)APD also has been observed in older adults, presumably due to nonpathologic neurologic changes associated with aging (Committee on Hearing, Bioacoustics and Biomechnaics [CHABA] Working Group on Speech Understanding and Aging, 1988; Gulya, 1991; Stach, Spretnjak, & Jerger, 1990). Atypical interhemispheric transfer of auditory information may be a factor contributing to the listening difficulties seen in some children and in aging adults (Bellis, Nicol, & Kraus, 2000; Bellis & Wilber, 2001; Chmiel & Jerger, 1996; Chmiel, Jerger, Murphy, Prozzolo, & Tooley-Young, 1997; Jerger, 1992; Jerger, Moncrieff, Greenwald, Wambacq, & Seipel, 2000; Jerger et al., 2002; Musiek, Gollegly, & Baran, 1984, Musiek, Pinheiro, & Wilson, 1980). Additional age-related changes in the CANS include less synchrony and time-locking, slower refractory periods, and decreased inhibition (Pichora-Fuller & Souza, 2003; Tremblay, Piskosz, & Souza, 2003; Willot, 1999; Woods & Clayworth, 1986).

A (C)APD manifests as a deficit in one or more of the following behaviors: sound localization and lateralization; auditory discrimination; auditory pattern recognition; temporal processing (e.g., temporal resolution, temporal masking, temporal integration, and temporal ordering); auditory performance with competing acoustic signals; and auditory performance with degraded acoustic signals (ASHA, 2005; Chermak & Musiek, 1997). Characteristically, patients with (C)APD have difficulty comprehending spoken language in competing speech or noise backgrounds

and in reverberation (Chermak & Musiek, 1997). Children with (C)APD ask frequently for repetitions, often misunderstand messages, have difficulty paying attention, have trouble following complex auditory directions or commands, and difficulty localizing sound (Bellis, 2003; Chermak & Musiek, 1997).

(C)APD is diagnosed on the basis of performance on a battery of auditory tests, which may include electrophysiologic as well as behavioral procedures, administered under acoustically controlled conditions (ASHA, 2005; Chermak & Musiek, 1997; Jerger & Musiek, 2000). The sensitivity and specificity of behavioral and electrophysiologic central auditory tests and procedures recommended for inclusion in the test battery (see Chapter 7) have been established on patients with known lesions of the CANS (e.g., Hendler, Squires, & Emmerich, 1990; Jerger et al., 2002; Musiek, Shinn, Jirsa, Bamiou, Baran, & Zaidan, 2005; Rappaport Gulliver, Phillips, van Dorpe, Maxner, & Bhan, 1994).

Prevalence data for (C)APD are sparse, particularly for children. Estimates of (C)APD in children range from 2 to 7%, with a 2:1 ratio between boys and girls (Bamiou, Musiek, & Luxon, 2001; Chermak & Musiek, 1997; Musiek, Gollegly, Lamb, & Lamb, 1990). Cooper & Gates (1991) estimated CAPD in 10 to 20% of older adults. Stach et al. (1990) reported (C)APD in 70% of clinical patients over age 60 years.

Attention Deficit Hyperactivity Disorder: An Overview

ADHD is characterized as the most common neurobehavioral disorder of childhood (Barkley, 1998). ADHD consists of a persistent pattern of inattention and/or hyperactivity-impulsivity that is more frequent and severe than is typically observed in individuals at a comparable level of development; manifests in at least two settings; interferes with developmentally appropriate social, academic, or occupational functions; and is present since before age 7 years (APA, 1994).

Patterns of inattention, hyperactivity, and impulsivity are used to differentiate ADHD into three subtypes. The predominantly inattentive type presents primary symptoms of inattention (APA, 1994). The predominantly hyperactive-impulsive type is considered a behavioral regulation disorder (APA, 1994; Barkley, 1994, 1998). The combined type is characterized by hyperactivity-impulsivity (i.e., behavioral regulation disorder) and inattention (APA, 1994). Different neuroanatomic loci are posited for the different subtypes. The combined and predominantly hyperactive-impulsive types might arise from problems in the prefrontal-limbic pathways, particularly the striatum (Lou et al., 1989). The predominantly inattentive type might involve more posterior associative cortical areas and/or cortical and subcortical feedback loops, perhaps involving the hippocampal system (Heilman, Voeller, & Nadeau, 1991; Hynd, Lorys, Semrud-Clikeman, Nieves, Huettner, & Lahey, 1991).

According to the DSM-IV, impulsivity is characterized by blurting out answers, failing to take turns, and interrupting or intruding on others. Hyperactivity is characterized by fidgeting with hands or feet or squirming in seat, difficulty remaining seated, running or climbing excessively in inappropriate contexts, difficulty engaging in quiet activity, constantly moving or engaging in activity, and talking excessively. Inattention in ADHD is marked by difficulties maintaining

focus, sustaining and shifting attention, concentrating, listening when spoken to, following through and completing tasks, engaging in tasks requiring sustained mental effort and persistence, organizing tasks, and ignoring extraneous stimuli, and is associated with careless mistakes in school work, losing things, and forgetfulness.

There are no empirical markers that identify ADHD. Diagnosis of ADHD is based on observational criteria defined as a cluster of behaviors involving impaired attention and distractibility, impulsivity, and hyperactivity (AAP, 2000; APA, 1994). The limited sensitivity and specificity of the rating scales used to identify ADHD can lead to misdiagnosis and overdiagnosis, possibly identifying some children with ADHD when in fact their primary deficit is (C)APD (Stein, 2001).

Many epidemiologic studies have been conducted to determine the prevalence of ADHD in children and adolescents, with estimates ranging from 2 to 14%. Based on their review of these studies, Scahill and Schwab-Stone (2000) concluded that the best estimate appears to be 5 to 10%. The prevalence of ADHD is higher among boys, with estimates ranging between 2:1 and 9:1, varying as a function of the age range sampled (Scahill & Schwab-Stone, 2000). The prevalence of ADHD is stable in girls across the range of 10 to 20 years; however, an age-related decline in ADHD is seen among boys (Scahill & Schwab-Stone, 2000).

Reconceptualization of ADHD

The recent shift in conceptualizing ADHD as a behavioral regulation disorder rather than a primary attention disorder differentiates (C)APD and ADHD (Chermak & Musiek, 1997). Symptoms of impulsivity and behavioral disinhibition are considered the result of neurologically based, developmental deficiencies in the regulation and maintenance of behavior by rules and consequences (Barkley, 1998). Deficits in rule-governed behavior, perhaps resulting from elevated arousal thresholds (Zentall, 1985) or elevated reinforcement thresholds (Haenlein & Caul, 1987), lead to problems initiating, inhibiting, or sustaining responses to tasks or stimuli (Barkley, 1998), which heretofore had been considered characteristics of attention deficits. Deficits in rule-governed behavior lead to problems in executive functioning and self-regulation (Barkley, 1998). Consistent with this reconceptualization, ADHD is seen, essentially, as a motivational deficit, rather than an attention deficit (Barkley, 1994, 1998). This reconceptualization of ADHD as one of poor rule-governed behavior may also explain the self-control problems, social skill deficits, and language disorders (e.g., difficulty topic-switching, turn-taking, and sustaining dialogue) so frequently observed in ADHD (Augustine & Damico, 1995).

Differentiating (C)APD and ADHD

Modeling Information Processing

Insofar as attention is essential to higher level processing, poor attention can compromise listening. Musiek & Chermak (1995) proposed that viewing the relationship between attention and auditory processing within the top-down and bottom-up information processing models provides a theoretical framework that clarifies the nature of the relationship

between ADHD and (C)APD. The inability to sustain sufficient attention to auditory stimuli might cause (i.e., top-down) auditory processing deficits; conversely, deficient auditory processing (i.e., bottom-up) might impair attention (Chermak & Musiek, 1997). Understanding the relationship between the attention deficits of ADHD and (C)APD hinges on the interaction between perception and higher-level cognitive processing (Chermak & Musiek, 1997). Most germane is whether an auditory processing deficit causes some attention deficit (as occurs in [C]APD) or whether a more global attention deficit impedes auditory processing (as occurs in ADHD).

Consistent with a bottom-up model, attention is driven by incoming sensory stimulation and garnered by properly integrated and processed sensory stimuli (Chermak & Musiek, 1997; Musiek & Chermak, 1995). If acoustic stimuli are not properly processed, as occurs in (C)APD, then optimal attention cannot be focused on these stimuli in a timely manner (Phillips, 1990). Attention deficits are seen as secondary to auditory perceptual processing deficits within the framework of a bottom-up model (Chermak & Musiek, 1997). In contrast, (C)APD would be seen as a manifestation of a global attention deficit within a top-down information processing model (Chermak & Musiek, 1997).

While it is likely that bidirectional interactions between central auditory processing and attention are necessary for optimal listening comprehension, experimental evidence from basic science supports a bottom-up view of attention deficits whereby deficiencies in auditory perceptual processes trigger attention deficits (Farah & Wallace, 1991; Harrison, Smith, Hagasawa, Stanton, & Mount,

1992; Hassamannova, Myslivecek, & Novakova, 1981; Irvine, Rajan, & Robertson, 1992; Mogdans & Knudsen, 1992, 1993, 1994; Phillips, 1995; Recanzone, Schreiner, & Merzenich, 1993; Robertson & Irvine, 1989). The known interactions between the auditory pathway and the reticular activating system at the brainstem level provide support for the bottom-up view of attention deficits (Koch, 1999). Experimental evidence regarding the plasticity of the CANS supports the bottom-up view of auditory perceptual deficits as causal to (C)APD. This evidence suggests that central changes are contingent on sensory function and experience (Moore, 1993). For example, cortical reorganization has been observed in young and adult mammals following induced cochlear lesions (Harrison et al., 1992; Irvine et al., 1992; Kilgard et al., 2001; Rajan & Irvine, 1998; Rajan, Irvine, Wise, & Heil, 1993; Robertson & Irvine, 1989; Schwaber, Garraghty, & Kaas, 1993; Willott, Aitkin, & McFadden, 1993).

Consistent with a bottom-up perspective, listening difficulties seen in (C)APD result from primarily auditory perceptual deficiencies rather than global attention deficits (ADHD predominantly inattention subtype) or behavioral regulation deficits (combined ADHD and predominantly hyperactive-impulsive ADHD subtypes) (Phillips, 1990, 1995; Tallal et al., 1996). As outlined in Table 15-1, (C)APD is considered an input disorder that

Table 15–1. Differentiating Attention Deficits in Attention Deficit Hyperactivity Disorder (ADHD) and (C)entral Auditory Processing Disorder ([C]APD)

ADHD Combined and Predominantly Hyperactive-Impulsive Subtypes
• Output (Behavioral Regulation) Disorder
• Sustained Attention (Vigilance) Deficit Secondary to Behavioral Disinhibition and Self-Regulation Deficit
• Executive Dysfunction Primary Source of Disorder
ADHD Predominantly Inattentive Subtype
• Input (Processing) Disorder
• Global (Supramodal) Attention Deficit
• Selective (Focused) Attention Deficit
• Reduced Speed of Information Processing Primary Source of Disorder
(C)APD
• Input (Processing) Disorder
• Primarily Auditory Modality Specific Perceptual Deficit
• Selective (Focused) and Divided Auditory Attention Deficits
• Executive Dysfunction as Secondary Source of Listening Problems

impedes selective and divided auditory attention. The combined and predominantly hyperactive-impulsive ADHD subtypes are seen as output disorders in response programming and execution that indirectly cause sustained attention deficits across modalities. Dual diagnoses of both (C)APD and ADHD may result, therefore, from comorbid attention deficits at different levels and primacy of sensory and global dysfunction (Chermak & Musiek, 1997).

Defining Attention and Types of Attention Deficits

Inattention is symptomatic of many psychiatric and medical conditions (Riccio, Reynolds, & Lowe, 2001). Symptoms of inattention unrelated to poor self-control (e.g., ADHD predominantly inattentive subtype) poses a particular diagnostic challenge (Chermak et al., 1999). In such cases, clinicians must rule out a range of possible disorders including anxiety, depression, obsessive-compulsive disorder, learning disabilities, and (C)APD. Although attention deficits may be seen to characterize (C)APD and ADHD (particularly the combined and predominantly inattentive subtypes), distinctions can be drawn regarding the *nature* of the inattention observed in the two disorders.

Consistent with the reconceptualization of ADHD as a behavioral regulation disorder, inattention in individuals with the hyperactive-impulsive and combined ADHD subtypes is reflected in behaviors of disorganization, distractibility, and lacking persistence (Barkley, 1994, 1998). Inattention attributed to individuals with the predominantly inattentive subtype of ADHD is reflected in their passive, sluggish, and *daydreamy* behavior (Barkley, 1998). In fact, individuals with (C)APD

are not truly *inattentive*. Rather, as noted above, deficits in auditory selective (focused) attention (or separation) and auditory divided attention (or integration) lead to difficulties understanding spoken language in competing noise and reverberant backgrounds, misunderstanding messages, and difficulty following directions in individuals with (C)APD (Chermak & Musiek, 1997). As outlined in Table 15-1, the attention deficits of ADHD typically are pervasive and supramodal, impacting more than one sensory modality (AAP, 2000; APA, 1994; Keller, 1992). In contrast, individuals with (C)APD experience attention deficits that may be restricted to the auditory modality or are at least more pronounced in the auditory modality (ASHA, 2005; Chermak & Musiek, 1997; Musiek, Bellis, & Chermak, 2005).

Different types of attention deficits may be seen in ADHD and (C)APD (Chermak & Musiek, 1997). Although the neural mechanisms underlying the different behaviors associated with various attention tasks are not fully known, research suggests that attention deficits associated with the combined and predominantly hyperactive-impulsive ADHD subtypes may be restricted to sustained attention, albeit in multiple modalities (Barkley, 1997a, 1997b; Hooks, Milich, & Lorch, 1994; Seidel & Joschko, 1990). Selective (multimodal) attention and speed of information processing deficits may characterize the predominantly inattentive ADHD subtype (Barkley, 1997a). Selective (focused) and divided auditory attention deficits characterize (C)APD (Cherry, 1980; Jerger & Jerger, 1984; Katz & Illmer, 1972; Keith, 1986; Lasky & Tobin, 1973) (See Table 15-1). Inclusion of tests of sustained attention (vigilance) in the central auditory test battery should prove helpful in substantiating the distinction discussed above regarding types of attention deficits (i.e., sustained, focused, and divided attention), aiding the differential diagnosis of (C)APD and ADHD (Chermak, 2004; Riccio et al., 2001; McPherson & Salamat, 2004; Salamat & McPherson, 1999).

Differentiating Behavioral Profiles

Despite some overlapping symptomatology, clinicians seem able to distinguish behavioral profiles for (C)APD and ADHD. Chermak, Somers, & Seikel (1998) found that pediatricians and audiologists view the predominant symptoms of ADHD and (C)APD as being rather distinct, with only two (i.e., inattention and distractibility) of the eleven most frequently cited behaviors reported as common to both conditions (see Table 15–2). Inattention and distractibility were ranked as

the first and second most typical behaviors characterizing ADHD. Audiologists ranked these same behaviors as seventh and sixth, respectively, in cases of (C)APD. (C)APD was characterized by a selective attention deficit and associated language processing and academic difficulties; ADHD was characterized by inappropriate motor activity, restlessness, and socially inappropriate interaction patterns. In a follow-up study, Chermak, Tucker, & Seikel (2002) found that pediatricians and audiologists can distinguish the primary symptoms of the predominantly inattentive subtype of ADHD and (C)APD. None of the four behaviors ranked two standard deviations above the grand means (i.e., inattention, academic difficulties, asking for things to be repeated, and poor listening skills) was ranked in common (see Table 15–3).

Other investigators have reported that behavior problems, such as difficulty waiting one's turn and playing quietly

Table 15–2. Rank Order of Behavioral Means Greater Than One Standard Deviation Above the Respective Grand Mean

ADHD		CAPD	
1. Inattentive	4.36	1. Difficulty hearing in background noise	4.40
2. Distracted	4.27	2. Difficulty following oral instructions	4.20
3. Hyperactive	4.14	3. Poor listening skills	4.10
4. Fidgety or restless	4.14	4. Academic difficulties	4.00
5. Hasty or impulsive	4.14	5. Poor auditory association skills	3.75
6. Interrupts or intrudes	3.86	6. Distracted	3.70
		7. Inattentive*	3.55
Grand mean	3.25		2.90
Standard deviation	0.55		0.66

*Note that inattentive was included based on "evens-down/odds-up" rounding rule; the standard deviation was 0.01 points below the criteria of +1 SD of the grand mean. (Reproduced with permission from "Behavioral signs of central auditory processing disorder and attention deficit hyperactivity disorder," by G. D. Cherman, E. K. *Academy of Auchology*, 9, 78–84. Copyright 1998 American Academy of Audiology.)

Table 15–3. Rank Order of Behavioral Means Greater Than One and Two (*) Standard Deviations Above the Respective Grand Mean

ADHD-PI	AVG.	C(APD)	AVG
Inattentive	4.45*	Asks for things to be repeated	4.39*
Academic difficulties	4.22*	Poor listening skills	4.39*
Daydreams	4.05	Difficulty following instructions given orally	4.33
Distracted	4.04		
Poor listening skills	3.86	Difficulty hearing in background/ambient noise	4.28
Disorganized	3.82		
Asks for things to be repeated	3.70	Academic difficulties	4.22
		Distracted	3.78
Auditory divided attention deficit	3.67	Reduced rate of information processing	3.78
Difficulty hearing in background/ambient noise	3.62	Auditory divided attention deficit	3.76
		Auditory selective attention deficit	3.76
		Auditory sustained attention deficit	3.71
		Poor memory	3.67
		Difficulty discriminating speech	3.65
Grand mean	3.11	Grand mean	2.93
Standard deviation	0.50	Standard deviation	0.72

Reprinted with permission from "Behavioral characteristics of auditory processing disorder and attention deficit disorder," by G. D. Chermak, E. Tucker, and J. A. Seikel, 2002. *Journal of the American Academy of Audiology, 13*, 332–338. Copyright 1992 American Academy of Audioloty.

and excessive talking, more often characterize children with ADHD than (C)APD (Newhoff et al., 1992). Similarly, severe socioemotional sequelae (i.e., conduct disorders, juvenile delinquency) are more common among children with ADHD (Newhoff et al., 1992). Interestingly, the predominantly inattentive ADHD subtype shares little if any comorbidity with disruptive behavior disorders, in contrast to the predominantly hyperactive-impulsive and combined ADHD subtypes (Barkley, 1997a). Wilens, Biederman, & Spencer (2002) noted that individuals with ADHD-combined subtype are most impaired, presenting more comorbid psychiatric diagnoses and more substance abuse

disorders. Individuals with ADHD combined subtype and ADHD-predominantly inattentive subtype experience greater academic problems, whereas individuals with ADHD-predominantly inattentive subtype experience fewer emotional and behavioral problems than other subtypes (Millstein, Wilens, Biederman, & Spencer, 1997; Wilens et al., 2002).

The distributed nature of information processing and underlying brain activation explains overlapping behavioral deficits; however, overlapping behavioral profiles do not necessarily implicate common antecedents. The sustained attention problems observed in ADHD probably result from a supramodal, cognitive deficit, deficiencies in behavioral regulation rather than attention per se. In contrast, the selective and divided auditory attention deficits of (C)APD result from deficient auditory perceptual processing. Similarly, difficulty following directions is commonly observed among individuals with ADHD and (C)APD; however, deficiencies in rule-governed behavior may underlie these difficulties in ADHD, whereas deficient central auditory processing of auditory signals may underlie the same performance deficit in (C)APD. Executive dysfunction, as discussed below, may also underlie the resemblance in clinical profiles seen across (C)APD and ADHD.

Summary

Although additional research is needed to clarify differences in the nature and type of attention deficits observed in ADHD and (C)APD, it is clear that the clinical inattention profiles differ significantly. The inattention profile of ADHD involves difficulty initiating, tracking, and remembering tasks (APA, 1994), in addition to sustaining allocation of attentional resources. The focused and divided attention deficits that characterize (C)APD impact monaural and binaural separation (i.e., selective attention), and binaural integration (i.e., divided attention) tasks (Chermak & Musiek, 1997). Most important, the inattentiveness seen in (C)APD is a primary deficit resulting from an input or information processing deficit. In contrast, the hyperactive-impulsive and combined ADHD subtypes are characterized as output or response programming and execution disorders (Barkley, 1997a, 1997b). Behavioral disinhibition ultimately results in poor goal-directed persistence and defective resistance to distraction subsequent

to poor self-regulation and executive control of behavior (Barkley, 1997a, 1997b; Goodyear & Hynd, 1992). Consistent with this conceptualization, inattention is a secondary deficit in the combined and predominantly hyperactive-impulsive ADHD subtypes (Barkley, 1997a, 1997b). As elaborated above, the ADHD inattention profile may implicate a primary executive control deficit, rather than an attention deficit per se. Differentiating the predominantly inattentive ADHD subtype from (C)APD is more challenging as the inattention in both disorders is considered to be a primary, input or information-processing deficit. Notwithstanding the challenge, differential diagnosis of (C)APD and the supramodal, predominantly inattentive ADHD subtype can be accomplished using a sensitized test battery of the CANS in combination with a comprehensive multidisciplinary evaluation. (See Test Batteries and Testing Strategies.)

Executive Function

Executive functioning provides a construct useful in understanding a wide range of symptoms observed across many disorders with overlapping clinical profiles (Pennington, Bennetto, McAleer, & Roberts, 1996), including ADHD and (C)APD. Because executive functions place significant demands on attention (both *sustained* and *selective attention* to enable sensory and perceptual processing of events) and memory to register, store, and make knowledge and experience available to the individual (Barkley, 1996; Butterfield & Albertson, 1995; Pennington, Bennetto, McAleer, & Roberts, 1996), executive dysfunction may be related to deficits characterizing ADHD and (C)APD.

Executive function is a component of metacognition that refers to a set of general control processes which ensure that an individual's behavior is adaptive, consistent with some goal, and beneficial to the individual (Borkowski, Milstead, & Hale, 1988; Brown, Bransford, Ferrara, & Campione, 1983; Denckla, 1996; Sternberg, 1985; Torgesen, 1996). Executive control processes coordinate knowledge (i.e., cognition) and metacognitive knowledge in support of task analyses, planning, and reflective decision-making, ultimately transforming this knowledge into behavioral strategies (Barkley, 1996; Butterfield & Albertson, 1995). They are crucial to the execution of novel behavioral sequences; learning and problem-solving; psychosocial function, including self-image, self-regulation of emotion and motivation; and goal-directed behaviors, including listening (Borkowski & Burke, 1996; Grattan, Bloomer, Archambault, & Eslinger, 1994; Grattan & Eslinger, 1992). Executive function may be assessed by a variety of procedures and tests, as noted later in this chapter.

Synchronized activation across multiple cortical and subcortical regions, including the frontal lobe, temporal lobe, parietal lobe, basal ganglia, and thalamus, subserves executive functioning (Eslinger & Grattan, 1993; Goldenberg, Oder, Spatt, & Podreka, 1992). Many of the neural networks thought to underlie executive function follow a prolonged course of postnatal development, extending into adolescence and perhaps continuing into adulthood (St. James-Roberts, 1979; Thatcher, 1991; Yakelov & Lecours, 1967); therefore, the system is highly vulnerable to disruption from a variety of causes, including neurobiologic stressors, as well as environmental deprivation (Barkley, 1996).

Executive function deficits have been described in a wide variety of clinical populations, often in association with brain disease or injury, and may underlie childhood neurologic disorders, in particular the academic problems experienced by children with learning disabilities or ADHD (Denckla, 1996; Fletcher, Taylor, Levin, & Satz, 1995; Graham & Harris, 1996; Pennington, 1991; Stanovich, 1986; Torgesen, 1994). Executive function deficits also have been identified in children who do not meet eligibility criteria for learning disabilities or ADHD but experience significant difficulties in school (Denckla, 1989). The prevalence of (C)APD in the latter group of children has not been determined (Chermak & Musiek, 1997).

Linkages among executive function, rule-governed behavior, and self-control (Hayes, Gifford, & Ruckstuhl, 1996) have led to suggestions that executive dysfunction is the source of the behavioral regulation and inattention problems, as well as the language problems exhibited in ADHD (Barkley, 1994; Denckla & Reader, 1993; Smith, Gould, Marsh, & Nichols, 1995; Tannock & Schachar, 1996). Recognizing that pragmatic and metacognitive behaviors associated with communication are both language-based and rule-governed, Westby and Cutler (1994) reasoned that executive dysfunction also may explain language deficits in ADHD, such as poor topic maintenance, inappropriate topic-switching, poor problem-solving, and difficulty producing coherent extended discourse such as stories and expository texts (Heyer, 1995), as well as contribute to the pragmatic problems observed in individuals with ADHD, which include excessive talking, interrupting others, blurting out answers, difficulty waiting one's turn, and difficulty negotiating peer interactions.

Although executive dysfunction in (C)APD has not been examined, it is reasonable to expect that auditory perceptual deficits impede operation of executive functions (Chermak & Musiek, 1997). Difficulty organizing, monitoring, and understanding acoustic signals may reflect limited use of executive function. In contrast to the proposed causal role of executive dysfunction in ADHD (Barkley, 1994; Denckla & Reader, 1993; Smith et al., 1995), and consistent with a bottom-up processing model, executive dysfunction in (C)APD would be considered a secondary feature, not a primary cause, of listening difficulties (Chermak & Musiek, 1997). These secondary deficits could compound auditory processing deficits, impede generalization of strategic listening behaviors across settings, and thereby jeopardize treatment effectiveness and efficacy (Borkowski & Burke, 1996; Chermak & Musiek, 1997).

Differential Diagnosis of ADHD and (C)APD

The Challenge

All auditory tasks, from pure tone detection to spoken language processing, are influenced by higher-order, nonmodality-specific factors such as attention, memory, motivation, and decision processes, and the underlying multimodal, cross-modal, and supramodal neural interfaces supporting performance of these behavioral tasks (Chermak, Hall, & Musiek, 1999; Chermak & Musiek,1997; Musiek, Bellis, & Chermak, 2005). For example, listening in noise activates auditory and nonauditory areas of the brain, including areas involved in attention, executive control, working memory, language processing, and motor planning (Salvi et al., 2002). Moreover, cognitive processes undergird basic perceptual events, as demonstrated by the integral role of working memory in numerous auditory processes, including localization, temporal resolution, and pattern recognition (Marler, Champlin, Gillam, 2002; Martinkauppi, Rama, Aronen, Korvenoja, & Carolson, 2002; Zattore, 2001). Indeed, the complex organization of the brain, involving interactive and interfacing sensory, cognitive, and linguistic networks, requires testing methods and careful interpretation of test outcomes that reduce the potential confound of factors not under direct examination in behavioral testing for (C)APD.

McFarland and Cacace (1995) discussed three categories of individuals who perform poorly on tests of auditory function: (1) those who represent (C)APD in its *purest* form and perform poorly solely on auditory tests; (2) those who exhibit auditory perceptual problems that coexist with other specific processing problems and, thus, present with a mixed or co-morbid pattern of deficits; and (3) those who perform poorly on auditory tests because of a global, supramodal problem involving, cognition, attention, language, memory, or related skills, and who perform poorly on both auditory and visual tasks. (C)APD is a deficit in neural processing of acoustic stimuli that *is not the result of* dysfunction in other modalities (ASHA, 2005). It would be inappropriate to apply the label of (C)APD to listening difficulties exhibited by individuals with higher-order, global, supramodal, or pansensory disorders (e.g., ADHD, autism, cognitive delay) *unless* a comorbid deficit in the CANS is documented. By combining multidisciplinary evaluation along with tests of central auditory function that have been demonstrated to be both sensitive and specific for disorders of the CANS, it is possible to differentiate the auditory deficits present in individuals falling into the first two categories whereas, at the same time, *ruling out* (C)APD in those individuals who fall into the third category (Musiek, Bellis, & Chermak, 2005).

Assessing Central Auditory Processing in Children with ADHD

Audiologic assessment of children with ADHD is clinically challenging. Valid behavioral measurement of auditory status requires that the child willingly cooperate in the assessment, understand the instructions, and attend to the task. Each of these requirements may be compromised in the ADHD population. The likelihood of successfully assessing CANS function in children with ADHD or suspected ADHD is enhanced by several practical modifications in the test strategy. However, when behavioral audiometric findings remain incomplete, inconclusive, or invalid despite the implementation of these modifications, one must rely more on electrophysiologic techniques (Chermak, et al., 1999; Chermak & Musiek, 1997).

Perhaps the single most important step in successful audiologic assessment of the child with diagnosed and medically managed ADHD is to ensure that the child received an effective dose of medication immediately before the test session (Cher-

mak, Hall, & Musiek, 1999).[1] Although this statement seems obvious, it is important to specifically instruct caregivers to follow the typical school day routine for medication on the day of the audiologic assessment. Some might argue that audiologic assessment should be conducted with the child in his or her natural state, for example, without medication. Others might express concerns about the possible confounding effects of the medication on test performance. Clinical experience suggests at least three responses to these arguments. First, if the child regularly is given medication on school days, then following the prescribed medication schedule will result in a typical state. Second, there is no evidence that the medications used in management of ADHD (e.g., Adderall, Ritalin, Strattera) have any influence on peripheral or central auditory nervous system function. Finally, for children with diagnosed ADHD who are treated medically, valid audiologic assessment would rarely be possible without medication. Therefore, it is advisable to verify that the child received appropriate medication on the test day. Also, the assessment is best scheduled to begin first thing in the morning (e.g., 8:30 or 9:00 AM). Frequent breaks during which the child is given the opportunity to move about should be provided during the test session. The child should be asked to repeat or paraphrase instructions and be given practice items. Furthermore, the child should be offered a verbal contract to discourage hyperactive and impulsive behavior and the child should be given positive reinforcement (e.g., frequent praise for his or her

---

[1]Certainly, one can imagine exceptions to this recommendation. For example, if questions arise regarding the effectiveness of medication, or if medication is not taken regularly, the audiologist might be asked to compare a child's auditory performance with and without medication.

efforts) to enhance motivation (Keller & Tillery, 2002).

Peripheral auditory function should be evaluated thoroughly, but expediently, prior to central auditory assessment. A feasible test sequence is: immittance measurement (tympanometry and both uncrossed and crossed acoustic reflexes), pure tone audiometry (including inter-octave frequencies of 3000 and 6000 Hz), speech reception thresholds, word recognition performance, and otoacoustic emissions (Chermak et al., 1999). As the overall objective is assessment of central auditory function, the evaluation of peripheral auditory function should be conducted as quickly as possible, without sacrificing vital information. To save test time, pure tone audiometry is limited to air conduction whenever immittance measurement yields findings consistent with normal middle ear function. As an aside, acoustic reflex thresholds should be measured very cautiously, or not at all, when history suggests the possibility of hyperacusis, or intolerance to loud sounds. Speech reception threshold measurement can be bypassed if pure tone audiometry is reliable and entirely normal. Word recognition performance can be evaluated with lists that include the 10 most difficult words first. The test can be stopped when the child responds correctly to these first 10 words. Otoacoustic emissions recording with a cooperative child will generally require less than 2 minutes per ear, even with a protocol that is sensitive to cochlear dysfunction (e.g., DPOAE with L1 = 65 dB and L2 = 55 dB or TEOAE with an 80-dB SPL click stimulus). By employing these test-time-saving strategies, the experienced audiologist can usually complete the peripheral assessment in less than 30 minutes.

Test Batteries and Testing Strategies

The overall objective of the central auditory test battery is to determine whether the individual has a deficit in one or more of the central auditory processes. Demonstration of distinctive *patterns* across multidisciplinary tests helps distinguish (C)APD from supramodal cognitive, language-based, and/or supramodal attention deficits. These patterns are derived from comparison of performance on behavioral tests of central auditory function and neurophysiologic results from auditory evoked potentials with behavioral and neurophysiologic measures of other sensory, language, and cognitive systems (Bellis, 2003; Bellis & Ferre, 1999; Chermak, 2004; Chermak et al., 1999; Chermak & Musiek, 1997; Musiek, Bellis, & Chermak, 2005).

Specific testing methods and interpretation strategies of test outcomes can reduce the potential confound of factors not under direct examination in behavioral testing for (C)APD. These methods and strategies, which employ patient-referenced (intrasubject) criteria as well as norm-referenced (intersubject) criteria, include: (1) use of nonverbal stimuli or, alternatively, stimuli that carry a light linguistic load; (2) employment of intrasubject comparisons, including ear differences, interhemispheric differences, intertest and cross-discipline (multimodal) analysis to explore supramodal effects; (3) use of binaural separation/integration tasks during dichotic listening (e.g., a consistent left-ear deficit, given symmetric hearing sensitivity, is unlikely to result from a supramodal deficit); and (4) use of a simple response mode (ASHA, 2005; Bellis, 2003; Bellis & Ferre, 1999; Chermak et al., 1999; Chermak & Musiek, 1997;

Jerger & Musiek, 2000; Musiek, Bellis, & Chermak, 2005).

Findings of asymmetric speech recognition deficits and/or speech recognition deficits seen only in the presence of either ipsilateral or contralateral competition would suggest a (C)APD rather than a supramodal attention deficit (Baran & Musiek, 1995), whereas poor performance across all measures suggests a more global deficit (e.g., attention, memory, anxiety, or motivation, among others). Phoneme processing difficulties in quiet are unlikely to be the result of a pervasive attention deficit (Jerger, Martin, & Jerger, 1987). Similarly, word recognition deficits in noise for phonemically similar words, but not for semantically similar words argues against a pervasive attention deficit as the cause of the abnormal performance (Jerger et al., 1987). Poor response consistency or reliability across trials also suggests a more global deficit, as do deficits that *resolve* with reinforcement. Finally, certain test paradigms and stimuli may be more resistant to alterations in laterality due to attention (e.g., dichotic fusion/Dichotic Rhyme Test) and particular dichotic test administration modes (e.g., directed report versus free recall) may minimize attention effects and thereby maximize the validity of observed laterality effects (Moncrieff & Musiek, 2002; Musiek et al., 2005; Shinn, Baran, Moncrieff, & Musiek, 2005).

Chermak (2003) outlined a test battery to aide the differential diagnosis of (C)APD and ADHD. In addition to the basic audiologic examination and central auditory test battery, Chermak (2003) suggested the use of analogous modality testing to examine multimodal, perceptual deficits and tests of cognitive or executive function to identify supramodal or pansensory deficits. Chermak (2003) noted that although use of analo-gous modality testing may identify sensory system deficits in other modalities, it still may be insufficient to assess fully cognitive and pansensory issues; therefore, she recommended assessment of executive function to evaluate more clearly supramodal or pansensory status versus multimodality function. Behavioral and electrophysiologic analog tests and procedures can be measured separately or simultaneously (e.g., auditory and visual (vigilance) continuous performance; event-related potentials; event-related potentials measured during auditory and visual gap detection) (Cacace & McFarland, 1998; Jerger et al., 2002; McFarland & Cacace, 1995; McPherson & Salamat, 2004). (Electrophysiologic measures may even differentiate performance of individuals with ADHD better than behavioral measures [McPherson & Salamat, 2004].) Measures of executive function assess the ability to sustain, focus, and shift attention (e.g., continuous performance tests, measures of verbal fluency, Matching Familiar Figures Test, Stroop tasks, Trail Making Test, and the Wisconsin Card Sort, among others) (Denckla, 1989).

Noting the limitations of multimodal (analog) tests that differ only in sensory stimulus, Musiek, Bellis, and Chermak (2005) encouraged the development of other approaches to examining multimodality function. Among the limitations they identified are: (1) questions of the equivalence and comparability of multimodal (analog) tests; (2) absence of data supporting the sensitivity and specificity of any multimodal analog tests to differentially identify known central auditory versus supramodal dysfunction; (3) practical and professional scope of practice issues (e.g., few professionals have the clinical education and training to assess multiple sensory modalities); and (4) many proposed multimodal tests are not currently available to clinicians engaged in diagnosing and treating (C)APD. These limitations suggest that it is more reasonable to adopt a multidisciplinary approach to differential diagnosis of (C)APD in which professionals with the relevant expertise and scope of practice (e.g., neuropsychologists, educational diagnosticians, speech-language pathologists) obtain validated measures of other modalities and of higher order cognitive, language, attention, and related function. Comprehensive multidisciplinary evaluation in combination with the sensitized test battery of the CANS will lead to accurate diagnoses that will guide treatment and management of (C)APD and ADHD. The reader is referred to other chapters in this volume for detailed discussion of (C)APD assessment procedures and protocols, as well as the analysis and interpretation of central auditory test findings.

Summary

Attention deficits, listening deficits, and poor academic achievement associated with both ADHD and (C)APD (APA, 1994; ASHA, 2005; Bellis, 2003; Chermak & Musiek, 1997) render differential diagnosis especially challenging and underscore the importance of thorough, multidisciplinary assessment with individuals suspected of these disorders. Differences in auditory areas of the brain, relative to normal controls, suggest a neuroanatomic basis for the frequently observed central auditory performance deficits among individuals diagnosed with ADHD. Listening difficulties seen in (C)APD result from auditory perceptual deficiencies rather than global attention deficits (ADHD predominantly inattention subtype) or behavioral regulation deficits

(combined ADHD and predominantly hyperactive-impulsive ADHD subtypes) (Phillips, 1990, 1995; Tallal et al., 1996). ADHD and (C)APD may differ in the extent of the attention deficit (i.e., cognitive and supramodal vs. sensory and restricted to the auditory modality), as well as the type of attention deficit (i.e., sustained vs. selective and divided attention). Within an information processing framework, the sustained attention problems observed in ADHD are seen as the consequence of a supramodal cognitive deficit whereas (C)APD results from a primarily modality-specific auditory perceptual deficit. Inattention in ADHD may reflect deficiencies in behavioral regulation rather than attention per se. In contrast, the selective auditory attention deficits of (C)APD result from deficient auditory perceptual processing.

Clinicians must use sensitive measures to evaluate the integrity of underlying perceptual and supramodal systems to determine the predominant and primary deficits, as well as secondary problems that may underlie these deficits (McFarland & Cacace, 1995). Such an approach requires the multidisciplinary efforts of audiologists, speech-language pathologists, educators, psychologists, and physicians for assessment, differential diagnosis, and for intervention.

Effective intervention for ADHD and (C)APD hinges on accurate diagnosis of these conditions and is detailed in Volume II of this Handbook.

References

Adesman, A. R., Altshuler, L., Lipkin, P., & Walco, G. (1990). Otitis media in children with learning disabilities and in children with attention deficit disorder with hyperactivity. *Pediatrics, 85*(Suppl.), 442–446.

American Academy of Pediatrics Committee on Quality Improvement, Subcommittee on Attention-Deficit/Hyperactivity Disorder. (2000). Clinical practice guideline: Diagnosis and evaluation of the child with attention-deficit/hyperactivity disorder. *Pediatrics, 105*(5),1158–1170.

American Psychiatric Association. (1994). *Diagnostic and statistical manual of mental disorders: DSM-IV* (4th ed.). Washington, DC: Author.

American Speech-Language-Hearing Association Task Force on Central Auditory Processing Consensus Development. (1996). Central auditory processing: Current status of research and implications for clinical practice. *American Journal of Audiology, 5*(2), 41–54.

American Speech-Language-Hearing Association. (2005). (Central) auditory processing disorders. Available at http://www.asha.org/members/deskref-journals/deskref/defaul

Augustine, L. E., & Damico, J. S. (1995). Attention deficit hyperactivity disorder: The scope of the problem. *Seminars in Speech and Language, 16*(4), 243–258.

Bamiou, D. E., Musiek, F. E., & Luxon, L. M. (2001). Aetiology and clinical presentation of auditory processing disorders—a review. *Archives of Disease in Childhood, 85,* 361–365.

Baran, J. A., & Musiek, F. E. (1995). Central auditory processing disorders in children and adults. In L. G. Wall (Ed.), *Hearing for the speech-language pathologist and health care professional* (pp. 415–440). Boston: Butterworth-Heinemann Medical Publishers.

Barkley, R. A. (1994). Delayed responding and response inhibition: Toward a unified theory of attention deficit hyperactivity disorder. In D. K. Routh (Ed.), *Disruptive behavior disorders in children: Essays in honor of Herbert Quay* (pp. 11–57). New York: Plenum.

Barkley, R. A. (1996). Linkages between attention and executive functions. In G. R. Lyon & N. A. Krasnegor (Eds.), *Attention, mem-* *ory, and executive function* (pp. 307–326). Baltimore: Paul H. Brookes.

Barkley, R. A. (1997a). Behavioral inhibition, sustained attention and executive functions: Constructing a unifying theory of ADHD. *Psychological Bulletin, 121*(1), 65–94.

Barkley, R. A. (1997b). *ADHD and the nature of self-control.* New York: Guilford Press.

Barkley, R. A. (1998). *Attention-deficit hyperactivity disorder: A handbook for diagnosis and treatment* (2nd ed.). New York: Guilford Press.

Baumgardner, T. L., Singer, H. S., Denckla, M. B., Rubin, M. A., Abrams, M. T., Colli, M. R., & Reiss, A. L. (1996). Corpus callosum morphology in children with Tourette syndrome and attention deficit hyperactivity disorder. *Neurology, 4,* 477–482.

Bellis, T. J. (2003). *Assessment and management of central auditory processing disorders in the educational setting: From science to practice* (2nd ed.). Clifton Park, NY: Thomson Learning.

Bellis, T. J., & Ferre, J. M. (1999). Multidimensional approach to the differential diagnosis of central auditory processing disorders in children. *Journal of the American Academy of Audiology, 10,* 319–328.

Bellis, T. J., Nicol, T., & Kraus, N. (2000). Aging affects hemispheric asymmetry in the neural representation of speech sounds. *Journal of Neuroscience, 20,* 791–797.

Bellis, T. J., & Wilber, L. A. (2001). Effects of aging and gender on interhemispheric function. *Journal of Speech, Language, and Hearing Research, 44,* 246–263.

Bishop, D. V. M., Carlyon, R. P., Deeks, J. M., & Bishop, S. J. (1999). Auditory temporal processing impairment: Neither necessary nor sufficient for causing language impairment in children. *Journal of Speech, Language, and Hearing Research, 42,* 1295–1310.

Borkowski, J., & Burke, J. (1996). Theories, models, and measurement of executive functioning: An information processing perspective. In G. R. Lyon & N. A. Krasnegor (Eds.), *Attention, memory, and exec-*

utive function (pp. 235–261). Baltimore: Paul H. Brookes.

Borkowski, J. G., Milstead, M., & Hale, C. (1988). Components of children's meta-memory: Implications for strategy generalization. In F. Weinert & M. Perlumutter (Eds.), *Memory development: Individual differences and universal changes* (pp. 73–100). Hillsdale, NJ: Lawrence Erlbaum.

Breedin, S. D., Martin, R. C., & Jerger, S. (1989). Distinguishing auditory and speech-specific perceptual deficits. *Ear and Hearing, 10*(5), 311–316.

Brown, A. L., Bransford, J., Ferrara, R. A., & Campione, J. C. (1983). Learning, remembering, and understanding. In J. Flavell & E. M. Markman (Eds.), *Carmichael's manual of child psychology.* (Vol. 1, pp. 77–166). New York: John Wiley & Sons.

Brown, D. P. (1994). Speech recognition in recurrent otitis media: Results in a set of identical twins. *Journal of the American Academy of Audiology, 5,* 1–6.

Burd, L., & Fisher, W. (1986). Central auditory processing disorder or attention deficit disorder? *Journal of Developmental and Behavioral Pediatrics, 7,* 215–216.

Butterfield, E. C., & Albertson, L. R. (1995). On making cognitive theory more general and developmentally pertinent. In F. Weinert & W. Schneider (Eds.), *Research on memory development* (pp. 73–99). Hillsdale, NJ: Lawrence Erlbaum.

Cacace, A. T., & McFarland, D. J. (1998). Central auditory processing disorder in school-aged children: A critical review. *Journal of Speech, Language, and Hearing Research, 41,* 355–373.

Campbell, T., & McNeil, M. (1985). Effects of presentation rate and divided attention on auditory comprehension in children with acquired language disorder. *Journal of Speech and Hearing Research, 28,* 513–520.

Castellanos, F. X. (1997). Towards a pathophysiology of attention-deficit/hyperactivity disorder. *Clinical Pediatrics, 36,* 381–393.

Castellanos, F. X., Giedd, J. N., Marsh, W. L., Hamburger, S. D., Vaituzis, A. C., Dickstein,

D. P., Sarfatti, S. E., Vauss, Y. C., Snell, J. W., Lange, N., Kaysen, D., Krain, A. L., Ritchie, G. F., Rajapakse, J. C., & Rapoport, J. L. (1996). Quantitative brain magnetic resonance imaging in attention-deficit hyperactivity disorder. *Archives of General Psychiatry, 53,* 607–616.

Chermak, G. D. (2003). It takes a team to differentially diagnose APD. *The Hearing Journal, 56*(4), 32.

Chermak, G. D. (2004). Neurobiological connections are key to APD. *The Hearing Journal, 57*(4), 58.

Chermak, G. D., Hall, J. W., & Musiek, F. E. (1999). Differential diagnosis and management of central auditory processing disorder and attention deficit hyperactivity disorder. *Journal of the American Academy of Audiology, 10,* 289–303.

Chermak, G. D., & Musiek, F. E. (1997). *Central auditory processing disorders: New perspectives.* San Diego, CA: Singular Publishing Group, Inc.

Chermak, G. D., Somers, E. K., & Seikel, J. A. (1998). Behavioral signs of central auditory processing disorder and attention deficit hyperactivity disorder. *Journal of the American Academy of Audiology, 9,* 78–84.

Chermak, G. D., Tucker, E., & Seikel, J. A. (2002). Behavioral characteristics of auditory processing disorder and attention deficit hyperactivity disorder: predominantly inattentive type. *Journal of the American Academy of Audiology, 13,* 332–338.

Chermak, G. D., Vonhof, M., & Bendel, R. B. (1989). Word identification performance in the presence of competing speech and noise in learning disabled adults. *Ear and Hearing, 10,* 90–93.

Cherry, R. S. (1980). *Selective Auditory Attention Test.* St. Louis, MO: Auditec.

Chmiel, R., & Jerger, J. (1996). Hearing aid use, central auditory disorder, and hearing handicap in elderly persons. *Journal of the American Academy of Audiology, 7,* 190–202.

Chmiel, R., Jerger, J., Murphy, E., Pirozzolo, G., & Tooley-Young, C. (1997). Unsuccessful use of binaural amplification by an elderly person. *Journal of the American Academy of Audiology, 8*, 1-10.

Committee on Hearing, Bioacoustics, and Biomechanics (CHABA) Working Group on Speech Understanding and Aging. (1988). Speech understanding and aging. *Journal of the Acoustical Society of America, 83*, 859-893.

Cook, J. R., Mausbach, T., Burd, L., Gascon, G. G., Slotnick, H. B., Patterson, B., Johnson, R. D., Hankey, B., & Reynolds, B.W. (1993). A preliminary study of the relationship between central auditory processing disorder and attention deficit disorder. *Journal of Psychiatry and Neuroscience, 18*(3), 130-137.

Cooper, J. C., Jr., & Gates, G. A. (1991). Hearing in the elderly—The Framingham Cohort, 1983-1985: Part II. Prevalence of central auditory processing disorders. *Ear and Hearing, 12*, 304-311.

Cunningham, J., Nicol, T., Zecker, S. G., Bradlow, A., & Kraus, N. (2001). Neurobiologic responses to speech in noise in children with learning problems: Deficits and strategies for improvement. *Clinical Neurophysiology, 112*, 758-767.

DeMarco, S., Harbour, A., Hume, W., & Givens, G. (1989). Perception of time-altered monosyllables in a specific group of phonologically disordered children. *Neuropsychologia, 27*, 753-757.

Denckla, M. B. (1989). Executive function, the overlap zone between attention deficit hyperactivity disorder and learning disabilities. *International Pediatrics, 4*, 155-160.

Denckla, M. B. (1996). A theory and model of executive function: A neuropsychological perspective. In G. R. Lyon & N. A. Krasnegor (Eds.), *Attention, memory, and executive function* (pp. 263-278). Baltimore: Paul H. Brookes.

Denckla, M. B., & Reader, M. (1993). Education and psychosocial interventions: Executive dysfunction and its consequences. In R. Kurlan (Ed.), *Handbook of Tourette's syndrome and related tic and behavioral disorders* (pp. 431-451). New York: Marcel Dekker.

Elliott, L. L., & Hammer, M. (1988). Longitudinal changes in auditory discrimination in normal children and children with language-learning problems. *Journal of Speech and Hearing Disorders, 53*, 467-474.

Eslinger, P. K., & Grattan, L. M. (1993). Frontal lobe and frontal-striatal substrates for different forms of human cognitive flexibility. *Neuropsychologica, 31*, 17-28.

Farah, M. J., & Wallace, M. A. (1991). Pure alexia as a visual impairment: A reconsideration. *Cognitive Neuropsychology, 8*(3/4), 313-334.

Feagans, L. V., Sanyal, M., Henderson, F., Collier, A., & Applebaum, M. (1987). Relationship of middle ear disease in early childhood to later narrative and attentional skills. *Journal of Pediatric Psychology, 12*, 581-594.

Ferguson, M. O., Cook, R. D., Hall, J. W., Grose, J. H., & Pillsbury, H. C. (1998). Chronic conductive hearing loss in adults. *Archives of Otolaryngology-Head and Neck Surgery, 124*, 678-685.

Ferre, J. M., & Wilber, L. A. (1986). Normal and learning disabled children's central auditory processing skills: An experimental test battery. *Ear and Hearing, 7*, 336-343.

Fletcher, J. M., Taylor, H. G., Levin, H. S., & Satz, P. (1995). Neuropsychological and intellectual assessment of children. In H. I. Kaplan & B. J. Sadock (Eds.), *Comprehensive textbook of psychiatry* (Vol. I, pp. 581-601). Baltimore: Williams & Wilkins.

Galaburda, A. M., & Eidelberg, D. (1982). Symmetry and asymmetry in the human posterior thalamus: II. Thalamic lesions in a case of developmental dyslexia. *Archives of Neurology, 39*, 333-336.

Galaburda, A. M., & Kemper, T. (1978). Cytoarchitectonic abnormalities in developmental dyslexia: A case study. *Annals of Neurology, 6*, 94-101.

Galaburda, A. M., Sherman, G. F., Rosen, G. D., Aboitiz, F., & Geschwind, N. (1985). Developmental dyslexia: Four consecutive patients with cortical anomalies. *Annuals of Neurology, 18*(2), 222-233.

Gallagher, M., & Schoenbaum, G. (1999). Function of the amygdala and related forebrain areas in attention and cognition. *Annals of the New York Academy of Sciences, 877*, 397-411.

Gascon, G. G., Johnson, R., & Burd, L. (1986). Central auditory processing in attention deficit disorders. *Journal of Child Neurology, 1*, 27-33.

Giedd, J., Castellanos, F. X., Casey, B., Kozuch, P., King, A.C., Hamburger, S., & Rapoport, J. (1994). Quantitative morphology of the corpus callosum in attention deficit hyperactivity disorder. *American Journal of Psychiatry, 151*(5), 665-669.

Goldenberg, G., Oder, W., Spatt, J., & Podreka, I. (1992). Cerebral correlates of disturbed executive function and memory in survivors of severe closed head injury: A SPECT study. *Journal of Neurology, Neurosurgery and Psychiatry, 55*, 362-368.

Goodyear, P., & Hynd, G.W. (1992). Attention-deficit disorder with (ADD/H) and without (ADD/WO) hyperactivity: Behavioral and neuropsychological differentiation. *Journal of Clinical Child Psychology, 21*, 273-305.

Graham, S., & Harris, K. R. (1996). Addressing problems in attention, memory, and executive functioning: An example from self-regulated strategy development. In G. R. Lyon & N. A. Krasnegor (Eds.), *Attention, memory, and executive function* (pp. 349-365). Baltimore: Paul Brookes.

Grattan, L. M., Bloomer, R., Archambault, F. X., & Eslinger, P. J. (1994). Cognitive flexibility and empathy after frontal lobe lesion. *Neuropsychiatry, Neurophyschology and Behavioral Neurology, 7*, 251-259.

Grattan, L. M., & Eslinger, P. J. (1992). Long-term psychological consequences of childhood frontal lobe lesion in patient DT. *Brain and Cognition, 20*, 185-195.

Gravel, J. S., & Wallace, I. F. (1992). Listening and language at four years of age: Effects of early otitis media. *Journal of Speech and Hearing Research, 35*, 588-595.

Gulya, J. (1991). Structural and physiological changes of the auditory and vestibular mechanisms with aging. In D. Ripich (Ed.), *Handbook of geriatric communication disorders* (pp. 39-54). Austin, TX: Pro-Ed.

Haenlein, M., & Caul, W. F. (1987). Attention deficit disorder with hyperactivity: A specific hypothesis of reward dysfunction. *Journal of the American Academy of Child and Adolescent Psychiatry, 26*, 356-362.

Hall, J. W., & Grose, J. H. (1993). The effect of otitis media with effusion on the masking level difference and the auditory brainstem response. *Journal of Speech and Hearing Research, 36*, 210-217.

Hall, J. W., & Grose, J. H. (1994). The effect of otitis media with effusion on comodulation masking release in children. *Journal of Speech and Hearing Research, 37*, 1441-1449.

Hall, J. W., Grose, J. H., & Pillsbury, H. C. (1994). Long-term effects of chronic otitis media on binaural hearing in children. *Archives of Otolaryngology—Head and Neck Surgery, 37*, 1441-1449.

Hall, J. W., Grose, J. H., & Pillsbury, H.C. (1995). Long-term effects of chronic otitis media on binaural hearing in children. *Archives of Otolaryngology—Head and Neck Surgery, 121*, 847-852.

Harrison, R. V., Smith, D. W., Hagasawa, A., Stanton, S., & Mount, R. J. (1992). Developmental plasticity of auditory cortex in cochlear hearing loss: Physiological and psychophysical findings. *Advances in the Biosciences, 83*, 625-633.

Hassamannova, J., Myslivecek, J., & Novakova, V. (1981). Effects of early auditory stimulation on cortical areas. In J. Syka & L. Aitkin (Eds.), *Neuronal mechanisms of hearing* (pp. 355-359). New York: Plenum Press.

Hayes, S. C., Gifford, E. V., & Ruckstuhl, L. E. (1996). Relational frame theory and executive function: A behavioral approach. In G. R. Lyon & N. A. Krasnegor (Eds.), *Attention, memory, and executive function* (pp. 279-326). Baltimore: Paul H. Brookes.

Heilman, K. M., Voeller, K. K. S., & Nadeau, S. E. (1991). A possible pathophysiological substrate of attention deficit hyperactivity disorder. *Journal of Child Neurology, 6*, 74–79.

Hendler, T., Squires, N., & Emmerich, D. (1990). Psychophysical measures of central auditory dysfunction in multiple sclerosis: Neurophysiological and neuroanatomical correlates. *Ear and Hearing, 11*(6), 403–416.

Heyer, J. (1995). The responsibilities of speech-language pathologists toward children with ADHD. *Seminars in Speech and Language, 16*(4), 275–288.

Hooks, K., Milich, R., & Lorch, E. P. (1994). Sustained and selective attention in boys with attention deficit hyperactivity disorder. *Journal of Clinical Child Psychology, 23*, 69–77.

Hutchings, M. E., Meyer, S. E., & Moore, D. R. (1992). Binaural masking level differences in infants with and without otitis media with effusion. *Hearing Research, 63*, 71–78.

Hynd, G. W., Lorys, A. R., Semrud-Clikeman, M., Nieves, N., Huettner, M. I. S., & Lahey, B. B. (1991). Attention deficit disorder without hyperactivity: A distinct behavioral and neurocognitive syndrome. *Journal of Child Neurology, 6*, S37–S43.

Hynd, G. W., & Semrud-Clikeman, M. (1989). Dyslexia and neurodevelopmental pathology: Relationships to cognition, intelligence, and reading acquisition. *Journal of Learning Disabilities, 22*, 204–216.

Hynd, G. W., Semrud-Clikeman, M., Lorys, A. R., Novey, E. S., & Eliopulos, D. (1990). Brain morphology in developmental dyslexia and attention deficit disorder/hyperactivity. *Archives of Neurology, 47*, 916–919.

Hynd, G. W., Semrud-Clikeman, M., Lorys, A. R., Novey, E. S., Eliopulos, D., & Lyytinen, H. (1991). Corpus callosum morphology in attention deficit-hyperactivity disorder: Morphometric analysis of MRI. *Journal of Learning Disabilities, 24*, 141–146.

Irvine, D. R. F., Rajan, R., & Robertson, D. (1992). Plasticity in auditory cortex of adult mammals with restricted cochlear lesions. In R. Naresh Singh (Ed.), *Nervous systems: Principles of design and function* (pp. 319–350). New Delhi: Wiley-Eastern Ltd.

Jerger, J. (1992). Can age-related decline in speech understanding be explained by peripheral hearing loss? *Journal of the American Academy of Audiology, 3*, 33–38.

Jerger, J., Moncrieff, D., Greenwald, R., Wambacq, I., & Seipel, A. (2000). Effect of age on interaural asymmetry of event-related potentials in a dichotic listening task. *Journal of the American Academy of Audiology, 11*, 383–389.

Jerger, J., & Musiek, F. (2000). Report of the Consensus Conference on the Diagnosis of Auditory Processing Disorders in School-Aged Children. *Journal of the American Academy of Audiology, 11*, 467–474.

Jerger, J., Thibodeau, L., Martin, J., Mehta, J., Tillman, G., Greenwald, R., Britt, L., Scott, J., & Overson, G. (2002). Behavioral and electrophysiologic evidence of auditory processing disorder: A twin study. *Journal of the American Academy of Audiology, 13*, 438–460.

Jerger, S., & Jerger, J. (1984). *Pediatric Speech Intelligibility Test: Manual for administration*. St. Louis, MO: Auditech.

Jerger, S., Jerger, J., Alford, B. R., & Abrams, S. (1983). Development of speech intelligibility in children with recurrent otitis media. *Ear and Hearing, 4*, 138–145.

Jerger, S., Martin, R. C., & Jerger, J. (1987). Specific auditory perceptual dysfunction in a learning disabled child. *Ear and Hearing, 8*(2), 78–86.

Jirsa, R. E., & Clontz, K. B. (1990). Long latency auditory event-related potentials from children with auditory processing disorders. *Ear and Hearing, 11*, 222–232.

Jonkman, L. M., Kemner, C., Verbaten, M. N., Koelega, H. A., Camfferman, G., van der Gaag, R. J., Buitelaar, J. K., & van Engeland, H. (1997). Event-related potentials and performance of Attention-Deficit Hyperactivity Disorder: Children and normal controls in auditory and visual selective attention tasks. *Biological Psychiatry, 41*, 595-611.

Katz, J. (1992). Classification of auditory processing disorders. In J. Katz, N. A. Stecker, & D. Henderson (Eds.), *Central auditory processing: A transdisciplinary view* (pp. 81-92). St. Louis, MO: Mosby Year Book.

Katz, J., & Illmer, R. (1972). Auditory perception in children with learning disabilities. In J. Katz (Ed.), *Handbook of clinical audiology* (pp. 540-563). Baltimore: Williams & Wilkins.

Keith, R. W. (1981). Audiological and auditory-language tests of central auditory function. In R. W. Keith (Ed.), *Central auditory and language disorders in children* (pp. 61-76). Houston, TX: College-Hill Press.

Keith, R. W. (1986). *SCAN: A screening test for auditory processing disorders.* San Antonio, TX: Psychological Corporation.

Keith, R. W., & Engineer, P. (1991). Effects of methylphenidate on the auditory processing abilities of children with attention deficit-hyperactivity disorder. *Journal of Learning Disabilities, 24*, 630-636.

Keller, W. D. (1992). Auditory processing disorder or attention-deficit disorder? In J. Katz, N. A. Stecker, & D. Henderson (Eds.), *Central auditory processing: A transdisciplinary view* (pp. 107-114). St. Louis, MO: Mosby Year Book.

Keller, W. D., & Tillery, K. L. (2002). Reliable differential diagnosis and effective management of auditory processing and attention deficit hyperactivity disorders. *Seminars in Hearing, 23*(4), 337-348.

Kilgard, M. P., Pandya, P. K., Vasques, J., Gehi, A., Schreiner, C. S., & Merzenich, M. M. (2001). Sensory input directs spatial and temporal plasticity in primary auditory cortex. *Journal of Neurophysiology, 86*(1), 326-338.

King, C., Warrier, C. M., Hayes, E., & Kraus, N. (2002). Deficits in auditory brainstem encoding of speech sounds in children with learning problems. *Neuroscience Letters, 319*, 111-115.

Klorman, R. (1991). Cognitive event-related potentials in attention deficit hyperactivity disorder. *Journal of Learning Disabilities, 24*, 130-140.

Knox, C., & Roeser, R. (1980). Cerebral dominance in auditory perceptual asymmetries in normal and dyslexic children. *Seminars in Speech, Language, and Hearing, 1*, 181-194.

Koch, M., (1999). The neurobiology of startle. *Progress in Neurobiology, 59*, 107-128.

Kraus, N. (2001). Auditory pathway encoding and neural plasticity in children with learning problems. *Audiology and Neuro-otology, 6*, 221-227.

Kraus, N., McGee, T. J., Carrell, T. D., Zecker, S. D., Nicol, T. G., & Koch, D. B. (1996). Auditory neurophysiologic responses and discrimination deficits in children with learning problems. *Science, 273*, 971-973.

Krishnamurti, S. (2001). P300 auditory event-related potential in binaural and competing noise conditions in adults with central auditory processing disorders. *Contemporary Issues in Communication Science and Disorders, 28*, 40-47.

Lahat, E., Avital, E., Barr, J., Berkovitch, M., Arlazoraff, A., & Aladjem, M. (1995). BAEP studies in children with attention deficit disorder. *Developmental Medicine and Child Neurology, 37*, 199-123.

Lasky, E. Z., & Tobin, H. (1973). Linguistic and nonlinguistic competing message effects. *Journal of Learning Disabilities, 6*, 243-250.

Lou, H. C., Henriksen, L., Bruhn, P., Borner, H., & Nielsen, J. B. (1989). Striatal dysfunction in attention deficit and hyperkinetic disorder. *Archives of Neurology, 46*, 48-52.

Lubert, N. (1981). Auditory perceptual impairment in children with specific language disorders. *Journal of Speech and Hearing Disorders, 46*, 3-9.

Mann, C. A., Lubar, J. F., Zimmerman, A. W., Miller, C. A., & Muenchen, R. A. (1992). Quantitiative analysis of EEG in boys with attention-deficit-hyperactivity disorder:

Controlled study with clinical implications. *Pediatric Neurology, 8*, 30-36.

Marler, J. A., Champlin, C. A., & Gillam, R. B. (2002). Auditory memory for backward masking signals in children with language impairment. *Psychophysiology, 39* (6), 767-780.

Martinkauppi, S., Rama, P., Aronen, H. J., Korvenoja, A., & Carolson, S. (2002). Working memory of auditory localization. *Cerebral Cortex, 10*, 889-898.

McFarland, D. J., & Cacace, A. T. (1995). Modality specificity as a criterion for diagnosing central auditory processing disorders. *American Journal of Audiology, 4*(3), 36-48.

McPherson, D. L., & Salamat, M. T. (2004). Interactions among variables in the P300 response to a continuous performance task in normal and ADHD adults. *Journal of the American Academy of Audiology, 15*, 666-677.

Merzenich, M., Schreiner, C., Jenkins, W., & Wang, X. (1993). Neural mechanisms underlying temporal integration, segmentation, and input sequence representations: Some implications for the origin of learning disabilities. *Annals of the New York Academy of Sciences, 682*, 1-22.

Merzenich, M., Wright, B., Jenkins, W., Xerri, C., Byl, N., Miller, S., & Tallal, P. (1996). Cortical plasticity underlying perceptual, motor, and cognitive skill development: Implications for neurorehabilitation. *Cold Spring Harbor Symposia on Quantitative Biology, 61*, 1-8. Cold Spring Harbor, NY: Cold Spring Harbor Laboratory Press.

Miller, C. A., Kail, R., Leonard, L. B., & Tomblin, J. B. (2001). Speed of processing in children with specific language impairment. *Journal of Speech, Language, and Hearing Research, 44*, 416-433.

Millstein, R. B., Wilens, T. E., Biederman, J., & Spencer, T. J. (1997). Presenting ADHD symptoms and subtypes in clinically referred adults with ADHD. *Journal of Attention Disorders, 2*(3), 159-166.

Mogdans, J., & Knudsen, E. I. (1992). Adaptive adjustment of unit tuning to sound localization cues in response to monaural occlusion in developing owl optic tectum. *Journal of Neuroscience, 12*(9), 3473-3484.

Mogdans, J., & Knudsen, E. I. (1993). Early monaural occlusion alters the neural map of interaural level differences in the inferior colliculus of the barn owl. *Brain Research, 619*, 29-38.

Mogdans, J., & Knudsen, E. I. (1994). Site of auditory plasticity in the brain stem (VLVp) of the owl revealed by early monaural occlusion. *Journal of Neurophysiology, 72*(6), 2875-2891.

Moncrieff, D., Jerger, J., Wambacq, I., Greenwald, R., & Black, J. (2004). ERP evidence of a dichotic left-ear deficit in some dyslexic children. *Journal of the American Academy of Audiology, 15*, 518-534.

Moncrieff, D. & Musiek, F. (2002). Interaural asymmetries revealed by dichotic listening tests in normal and dyslexic children. *Journal of the American Academy of Audiology, 13*, 428-437.

Moore, D. R. (1993). Plasticity of binaural hearing and some possible mechanisms following late-onset deprivation. *Journal of the American Academy of Audiology, 4*(5), 227-283.

Moore, D. R., Hutchings, M. E., & Meyer, S. E. (1991). Binaural masking level differences in children with a history of otitis media. *Audiology, 30*, 91-101.

Musiek, F. E., Baran, J. A., & Pinheiro, M. L. (1992). P300 results in patients with lesions of the auditory areas of the cerebrum. *Journal of the American Academy of Audiology, 3*, 5-15.

Musiek, F. E., Baran, J. A., & Pinheiro, M. L. (1994). *Neuroaudiology: Case studies*. San Diego, CA: Singular Publishing Group.

Musiek, F. E., Bellis, T. J., & Chermak, G. D. (2005). Nonmodularity of the CANS: Implications for (central) auditory processing disorder. *American Journal of Audiology, 14*, 128-138.

Musiek, F., Charette, L., Kelly, T., Lee, W. & Musiek, E. (1999). Hit and false-positive rates for the middle latency response in patients with central nervous system involvement. *Journal of the American Academy of Audiology, 10*(3), 124–132.

Musiek, F. E., & Chermak, G. D. (1995). Three commonly asked questions about central auditory processing disorders: Management. *American Journal of Audiology, 4*(1), 15–18.

Musiek, F. E., Gollegly, K. M., & Baran, J. A. (1984). Myelination of the corpus callosum and auditory processing problems in children: Theoretical and clinical correlates. *Seminars in Hearing, 5,* 231–241.

Musiek, F. E., Gollegly, K., Lamb, L., & Lamb, P. (1990). Selected issues in screening for central auditory processing dysfunction. *Seminars in Hearing, 11,* 372–384.

Musiek, F. L., & Lee, W. W. (1995). The auditory brain stem response in patients with brain stem or cochlear pathology. *Ear and Hearing, 16,* 631–636.

Musiek, F. E., Pinheiro, M. L., & Wilson, D. (1980). Auditory pattern perception in split-brain patients. *Archives of Otolaryngology —Head and Neck Surgery, 106,* 610–612.

Musiek, F. E., Shinn, J., Jirsa, R., Bamiou, D., Baran, J., & Zaidan, E. (2005). The GIN (Gaps In Noise) test performance in subjects with and without confirmed central auditory nervous system involvement. *Ear and Hearing, 26,* 608–618.

Newhoff, M., Cohen, M. J., Hynd, G. W., Gonzalez, J. J., & Riccio, C. A. (1992). *Etiological, educational and behavioral correlates of ADHD and language disabilities.* Presented at the annual convention of the American Speech-Language-Hearing Association, San Antonio, TX.

Nittrouer, S. (1999). Do temporal processing deficits cause phonological processing problems? *Journal of Speech, Language, and Hearing Research, 42,* 925–942.

Paus, T. (2000). Functional anatomy of arousal and attention systems in the human brain. In H. B. M. Uylings, et al. (Eds.), *Progress in brain research: Cognition, emotion, and autonomic responses: The integrative role of the pre-frontal cortex and limbic structures* (Vol. 126, pp. 65–77). Amsterdam: Elseiver.

Pennington, B. F. (1991). *Diagnosing learning disorders: A neuropsychological framework.* New York: Guilford.

Pennington, B. F., Bennetto, L., McAleer, O., & Roberts, R. J. (1996). Executive functions and working memory: Theoretical and measurement issues. In G. R. Lyon & N. A. Krasnegor (Eds.), *Attention, memory, and executive function* (pp. 327–348). Baltimore: Paul H. Brookes.

Phillips, D. (1990). Neural representation of sound amplitude in the auditory cortex: Effects of noise masking. *Behavioral Brain Research, 37,* 197–214.

Phillips, D. P. (1995). Central auditory processing: A view from auditory neuroscience. *The American Journal of Otology, 16*(3), 338–352.

Pichora-Fuller, M., & Souza, P. (2003). Effects of aging on auditory processing of speech. *International Journal of Audiology, 42*(2), 2S11–2S16.

Pillsbury, H. C., Grose, J. H., Coleman, W. L., Conners, C. K., & Hall, J. W. (1995). Binaural function in children with attention-deficit hyperactivity disorder. *Archives of Otolaryngology—Head and Neck Surgery, 121,* 1345–1350.

Pillsbury, H. C., Grose, J. H., & Hall, J. W. (1991). Otitis media with effusion in children: Binaural hearing before and after corrective surgery. *Archives of Otolaryngology—Head and Neck Surgery, 117,* 718–723.

Poremba, A., Saunders, R. C., Crane, A. M., Cook, M., Sokoloff, L., & Mishkin, M. (2003). Functional mapping of the primate auditory system. *Science, 299,* 568–571.

Purdy, S., Kelly, A., & Davies, M. (2002). Auditory brainstem response, middle latency response, and late cortical evoked potentials in children with learning disabilities. *Journal of the American Academy of Audiology, 13,* 367–382.

Rajan, R., & Irvine, D. R. (1998). Neuronal responses across cortical field A1 in plasticity induced by peripheral auditory organ damage. *Audiology and Neurootology, 3*(2-3), 123–144.

Rajan, R., Irvine, D. R. F., Wise, L. Z., & Heil, P. (1993). Effect of unilateral partial cochlear lesions in adult cats on the representation of lesioned and unlesioned cochleas in primary auditory cortex. *Journal of Comparative Neurology, 338,* 17-49.

Rappaport, J., Gulliver, M., Phillips, D., Van Dorpe, R., Maxner, C., & Bhan, V. (1994). Auditory temporal resolution in multiple sclerosis. *The Journal of Otolaryngology, 23*(5), 307-324.

Recanzone, G. H., Schreiner, C. E., & Merzenich, M. M. (1993). Plasticity in the frequency representation of primary auditory cortex following discrimination training in adult owl monkeys. *Journal of Neuroscience, 13,* 87-103.

Rey, V., De Martino, S., Espesser, R., & Habib, M. (2002). Temporal processing and phonological impairment in dyslexia: Effect of phoneme lengthening on order judgment of two consonants. *Brain and Language, 80,* 576-591.

Riccio, C. A., Cohen, M. J., Garrison, T., & Smith, B. (2005). Auditory processing measures: Correlation with neuropsychological measures of attention, memory, and behavior. *Child Neuropsychology, 11,* 363-372.

Riccio, C. A., Hynd, G. W., Cohen, M. J., & Gonzalez, J. J. (1993). Neurological basis of attention deficit hyperactivity disorder. *Exceptional Children, 60*(2), 118-124.

Riccio, C. A., Hynd, G. W., Cohen, M. J., & Molt, L. (1996). The Staggered Spondaic Word Test: Performance of children with attention-deficit hyperactivity disorder. *American Journal of Audiology, 5*(2), 55-62.

Riccio, C. A., Reynolds, C. R., & Lowe, P. A. (2001). *Clinical applications of continuous performance tests.* New York: John Wiley & Sons.

Roberts, J. E., Burchinal, M. R., Collier, A. M., Ramey, C. T., Koch, M. A., & Henderson, F. W. (1989). Otitis media in early childhood, and cognitive, academic, and classroom performance of the school-aged child. *Pediatrics, 83,* 477-485.

Robertson, D., & Irvine, D. R. F. (1989). Plasticity of frequency organization in auditory cortex of guinea pigs with partial unilateral deafness. *Journal of Comparative Neurology, 282,* 456-471.

Robin, D. A., Tomblin, J. B., Kearney, A., & Hugg, L. N. (1989). Auditory temporal pattern learning in children with speech and language impairments. *Brain and Language, 36*(4), 604-613.

Salamat, M. T., & McPherson, D. L. (1999). Interactions among variables in the P_{300} response to a continuous performance task. *Journal of the American Academy of Audiology, 10,* 379-387.

Salvi, R. J., Lockwood, A. H., Frisina, R. D., Coad, M. L., Wack, D. S., & Frisina, D. R. (2002). PET imaging of the normal human auditory system: Responses to speech in quiet and in background noise. *Hearing Research, 170,* 96-106.

Scahill. L., & Schwab-Stone, M. (2000). Epidemiology of ADHD in school-aged children. *Child and Adolescent Psychiatric Clinics of North America, 9*(3), 541-555.

Schwaber, M. K., Garraghty, P. E., & Kaas, J. H. (1993). Neuroplasticity of the adult primate auditory cortex following cochlear hearing loss. *American Journal of Otolaryngology, 14,* 252-258.

Seidel, W. T., & Joschko, M. (1990). Evidence of difficulties in sustained attention in children with ADDH. *Journal of Abnormal Child Psychology, 18,* 217-229.

Semrud-Clikeman, M., Filipek, P., Biederman, J., Steingard, R., Kennedy, D., Renshaw, P., & Bekken, K. (1994). Attention-deficit hyperactivity disorder: Magnetic resonance imaging morphometric analysis of the corpus callosum. *Journal of the American Academy of Child and Adolescent Psychiatry, 33*(6), 875-881.

Shinn, J., Baran, J., Moncrieff, D., & Musiek, F. (2005). Differential attention effects on dichotic listening. *Journal of the American Academy of Audiology, 16,* 205-218.

Silva, P. A., Chalmers, D., & Stewart, I. (1986). Some audiological, psychological, educational and behavioral characteristics of children with bilateral otitis media with effusion: A longitudinal study. *Journal of Learning Disabilities, 19*, 165-169.

Silva, P. A., Kirkland, C., Simpson, A., Stewart, I. A., & Williams, S.M. (1982). Some developmental and behavioral problems associated with bilateral otitis media with effusion. *Journal of Learning Disabilities, 15*, 417-421.

Sloan, C. (1980). Auditory processing disorders and language development. In P. J. Levinson & C. Sloan (Eds.), *Auditory processing and language: Clinical and research perspectives* (pp. 101-116). New York: Grune & Stratton.

Smith, M. D., Gould, D., Marsh, L., & Nichols, A. (1995). The metaphysics of ADHD: A unifying case scenario. *Seminars in Speech and Language, 16*(4), 303-313.

Sowell, E., Thompson, P., Welcome, S., Henkenius, A., Toga, A., & Peterson, B. (2003). Cortical abnormalities in children and adolescents with attention-deficit hyperactivity disorder. *The Lancet, 362*, 1699-1707.

St. James-Roberts, I. (1979). Neurological plasticity, recovery from brain insult, and child development. *Advances in Child Development and Behavior, 14*, 253-319.

Stach, B. A., Spretnjak, M. L., & Jerger, J. (1990). The prevalence of central presbycusis in a clinical population. *Journal of the American Academy of Audiology, 1*(2), 109-115.

Stanovich, K. E. (1986). Cognitive process and the reading problems of learning disabled children: Evaluating the assumption of specificity. In J. K. Torgesen & B. L. Wong (Eds.), *Psychological and educational perspectives on reading disabilities* (pp. 87-131). New York: Academic Press.

Stein, M. A. (2001). ADHD in primary care: Overdiagnosed, under-treated, and frequently misunderstood. In B. Rogers, T. Montgomery, T. Lock, & P. Accardo (Eds.), *Attention deficit hyperactivity disorder: The clinical spectrum* (pp. 51-71). Baltimore: York Press.

Sternberg, R. (1985). *Beyond I.Q.: A triarchic theory of intelligence.* New York: Cambridge University Press.

Streitfeld, B. (1980). The fiber connections of the temporal lobe with emphasis on Rhesus monkey. *International Journal of Neuroscience, 11*, 51-71.

Studdert-Kennedy, M., & Mody, M. (1995). Auditory temporal perception deficits in the reading-impaired: A critical review of the evidence. *Psychonomic Bulletin and Review, 2*, 508-514.

Tallal, P. (1980a). Auditory processing disorders in children. In P. J. Levinson & C. Sloan (Eds.), *Auditory processing and language: clinical and research perspectives* (pp. 81-100). New York: Grune & Stratton.

Tallal, P. (1980b). Auditory temporal perception, phonics and reading disabilities in children. *Brain and Language, 9*, 1982-1988.

Tallal, P., Miller, S., Bedi, G., Byma, G. Wang, X., Nagarajan, S. S., Schreiner, C., Jenkins, W. M., & Merzenich, M. H. (1996). Language comprehension in language-learning impaired children improved with acoustically modified speech. *Science, 271*, 81-84.

Tallal, P., & Piercy, M. (1973). Defects of nonverbal auditory perception in children with developmental aphasia. *Nature, 241*, 468-469.

Tallal, P., Stark, R. E., & Mellits, D. (1985). Identification of language-impaired children on the basis of rapid perception and production skills. *Brain and Language, 25*, 314-322.

Tannock, R. (1998). Attention deficit hyperactivity disorder: Advances in cognitive, neurobiological, and genetic research. *Journal of Child Psychology and Psychiatry, 39*, 65-99.

Tannock, R., & Schachar, R. (1996). Executive dysfunction as an underlying mechanism of behavior and language problems in attention deficit hyperactivity disorder. In J. H. Beitchman, N. Cohen, M. M. Konstantareas, & R. Tannock (Eds.), *Language, learning, and behavior disorders: Developmental, biological, and clinical perspectives* (pp. 128-155). New York: Cambridge University Press.

Thatcher, R. (1991). Maturation of the human frontal lobes: Physiological evidence for staging. *Developmental Neuropsychology*, 7, 397-419.

Torgesen, J. K. (1994). Issues in the assessment of executive function: An information-processing perspective. In G. R. Lyon (Ed.), *Frames of reference for the assessment of learning disabilities* (pp. 143-162). Baltimore: Paul H. Brookes.

Torgesen, J. K. (1996). A model of memory from an information processing perspective: The special case of phonological memory. In G. R. Lyon & N. A. Krasnegor (Eds.), *Attention, memory, and executive function* (pp. 157-184). Baltimore: Paul H. Brookes.

Tremblay, K., Piskosz, M., & Souza, P. (2003). Effects of age and age-related hearing loss on the neural representation of speech cues. *Clinical Neurophysiology*, *114*, 1332-1343.

Voeller, K. K. (1991). Toward a neurobiologic nosology of attention deficit hyperactivity disorder. *Journal of Clinical Neurology*, *6*(Suppl.), S2-S8.

Warrier, C. M., Johnson, K. L., Hayes, E. A., Nicol, T., & Kraus, N. (2004). Learning impaired children exhibit timing deficits and training-related improvements in auditory cortical responses to speech in noise. *Experimental Brain Research*, *157*, 431-441.

Westby, C. E., & Cutler, S. K. (1994). Language and ADHD: Understanding the bases and treatment of self-regulatory deficits. *Topics in Language Disorders*, *14*(4), 58-76.

Wible, B., Nicol, T. G., & Kraus, N. (2002). Abnormal neural encoding of repeated speech stimuli in noise in children with learning problems. *Clinical Neurophysiology*, *113*, 485-494.

Wilens, T. E., Biederman, J., & Spencer, T. J. (2002). Attention deficit/hyperactivity disorder across the lifespan. *Annual Review of Medicine*, *53*, 113-131.

Willott, J. F. (1999). *Neurogerontology: Aging and the nervous system.* New York: Springer.

Willott, J. F., Aitkin, L. M., & McFadden, S. L. (1993). Plasticity of auditory cortex associated with sensorineural hearing loss in adult C57BL/6J mice. *Journal of Comparative Neurology*, *329*, 402-411.

Woods, D. L., & Clayworth, C. C. (1986). Age-related changes in human middle latency auditory evoked potentials. *Electroencephalography and Clinical Neurophysiology*, *65*, 297-303.

Yakelov, P. I., & Lecours, A. R. (1967). Myelogenetic cycles of regional maturation of the brain. In A. Minkiniwski (Ed.), *Regional development of the brain in early life* (pp. 3-70). Oxford: Blackwell Press.

Zametkin, A. J., Nordahl, T. E., Gross, J., King, C. A., Semple, W. E., Rumsey, J., Hamberger, M. A., & Cohen, R. M. (1990). Cerebral glucose metabolism in adults with hyperactivity of childhood onset. *New England Journal of Medicine*, *323*, 1361-1366.

Zatorre, R. J. (2001). Neural specialization for tonal processing. *Annals of the New York Academy of Sciences*, *930*, 193-210.

Zentall, S. S. (1985). A context for hyperactivity. In K. D. Gadow & I. Bailer (Eds.), *Advances in learning and behavioral disabilities* (Vol. 4, pp. 273-343). Greenwich, CT: JAI Press.

SECTION IV

Multidisciplinary Perspectives

CHAPTER 16

COGNITIVE-COMMUNICATIVE AND LANGUAGE FACTORS ASSOCIATED WITH (CENTRAL) AUDITORY PROCESSING DISORDER: A SPEECH-LANGUAGE PATHOLOGY PERSPECTIVE

GAIL J. RICHARD

Assessment of Cognitive-Communicative and Language Factors in (Central) Auditory Processing Disorder

The ability to process auditory information requires exquisite neurological coordination between multiple anatomic and physiologic structures. Although the central auditory nervous system (CANS) has extensive redundancy, it is also incredibly complex. The complexity and redundancy can be both a positive and negative influence on the ability to attach meaning to acoustic stimuli. Those two variables also create a significant challenge for the professionals responsible for assessment.

Dual structures in each hemisphere, with multiple crossover points in the central auditory nervous system, create a system of checks and balances for acoustic information. The brain seeks patterns and matches in the acoustic stimuli received. The two hemispheres usually receive acoustic information in a diotic manner—both ears receive similar stimuli at the same time (Willeford & Burleigh, 1985). If background noise compromises the signal on one side, the crossover points and interhemispheric communication via the corpus callosum can fill in the missing pieces to ensure reception of an intact acoustic signal at the cortical level (Young, 1983). This is the positive aspect of the neurological complexity and redundancy of the central auditory nervous system.

The same dual structure with multiple crossover points that introduces neurological redundancy (Protti, 1983), creates a significant challenge for the audiologist responsible for evaluating integrity of the CANS. It becomes very difficult to functionally isolate or separate those finely integrated structures to conduct discrete assessment of the component parts within the CANS. Compensatory overlap within neurological and cortical functions can result in inaccurate or misleading assessment results. A behavioral response that suggests a problem or dysfunction within the central auditory system can be due to a variety of different reasons.

For example, an individual is verbally presented with an instruction to follow. A specific behavioral response occurs— the individual ignores the instruction. The diagnostic challenge is to determine why that behavioral response occurred. A variety of possibilities could account for the response. Consider the following:

- The individual ignored the instruction because the signal was blocked by a sudden, loud noise outside the room (i.e., competing signal that interfered with primary stimulus).
- The individual ignored the instruction because it was presented in a language or linguistic code that was unfamiliar (i.e., foreign language).
- The individual ignored the instruction because he or she chose not to comply (i.e., choice).
- The individual ignored the instruction because he or she could not remember it long enough to comply (i.e., memory).
- The individual ignored the instruction because he or she was not sure what the instruction meant (i.e., language).

- The individual ignored the instruction because he or she was not neurologically capable of producing the required motor response (i.e., apraxia).
- The individual ignored the instruction because the acoustic signal was not received (i.e., deaf).
- The individual ignored the instruction because he or she was thinking about something else (i.e., attention deficit).
- The individual ignored the instruction because the acoustic signal was compromised and not clear (i.e., [central] auditory processing disorder [C]APD).

In all cases, the person failed to respond appropriately to a presented auditory stimulus. However, a (C)APD would account for only the last scenario. Even though the behavioral response in each instance suggested the possibility of a (C)APD, further evaluation would support a different cause for the inaccurate behavioral response.

In the first eight of nine examples, intervention for a (C)APD would be ineffective; the primary source of the problem has not been accurately assessed. Intervention strategies consistent with (C)APD would not improve performance of the individual. In fact, the individual would probably become very frustrated if the cause of the aberrant behavioral response was among the first examples and the recommended intervention was an FM system. Amplification of the signal will not help a person produce a more appropriate response if the disorder is verbal apraxia. Repeating the stimulus will not facilitate comprehension for a person who does not know the language in which the stimulus is spoken. Allowing more time will not help the person who has a memory deficit; however, repetition of the signal might be very helpful.

A careful and thorough evaluation is essential to diagnose (C)APD. There are many deficits that can mirror or parallel the symptomatic characteristics of (C)APD. Intervention can only be effective if careful assessment procedures precede treatment. Professionals should not jump to the conclusion that a (C)APD is the cause of a child's listening problems in a classroom setting. The professional conducting the evaluation needs to carefully differentiate the various contributing components to effective attachment of meaning to an auditory stimulus.

Differential Diagnosis of (C)APD

The previous example illustrates the challenge that confronts an audiologist conducting a central auditory processing evaluation. Consequently, it is important to differentiate discrete primary aspects of the auditory processing continuum so the resulting diagnosis can be as specific as possible.

It has been established that attaching meaning to an auditory stimulus involves multiple neurological structures. The audiologic hierarchy for central auditory processing has been fairly well delineated (Noback, 1985). Audiologists and speech-language pathologists are familiar with differentiation of the peripheral auditory system (i.e., external ear, middle ear, inner ear), CANS (e.g., superior olivary, inferior colliculus, medial geniculate body, etc.) to the temporal lobe auditory cortex at Heschl's gyrus. The differentiation becomes anatomically more difficult at the

level of the cortex, due to the integration of cortical structures and areas. However, the auditory processing hierarchy can be further delineated using functional aspects for processing the auditory signal.

The Bellis/Ferre model (Bellis, 2006) identifies three primary subtypes of (C)APD. The subtype titles are descriptive of the deficits observed and include the presumed site of dysfunction for each. They include the following:

- Auditory decoding deficit: (deficit in primary auditory cortex—left hemisphere) problems in sound discrimination, reading, spelling, speech-in-noise, and phonological awareness.
- Prosodic deficit: (deficit in right hemisphere) problems in understanding prosodic aspects of speech that can impact pragmatic language, reading, spelling, and speaking.
- Integration deficit: (deficit in corpus callosum) problems coordinating auditory discrimination with prosodic aspects of speech; difficulty linking prosodic and linguistic speech components.

The Bellis/Ferre model begins to differentiate the aspects of auditory processing that occur cortically, but lacks the structured hierarchy that exists in the CANS model. The subtypes are differentiated functionally by the tasks in which the individual experiences difficulty; however, it is important to note that most of the descriptions begin to include language-based skills. It becomes apparent that once the model enters the upper cortex, it is almost impossible to exclude linguistic aspects from auditory processing (Rees, 1981; Rice & Kemper, 1984).

Kamhi (1981) concluded that the "auditory nature of linguistic input coupled with its symbolic aspects accounts for much of the difficulty language-impaired children encounter learning the linguistic system" (p. 452). He further stated that "By themselves, neither a symbolic deficit nor auditory processing difficulties seem able to explain the extent and nature of the linguistic deficiencies demonstrated by language-impaired children" (p. 452). In other words, to differentially assess auditory processing disorders, it becomes important for the audiologist to focus on acoustic versus linguistic aspects within the evaluation.

Auditory Processing Continuum

The CANS is responsible for transferring an acoustic signal through the brainstem to the upper cortex. Once the signal reaches Heschl's gyrus, linguistic factors begin to influence the acoustic signal, leading to comprehension in a language symbol system (Richard, 2001). Auditory processing begins to transition from primarily an acoustic phenomenon to a linguistic phenomenon. The differential assessment model needs to be extended into the cortex if evaluation of (C)APD is going to be clinically relevant, that is, lead to specific treatment that addresses the presenting deficits.

Auditory processing was defined by Massaro (1975) as "the ability to abstract meaning from an acoustic stimulus." Some aspects of auditory processing are very acoustic-based, whereas other aspects are very language-based. Norma Rees (1973) questioned the influence of "auditory" versus "language" in what was defined as "auditory processing."

A functional division that assists in differential diagnosis of (C)APD is to think of auditory processing as a continuum that moves through a neurological hierarchy in the central nervous system and brain (Richard, 2001). The peripheral system takes in the acoustic stimulus and conducts it to the CANS, which transfers the acoustic signal through the brainstem to the cortex. The primary auditory cortical structure is Heschl's gyrus in the temporal lobe, where discrimination of the acoustic aspects of the signal begins to occur (Gaddes, 1980; Protti, 1983). Meaning is attached once the acoustic characteristics are interpreted through use of a phonemic sound-symbol system associated with a linguistic system. Meaning cannot be attached to the signal without language knowledge. A summary of the auditory processing continuum is presented in Table 16-1.

Differential assessment needs to consider the major divisions in the type of processing that occurs (as delineated in Table 16-1) along the continuum. If an audiologist assumes responsibility for assessment of the entire continuum, problems in language, motor coordination, attention, or phonic/phonemic awareness all could be diagnosed as a (C)APD. This is very misleading for the professionals responsible for intervention, as well as for family members and adjunct professionals who are trying to understand the disability.

A more effective way to assess the continuum of auditory processing is to use the neurological hierarchy to differentiate primary responsibilities along the continuum. Figure 16-1 presents a graphic representation of how the continuum could be divided.

Assessment of the peripheral system and the CANS is the primary responsibility of the audiologist. Typical evaluation procedures of the peripheral system include

Table 16–1. Neurologic Continuum of Auditory Processing

	Anatomic Structures/Site	Type of Processing
Peripheral Auditory System	External ear	Auditory acuity
	Middle ear	Perception/Reception of acoustic of signal
	Inner ear/cochlea	
Central Auditory Processing	Central auditory nervous system	Neurologic transference of acoustic signal
	Auditory nerve/Brainstem	Discrimination of acoustic characteristics of signal
Phonemic Processing	Heschl's gyrus—Temporal lobe	Discrimination of phonemic characteristics of signal
Language Processing	Wernicke's area—Temporal lobe	Discrimination of linguistic characteristics of signal
	Angular gyrus	Attaching meaning in linguistic code
		Integrating aspects of signal
Executive Functions	Prefrontal /Frontal lobe	Planning and executing response
	Motor Strip	

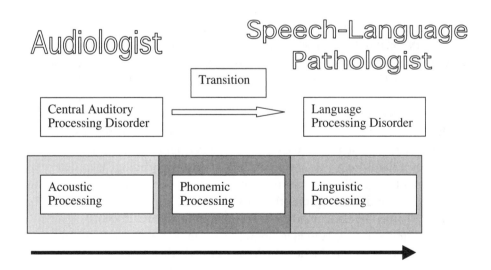

Figure 16–1. Auditory processing continuum.

pure-tone screening, air-bone conduction, otoacoustic emissions, and tympanometry. Peripheral assessment for auditory acuity would be prerequisite to central auditory processing assessment.

The purpose of central auditory processing assessment is usually to stress the CANS by reducing or eliminating redundancy. This is typically accomplished with dichotic evaluation procedures, in which a competing signal is introduced using tones, digits, syllables, words, or sentences. Acoustic integrity for transference of the signal is also evaluated using filtered speech, speech in noise, and timing modification tasks. Electrophysiological measures also can be used. Maintaining integrity of the acoustic signal as it is transferred through the brainstem to the cortex is the focus of assessment tasks in this part of the continuum. Evaluation tasks are discrete and focused; tasks are also usually controlled to minimize memory and language as confounding variables. This type of assessment is the responsibility of the audiologist and is encompassed within the more traditional definition of (C)APD.

As the acoustic signal enters the temporal lobe at Heschl's gyrus, interpretation of the acoustic signal begins to take on a phonemic focus, using the sound-symbol system of a designated language or linguistic code. The phonemic discrimination of sounds (e.g., "d" versus "t"), and segments (e.g., first sound in word, number of sounds) transitions the processing task into linguistic building blocks of preliteracy skills. A language sound-symbol system is required when the individual is asked to discriminate the phonic representation of a sound with the corresponding grapheme symbol. In other words, an individual transitions from

recognition that spoken words are composed of discrete sound units called phonemes, to a visual-orthographic representation of sound-symbol recognition (Mody, 2004).

Phonemic processing of the auditory signal is an area of overlap within audiology and speech-language pathology (Richard, 2006). Audiology evaluations typically include sound and speech discrimination tasks. At the same time, most speech-language pathologists conduct assessment of phonemic awareness skills to determine preliteracy skills for spelling, reading, and writing. Phonemic awareness is the ability to identify the sound units which comprise syllables and words (Ball, 1993). Phonemic segmentation and synthesis are two major aspects encompassed within phonemic awareness (Bernthal & Bankson, 2004). This part of the auditory processing continuum is a transition from acoustic processing into phonemic processing; assessment tasks in both disciplines will evaluate specific skills in this aspect of auditory processing. Ideally, this would be the aspect where audiology evaluations terminate and speech-language pathology evaluations begin. Both disciplines need information about this aspect of auditory processing—audiologists to determine if the acoustic characteristics are transferred and received accurately; speech-language pathologists to determine if the acoustic characteristics are being interpreted accurately within a linguistic code (Richard, 2006).

Once the sound characteristics are coded into a phonic-symbol system at the word level, then linguistic meaning is attached to the auditory stimulus. Auditory processing is now actually language processing, in that the acoustic signal should be translated into a visual representation of an idea, object, or event, at a cognitive level. The ability to meaningfully interpret an auditory signal is not an acoustic task, it is a linguistic task. If an individual cannot meaningfully interpret an auditory signal at this level, it is not an acoustic problem; it is a language-based problem. When an audiologist diagnoses an auditory processing problem, the usual intervention is to focus on enhancing or maximizing the auditory signal. That will not be beneficial for a person who is encountering difficulty at the linguistic level of the auditory processing continuum. Once auditory processing has transitioned into linguistic interpretation of meaning, it is the responsibility of the speech-language pathologist to use knowledge of language disorders to determine the primary deficits present.

Figure 16-1 illustrates the auditory processing continuum for differential analysis of the primary components in the hierarchy. It is important to consider the major divisions within the continuum of auditory processing when attempting to determine if a disorder is present. The ramifications of overstepping professional boundaries when conducting assessment can result in confusion, frustration, and wasted time and energy if differential diagnosis is not carefully done.

The diagram is not intended to imply a simple linear attachment of meaning along the auditory processing continuum. In *Thought and Language*, Vygotsky (1962) introduced the concept of process being a continual back-and-forth movement between words and thoughts. Processing is the ability to integrate the auditory aspect of listening with the language aspects of speaking, reading, and writing (American Speech-Language-Hearing Association, 1996). Differential assessment must take into consideration that multiple aspects of speech and language are encompassed within the area of auditory processing.

Language Factors to Consider

Just as peripheral auditory acuity is prerequisite to initiating an auditory processing evaluation along the continuum, it is important to consider aspects of auditory processing that occur following completion of an evaluation along the main continuum. The prefrontal and frontal cortical areas are involved in planning, organizing, and executing an appropriate motor response to the received auditory stimulus (Richard & Fahy, 2005). The ability to process prosodic features of an acoustic stimulus is also mediated in the prefrontal cortex. Deficits in executive function can contribute to poor performance on assessment procedures that require interpretation of an acoustic stimulus.

For example, a person with Asperger syndrome or nonverbal learning disorder may ignore facial expression or tone of vocal delivery, resulting in a literal interpretation of the auditory stimulus. Diagnosing a (C)APD rather than Asperger syndrome or nonverbal learning disorder would be misleading. One symptomatic aspect should not be diagnosed as the primary disorder, when in reality, a much broader disorder is present that accounts for the auditory processing deficits.

(C)APD should not be diagnosed in the absence of language assessment or information. A (C)APD could exist in isolation, but it is likely to have ramifications for language development. It is also possible for language deficits to significantly influence results on assessment tasks in a central auditory processing evaluation. The continuum illustrated in Figure 16-1 helps identify the primary language factors that should be considered when interpreting central auditory processing assessment results. Deficits in the three main aspects of auditory processing could occur in isolation, or in combination with each other. Possible deficits that could be present are illustrated in Figure 16-2.

The three circles in Figure 16-2 represent the primary differential aspects encompassed along the continuum of auditory processing—central auditory processing, phonemic processing, and language processing. The letters represent possible configurations of disorders that could occur. Each is discussed briefly in the following section.

A. **Central auditory processing disorder (CAPD) only.** The individual is not receiving an intact auditory signal at a cortical level. Acoustic characteristics of the stimulus are being compromised during neurological transfer and processing in the CANS, so that the signal perceived by the listener is distorted, resulting in misrepresentation, inaccuracy, and confusion. Intervention will focus primarily on signal enhancement and the audiologist will be the primary diagnostician.

B. **Language processing disorder (LPD) only.** The individual is receiving an intact auditory signal at the cortical level, but is unable to attach linguistic meaning to decode the intended message. The person might even be able to repeat or echo the auditory stimulus, but cannot

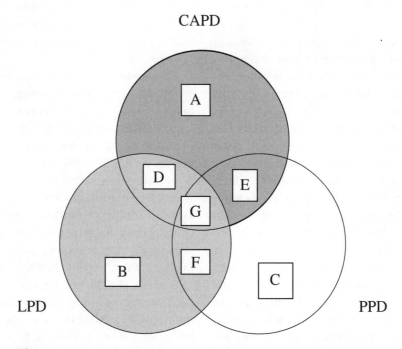

Figure 16-2. Confluence of (C)APD, phonemic processing disorders (PPD), and language processing disorders (LPD).

understand what it means to then mediate a response. The speech-language pathologist will be the primary diagnostician.

C. **Phonemic processing disorder (PPD) only.** The acoustic signal is being transferred intact to the cortical level, but the individual is unable to phonemically discriminate segments within the signal. The person might be able to repeat the stimulus, but cannot determine specific sound segments at a phonemic or phonic (grapheme representation) level. Aspects of both the audiologist's and speech-language pathologist's assessment tasks should be used to diagnose.

D. **Central auditory processing and language processing disorders co-occurring ([C]APD & LPD).** As a result of a (C)APD, the distorted auditory signal is negatively influencing the ability to attach meaning within a language code. The individual hears a garbled or unintelligible auditory stimulus, further compromising development of linguistic interpretation skills. Aspects of both the audiologist's and speech-language pathologist's assessment tasks should be used for diagnosis.

E. **Central auditory processing and phonemic processing disorders co-occurring ([C]APD & PPD).** The compromised auditory signal ([C]APD) leads to difficulty in developing the ability to discriminate and represent sounds in a phoneme-grapheme/sound-symbol relationship. The acoustic signal needs to be enhanced to facilitate a foundation for literacy skills. Aspects of both the audiologist's and speech-language pathologist's assessment tasks should be used to determine the diagnosis.

F. **Phonemic processing and language processing disorders co-occurring (PPD & LPD).** Poor discrimination of the sound aspects of the auditory signal (PPD) results in problems understanding and interpreting language presented in an auditory modality. Individuals tend to rely on concrete visual stimuli when there are problems in the phonemic/phonic preliteracy skills. The written presentation of information does not correspond to the auditory, so reading comprehension is significantly affected. Aspects of both the audiologist's and speech-language pathologist's assessment tasks should be used to diagnose.

G. **Central auditory processing, phonemic processing, and language processing disorders all present ([C]APD & PPD & LPD).** This scenario is a classic domino-effect, where a problem in signal reception has a negative and dramatic impact on all subsequent levels along the auditory processing continuum. Aspects of both the audiologist's and speech-language pathologist's assessment tasks will be necessary to diagnose deficits in all areas of the processing continuum.

Variables to Control

An audiologist is not always well-versed in knowing how to discriminate and control the influence of language variables in central auditory processing assessment procedures. A further confounding factor is the transference of responsibility between assessment and treatment. An audiologist is the primary professional responsible for assessment and diagnosis of (C)APD; treatment is usually provided by a speech-language pathologist. Therefore, a (C)APD may be diagnosed in the absence of any language tests. However, certain types of language deficits could significantly influence results on the central auditory assessment tasks.

Consider the following instructions that a child might receive for completing a dichotic listening assessment task: "You are going to hear a word in your left ear. You will hear a different word at the same time in your right ear. I want you to tell me the word you heard first in your left ear, then the word that you heard in your right ear." What are the language variables that could negatively influence the child's ability to respond appropriately on this dichotic test?

Language needs to be fairly well developed to comply with these instructions. The child must understand concepts of same/different, left/right, and first/second. In addition, the child must possess adequate attention and short-term memory to listen and retain the instructions given by the examiner. Any motor programming or production problems in articulation/phonology could influence the examiner's interpretation of which word the child reports hearing. A certain level of cognitive ability is required for the child even to be able to respond to the task.

Finally, there has been much debate regarding maturation of the CANS. Myelination is only partially completed at birth and structures related to higher-level auditory processing, corpus callosum, and executive function continue to myelinate into adolescence (Whitelaw & Yuskow, 2006). Evaluating a young child for deficits in central auditory processing could result in diagnosing a disorder when, in reality, there is a maturational delay in development of the central auditory system that will resolve over time.

Variables which the audiologist needs to control for, or consider the influence of, during assessment of auditory processing include the following: general language development/cognitive ability; memory; attention; and neurological maturation. Cognitive ability or general language development needs to approximate 5 to 6 years of age. The language skills to understand and comply with directions in most central auditory processing evaluations require at least a kindergarten level of conceptual development.

Auditory processing assessment tasks are usually fairly discrete and brief in their presentation format. However, a certain amount of memory is required for the individual to comply with presented directions. Many of the tasks presume that the individual being evaluated has the ability to retain auditory stimuli long enough to repeat, synthesize, integrate, or discriminate, whatever the task might be.

The assessment tasks within a central auditory processing evaluation battery require careful listening and attention. It can be tiring and frustrating for an individual to sit and listen to sounds, tones, or words under headset conditions for an extended period of time. Individuals with poor attention may not focus on the stimulus presentation, resulting in inaccurate responses. Performance may diminish over time, suggesting poor attention rather than processing ability.

Many audiologists refrain from conducting central auditory processing evaluations until a child is at least 6 years of age. Research on neurological maturation of the auditory system suggests that the CANS continues developing through the preschool years and later for higher levels of the CANS. Poor performance results in a four-year-old child might not be indicative of an auditory processing problem; it could be a child whose neurological maturation is delayed.

Assessment Instruments

"What's in a name? That which we call a rose by any other word would smell as sweet."
(*Romeo and Juliet*, Act II, Scene II)

There are numerous assessment instruments that are commercially available for assessment in the area of auditory processing. It is important for the professional conducting the evaluation to carefully evaluate the actual task required. The previous section discussed some of the variables that could negatively impact assessment results, leading to invalid diagnostic conclusions. The same is true when looking at the name or title of a test or subtest task.

Most assessment instruments include multiple subtest tasks. The title of the composite test may suggest that it is evaluating auditory processing, but several of the subtests may actually be more phonemic or linguistic in nature than acoustic. There is not good agreement within the disciplines of audiology and speech-language pathology when defining auditory processing disorders. An author's perspective can differ dramatically from accepted practice, resulting in an assessment instrument that is misleading by its title. The title of a test should not necessarily be the determining factor in a diagnostic label. For example, a test may be called a test of auditory processing, when in reality it evaluates auditory memory or phonemic awareness. The term "auditory processing" encompasses many skills, some of which are acoustic, many that are linguistic-based. The professional administering the assessment instrument needs to make a determination as to what skills an instrument actually evaluates, regardless of its title.

The professional conducting assessment should analyze the stimuli presented, the task required of the individual being evaluated, and the type of response expected. The continuum of auditory processing (see Figure 16–2) should be used to evaluate whether the task is primarily acoustic, phonemic, or linguistic in nature. Confounding variables that could affect results, such as poor attention, a phonological disorder, or cognitive impairment, should also be considered.

The human neurology and cortical structures are highly coordinated and function in a systematic fashion; they will also dysfunction in a systematic pattern (Gaddes, 1980). An individual can rarely fake correct responses on central auditory processing assessment tasks. If a person performs well on multiple similar tasks with one exception, the exception should not necessarily result in diagnosis of (C)APD. The other results might need to be weighed more heavily in the diagnostic process. Tests results must always be carefully interpreted by an individual with clinical experience in the area of central auditory processing. An inexperienced evaluator may have a difficult time differentiating the various aspects that are encompassed within processing, as well as possible confounding variables. The diagnostic process should not be driven by test results, but by professionals experienced in interpreting test results.

For this reason, it is important to conduct a battery of tests when assessing auditory processing skills. The complexity of the CANS and variety of skills along the auditory processing continuum necessitate sampling multiple types of processing ability. The examiner should ask a series of questions regarding what the individual can and cannot do in regard to processing. Sometimes knowing what a person is able to do is more valuable information than what he or she is unable to accurately demonstrate. The auditory processing continuum provides landmarks for minimally three major assessment areas—acoustic, phonemic, and linguistic. Each of those primary aspects of auditory processing can be further delineated in specific tasks. A diagnostic assessment is not complete until the examiner has information to address multiple aspects of auditory processing.

Language Impairment

Language encompasses phonology, morphology, syntax, semantics, and pragmatics. Another division of major language components is form (phonology, morphology, syntax), content (semantics), and use (pragmatics). In relation to (C)APD, the "form" aspect of phonology is probably the most pertinent to early levels of the auditory processing continuum. Bloom and Lahey (1978) defined the form of an utterance in terms of the acoustic, phonetic shape.

An individual with impairment in the "form" aspect of language is likely to have difficulty with central auditory processing assessment tasks. A significant phonological deficit suggests that development of sound recognition and production is delayed. Consequently, the individual will struggle to reproduce or

discriminate acoustic stimuli presented during a central auditory processing evaluation. It would be erroneous on the part of an audiologist to diagnose a (C)APD in addition to the phonological disorder, based only on phoneme task results. Evaluation procedures might need to modify the response modality to picture-pointing to circumvent difficulty with production of a verbal response. Assessment tasks in the battery should focus more on tone/pitch, numbers/digits, or non-phonemic/non-linguistic stimuli to avoid evaluating for a central auditory processing problem through an already identified deficit area, that is, phonology. Deficits in higher levels of "form" (morphology and syntax) could influence results on tests of binaural integration and dichotic competing sentences.

The portion of the auditory processing continuum that is primarily the responsibility of the audiologist includes "form" aspects of language. Consequently, the audiologist must consult with the speech-language pathologist or be cognizant of any existing deficits in this area. The first portion of the continuum focuses primarily on acoustic features, but the transition area that introduces phonemic awareness must be carefully evaluated and interpreted so that confounding factors do not result in misdiagnosis of a (C)APD.

The overlap transition area on the continuum allows for input by the speech-language pathologist regarding phonemic aspects of language. Content (semantics) and use (pragmatics) become factors at the latter end of the continuum in levels of language processing. However, deficits in semantic language could influence results on assessment tasks that are intended to evaluate earlier acoustic levels on the continuum. The example presented earlier in this chapter illustrated how poor concept development (e.g., left/right, same/different, first/second) could result in failure to understand and comply with directions for dichotic tasks intended to assess central auditory processing.

One other language impairment that should be considered by an audiologist when conducting assessment would be oral apraxia. Children and adults who present with difficulty neurologically programming speech output will struggle with "on demand" verbal production. Their errors will be inconsistent, as they reprogram each attempt at speech. An audiologist might interpret the variable verbal output as guessing or incorrect responses, when the actual problem is an inability to program the speech musculature to reproduce the desired response. Hearing might be accurate; the ability to verbally represent what was heard is in deficit. Once again, it will be important for the audiologist assessing central auditory processing to have information regarding any language or motor impairments that might necessitate modifications in evaluation procedures (e.g., nonverbal response) or interpretation of performance.

Learning Disability

A learning disability exists when an individual presents with normal cognitive ability that is not realized within actual performance. The discrepancy can be a significant gap between verbal and performance intelligence tasks, or an inconsistent, splintered learning profile. The learning disability results in an individual having difficulty being able to interpret what he sees or hears.

The Individuals with Disabilities Education Act (IDEA '97) defines a learning disability as a "disorder in one or more of the basic psychological processes involved in understanding or in using spoken or written language, which may manifest itself in an imperfect ability to listen, think, speak, read, write, spell, or to do mathematical calculations." According to the *Diagnostic and Statistical Manual of Mental Disorders* (APA 2000), a learning disability is diagnosed when an individual's achievement is below expectations, based on age, education, and intelligence.

The subtypes of learning disabilities have been researched with mixed results, due to discrepancies and inconsistencies in diagnostic criteria (Rourke, 1985). The *DSM-IV-TR* (2000) differentiates learning disabilities by the academic skills which are deficient, defining a Reading Disorder, Mathematics Disorder, and Disorder of Written Expression. However, classifying the resulting secondary academic deficit does little to differentiate the primary cause of the learning problems. Experience-based professionals have used incidence figures of diagnostic labels and special services provided in the public schools to derive a theoretical differentiation within the learning disabilities category.

As depicted in Figure 16–3, approximately 80% of learning disabilities are referred to as language-learning disorders (LLD), because the difficulty is presumed to be primarily in the temporal lobe, dealing with interpretation of stimuli. The level of difficulty is within the linguistic aspect of attaching meaning to what has been visually or auditorily presented for processing. Individuals hear what is said, but struggle to understand the message or integrate it with other

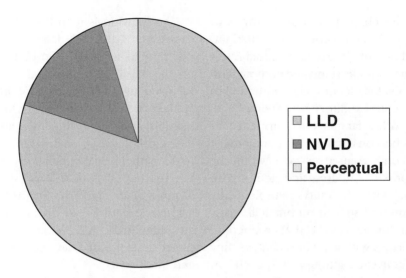

Figure 16–3. Types of learning disabilities.

stored information. The phonemic and linguistic aspects of auditory processing disorders would be within this category of learning disabilities. Obvious areas of academic impact would be deficits in reading and written language, but additional academic subjects could also be affected.

Approximately 15% of learning disabilities are classified as nonverbal learning disorders (NVLD), which are presumed to be based in the frontal lobe and prefrontal cortex where executive functions are coordinated. The primary difficulty in this type of learning disability is "reading between the lines." Individuals tend to literally interpret verbal communication and miss subtle nuances that alter the message, such as facial expression or gestures, and tone of voice indicating sarcasm or teasing. Prosodic features embedded in an acoustic stimulus are usually ignored or overlooked. Poor planning and organization are also characteristics of a nonverbal learning disability. Higher-level language processing

disorders and deficits in executive functions would be included within this category, including social-pragmatic deficits.

The remaining 5 to 7% of learning disabilities is thought to be modality-based, primarily in the area of visual-perceptual problems. Symptoms could include letter reversals and poor interpretation of visual stimuli.

Learning disabilities are attributed to subtle neurological differences. The nature of the deficit could be a biochemical neurological interaction that results in inefficient functioning at the cortical level. The subtle deficits in the central nervous system also contribute to co-morbid conditions that often accompany a learning disability. These can include attention deficit hyperactivity disorder (ADHD), attention deficit disorder (ADD), long and short-term memory deficits, and word retrieval problems.

The components of a learning disability can significantly influence results of central auditory processing assessment. An individual with a learning disability may not process directions presented by an examiner, due to language processing deficits, attention deficits, or memory problems. The individual may be easily distracted or unable to pay attention to auditory stimuli except for brief periods of time. The audiologist conducting central auditory processing assessment needs to be aware of any learning disability and its characteristics so evaluation procedures can be adjusted or modified to ensure valid and reliable results.

Interpretation of test performance also needs to take into account variables of attention, memory, and retrieval. Inconsistencies are typical in the performance of individuals with learning disabilities. The battery of tests should be carefully evaluated to ensure that skills evidenced on one test are not minimized or ignored because they were deficient on a second test. It is difficult to fake positive results if the central auditory system is truly dysfunctional. Test results should not be interpreted as independent, irrefutable documentation that substantiates a (C)APD. Test results within a battery of evaluation tasks should be carefully interpreted by an experienced audiologist with knowledge and understanding of how a specific learning disability might impact auditory test performance. Potential confounding factors related to the behavioral characteristics of a learning disability (e.g., issues related to language processing, attention, working memory, etc.), should be identified and test performance should be interpreted with consideration for these factors before reaching any diagnostic conclusions.

Perhaps the most important variables that must be considered by all clinicians administering diagnostic tests are test sensitivity and specificity (i.e., efficiency). The diagnostic power of any test (whether auditory, language, memory, or other) is contingent on its ability to identify correctly those individuals who have the dysfunction (i.e., sensitivity) and identify correctly those individuals who do not have the dysfunction (i.e., specificity). In terms of (C)APD, the audiologist must carefully analyze the test instruments included in the diagnostic battery with knowledge of each test's capability to detect central auditory dysfunction when in fact it does exist (i.e., sensitivity) and to define normal central auditory function when that is the case (i.e., specificity). Test efficiency is a major consideration in determining an appropriate test battery for a particular client.

Primary Intervention Strategies

Intervention strategies should be tailored to address specific deficits along the auditory processing continuum. The diagnostic process needs to differentiate aspects that are problematic so treatment can focus on resolving or compensating for specific aspects of the disorder. If the diagnostic process lacks discrete analysis of auditory processing components, then intervention is likely to be too global or generic to be effective.

Primary intervention strategies will address the three main delineations along the auditory processing continuum—acoustic, phonemic, linguistic. Goals should consider both compensatory techniques and development of specific skills in each area. General examples of a primary intervention focus for each aspect of auditory processing are summarized in the following section.

Acoustic Processing—(C)APD

Purpose: The primary focus of intervention for central auditory processing is auditory training and signal enhancement to ensure accurate reception and transfer of the auditory stimulus from the peripheral system to the upper cortex.

Goals: Strategies that address the signal-to noise ratio environmentally through techniques such as an FM system, preferential seating, acoustic tiles in the classroom, and so forth are examples of compensatory techniques. Providing visual backup and auditory repetition would be additional strategies for compensating for a compromised auditory signal. The specific discrete tasks used for assessment can be incorporated in treatment (i.e., auditory training) to teach the individual to "fill in" missing signal components. Types of tasks could include tone discrimination (e.g., low versus high), figure-ground (e.g., primary message in static background), lip reading (i.e., using visual cues to supplement distorted auditory information), and auditory closure (i.e., fill in missing acoustic information).

Phonemic Processing

Purpose: The primary focus of intervention for phonemic processing is to develop awareness and discrimination of sound segments, gradually introducing the grapheme representation of sounds to build a preliteracy foundation.

Goals: A variety of sound analysis tasks focused on phonemic awareness should be introduced initially.

The individual needs to develop the ability to discriminate one sound from another; identify the first or last sound; replace, add or delete sounds, and so forth. Once the individual can identify sound segments from the auditory presentation, sound-symbol correspondence should be introduced with the use of graphemes representing the sounds. Phonemic awareness tasks should gradually transition to phonic-based tasks to facilitate development of literacy skills for reading, spelling, and written language.

Language Processing

Purpose: The primary focus for addressing language processing is the attachment of meaning to auditory stimuli. Language processing begins with simple discrete vocabulary development and gradually progresses in semantic complexity to concepts, nonliteral meaning, and problem-solving.

Goals: Visual stimuli can be used in early stages of language processing to complement and supplement the acoustic signal. Additional compensatory strategies could include cueing techniques to facilitate comprehension and retrieval within contexts. Specific skills should address major semantic language abilities, such as categorization, the ability to compare and contrast, multiple meanings, idiomatic expressions, and so forth.

Concluding Comments and Impressions

Auditory processing disorders have been identified as a clinical entity since early in the history of the professions of audiology and speech-language pathology. However, the definition and scope of functional skills encompassed within the disorder area has been a changing and evolving entity.

The term "auditory processing" initially referred to all aspects of dealing with an auditory stimulus. In the 1970s, audiology introduced the term central auditory processing to clarify the specific aspect of moving the acoustic stimulus through the CANS; however, the general term of auditory processing continued to be used by both speech-language pathologists and audiologists.

As aspects of language became better defined and differentiated beyond structural forms, the terms "information processing" and "language processing" were introduced within the scope of speech-language pathology. A hierarchy of language skills encompassed within language processing was identified and extended to include problem-solving, reasoning, and executive functions. This resulted in further confusion regarding exactly what was encompassed within auditory processing. In the 1990s, phonological awareness evolved into preliteracy skills that provided the foundation for reading, spelling, and written language. The ability to discriminate, segment, and manipulate sounds and their symbols grew within the scope of practice assigned to speech-language pathologists.

Audiology retained the diagnostic responsibility for assessing and diagnosing auditory processing disorders, despite the expanding breadth of what was sometimes included within the functional definition. The historical treatment for auditory processing disorders was primarily compensatory in nature, modifying the environment in ways to enhance the signal and ensure accurate reception and transfer of the acoustic stimulus. But as the definition expanded to include phonemic and linguistic aspects of processing, the diagnostic and treatment issues became confused. The deficits encompassed under "auditory processing disorder" were more involved than ensuring an intact signal. As a result, speech-language pathologists became the primary professionals responsible for providing treatment in the area of auditory processing disorders, despite not being involved in the assessment procedures that resulted in the diagnosis.

The present day dilemma continues to some extent. Auditory processing disorders continue to be defined in various ways within the professions of audiology and speech-language pathology, despite attempts by professional groups to codify the term in position papers and technical reports. The dichotomy between diagnosis and treatment responsibilities contributes to the professional challenge. The issue more important than professional autonomy and responsibility within aspects of auditory processing, is the clinical implication. When an auditory processing disorder is diagnosed, what exactly does it mean? What specifically is the deficit or problem being exhibited by the individual that resulted in the diagnosis? What treatment methodology might address the deficits?

Summary

This chapter attempted to delineate a clinical continuum for analyzing auditory processing disorders to provide functional diagnostic information. The audiologist is responsible for assessment, but should never work in a vacuum when evaluating this disorder. The influence of language, both phonetic and linguistic parameters, on performance on central auditory processing evaluation tasks must be considered by the audiologist. Diagnostic tests need to be discrete, identifying as specifically as possible, adequate capabilities and areas of deficit. Multiple factors and language variables must be considered when conducting the evaluation and interpreting test results.

References

American Psychiatric Association (2000). *Diagnostic and statistical manual of mental disorders* (4th ed., text revision). Washington, DC: Author.

American Speech-Language-Hearing Association. (1996). Central auditory processing: Current status of research and implications for clinical practice. *American Journal of Audiology, 5*(2), 41-54.

Ball, E. (1993). Assessing phoneme awareness. *Language Speech and Hearing Services in Schools, 24*, 130-139.

Bellis, T. (2006), Interpretation of APD tests results. In T. K. Parthasarathy (Ed.), *An introduction to auditory processing disorders in children* (pp. 145-160). Mahwah, NJ: Lawrence Erlbaum Associates.

Bernthal, J., & Bankson, N. (2004). *Articulation and phonological disorders* (5th ed.). Boston: Allyn & Bacon.

Bloom, L., & Lahey, M. (1978). *Language development and language disorders*. New York: Macmillan Publishing Co.

Gaddes, W. (1980). *Learning disabilities and brain function—A neuropsychological approach*. New York: Springer-Verlag.

Kamhi, A. (1981). Nonlinguistic symbolic and conceptual abilities of language-impaired and normally developing children. *Journal of Speech and Hearing Research, 24*, 446-453.

Massaro, D. (1975). *Understanding language: An information-processing analysis of speech perception, reading, and psycholinguistics*. New York: Academic Press.

Mody, M. (2004). Neurobiological correlates of language and reading impairments. In C. Stone, E. Silliman, B. Ehren, & K. Apel (Eds.), *Handbook of language and literacy* (pp. 49-72). New York: The Guilford Press.

Noback, C. (1985). Neuroanatomical correlates of central auditory function. In M. Pinheiro & F. Musiek (Eds.), *Assessment of central auditory dysfunction* (pp.7-21). Baltimore: Williams & Wilkins.

Protti, E. (1983). Brainstem auditory pathways and auditory processing disorders. In E. Lasky & J. Katz (Eds.), *Central auditory processing disorders* (pp.117-139). Baltimore: University Park Press.

Rees, N. (1973), Auditory processing factors in language disorders: The view from Procrustes' bed. *Journal of Speech and Hearing Disorders, 38*(3), 304-315.

Rees, N. (1981). Saying more than we know: Is auditory processing disorder a meaningful concept? In R. Keith (Ed.), *Central auditory and language disorders in children*. San Diego, CA: College-Hill Press.

Rice, M., & Kemper, S. (1984). *Child language and cognition*. Baltimore: University Park Press.

Richard, G. (2001). *The source for processing disorders*. East Moline, IL: LinguiSystems.

Richard, G. (2006). Language based assessment and intervention of APD. In T. K. Parthasarathy (Ed.), *An introduction to auditory processing disorders in children* (pp. 95-108). Mahwah, NJ: Lawrence Erlbaum Associates.

Richard, G., & Fahy, J. (2005). *The source for development of executive functions*. East Moline, IL: LinguiSystems.

Rourke, B. (1985). *Neuropsychology of learning disabilities*. New York: The Guilford Press.

Shakespeare, W. From *Romeo and Juliet* (II, ii).

Vygotsky, L. (1962). *Thought and language.* Cambridge, MA: MIT Press.

Whitelaw, G., & Yuskow, K. (2006) Neuromaturation and neuroplasticity of the central auditory system. In T. K. Parthasarathy (Ed.), *An introduction to auditory processing disorders in children* (pp. 21–38). Mahwah, NJ: Lawrence Erlbaum Associates.

Willeford, J., & Burleigh, J. (1985). *Handbook of central auditory processing disorders in children.* Orlando, FL: Grune & Stratton.

Young, M. (1983). Neuroscience, pragmatic competence, and auditory processing. In E. Lasky & J. Katz (Eds.), *Central auditory processing disorders* (pp. 141–161). Baltimore: University Park Press.

CHAPTER 17

(CENTRAL) AUDITORY PROCESSING DISORDER AND ATTENTION DEFICIT HYPERACTIVITY DISORDER

A Psychological Perspective

ART MAERLENDER

Introduction

Central auditory processing disorder ([C]APD) is defined as "deficits in the information processing of audible signals not attributed to impaired peripheral hearing sensitivity or intellectual impairment" (Jerger & Musiek, 2000). This disorder is thought to disrupt the continuous auditory processing of acoustic, phonetic, and linguistic information; however, little is known about this symptom cluster from a neuropsychological perspective. In children, this disruption has been associated with a variety of functional problems, including difficulties with selective attention, temporal processing problems, auditory memory, and sound blending (Jerger & Musiek, 2000). In addition, the relationship between auditory-

sensory deficits and better known clinical and psychiatric disorders has not been clearly demonstrated (Chermak, 1996). For example, two studies examining the comorbidity of (C)APD and attention deficit hyperactivity disorder (ADHD) demonstrated substantial overlap of clinical profiles, but independence of diagnoses (Chermak, 1996; Riccio, Hynd, Cohen, Hall, & Molt, 1994); however, little follow-up work has been completed.

Research to bridge the gap between audiology and psychology has been limited to making it difficult for psychologists to incorporate the putative (C)APD construct into their own theoretical frameworks. Because there is overlap in symptoms in ADHD and (C)APD, this is a point at which clinical audiology and clinical behavioral neurosciences appear to intersect. Thus, ADHD is an appropriate clinical entity to study in regard to relationships between these disciplines and their different ways of understanding. In this chapter we discuss the clinical entity of ADHD from neurologic and behavioral perspectives and then report on studies from our clinical neuropsychology laboratory assessing (C)APD from a neuropsychological perspective. Specific inquiry into the relationship of (C)APD and ADHD is reported. Some of that work has been previously published (Maerlender, Wallis, & Isquith, 2004), and some is in the publication process (Maerlender, 2006).

The literature on ADHD is quite extensive. The discussion presented here is an attempt to synthesize some of the important work that has been done in this area, but it is by no means complete.

The Diagnostic Construct of ADHD

ADHD is a well-characterized, and relatively common behavior disorder of development (American Psychiatric Association, 2000). However, controversies about its diagnostic consistency (purity) remain. The name of the disorder suggests that it is primarily related to attentional functioning. Because of the similarity in symptom presentation between ADHD and traumatic brain injured patients, a relationship with executive functioning (EF) has long been posited (EF representing those behaviors necessary for planning and carrying out complex behaviors; Barkley, 1997). Willcutt, Doyle, Nigg, Faraone, and Pennington (2005) have challenged the idea that EF is a core construct of ADHD because of the moderate effect sizes of EF measures in explaining symptoms of ADHD, and in part because of

the typical failure to control for covariates such as IQ and reading ability. However, a good deal of literature confirms that a relationship exists (e.g., see Weyandt, 2005).

Over the past two decades there have been as many as 19 community-based studies offering estimates of prevalence ranging from 2 to 17% (Scahill & Schwab-Stone, 2000). The dramatic differences in these estimates are due to the choice of informant, methods of sampling and data collection, and the diagnostic definition. Based on the 19 studies reviewed by Scahill and Schwab-Stone, the best estimate of prevalence of ADHD is 5 to 10% in general school-aged children.

As a diagnostic category, current conceptualization of ADHD identifies three primary subtypes (American Psychiatric Association, 2000): symptoms of inattentive behaviors (including difficulty sustaining attention in tasks or play activities, and not seeming to listen when spoken to directly); hyperactive-impulsive behaviors (excessive motor behaviors, fidgeting, and difficulty sitting still); and a combined type. A "sluggish-cognitive tempo" type has also been discussed as a specific subtype of the Inattentive type (Hartman, Willcutt, Rhee, & Pennington, 2004). In this research category subtype, symptoms of daydreaming, a tendency to become confused, a lack of mental alertness, and physical hypoactivity are felt to be representative.

Besides the presence of specific symptom clusters, other qualitative factors must be documented to diagnose ADHD. Some of the symptoms must be present before the age of 7 in a manner that is inconsistent with normal development. There must be clear indication that the symptoms cause functional impairment; the symptoms must cause impairment across settings to rule out the effect of specific environments or demands. The symptoms must also not be better explained by other developmental or psychiatric disorders, such as autism, anxiety, or a dissociative disorder (American Psychiatric Association, 2000). The standard for diagnosis rests on functional behaviors (across settings) and identified history of problems (to establish the developmental nature of the behaviors). Although specific neuropsychological tests have been shown to differentiate ADHD from normal controls (Kelly, 2000; Lovejoy et al., 1999) the clinical diagnosis of ADHD does not require such testing.

In addition, the subtyping of ADHD is still open to question. Nigg (2005) asserts that the issue of heterogeneity of presentation has not been adequately studied, and that most of the neuropsychological literature is focused on the combined subtype (ADHD-Combined) that includes symptoms of both inattention and hyperactivity-impulsivity. His study in 2002 (Nigg, Blaskey, Huang-Pollack, & Rappley) assessed 46 children aged 7 to 12 with diagnoses of ADHD-C (Combined type), 18 children with ADHD-I (Inattentive type), and compared them to 41 community control children. Few differences were found between the ADHD-C and ADHD-I groups and the authors concluded that ADHD-I shared neuropsychological deficits with ADHD-C in the domain of output speed, although boys with ADHD-C differed from boys with ADHD-I in motor inhibition (ADHD-C being more disinhibited). There was no difference between the girls in this study.

The findings of Nigg et al. (2002) were generally consistent with an earlier study by Chhabildas, Pennington, and Willcutt (2001) who also did not find different neuropsychological profiles in a large sample of children with inattentive, hyperactive-impulsive, or combined subtypes of ADHD as compared to controls. That study compared the neuropsychological profiles of children without ADHD ($n = 82$) and children who met symptom criteria for *DSM-IV* Predominantly Inattentive subtype (ADHD-I; $n = 67$), Predominantly Hyperactive Impulsive subtype (ADHD-HI; $n = 14$), and Combined subtype (ADHD-C; $n = 33$) in the areas of processing speed, vigilance, and inhibition. Contrary to their prediction, symptoms of inattention best predicted performance on all dependent measures, and children with ADHD-I and ADHD-C had similar impairment profiles. Children with ADHD-HI were not significantly impaired on any of the dependent measures once subclinical symptoms of inattention were controlled. However, despite the questionable validity, diagnostic nomenclature continues to specify these subtypes in clinical practice. Furthermore, both Clarke, Barry, McCarthy, and Selikowitz (2002) and Stewart, Steffler, Lemoine, and Leps (2001) have provided evidence that both ADHD-C and ADHD-I share similar EEG profiles that are indicative of hypoarousal. Thus, although accepted in clinical practice, the diagnostic descriptions of ADHD and the specificity of its subtypes remain a point of some discussion.

The Neurobiology of ADHD

Although the pathophysiology of ADHD is not completely understood, ADHD is thought to be due to dysfunctional catecholamine neurotransmission in several key brain regions (especially norepinephrine and dopamine). Catecholamines are involved in attention, various aspects of inhibition and response in the motor system, motivated behaviors, reward systems, and spatial working memory functions (Arnsten, Steere, & Hunt, 1996; Calderon-Gonzalez, 1993). The catecholamines norepinephrine and dopamine are involved in attention-deficit disorders (Himelstein, Newcorn, & Halperin, 2000). Both neurotransmitter systems modulate the transfer of information through different regions of the brain, including the thalamus, prefrontal cortex (PFC), and basal ganglia (Russell, 2002).

Converging evidence from studies of the neuropharmacology, genetics, neuropsychology, and neuroimaging of ADHD imply the involvement of frontostriatal circuitry in ADHD (Durston, 2003; Durston et al., 2003; Sowell et al., 2003; Tannock, 1998). Although a significant amount of progress has been made investigating the neurobiology of this disorder, its precise etiology still remains unclear. However, although it does appear that poor inhibitory control and the deficits in frontostriatal circuitry associated with it are central to the expression of ADHD, there is evidence to suggest that more posterior cerebral areas are also implicated in this disorder (Castellanos et al., 2002). Anatomic studies suggest widespread reductions in volume throughout the cerebrum and cerebellum, whereas functional imaging studies suggest that affected individuals activate more diffuse areas than controls during the performance of cognitive tasks (Durston et al., 2003).

Quantitative electroencephalogram (qEEG) studies have supported much of the imaging research, and have also identified subcortical structures involved in ADHD, including hippocampal involvement and thalamocortico circuits (Chabot et al., 1999). The latter circuits are in-

volved with cognitive control, and thus are important in understanding the neurobiology of ADHD (Luu & Tucker, 2003).

Correlating clinical conditions with cognitive deficits of attention has been a long-standing area of difficulty for researchers. Imaging studies of brain anomalies in ADHD have shed considerable light on the biological bases of ADHD. To be sure, functional differences between ADHD groups and control subjects have been demonstrated, both with functional and structural magnetic resonance imaging (MRI). The link between response inhibition and frontal lobe functioning in children with ADHD has been well documented in many recent studies (for examples, see Casey et al., 1997, Castellanos et al., 2002; Durston et al., 2003; Rubia, Smith, Brammer, Toone, & Taylor, 2005; Rubia et al., 2001, Schulz et al., 2004; Vaidya et al., 1998; Vaidya et al., 2005). For instance, differential activation of regions such as right frontal lobe and caudate nucleus has been documented (Rubia et al., 2001; Vaidya et al., 2005). Rubia et al., combined specific motor timing and inhibition tasks with fMRI, comparing ADHD and psychiatric control children. They noted that: "(t)he impairments in hyperactive children were thus specific to the more demanding inhibition tasks requiring inhibition of discrete motor responses and were not due to generalized impairments in the interruption of automatic activities nor motor timing" (p. 141).

Although the bulk of focus in the attention literature has been on the frontostriatal circuits, other brain structures have been identified as important in the process of attention. Mirsky, Anthony, Duncan, Ahearn, & Kellam. (1991) identified brainstem regions (i.e., the mesopontine brainstem reticular formation), as well as other subcortical midline brain regions (i.e., midline thalamus, and reticular nuclei of the thalamus) as critical for sustaining attentional focus. Mirsky asserted that "all patients whose symptoms include disturbances in vigilance or sustained attention, no matter what the diagnosis, share some pathological involvement or disturbance in this corticoreticular system. This would include persons with the diagnosis of ADHD" (Mirsky, Pascualvaca, Duncan, & French, 1999, p. 171). The brainstem region of the locus coeruleus is known to be the origin of serotonergic neurons, which are closely linked to dopaminergic neurons. Arnsten et al. (1996) argued that diminished brainstem norepinepherine activity and release caused a partial denervation of postsynaptic alpha-2 receptors in the prefrontal cortex, which in turn disrupts the inhibitory control functions of the PFC. This, then, produces the deficits in behavioral inhibition characteristic of children with ADHD. Thus, neurophysiologic mechanisms originating in the brainstem are also important contributors to the attentional process.

A genetic component to ADHD has long been noted. A recent review of genetic studies conducted between 1991 and 2004 found evidence of association between the presence of ADHD and four genes: the dopamine D4 and D5 receptors, and the dopamine and serotonin transporters (Bobb, Castellanos, Addington, & Rapoport, 2005). Thus, a genetic predisposition is well established as one factor in the etiology of ADHD. As the authors noted, studies continue to suffer from low power and modest odds ratios. More promising approaches have been the investigations of specific alleles and enzymes related to cognitive performance. Considerable work investigating

the genes expressed in the prefrontal cortex has been accomplished thanks to the fruits of the genome project and advances in molecular and computational technology. The COMT enzyme (catechol-O-methyltransferase) appears to regulate dopamine activity in the prefrontal cortex, and several studies have implicated the valine-methione (val158met) protein sequence SNP (single nucleotide polymorphism) in specific aspects of cognition, such as inhibitory control and working memory (for review, see Savitz, Solms, & Ramesar, 2006). Although these studies do not all address ADHD, the genetics of dopamine catabolism appears to have a role in the cognitive functions associated with this disorder.

There seems to be agreement that ADHD is characterized by slightly smaller brain volume, involving both gray and white matter (about 4% total brain volume reduction) (Durston, 2003). However, regional enlargements have also been identified. Both Swanson and colleagues (2004) and Durston and colleagues (2003) have identified occipital lobe size increases that are in conjunction with reduced frontal lobe sizes.

As noted, the striatum has been implicated in many studies. The striatum is a part of the basal ganglia, which is a group of neurons in the basal forebrain with rich connections to the premotor frontal areas. These neurons are involved with the modulation of movement, including the force of movement (Parent & Hazrati, 1995; Teicher et al., 2000). In addition, there appears to be a 15% decrease in the size of the posterior cerebellum (Castellanos et al., 2002). The cerebellum also is involved in motor movements; specifically, it appears to be involved in the acquisition and maintenance of motor skills. One function of the cerebellum appears to involve a timing mechanism. Another is for making adjustments to keep movements accurate. Error correction and feedback to the cortex are critical. These structural abnormalities in ADHD do not appear to progress with age. Thus, it is not a degenerating disorder, and some level of accommodative abilities can be obtained (Castellanos et al., 2002).

Sowell and colleagues (2003) observed significant differences in brain structure in the bilateral frontal cortices of brains of children with ADHD relative to normal children, with reduced regional brain size mainly confined to small areas of the dorsal prefrontal cortices. Reduced brain size in anterior temporal areas bilaterally was also noted in the children with ADHD. In addition, substantial increases were noted in the volume of gray matter in large areas of the posterior temporal and inferior parietal cortices of children with ADHD, compared with children in the control group. The increased presence of gray matter suggests a decrease in white matter, or connective tissue. There was a statistical trend toward total white matter reduction. These more specific findings indicated smaller and hypofunctional lateral prefrontal cortices in children with ADHD. The Sowell study (2003) found no differences between boys and girls, although other studies have shown such differences. Durston and colleagues found somewhat similar differences when comparing boys with ADHD and their unaffected siblings (2003).

Given the etiologic theories suggesting that ADHD involves a deficit in corticostriatal circuits, particularly circuits modulated by dopamine, Teicher and colleagues (2000) devised a series of functional magnetic resonance imaging (fMRI) experiments to test the hypothe-

sis that the activity of the putamen was related to ADHD symptoms. The putamen is rich in dopaminergic neurons. In their functional imaging studies of ADHD and normal boys, there was significant evidence for deficit in boys with ADHD. In addition, the physiologic findings were strongly correlated with the child's capacity to sit still and his accuracy in accomplishing a computerized attention task. They concluded that ADHD symptoms may be closely tied to functional abnormalities in the putamen, which is mainly involved in the regulation of motor behavior.

Willis and Weiler (2005) recently reviewed the literature on electroencephalography (EEG) and MRI findings in children with ADHD. They concluded that, collectively, studies support theories implicating frontal-striatal cortical networks. Unfortunately, they note, these physiologic procedures have not yet reached a point where diagnostic utility can be provided.

In summary, general consensus about the neurobiology of ADHD appears to include the following: (1) specific regions of the brain that are high in dopamine reception density are smaller in ADHD groups than control groups; (2) there appears to be a frontal-posterior dimension of difference, with ADHD groups having smaller frontal lobes and larger posterior structures (i.e., occipital lobes); and (3) areas that are necessary for the coordination and timing of activities from multiple brain regions have smaller subregions in ADHD groups (i.e., the corpus callosum, cerebellum) (Swanson et al., 2004). Pacing of electrical activity (especially theta) implicates hippocampal nuclei, whereas generation of alpha activity suggests thalamic nuclei involvement (Luu & Tucker, 2003). Although a genetic link to ADHD has been established (Bobb et al., 2005), the precise genetic mechanisms have not been worked out; clearly, dopamine receptors appear to play a role.

ADHD, Attention, and Executive Function (EF)

Attention

One of the difficulties in discussing ADHD has been the tendency to conflate the clinical manifestations of the *DSM-IV* diagnostic category of ADHD with the cognitive concepts of attention (Swanson et al., 2004). It seems logical that ADHD should be about attention. From a cognitive perspective, attention is a complex neurologic phenomenon involving multiple coordinated pathways and structures (e.g., Posner & Peterson, 1990; Posner & Rothbart, 1998). Posner describes orienting, alerting, focusing, and shifting as key components. Posner's studies have demonstrated cortical networks that underlie these functions, which include dorsal parietal, subcortical, and frontal networks.

The term executive function (EF) refers to a collection of interrelated functions that are responsible for purposeful activity that is goal-directed and typically involves some level of problem-solving. EF was originally defined by Luria (1973) as those functions that are involved in the planning, regulation, and verification of an action. Stuss and Benson (1986) described EF as a directive, control-type of mechanisms that included anticipation, goal selection, planning, monitoring, and use of feedback. Some of the cognitive abilities included in this domain are self-

regulation, set maintenance, response organization, and cognitive flexibility (Gioia, Isquith, Guy, & Kenworthy, 2001). However, this term is problematic: Pennington and Ozonoff (1966) stated that the term EF is "provisional and under-specified" (p. 55). Results of studies vary as to the specific measures used, and the operationalization of the term (see, for example, Fletcher, 1996). Nevertheless, the term EF enjoys widespread clinical use.

One difficulty in describing "attention" from a sensory perspective is the complexity of attentional processing. As described by Posner (Posner & Peterson, 1990; Posner & Rothbart, 1998), attention is a process and not a site-specific activity. The process of attention serves to connect the individual to the immediate world, with obvious survival (and likely evolutionary) value. The process includes some sort of monitoring or scanning of the environment (awareness), focusing on target stimuli, appropriately processing the information provided, disengaging or shifting to other relevant stimuli (but not irrelevant stimuli), all the while maintaining sufficient cortical arousal to process the information (Posner & Peterson, 1990; Posner & Rothbart, 1998). Much of this process has been well identified in the visual domain. It is noteworthy that only 2 of 32 chapters address audition or auditory processes in Posner's recent textbook *The Cognitive Neuroscience of Attention* (2004). However, in clinical studies, temporal lobe processing has been implicated in attentional processing and ADHD (Kelly, 2000; Mirsky et al.,1991; Mirsky et al., 1999; Posner & Peterson, 1990). An encoding function has been included in these models, based on performance on the auditory Digit Span task (Wechsler Intelligence Scale for Children, [Wechsler,

1991] and Wechsler Adult Intelligence Scales [Wechsler, 1981]).

Attention also is a complex process. (Posner refers to it as an "organ system:" 2004, p.3). Constructs such as "selective" attention and "divided" attention have been well-described in the experimental literature (see for example (Corbetta, Miezin, Dobmeyer, Shulman, & Petersen, 1991; Craik, Govoni, Naveh-Benjamin, & Anderson, 1996; Luck & Ford, 1998).

Tzourio et al. (1997) confirmed the activation of temporal lobes in a series of selective attention experiments using neuroimaging (positron emission tomography: PET) and event-related potentials (ERPs). Based on subjects listening to various tonal frequencies, they documented activation in Heschl's gyri and planum temporale cortical areas bilaterally when compared to a resting baseline, with a right asymmetry noted. When deviations in stimuli were presented, frontal activation was observed. They concluded that two major networks seemed to be involved during selective auditory attention: a local temporal lobe network and a frontal network that could mediate the temporal cortex modulation by attention.

Näätänen and colleagues have presented data to support the theory that there are two types of selective attention processes in audition (for review, see Näätänen & Ahlo, 2004). One aspect is associated with a course selection of sounds (e.g., right versus left) when stimulus rates are high and focused attention is strong; one process that is more similar to the processing of unattended sounds selects sounds at lower stimulus rates. Selected sounds are gradually matched to what is termed the "attentional trace." This trace is actively maintained in cortical representation. Mismatched sounds are rejected, whereas matched sounds generate enhanced cortical activity. This attentional trace is formed in the auditory cortex and is composed of actively rehearsed sensory-memory representations. Näätänen and Ahlo go on to argue that a later response identified in the frontal lobes is generated by the active rehearsal of the attentional trace after each occurrence of an attended sound (2004). Thus, the frontal lobes have an active role in maintaining selective auditory attention.

In studies of lesioned patients, Zatorre (Zatorre & Penhume, 2001) concluded that, contrary to hypotheses derived from animal studies, human auditory spatial processes are dependent primarily on cortical areas within the right superior temporal cortex. Later experiments on normal adults described activation of posterior temporal lobes and inferior parietal lobes in the auditory identification of spatial cues (Zatorre, Bouffard, Ahad, & Belin, 2002). Thus, the temporal lobe network seems critical for various attentional processes in the auditory modality.

The Neuropsychology of ADHD and Executive Functions

The neuropsychological study of ADHD has been based on the neurologic findings, and particularly the work of Posner (Posner & Peterson, 1990; Posner & Rothbart, 1998) and Mirsky and colleagues (1991, 1999). Barkley's description of the role of executive functioning as a hallmark of ADHD has further informed neuropsychology. Neuropsychological test findings support anatomic and behavioral conclusions, for both attentional and EF deficits, although the specification of diverse sensory processes is still quite crude (see Kelly, 2000, and Perugini, Harvey, Lovejoy, Sanstron, & Webb, 2000).

Although diagnostic requirements do not include neuropsychological testing, neuropsychological tests have shown considerable sensitivity to attentional and executive functioning (EF) processes (Kelly, 2000; Lovejoy et al., 1999; Muir-Broaddus, Rosenstein, Medina, & Soderberg, 2002; Perugini, Harvey, Lovejoy, Sanstron, & Webb, 2000).

Mirsky's group (1991, 1999) developed a general neuropsychological model for conceptualizing the components of attention. Neuropsychological test scores obtained from two samples, the first consisting of 203 adult neuropsychiatric patients and normal control subjects, and the second, an epidemiologically based sample of 435 elementary schoolchildren, were submitted to principal components analyses. Each sample yielded similar results with a set of independent elements of attention assayed by different tests. Based on their studies, they proposed a taxonomy of attentive functions that included functions labeled focus, execute, sustain, and stabilize, shift, and encode. This taxonomy was based, in part, on the results of a factor analysis of their neuropsychological test data. The tests selected were thought to be especially sensitive to the effects of poor attention. Relevant to our later discussion, the Mirsky group found that variability of reaction time (RT) for the auditory continuous performance test (CPT) (stabilize function) differentiated the ADHD sample from controls, whereas the Digit Span (encode function) did not differentiate groups.

Kelly (2000) submitted neuropsychological results to a factor analysis from a series of 100 children diagnosed with ADHD. He obtained results very similar

to Mirsky et al. (1991), with the exception of a factor reflecting impulsivity. Kelly labeled his factors information processing, impulsivity, sustaining, and shifting. Information processing reflected a speed of processing factor that used primarily visual tests, all with time elements. Impulsivity reflected errors made on some of the timed test; sustaining reflected visual vigilance over time, whereas shifting reflected cognitive flexibility.

Nigg, Blaskey, Huang-Pollack, and Rappley (2002) attempted to differentiate children with *DSM-IV* attention-deficit/hyperactivity disorder combined (ADHD-C) and inattentive (ADHD-I) subtypes. They administered a battery of neuropsychological tests of EF to 64 boys and girls with ADHD compared to 41 community controls. Both subtypes had deficits on output speed, with one motor response inhibition test differentiating ADHD-C boys from ADHD-I boys. In general, the ADHD-C group demonstrated a deficit in planning. Neither ADHD group had a deficit in interference control per se, although they were slower than controls on one speeded task. Nigg et al. (2002) concluded that children with ADHD-I shared neuropsychological deficits with children with ADHD-C in the domain of output speed; however, in most domains the subtypes did not differ.

Weyandt and Willis (1994) were able to classify 77% of a sample of 115 children using a battery of executive and nonexecutive function tests. Children were identified as either ADHD, developmental language disorder, or nondisabled. Children with ADHD demonstrated significant differences in executive functions relative to the normal controls, but nonexecutive tasks did not differentiate these groups. Only two executive tasks were more impaired in the ADHD group: a visual search and impulse control task, and a planning task. No difference between ADHD and language impaired were found on these tests. However, the ADHD group performed more poorly on a maze finding test.

Perugini et al. (2000) compared 21 boys with Hyperactive-Impulsive or Combined types of ADHD to 22 normal controls using a battery of neuropsychological tests (many the same as in the Mirsky and Kelly batteries). Only a visual CPT accurately differentiated the two groups, although a visual speeded sequencing test and the Digit Span test were also sensitive to ADHD. Sensitivity of the CPT was moderate (0.62) but strongly specific (0.91). These outcomes are somewhat different from other studies of CPTs in that sensitivity is usually higher.

Sergeant, Guertz, and Oosterlaan (2002) reviewed tests of EF across several psychiatric disorders including ADHD, oppositional defiant disorder, conduct disorder, higher functioning autism, and Tourette syndrome. They noted some specificity of tests for ADHD relative to the other disorders, particularly those requiring behavioral inhibition.

Although most neuropsychological studies of attention/ADHD in research and clinical practice involve visual CPTs, one exception was a study by Benedict et al. (1998). They were able to adapt a CPT for auditory assessment to be obtained concurrent with fMRI imaging. They also acquired positron emission tomography (PET) scans to corroborate activation patterns. Scans were acquired in normal young adults. They demonstrated that simple attention caused a large region of activation involving the anterior cingulate gyrus and the right anterior/mesial frontal lobe. There were few differences between focused and divided attention. The findings were felt to be consistent with activation of an anterior attention network during auditory attention, without involvement of posterior attention structures. Mirsky et al. (1999) also obtained evidence that the variability of response-time to an auditory CPT stimulus differentiated ADHD children from controls.

Barkley and others have noted that the cognitive correlates of ADHD are principally accounted for by deficits in EF (Anderson, 2002; see also Barkley, 1997). The anterior regions of the brain are thought to mediate executive functions. Deficits in EF often follow damage to prefrontal regions (e.g., Stuss & Benson, 1986). Imaging studies have supported these expectations, documenting prefrontal activation in this region while individuals perform EF tasks (e.g., Baker et al., 1996; Morris, Ahmed, Syed, & Toone, 1993).

Significant protective and proactive functionality is associated with well-functioning attentional networks. Barkley's influential summary and theoretical formulation of ADHD described a model that linked inhibition to executive neuropsychological functions (1997). The four functions identified were: (a) working memory, (b) self-regulation of affect-motivation-arousal, (c) internalization of speech, and (d) reconstitution (behavioral analysis and synthesis).

As discussed previously, response inhibition is seen as a functional hallmark of ADHD. From a neuropsychological perspective, significant findings of (response) inhibitory dyscontrol in children with ADHD-C were noted by Gioia using an executive function rating scale (Gioia et al., 2002). Muir-Broaddus et al. (2002) confirmed findings of EF difficulties on a sample of students with ADHD. Tests of attention span, sustained attention, response inhibition, and working memory were low relative to normative standards. These tests implicated fronto-executive functioning, as well as subcortical functioning relative to the free recall of verbal information. In addition, higher levels of inattention or hyperactivity as assessed from parent reports were associated with poorer performance on neuropsychological tests.

In summary, although there are difficulties in definitions of ADHD and in operationalizing the constructs of attention and executive functions, there is a large literature that converges implicating poor inhibitory control as a hallmark of ADHD. Inhibitory control is one function of the executive system that is needed for managing attention and sensory input.

The Relationship of ADHD to (C)APD: Empirical Findings

The question of (C)APD and ADHD comorbidity has received considerable attention (Chermak, Hall, & Musiek, 1999; Keller & Tillery, 2002; Moss & Sheiffele, 1994; Riccio et al., 1994). In these studies, ADHD was associated with more global disruption of sensory information processing, whereas (C)APD was only associated with disruption of auditory information processing. The differentiation has also been based on the observation that not all children with ADHD demonstrate auditory difficulties (Chermak et al., 1999).

Riccio, Cohen, Garrison, and Smith (2005) extended Riccio et al.'s earlier work (1994) to identify relationships between

audiometric tests and neuropsychological tests and rating scales for attentional processes. Thirty-six children underwent a neuropsychological test battery and then audiometric testing for (C)APD. Correlational analysis revealed only one significant correlation: between the right ear score of the Staggered Spondaic Word (SSW) test and a memory for sentences test (Clinical Evaluation of Language Fundamentals [3rd ed.] Sentence Repetition). They concluded that auditory measures tap some element of auditory memory, and that (C)APD and ADHD may be overlapping but independent disorders.

Tillery, Katz, and Keller (2000) attempted to assess the effects of stimulant medication on 32 children diagnosed with both (C)APD and ADHD. In a double-blind, placebo-controlled study, they found no effects of methylphenidate on audiometric test scores, although scores on an auditory CPT did improve.

The following sections describe results from our neuropsychological laboratory. We completed several studies using psychometric tests that are often used in the characterization of ADHD, but which show specificity for identification of (C)APD.

Auditory Short-Term Memory and Working Memory

Forward span capacity has a long history in psychology as a measure of auditory short-term, or immediate memory. Although there is much evidence demonstrating that forward and backward span performances and operations are correlated (Daneman & Merikle, 1996; Groeger, Field, & Hammond, 1999), the two span tasks are dissociable (Engle, Tuholski, Laughlin, & Conway, 1999). The forward span process is language related (Paulesu,

Frith, & Frackoviak, 1993) and has been described as the "phonological loop" or "articulatory loop" (Baddeley, 1992). This loop theoretically maintains information in short-term or immediate memory store. The digits reversed or backward procedure requires additional processing demands to manipulate the information, scaffolding onto the forward process (Torgesen, 1996). Rudel and Denckla (1974) hypothesized that the digits forward procedure makes greater demands on auditory processes than does the reverse procedure. It was postulated that the reverse procedure utilizes other processing, such as visualization of the numbers.

The need to assess span tasks as separate cognitive functions has long been suggested (Kaplan, Fein, Morris, & Delis, 1991; Rudel & Denckla, 1974). Farrand and Jones (1996) experimentally demonstrated the involvement of different processes in forward versus backward digit recall across several modalities, noting that recall for digits in reverse order was significantly worse than forward order in both spatial and verbal modalities. Groeger et al. (1999) examined processes underlying forward and reverse auditory, visual, and motor span tasks. They found that forward and reverse span performances were highly correlated regardless of presentation modality. Although forward span performance was related to reverse span performance, only reverse span performance was strongly related to other factors, such as general intellectual ability and EF. Hale, Hoeppner, and Fiorello (2002) found that reverse digit span was substantially more predictive of attention and EF than forward digit span, and Reynolds (1997) demonstrated that forward and backward digit span tasks load onto separate factors. In addition to psychometrically based support for separating forward from backward span tasks, functional imaging studies have demonstrated different areas of activation for these tasks, with dorsolateral prefrontal activation obtained during backward span tasks but not for forward span tasks, suggesting greater working memory demand in the former (Larrabee & Kane, 1986).

On the surface, there is considerable overlap in functional demand between one of the most robust tests of (C)APD (dichotic listening) and digit span tasks. Both are auditory tasks, frequently presenting numbers for stimuli, and relying on verbal confirmation of the stimuli. Some element of short-term memory is required for both. However, the dichotic listening task (Dichotic Digits test: Musiek, 1983), often used in audiologic evaluation for (C)APD, requires a maximum span of four numbers presented within 2 seconds. Digit span tasks used in psychometric assessment typically increase the span length with each successful trial. Thus, although similar, there are significant differences in processing demands between the two. Reverse digit span tasks likely place the greatest demand on function, requiring mental manipulation in working memory along with increasing reliance on span and on verbal responses.

Series 1: Initial Findings

In the first series of studies, archival data of children diagnosed with (C)APD were analyzed to demonstrate the relationship of Wechsler Intelligence Scale for Children, third edition (WISC-III) Digit Span (Wechlser et al., 2004) to (C)APD ($n = 74$; Maerlender et al., 2004). Mean Digit Span

(DS) scores for children diagnosed with (C)APD were compared with DS scores for children evaluated but who did not meet criteria for diagnosis of (C)APD. Analysis of variance revealed a significant difference between groups on DS scores, $F(1, 72) = 7.34, p = .008; \eta^2 = 0.092$. Children diagnosed with (C)APD had lower DS scores ($M = 7.81, SD = 2.86$) than children who did not meet diagnostic criteria ($M = 9.65, SD = 2.67$. Eighty-one percent (81%) of children with Digit Span scores below 7 (<16th percentile) had positive (C)APD diagnoses, whereas only 40% of those not identified as (C)APD had scaled scores below 7.

It appeared that poor performance on Digit Span was a robust characteristic of children diagnosed with (C)APD. Moreover, children with impaired performance on the Dichotic Digits test had lower scores on DS than children with normal DD performances, and DS scores were significantly worse for children with bilateral DD performance deficits than for those with only unilateral or no deficits.

A second study from that series analyzed DS and Dichotic Digits (DD) data from a cohort of children referred for neuropsychological evaluation ($n = 51$). In this study we did not have diagnostic results, so the independent factor was based on performance on the DD test (Pass Both ears, Fail Left ear; Fail Both ears). Z-scores for maximum forward digit span (DSFm) and maximum backward digit span (DSBm) were entered as dependent variables in a MANOVA with DD group as the between subjects factor. The multivariate test was significant, $F(2, 48) = 8.45, p = .001, \eta^2 = 0.27$. Examination of the univariate results revealed a significant difference between groups on both DSFm, $F(2, 48) = 6.78, p = .003, \eta^2 = 0.22$, and DSBm, $F(2, 48) = 3.63$,

$p = .043, \eta^2 = 0.12$. Planned contrasts revealed a different pattern of performance on DSFm and DSBm by DD performance. For DSFm, both the Fail Both and Fail Left groups had significantly lower scores than the Pass Both group ($p < .01$). Although the Fail Both group was somewhat lower than the Fail Left group, the difference was not significant. For DSBm scores, there was no difference between the Fail Left and Pass Both groups; however, the Fail Both group was significantly lower than the Pass Both group ($p = .023$). Thus, individuals with left ear deficits on a dichotic listening task had lower forward span scores than normal controls, but not lower reverse span scores. Groups with bilateral impairments, however, showed deficits on both forward span and reverse span tasks (Maerlender et al., 2004).

Series 2: The Neuropsychology of (C)APD

The previous findings led us to study neuropsychological test results in children who had recently undergone (C)APD testing. In this second series of studies we hoped to determine the diagnostic utility of specific neuropsychological tests. These data are fully described in Maerlender (2006). Although the neuropsychological battery was composed of primarily auditory tests, two tests related specifically to ADHD also were included: one was a visual CPT (see Perugini et al., 2000 for diagnostic efficiency data), and the other was the Behavioral Rating Inventory of Executive Function (BRIEF: Gioia et al., 2001) rating scale, which has also been shown to have sensitivity to ADHD (Gioia, Isquith, Kenworthy, & Barton, 2002).

Thirty-six consecutive referrals for central auditory processing testing were followed with a battery of neuropsychological tests, although our laboratory received diagnostic information after the neuropsychological battery had been completed. Children who had undergone (C)APD evaluations and diagnosis by an expert in (C)APD (Frank Musiek, Ph.D.) were identified and contacted to participate in the neuropsychological test battery (human subjects approval was obtained). The neuropsychological battery included auditory and visual continuous performance tests (CPTs), as well as many tests thought to measure auditory processes (see Table 17–1). Diagnosis of (C)APD was based on standard clinical practice of two or more tests showing performance more than 2 standard deviations below normal.

Test scores were grouped by test and multivariate analyses of variance (MANOVA) were conducted for each test

Table 17–1. Cognitive Tests Administered

Tests/subtests
WISC-IV Subtests
Arithmetic
Digit Span Forward (DSF)
Digit Span Reverse (DSB)
Coding (CODE)
Letter Span (Rhyming: LSR; Nonrhyming: LSNR)
CELF-III Subtests
Recalling Sentences (CELFRS)
Listening to Paragraphs
Concepts and Directions (CELFCD)
Comprehensive Test of Phonologic Processing (CTOPP)
Rapid Naming (Digits: CTOPPRD; Letters CTOPPRL)
Phonologic Awareness (Nonword Blending, Nonword Segmenting)
Continuous Performance Test: Visual and Auditory
Lindamood Auditory Conceptualization Test (LAC) (part 1 only)
Woodcock Johnson III Tests of Cognitive Ability
Sound Blending
Auditory Attention
Incomplete Words
Auditory Perception
Behavioral Rating Inventory of Executive Function (BRIEF)

(i.e., Wechsler Intelligence Scale for Children, 4th ed., WISC-IV; Clinical Evaluation of Language Fundamentals, 3rd ed., CELF-III subtests; etc.) by diagnosis ([C]APD vs. no [C]APD). Five variables were significant ($p < .01$): Digit Span forward (DSF), Letter Span Non-Rhyming (LSNR), Comprehensive test of Phonologic processing Rapid Digit Naming (CTOPPRD), CELF-III Recalling Sentences (CELFRS), CELF-III Concepts and Directions (CELFCD). Of note, none of the visual or auditory CPT measures, nor the BRIEF scales were significantly different between groups. Three of the five variables demonstrating significance related to short-term memory span (DSF, LSNR, and CELFRS). It was less clear why Concepts and Directions and a rapid naming task would differentiate groups.

To better characterize the diagnostic potential of these subtests, the test scores were entered into several logistic regression analyses (by test grouping). Tests that significantly predicted diagnosis of (C)APD within each group were then entered together (forward conditional entry) to identify predictors of (C)APD. The results found Digit Span forward (DSF) to be the best predictor of (C)APD from the battery of tests, with all other tests dropping out of the regression. For this sample, DSF had a sensitivity of 85.7%, specificity of 71.4%, positive predictive power of 83%, and negative predictive power of 77%.

In support of the earlier study, DSF and Dichotic Digits showed significant relationships, primarily for left-ear scores. To look at the relative contribution of the most sensitive auditory variables relative to the most robust cognitive variable, DSF, Dichotic Digits—left ear, Frequency Pattern—right ear, and Low-Pass Filtered Speech—right ear scores from the (C)APD battery were entered into a logistic

regression to predict diagnosis. A forward conditional entry was chosen to allow the strongest variables to emerge. Only DSF predicted group membership ($\beta = -0.56499$, $p = .005$), indicating that, in this data set, DSF was a better single predictor of diagnostic group membership than the auditory variables.

Series 3: (C)APD and ADHD Findings

Although these studies provided strong support for the role of DSF in identification of (C)APD, it had not been possible to compare specific clinical groups such as ADHD. In an attempt to answer the specific question of relationships between (C)APD and ADHD, we were able to obtain and analyze data sets for the same span tasks from the (C)APD children above (Series 2) and the ADHD cases from the clinical standardization sample from the WISC-IV database. All children were aged 7 to 14. Cases with positive diagnoses for (C)APD from the studies in Series 2 ($n = 22$; 14 males and 8 females) were combined with the ADHD cases ($n = 40$; 27 males and 13 females: Wechsler et al., 2004). DSF, DSB, LSR, and LSNR were analyzed. Means and standard deviations of the variables appear in Table 17–2.

Between Group Differences

There was no difference between groups on Verbal IQ (F[1, 58] - 3.23, $p = .0770$, and there was no difference in the distribution of gender by diagnostic groups (*chi square* = 0.094, $p = .785$). Multivariate analysis of variance of the variables of interest by clinical group found significant differences among all the variables,

Table 17–2. Means and Standard Deviations (SD) for Span Variables by Diagnostic Group

	(C)APD	ADHD
DSF	6.10 (1.77)	10.48 (3.12)
DSB	7.65 (2.64)	11.00 (2.53)
LSNR	7.50 (2.19)	9.88 (2.86)
LSR	7.80 (2.67)	9.88 (3.14)

ADHD—Attention Deficit/Hyperactivity Disorder; (C)APD—(Central) Auditory Processing Disorder; DSB—Digit Span Backward; DSF—Digit Span Forward; LSNR—Letter Span Nonrhyming; LSR—Letter Span Rhyming.

Table 17–3. Logistic Regression Classification Rates of Diagnostic Group by DSF Score

	Predicted	
Observed	ADHD	(C)APD
ADHD	35	5
(C)APD	4	16

ADHD—Attention Deficit/Hyperactivity Disorder; (C)APD—(Central) Auditory Processing Disorder.

$F(1,58) = 10.362, p = .000$. Univariate results demonstrated significant differences for each, with DSF having the largest effect: DSF, $F(1,58) = 33.66$, $p = 0.000$, $\eta^2 = 0.37$; DSB,. $F(1,58) = 22.68$, $p = 0.000$, $\eta^2 = 0.28$; LSNR, $F(1,58) = 10.66$, $p = .002$, $\eta^2 = 0.16$; LSR, $F(1,58) = 6.41$, $p = .014$, $\eta^2 = 0.10$.

To determine which variable was best at predicting diagnostic membership, the four variables were entered into logistic regression with conditional entry. Of the four variables identified, only DSF functioned as a significant variable for identifying diagnostic groups ($\beta = -0.900$, $p = .000$). Diagnostic efficiency statistics were quite robust: sensitivity = 90%, specificity = 76%; positive predictive power (PPP) = 88%; and negative predictive power (NPP) = 80%. Classification rates are presented in Table 17–3.

Would specific scores on these measures help to differentiate between the two groups? In order to determine cutoff scores for DSF in identification of diagnoses of (C)APD and ADHD, a series of

Receiver Operator Characteristics (ROC) curves were fitted to the data for both DSF. Inspection of the test results identified optimal cutoff scores based on specificity and sensitivity. For differentiated (C)APD from ADHD, a DSF scaled score of 7 provided a sensitivity of 0.773 and specificity of 0.875; a scaled score of 8 provided sensitivity of 0.864 and specificity of 0.70. (See Chapter 6 for discussion of the importance of sensitivity and specificity for screening and diagnosis.)

Within Group Differences

The strength of DSF in identifying (C)APD in this study is consistent with the previous work. However, DSB has also shown some ability to differentiate groups. The relationship between these two variables is of interest. In all previous studies (including the normative studies of the WISC-IV), there is a strong correlation between DSF and DSB. In this clinical standardization sample, the correlation was $r = .622$ ($p = .000$). The question arises: is there a systematic difference in the relationship of DSF and DSR between these two clinical groups? To answer this, we computed paired samples t-tests to determine differences between DSF and DSB, as well as between LSNR and LSR for each of the groups. The difference between DSB and DSF was significantly different for the (C)APD group [t (21) = 2.61, p = .01], indicating that, on average (mean = 1.45, SD = 2.61), DSF is significantly lower than DSB in the (C)APD sample, but not in the ADHD sample. This difference suggests another possible marker for differentiating the groups.

Summary of Empiric Studies

In two previous series of studies, we demonstrated that DSF was a robust marker of (C)APD (Maerlender, 2006; Maerlender, Wallis & Isquith, 2004). In a third study reported here, the earlier findings are supported and extended to differentiating (C)APD and ADHD. This combined data set provided a unique opportunity to compare specific test results as they pertain to these diagnostic groups. Significant differences between the two groups for three of four auditory span tasks (i.e., DSF, DSB, LSNR) support the inference that (C)APD and ADHD are indeed independent entities. As predicted, DSF was a robust predictor of group membership between the two diagnostic groups. Furthermore, identification of cutoff scores should provide some guidance for helping to differentiate these two groups. There was also evidence that the absolute difference between DSF and DSB is unique to the (C)APD group. It appears that children with (C)APD demonstrate consistently weak auditory short-term memory span. The difference between short-term and working memory scores indicates that it is the short-term span that is most impaired.

Conclusions: Relevance to Clinical Practice

The identification of short-term memory impairments as a marker for (C)APD is important for clinical practice. Because accurate diagnoses of either ADHD or (C)APD cannot be made on one test alone, these findings help to generate hypotheses regarding diagnostic possibilities. It must be noted that at a functional level, an individual's short-term span limits their working memory span. Longer forward spans than backward spans are highly unusual (Wechsler et al., 2004). However, scaled scores are age adjusted and do not accurately reflect the maximum span for any one individual. Thus, a forward span-scaled score that is lower than a backward span-scaled score may also suggest central auditory difficulties.

The data presented here suggest that for children with suspected (C)APD, a Digit Span forward (DSF)-scaled score of less than 8 points may corroborate those suspicions. Furthermore, DSF scaled scores that are more than 2 scaled-score points lower than the Digit Span backward (DSB)-scaled score also raises suspicion of (C)APD. In practice, it is important to look for other markers of (C)APD versus ADHD. A developmental history that is positive for recurrent, chronic chronic otitis media, high-risk neurologic factors such as prematurity, asphyxia, hyperbilirubinemia, cortical lesion, or vascular changes in the brain can be risk factors (Jerger & Musiek, 2000). Specific functional symptoms can include poor attentiveness, particularly in complex listening environments, and/or difficulty discriminating and retaining auditory information. However, it is important to note that depressed DSF or even the DSF less than DSB, even though sensitive in these studies, is probably a nonspecific finding. Hence, the use of the efficient central auditory test battery remains the most efficient (sensitive/specific) approach to diagnosing (C)APD (ASHA, 2005; Jerger & Musiek, 2000).

These data also suggest that (C)APD is an independent entity relative to ADHD, supporting the earlier contention of Chermak et al. (1999) that (C)APD is likely a more specific disorder than ADHD in that it involves only one or primarily one sensory modality (ASHA, 2005). DSF has been linked to hypoperfusion of the auditory cortex. If, as we suspect, good DSF performance requires intact audiologic processes from the peripheral ear to the auditory cortex, it seems reasonable to suspect that DSF is in fact a global indicator of impairment somewhere along the aural pathway, if not the cortex itself. ADHD is known to involve higher level processing that implicates frontal lobes. As the "executive," the frontal lobes depend on accurate information from lower structures and processes. Impairments up to and including the auditory cortex would necessarily impinge on frontal functioning. Thus, executive difficulties (including working memory) are likely secondary effects of more basic sensory dysfunctions. The accurate identification of auditory processing difficulty, whether in the context of ADHD or not, leads to more informed remedial strategies.

Absent a complete central auditory evaluation, recommendations for treatment are based only on symptoms and, therefore, are of questionable value and of uncertain potential for effectiveness. As therapeutic strategies are developed and standardized, it will be interesting to see if short-term auditory span lengths can improve, over and above practice effects. Confirmation through neuroimaging also will be helpful for validating short-term memory as a final common pathway of central auditory impairments. (Rehabilitation approaches for individuals diagnosed with (C)APD are described in Volume II of this Handbook.)

Finally, it is important to reiterate that the clinical practice of reporting only Digit Span (total) scores is a problematic practice. Psychologists are well advised to include both forward and backward scores in their reporting, and to be familiar with the possible implications of low scores.

References

American Psychiatric Association. (2000). *Diagnostic and statistical manual of mental disorders* (4th ed., text revision) (DSM-IV-TR). Washington, DC: Author.

American Speech-Language-Hearing Association. (2005). *(Central) auditory processing disorders.* Available at http://www.asha.org/members/deskref-journals/deskref/default.

Anderson, P. (2002). Assessment and development of executive function (EF) during childhood. *Child Neuropsychology, 8,* 71–82.

Arnsten, A. F., Steere, J. C., & Hunt, R. D. (1996). The contribution of alpha 2-noradrenergic mechanisms of prefrontal cortical cognitive function: Potential significance for attention-deficit hyperactivity disorder. *Archives of General Psychiatry, 53,* 448–455.

Baddeley, A. D. (1992). Working memory. *Science, 255,* 556–559.

Baker, S. C., Rogers, R. D., Owen, A. M., Frith, C. D., Dolan, R. J., Frackowiak, R. S. J., & Robbins T. W. (1996). Neural systems engaged by planning: A PET study of the

Tower of London task. *Neuropsychologia, 34,* 531-526.

Barkley, R. A. (1997). Behavioral inhibition, sustained attention, and executive functions: Constructing a unifying theory of ADHD. *Psychological Bulletin, 121,* 65-94.

Benedict, R. H. B., Lockwood, A. H., Shucard, J., Shucard, D. W., Wack, D., & Murphy, B. W. (1998). Functional neuroimaging of attention in the auditory modality. *NeuroReport, 5,* 121-126.

Bobb, A. J., Castellanos, F. X., Addington, A. M., & Rapoport, J. L. (2005). Molecular genetic studies of ADHD: 1991 to 2004. *American Journal of Medical Genetics: Neuropsychiatic Genetics, 132,* 109-125.

Calderon-Gonzalez, R. (1993). Attention deficit disorders spectrum: Neurological and neuropsychological basis. *International Pediatrics, 8,* 189-198.

Casey, B. J., Castellanos, F. X., Giedd, J. N., Marsh, W. L., Hamburger, S. D., Schubert, A. B., Vauss, Y. C., Vaituzis, A. C., Dickstein, D. P., Sarfatti, S. E., & Rapoport, J. L. (1997). Implication of right frontostriatal circuitry in response inhibition and attention-deficit/hyperactivity disorder. *Journal of the American Academy of Child and Adolescent Psychiatry, 363,* 374-383.

Castellanos, F. X., Lee, P. P., Sharp, W., Jeffries, N. O., Greenstein, D. K., Classsen, L. V., Blumenthal, J. D., James, R.S., Ebbens, C. L., Walter, J. M., Zijdenbos, A., Evans, A. C., Geidd, J. N., & Rapoport, J. L. (2002). Developmental trajectories of brain volume abnormalities in children and adolescents with Attention Deficit/Hyperactivity Disorder. *Journal of the American Medical Association, 288,* 1740-1748.

Chabot, R. J., Orgill, A. A., Crawford, G., Harris, M. J., & Serfontein, G. (1999). Behavioral and electrophysiological predictors of treatment response to stimulants in children with attention disorders. *Journal of Child Neurology, 14,* 343-351.

Chermak, G. D. (1996). Central auditory testing. In S. E. Gerber (Ed.), *Handbook of pediatric audiology.* Washington, DC: Gallaudet University Press.

Chermak, G. D., Hall, J. W. III, & Musiek, F. E. (1999). Differential diagnosis and management of central auditory processing disorder and attention deficit hyperactivity disorder. *Journal of the American Academy of Audiology, 10*(6), 289-303.

Chhabildas, N., Pennington, B., F., & Willcutt, E. (2001). A comparison of the neuropsychological profiles of the DSM-IV subtypes of ADHD. *Journal of Abnormal Child Psychology, 29*(6), 529-540.

Clarke, A. R., Barry, R. J., McCarthy, R., & Selikowitz, M. (2002). Children with attention-deficit/hyperactivity disorder and co-morbid oppositional defiant disorder: An EEG analysis. *Psychiatry Research, 111,* 181-190.

Corbetta, M., Miezin, F., Dobmeyer, S., Shulman, G., & Petersen, S. (1991). Selective and divided attention during visual discriminations of shape, color, and speed: Functional anatomy by positron emission tomography. *Journal of Neuroscience, 11*(8), 2383-2402.

Craik, F. I. M., Govoni, R., Naveh-Benjamin, M., & Anderson, N. D. (1996). The effects of divided attention on encoding and retrieval processes in human memory. *Journal of Experimental Psychology: General, 125,* 159-180.

Daneman, M., & Merikle, P. M. (1996). Working memory and language comprehension: A meta-analysis. *Psychonomic Bulletin and Review, 3,* 422-433.

Durston, S. (2003). A review of the biological bases of ADHD: What have we learned from imaging studies? *Mental Retardation and Developmental Disabilities Research Review, 9,* 184-195.

Durston, S., Tottenham, N. T. Thomas, K. M., Davidson, M. C., Eigsti, I. M., Yang, Y., Ulug, A. M., & Casey, B. J. (2003). Differential patterns of striatal activation in young children with and without ADHD. *Biological Psychiatry, 53,* 871-878.

Engle, R. W., Tuholski, S. W., Laughlin, J. E., & Conway, A. R. A. (1999). Working memory, short-term memory, and general fluid intelligence: A latent variable approach. *Journal of Experimental Psychology: General, 128*, 309-331.

Farrand, P., & Jones, D. (1996). Direction of report in spatial and verbal serial short-term memory. *Quarterly Journal of Experimental Psychology, 20*, 80-115.

Fletcher, J. M. (1996). Executive functions in children: Introduction to the special series. *Developmental Neuropsychology, 12*, 1-3.

Gioia, G., Isquith, P., Guy, S., & Kenworthy, L. (2001). *Behavior rating inventory of executive function (BRIEF) manual.* Odessa, FL: Psychological Assessment Resources, Inc.

Gioia, G. A., Isquith, P. K., Kenworthy, L., & Barton, R. M. (2002). Profiles of everyday executive function in acquired and developmental disorders. *Child Neuropsychology, 8*, 121-137.

Groeger, J. A., Field, D., & Hammond, S. M. (1999). Measuring memory span. *International Journal of Psychology, 34*, 359-363.

Hale, J. B., Hoeppner, J. B., & Fiorello, C. A. (2002). Analyzing digit span components for assessment of attention processes. *Journal of Psychoeducational Assessment, 20*, 128-143.

Hartman, C. A., Willcutt, E. G., Rhee, S. H., & Pennington, B. F. (2004). The relation between sluggish cognitive tempo and *DSM-IV* ADHD. *Journal of Abnormal Child Psychology, 32*(5), 491-503.

Himelstein, J., Newcorn, J. H., & Halperin, J. M. (2000). The neurobiology of attention-deficit hyperactivity disorder. *Frontiers in Bioscience, 53*, D461-D478.

Jerger, J., & Musiek, F. (2000). Report of the consensus conference on the diagnosis of auditory processing disorders in school-aged children. *Journal of the American Academy of Audiology, 11*, 467-474.

Kaplan, E., Fein, D., Morris, R., & Delis, D. (1991). *WAIS-R as a neuropsychological instrument.* San Antonio, TX: The Psychological Corporation.

Keller, W. D., & Tillery, K. L. (2002). Reliable differential diagnosis and effective management of auditory processing and attention deficit hyperactivity disorders. *Seminars in Hearing, 23*, 337-348.

Kelly, T. P. (2000). The clinical neuropsychology of attention in school-aged children. *Child Neuropsychology, 6*(1), 24-36.

Larrabee, G. J., & Kane, R. L. (1986). Reversed digit repetition involves visual and verbal processes. *International Journal of Neuroscience, 30*, 11-15.

Lovejoy, D. W., Ball, J. D., Keats, M., Stutts, M. L., Spain, E. H., Janda, L., & Janusz, J. (1999). Neuropsychological performance of adults with attention deficit hyperactivity disorder (ADHD): Diagnostic classification estimates for measures of frontal lobe/executive functioning. *Journal of the International Neuropsychological Society, 5*, 222-233.

Luck, S. J., & Ford, M. A. (1998). On the role of selective attention in visual perception. *Proceedings of the National Academy of Sciences, USA, 95*(3), 825-830.

Luria, A. R. (1973). *The working brain: An introduction to neuropsychology.* New York: Basic Books.

Luu, P., & Tucker, D. M. (2003). Self-regulation and the executive functions: Electrophysiological clues. In A. Zani & A. M. Proverbio (Eds.), *The cognitive electrophysiology of mind and brain* (pp. 199-223). San Diego, CA: Academic Press.

Maerlender, A. (2006). *Auditory short-term memory and CAPD: Neuropsychological findings.* Manuscript submitted for publication.

Maerlender, A., Isquith, P., & Wallis, D. (2004). Psychometric and behavioral measures of central auditory function: The relationship of dichotic listening and digit span tasks. *Child Neuropsychology, 10*, 318-327.

Mirsky, A. F., Anthony, B. J., Duncan, C. C., Ahearn, M. B., & Kellam, S. G. (1991). Analysis of the elements of attention: A neuropsychological approach. *Neuropsychology Review (Historical Archive), 2*(2), 109-145.

Mirsky, A. F., Pascualvaca, D. M., Duncan, C. C., & French, L. M. (1999). A model of attention and its relation to ADHD. *Mental*

Retardation and Developmental Disabilities Reviews, 5, 169-176.

Morris, R. G., Ahmed, S., Syed, G. M., & Toone, B. K. (1993). Neural correlates of planning ability: Frontal lobe activation during the Tower of London test. *Neuropsychologia*, *31*, 1367-1378.

Moss, W. L., & Sheiffele, W. A. (1994). Can we differentially diagnose an attention deficit disorder without hyperactivity from a central auditory processing problem? *Child Psychiatry and Human Development*, 25(2), 85-96.

Muir-Broaddus, J. E., Rosenstein, L. D., Medina, D. E., & Soderberg, C. (2002). Neuropsychological test performance of children with ADHD relative to test norms and parent behavioral ratings. *Archives of Clinical Neuropsychology*, 17(7), 671-689.

Musiek, F. E. (1983). Assessment of central auditory dysfunction: The dichotic digit test revisited. *Ear and Hearing*, *4*, 79-83.

Näätänen, R., & Alho, K. (2004). Mechanisms of attention in audition as revealed by event-related potentials of the brain. In M. I. Posner (Ed.), *Cognitive neuroscience of attention* (pp. 194-206). New York: Guilford Press.

Nigg, J. T. (2005). Neuropsychological theory and findings in Attention Deficit Hyperactivity Disorder: The state of the field and salient challenges for the coming decade. *Biological Psychiatry*, *57*, 1425-1435.

Nigg, J. T., Blaskey, L. G., Huang-Pollack, C. L., & Rappley, M. D. (2002). Neuropsychological executive functions and DSM-IV ADHD subtypes. *Journal of the American Academy of Child and Adolescent Psychiatry*, *41*, 59-66.

Parent, A., & Hazrati, L.-N. (1995). The functional anatomy of the basal ganglia. II. *Brain Research Review*, *20*, 128-154.

Paulesu, E., Frith, C. D., & Frackoviak, R. S. J. (1993). The neural correlates of the verbal component of working memory. *Nature*, *362*, 342-345.

Pennington, B. F., & Ozonoff, S. (1996). Executive functions and developmental psychopathology. *Journal of Child Psychology and Psychiatry*, *37*, 51-87.

Perugini, A. M., Harvey, E. A., Lovejoy, D. W., Sanstron, K., & Webb, A. H. (2000). The predictive power of combined neuropsychological measures of Attention Deficit/Hyperactivity Disorder in children. *Child Neuropsychology*, *6*, 101-114.

Posner, M. I. (Ed.). (2004). *Cognitive neuroscience of attention*. New York: Guilford.

Posner, M. I., & Petersen, S. E. (1990). The attention system of the human brain. *Annual Review of Neuroscience*, *13*(1), 25-42.

Posner, M. I., & Rothbart, M. K. (1998). Attention, self-regulation and consciousness. *Philosophical Transactions of the Royal Society of London Biological Sciences*, *353*, 1915-1927.

Reynolds, C. R. (1997). Forward and backward memory span should not be combined for clinical analysis. *Archives of Clinical Neuropsychology*, *12*(1), 29-40.

Riccio, C. A., Cohen, M. J., Garrison, T., & Smith, B. (2005). Auditory processing measures: Correlation with neuropsychological measures of attention, memory and behavior. *Child Neuropsychology*, *11*, 363-372.

Riccio, C. A., Hynd, G. W., Cohen, M. J., Hall, J., & Molt, L. (1994). Comorbidity of central auditory processing disorder and attention-deficit hyperactivity disorder. *Journal of the American Academy of Child and Adolescent Psychiatry*, *33*, 849-857.

Rubia, K., Smith, A. B., Brammer, M. J., Toone, B., & Taylor, E. (2005). Abnormal brain activation during inhibition and error detection in medication-naive adolescents with ADHD. *American Journal of Psychiatry*, *162*, 1067-1075.

Rubia, K., Taylor, E., Smith, A. B., Oksannen, H., Overmeyer, S., & Newman, S. (2001). Neuropsychological analyses of impulsiveness in childhood hyperactivity. *British Journal of Psychiatry*, *179*, 138-143.

Rudel, R. G., & Denckla, M. B. (1974). Relation of forward and backward digit span repetition to neurological impairment in children with learning disabilities. *Neuropsychologia*, *12*, 109–118.

Russell, V. A. (2002). Hypodopaminergic and hypernoradrenergic activity in prefrontal cortex slices of an animal model for attention-deficit hyperactivity disorder—the spontaneously hypertensive rat. *Behavior and Brain Research*, *130*, 191–196.

Savitz, J., Solms, M., & Ramesar, R. (2006). The molecular genetics of cognition: dopamine, COMT and BDNF. *Genes, Brain, and Behavior*, *5*(4), 311–328.

Scahill, L., & Schwab-Stone, M. (2000). Epidemiology of ADHD in school-aged children. *Child and Adolescent Psychiatric Clinics of North America*, *9*(3), 541–555.

Schulz, K. P., Fan, J., Tang, C. Y., Newcorn, J. H., Buchsbaum, M. S., Cheung, A. M., & Halperin, J. M. (2004). Response inhibition in adolescents diagnosed with Attention Deficit Hyperactivity Disorder during childhood: An event-related fMRI study. *American Journal of Psychiatry*, *161*, 1650–1657.

Sergeant, J. A., Guertz, H., & Oosterlaan, J. (2002). How specific is a deficit of executive functioning for attention-deficit/hyperactivity disorder? *Behavioral and Brain Research*, *130*, 3–28.

Sowell, E. R., Thompson, P. M., Welcome, S. E., Henkenius, A. L., Toga, A. W., & Peterson, B. S. (2003). Cortical abnormalities in children and adolescents with attention-deficit hyperactivity disorder. *The Lancet*, *363*, 1699–1707.

Stewart, G. A., Steffler, D. J., Lemoine, D. E., & Leps, J. D. (2001). Do quantitative EEG measures differentiate hyperactivity in attention-deficit/hyperactivity disorder? *Child Study Journal*, *31*, 103–121.

Stuss, D. T., & Benson, D. F. (1986). *The frontal lobes*. New York: Raven Press.

Swanson, J. M., Casey, J. B., Nigg, J., Catellanos, F. X., Volkow, N. D., & Taylor, E. (2004). Clinical and cognitive definitions of attention deficits in children with Attention Deficit/Hyperactivity Disorder. In M. I. Posner (Ed.), *Cognitive neuroscience of attention*. New York: Guilford.

Tannock, R. (1998). Attention deficit hyperactivity disorder: Advances in cognitive, neurobiological and genetic research. *Journal of Child Psychology and Psychiatry*, *39*, 65–99.

Teicher, M. H., Anderson, C. M., Polcari, A., Glod, C. A., Maas, L. C., & Renshaw, P. F. (2000). Functional deficits in basal ganglia of children with attention-deficit/hyperactivity disorder shown. *Nature Medicine*, *6*(4), 470–473.

Tillery, K. L., Katz, J., & Keller, W. D. (2000). Effects of methylphenidate (Ritalin) on auditory performance in children with attention and auditory processing disorders. *Journal of Speech, Language and Hearing Research*, *43*, 893–901.

Torgesen, J. K. (1996). A model of memory from an information processing perspective: The special case of phonological memory. In G. R. Lyon & N. A. Krasnegor (Eds.), *Attention, memory and executive function* (pp. 157–184). Baltimore: Brookes.

Tzourio, N., El Massioui, F., Crivello, F., Joliot, M., Renault, B., & Mazoyer, B. (1997). Functional anatomy of human auditory attention studied with PET. *NeuroImage*, *5*(1), 63–77.

Vaidya, C. J., Austin, G., Kirkorian, G., Ridlehuber, H. W., Desmond, J. E., Glover, G. H., & Gabrieli, J. D. (1998). Selective effects of methylphenidate in attention deficit hyperactivity disorder: A functional magnetic resonance study. *Proceedings of the National Academy of Sciences, USA*, *24*, 14494–14499.

Vaidya, C. J., Bunge, S. A., Dudukovic, N. M., Zalecki, C. A., Elliott, G. R., & Gabrieli, J. D. E. (2005). Altered neural substrates of cognitive control in childhood ADHD: Evidence from functional magnetic resonance imaging. *American Journal of Psychiatry*, *162*, 1605–1613.

Wechsler, D. (1981). *Wechsler Adult Intelligence Scale (revised) (WAIS-R) manual*. New York: The Psychological Corporation.

Wechsler, D. (1991). *Wechsler Intelligence Scale for Children manual* (3rd ed.). San Antonio, TX: The Psychological Corporation.

Wechsler, D., Kaplan, E., Fein, D., Kramer, J., Delis, D., Morris, R., & Maerlender, A. (2004). *Manual for the Wechsler Intelligence Scale for Children* (4th ed.) *Integrated (WISC-IV)*. San Antonio, TX: Psychological Corporation.

Weyandt, L. L. (2005). Executive function in children, adolescents, and adults with attention deficit hyperactivity disorder: Introduction to the special issue. *Developmental Neuropsychology*, *27*, 1-10.

Weyandt, L. L., & Willis, W. G. (1994). Executive functions in school-aged children: Potential efficacy of tasks in discriminating clinical groups. *Developmental Neuropsychology*, *10*, 27-38.

Willcutt, E. G., Doyle, A.E., Nigg, J. T., Faraone, S. V., & Pennington, B. F. (2005). Validity of the executive function theory of Attention Deficit/Hyperactivity Disorder: A meta-analytic review. *Biological Psychiatry*, *57*, 1336-1446.

Willis, W. G., & Weiler, M. D. (2005). Neural substrates of Attention Deficit Hyperactivity Disorder: Electroencephalagraphic and magnetic resonance imaging evidence. *Developmental Neuropsychology*, *27*, 135-182.

Zatorre, R. J., Bouffard, M., Ahad, P., & Belin, P. (2002). Where is "where" in human auditory cortex? *Nature Neuroscience*, *5*, 905-909.

Zatorre, R. J., & Penhume, V. B. (2001). Spatial localization after excision of human auditory cortex. *Journal of Neuroscience*, *21*, 6321-6328.

CHAPTER 18

ASSESSMENT OF INDIVIDUALS SUSPECTED OF OR DIAGNOSED WITH (CENTRAL) AUDITORY PROCESSING DISORDER: A MEDICAL PERSPECTIVE

REBEKAH CLEMEN and DOUGLAS D. BACKOUS

Introduction

(Central) auditory processing disorder ([C]APD) was first defined in 1996 by a task force from the American Speech-Language-Hearing Association (ASHA) and later refined to auditory processing disorder (APD) by the Bruton Conference in 2000. In 2005, an ASHA work group issued a technical report further refining the definition, nature, diagnosis, and treatment of the disorder and suggesting the disorder be labeled as (central) auditory processing disorder ([C]APD) reflecting the origins of the disorder in the central auditory nervous system (CANS). (C)APD represents a spectrum of disordered processing of auditory information despite normal auditory thresholds (Chermak, 2002).

The abnormality is characterized by one or more of the following: deficiency in sound localization and lateralization; auditory discrimination; auditory pattern recognition; temporal aspects of audition, including temporal integration, temporal discrimination (e.g., temporal gap detection), temporal ordering, and temporal masking; auditory performance in competing acoustic signals (including dichotic listening); and auditory performance with degraded acoustic signals (Demanez, Boniver, Dony-Closon, Lhonnex-Ledoux, & Demanez, 2003). Recent studies have shown a correlation between (C)APD and other disorders involving developmental language delay, attention deficit, and learning disabilities (Strauss, Delb & Plinkert, 2004). The prevalence of (C)APD is estimated between 2 and 3% in children (2:1 boys to girls) and 17

441

to 20% in adult populations (Demanez et al., 2003).

Patients with (C)APD often complain of difficulty understanding speech in the presence of background noise, which may result from a deficit in phonetic decoding, binaural separation, binaural integration, or monaural interaction disorder (Masquelier, 2003). The phonetic decoding process, also called auditory closure, involves the aptitude of a normal listener to utilize intrinsic or extrinsic redundancy to fill in missing and distorted portions of the auditory signal and thereby recognize the totality of the message. Binaural separation allows for the processing of an auditory message coming into one ear while ignoring a separate message being presented to the opposite ear at the same time. Binaural integration is the ability to process dissimilar information being presented to both ears simultaneously. Finally, monaural separation is the ability to listen to a target stimulus in the presence of a competing signal delivered to the same ear. Injury or maldevelopment in the central auditory pathway can disrupt the complex neural network necessary to perform fundamental listening tasks (Demanez et al., 2003).

The assessment of (C)APD requires a multidisciplinary approach including medical, audiologic, and often speech-language evaluations. The goal of the medical evaluation is to examine the auditory pathway with the intent to elucidate possible etiologies for (C)APD and to identify medically or surgically treatable conditions. This chapter focuses on the medical evaluation inclusive of patient history, physical examination, laboratory testing, and neuroimaging. A cursory sketch of the anatomy of the CANS precedes discussion of the four components of medical evaluation.

Anatomy

The CANS is an intricate arrangement of neural pathways (Figure 18–1). Sound pressure enters the external ear, passes through the tympanic membrane and ossicles, and undergoes transformation into a coded signal in the auditory nerve. After passing through the cochlear nucleus (dorsal or ventral), the signal ascends through the superior olivary nucleus, lateral lemniscus to the inferior colliculus, medial geniculate body, terminating in the auditory cortex in the transverse temporal gyrus. Some fibers ascend the brainstem ipsilaterally, but the majority cross the midline (i.e., decussate) and ascend along the contralateral pathway. Crossover from the ipsilateral to contralateral side occurs via three stria: at the cochlear nucleus, the commisure of Probst at the lateral lemniscus, and the commissure of the inferior colliculus. This provides the system with both ipsilateral and (a relatively stronger) contralateral pathways to the cortex, where signals again cross over via the corpus callosum. (Bamiou, Musiek, & Luxon, 2001).

Sensory information is processed in both a sequential and a parallel manner as it travels within the highly efficient CANS. Due to the extensive interaction of its structures, the CANS is characterized by an *intrinsic redundancy*, phenomenon responsible for the ability of the system to resist displaying deficits on standard auditory testing despite the presence of a lesion (Bamiou et al, 2001). Therefore, a diagnostic examination surveying both peripheral (auditory nerve, cochlea, middle ear, tympanic membrane, and ear canal) and central (brainstem to cortex) lesions is necessary. Damage to any part of the central pathway can result in (C)APD.

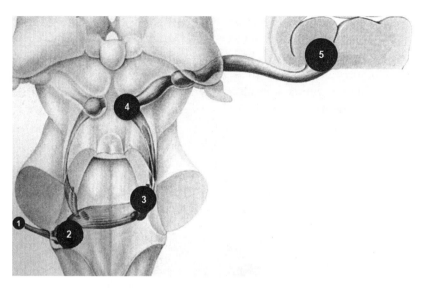

Figure 18–1. Schematic of the auditory pathway pertinent to physical examination: (1) peripheral auditory system (external and middle ear, cochlea, and auditory nerve); (2) ventral and dorsal cochlear nuclei; (3) superior olivary nucleus; (4) inferior colliculus; and (5) auditory cortex in the temporal lobe.

History

The onset of (C)APD can be observed at every stage of life. Perinatal risk factors include low birth weight, prematurity, hyperbilirubinemia, sepsis, ototoxic medications, and birth hypoxia. Postnatal viral infections (mumps, measles), meningitis, head injury, metabolic disorders, and the report of affected siblings may direct diagnostic testing. A family history of affected first- or second-degree relatives, consanguinity, or other indicators of genetic sources for developmental abnormalities should be elicited.

Children with (C)APD typically fail to develop speech appropriate to age or dialect. School-aged children are easily upset by noisy environments and find it difficult to follow conversations. Although performance and behavior improves in a quieter setting, children with (C)APD have difficulty following directions, regardless of the degree of difficulty. Reading, spelling, writing, and other speech-language difficulties are especially apparent in the classroom or other boisterous group environments. Abstract information, such as math verbal problems, are often challenging for the child to comprehend. Children with (C)APD can be disorganized and forgetful. A family history of learning disability or other relatives with (C)APD should be sought. Careful history should be gathered from parents, caregivers, teachers, therapists, and the child, when appropriate, to ensure the best information is factored into formulating an accurate diagnosis.

In noisy environments, 17 to 90% of adults can exhibit degraded speech recognition despite normal tonal audiometry (Demanez & Demanez, 2003). The most common complaint of patients with (C)APD is difficulty understanding speech in the presence of background noise. Many patients exhibit difficulty following long conversations, hearing dialogue while talking on the telephone, sounding out words, or following multistep directions. These individuals will often confuse similar-sounding words and need continual verbal clarification. Other problems include inability to process nonverbal information (e.g., lack of music appreciation), as well as poor organizational and memorization skills. It is particularly difficult for individuals to direct, sustain, or divide attention. Stroke, seizures, otologic disease, meningitis, drug and alcohol use, central demyelinating conditions, exposure to neurotoxic substances, and intracranial injury or pathology should be examined as potential explanations. Risk factors from the pediatric history should be examined as some patients may have struggled through the education process without having been diagnosed with (C)APD in childhood. Furthermore, changes in the ability to understand speech may identify a sentinel event leading to late onset (C)APD.

Dissatisfaction with hearing aids is a common phenomenon in adults and children. A history of multiple sets of hearing aids or the ability to hear sound but not understand speech clearly may indicate (C)APD. Diagnostic workup often emphasizes a search for peripheral hearing loss rather than the possible effects of (C)APD. A high index of suspicion is essential to include (C)APD in the differential diagnosis in affected patients. Findings and conditions that may be associated with (C)APD are presented in Table 18-1.

Dysfunction in the vestibular system, characterized by imbalance, vertigo, and disequilibrium in adults and delayed attainment of motor developmental milestones such as rolling over, crawling, and

Table 18-1. Differential Diagnosis for the Medical Evaluation of (C)APD

Attention deficit and hyperactivity disorder (ADHD)
Autism spectrum
Dyslexia
Learning disability (LD)
Nonspecific developmental delay
Elevated intracranial pressure
Normal pressure hydrocephalus
Dementia
Cerebrovascular accident (CVA or stroke)
Congenital malformation of the auditory pathway
Peripheral abnormalities (fluctuating hearing loss; otitis media)

walking in children may indicate brainstem or cortical deficits or malformations and guide the clinician to localizing a source for central auditory dysfunction. Diagnostic workup of vertigo is driven by the characterization of the symptoms outlined by the patient or description rendered from the parent.

Physical Examination

The physical examination begins with an overall assessment of the patient's condition, gait, and ability to understand questioning by the examiner. Symmetric eye color, the presence of a white forelock (Waardenburg syndrome), the presence of a goiter (Penderd's syndrome or other thyroid dysfunction), preauricular pits, skull shape, and skin pigmentary abnormalities (neurofibromatosis) should be noted. Deformities of the auricle or facial skeleton may indicate syndromic features.

Otoscopic examination evaluates the external ear canal, tympanic membrane, and portions of the middle ear. External auditory canal exostoses, cerumen impaction, tympanic membrane perforations, middle ear effusion, or middle ear masses may direct the clinician to explore more closely for peripheral pathology. Middle ear fluid and recurrent otitis media can cause hearing loss and subsequent speech delay in young children (Lehmann, Charron, Kummer, & Keith, 1979). Deprivation of sound to the CANS during critical periods of language development may lead to signs of (C)APD. Acute otitis media is treated with antibiotics. In cases where middle ear fluid persists for more than 3 months or there is detection of speech delay, tympanostomy tube placement is indicated.

Tympanic membrane perforations can occur in the inferior drum (pars tensa) or in the superior pars flaccida (Figure 18–2).

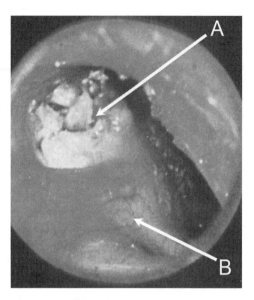

Figure 18–3. Otoscopic view of right tympanic membrane notable for a pars flaccida cholesteatoma extending through Prussak's space into the epitympanum: *(A)* cholesteatoma; *(B)* opaque tympanic membrane secondary to middle ear fluid.

The entire tympanic membrane should be visualized to rule out subtle findings of cholesteatoma in the difficult to view pars flaccida. (Figure 18–3) Traditional teaching holds that a normal light reflex (reflection of a cone of light from the umbo to the anterior-inferior tympanic membrane) indicates a normal ear. This is inaccurate, however, as a normal cone of light can be seen in cases of significant middle ear inflammation or effusion (Davies, 2004).

Cranial Nerve Examination

Cranial nerves II to XII should be evaluated to identify concomitant brainstem pathology (see Table 18-2). Assessment of the auditory portion of the VIIIth nerve is discussed in further detail in other chapters of this text and will not

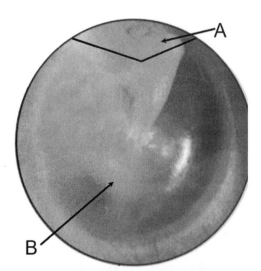

Figure 18–2. Otoscopic view of the normal (right) tympanic membrane: *(A)* pars flaccida; *(B)* pars tensa.

Table 18–2. Screening Cranial Nerve Exam

Cranial Nerve	Clinical Examination
I (olfactory)	testing sense of smell
II (optic)	vision screening
III (oculomotor)	ptosis, papillary light reflex, extraocular movements
IV (trochlear)	downward gaze with intorsion, abduction
V (trigeminal)	sensation of forehead, face, and upper neck, chewing and mastication
VI (abducens)	eye abduction
VII (facial)	motor movement of face, Schirmer test taste of anterior 2/3 tongue
VIII (vestibulocochlear)	see text
IX (glossopharyngeal)	gag reflex
X (vagus)	gag reflex, phonation
XI (spinal accessory)	neck muscle strength
XII (hypoglossal)	tongue movement

be covered here. Traditional "bedside" tests of finger rubbing, whispering, and talking to patients at varied volumes are ineffective as they are inaccurate and unreliable even in patients with severe losses. Hearing screening is done with tuning forks (256 Hz, 512 Hz, and 1028 Hz), but the definitive evaluation of hearing is done by the audiologist (i.e., audiometry, auditory brainstem response (ABR), otoacoustic emissions (OAE), etc.). The vestibular component of the VIIIth nerve is screened by observing the function of the vestibulo-ocular reflex (VOR), a three-neuron reflex arc designed to stabilize objects of visual interest on the fovea of the retina.

Bedside testing of the VOR includes observation of spontaneous nystagmus, head shake nystagmus, and corrective saccades on head impulse testing. Nystagmus is defined as to-and-fro, jerking, eye movements. The fast phase of nystagmus is a compensatory eye movement equal and opposite to the physiologic slow phase. The fast phase is typically described as it is easier to visualize. Nystagmus can occur in the horizontal, vertical, or torsional planes. Peripheral nystagmus typically is present without visual fixation and is suppressed with visual fixation. Suppression is obtained with the use of Fresnel glasses (20-diopter lenses with an internal light source) (Figure 18–4). Nystagmus is a nonlocalizing finding and can occur with central (brainstem and cortex) and peripheral (inner ear) lesions.

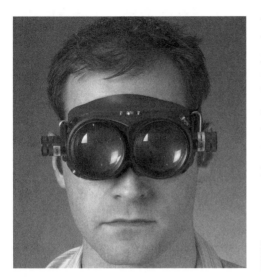

Figure 18–4. Fresnel glasses used to remove visual fixation for VOR testing. These 20-diopter lenses can also magnify fine nystagmus during clinical examination.

The majority of VOR testing examines the horizontal canal. Placing the head in a 30 degree, nose-down position places the horizontal semicircular canal in the optimum plane for stimulation. Completing 25 large amplitude head shakes with Fresnel glasses in place will induce a nystagmus in patients with vestibular dysfunction. This is due to an asymmetry in the storage mechanism in the brainstem for velocity information. This nystagmus is indicative of vestibular pathology, but cannot differentiate central versus peripheral etiologies. Notation of jerking eye movements of any kind should prompt otoneurologic evaluation.

The head impulse test can diagnose a peripheral deficit, even in patients who have compensated for their inner ear deficit. The examiner sits 24 to 36 inches away from the patient and has the patient fixate on part of the examiner's face (e.g., nose). The examiner then pro-

vides a low amplitude but brisk head thrust to the right and to the left. The patient's eye should stay fixed on the examiner's nose. If the eye moves with the head and then a quick corrective eye movement back to the target is identified, then a peripheral lesion is present. Head impulse testing is localized to a peripheral (inner ear) lesion and can be tested in children (Phillps & Backous, 2002).

Laboratory Testing

Hematologic testing should be utilized prudently in patients with (C)APD. The history and physical examination will determine which studies to complete. Global "testing batteries" should be discouraged. Screening studies like complete blood counts, thyroid function tests, erythrocyte sedimentation rate, Syphilis testing, Lyme titers, and tests for evidence of inflammation and autoimmunity may lead to referral to endocrinologists or rheumatologists for more specific testing and evaluation as needed.

Since the 1997 discovery that mutations on the gene coding for connexin 26 (Cx 26) are responsible for up to 50% of cases of autosomal recessive, nonsyndromic, sensorineural hearing loss, genetic testing and counseling have become integral parts of the evaluation of patients with hearing deficits (Kelsell et al., 1997). Cx 26 screening is now available in laboratories around the world. The number of tests available will likely increase as more genes related to hearing loss are discovered. Although the relationship between genetic forms of hearing loss and (C)APD has not yet been clearly established, genetic testing should be considered in patients with positive family histories of (C)APD, auditory deficits, or other neurologic abnormalities. Genetic counseling is essential for patients and for parents of children who screen positive for genetic sensorineural hearing loss. Types of assays and the major associated disorders for which they screen are listed in Table 18–3.

Electrocardiograms (EKG) can rule out long Q-T interval (Jervelle and Lange-Nielsen) syndrome. Ophthalmologic consultation may be necessary in cases of congenital hearing losses (Hone & Smith, 2002). Lumbar puncture with subsequent serologic testing of cerebrospinal fluid can yield diagnostic clues to causes of (C)APD, such as multiple sclerosis, neural syphilis, or elevated CSF pressure syndromes.

Electronystagmography (ENG) quantifies horizontal semicircular canal function.

The test battery varies between laboratories, but typically includes testing of gaze, saccades, and smooth pursuit, and positional testing and Dix-Hallpike testing. Calculation of unilateral weakness and directional preponderance from bithermal caloric testing remains the gold standard for laboratory verification of the side of a peripheral lesion. The rotational chair tests the horizontal VOR in a more physiologic range than the ENG and calorics. Velocity steps and sinusoids can uncover asymmetries in vestibular function. Although more sensitive to vestibular dysfunction, isolated chair testing rarely renders a differentiation between central versus peripheral lesions and does not define the side of loss in cases of inner ear dysfunction. Electronystagmography and rotational chair testing should be ordered in patients with a history of imbalance, ver-

Table 18–3. Screening Laboratory Testing in the Evaluation of (C)APD

Assay	Disorder
Complete blood count	Anemia, screen for white cell elevation
Blood smear	Thalassemia, Sickle cell disease
Platelets	Syndromic deafness (Fechtner and Epstein syndromes)
Electrolytes, urinalysis	Alport's syndrome
Thyroid functions (TSH, T4, T3)	Hypothyroidism
FTA-ABS, RPR	Syphilis
Lyme titers	Lyme disease
Rheumatoid factor (RF), Antineutrophil autoantibody (ANA), Erythrocyte sedimentation rate (ESR)	Autoimmune etiologies
68-kD protein analysis	Autoimmune inner ear disease
Connexin 26 (35delG) mutation	Genetic sensorineural hearing loss

tigo, or disequilibrium. Young children often have difficulty tolerating caloric testing, leaving rotational chair testing as the staple assessment tool (Phillips & Backous, 2002).

Radiographic Evaluation

Neuroimaging is the final component of the medical evaluation process. Computerized tomography (CT) scanning images bony structures, whereas magnetic resonance imaging (MRI) images soft tissues and fluids. The study chosen depends on the findings from the history and physical examination. CT scanning can identify fluid or soft tissue densities in the mastoids and middle ears in cases of chronic otitis media with or without cholesteatoma. The labyrinth, endolymphatic sac, cochlear aqueduct, and surrounding structures are visualized by bony detail. Congenital labyrinthine deformities, like Mondini malformations or

enlarged vestibular aqueduct syndrome, can lead to hearing loss and balance abnormalities (See Figure 18–5).

MRI remains the gold standard for assessing central or intracranial pathology. High-resolution T2-weighted images are now commonly used to screen patients for malformations, microvascular loops in the internal auditory canal, and for vestibular schwannomas which could cause hearing loss or abnormal central processing of auditory signals. Their advantage over standard brain MRI is a shorter study without contrast (gadolinium). The downfall of the T2 screening study is the limited amount of the brain imaged (Figure 18–6).

The standard, gadolinium-enhanced brain MRI gives full and multiplanar views of the brainstem, cortex, internal auditory canal, and neurovascular structures. Demyelination, strokes, tumors, acute and chronic changes from hydrocephalus, and developmental anomalies can be identified with this comprehensive imaging study (Figure 18–7).

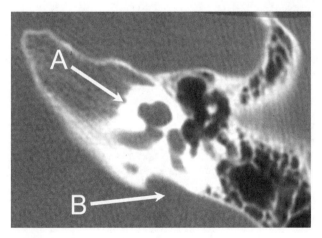

Figure 18–5. Axial CT scan of the left temporal bone: *(A)* cochlea with only 1.5 turns (Mondini malformation); *(B)* enlarged vestibular aqueduct.

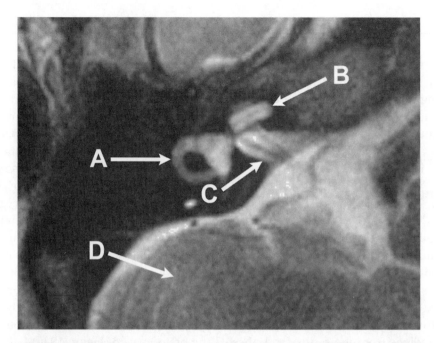

Figure 18–6. Axial cut of a T2-weighted, noncontrast, MRI scan of the temporal bone structures. Fluid enhances and bone are black. *(A)* Lateral semicircular canal of vestibular labyrinth; *(B)* cochlea; *(C)* internal auditory canal with the vestibular and cochlear nerves present; *(D)* cerebellum.

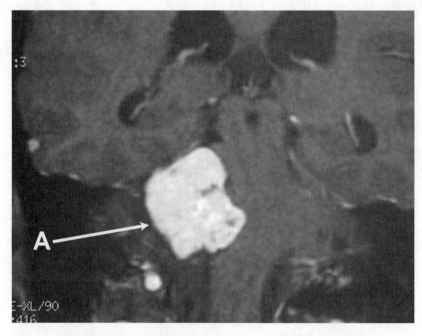

Figure 18–7. Coronal MRI of the brain, with gadolinium enhancement, visualizing the cerebellopontine angle: *(A)* a large enhancing mass in the right CPA, verified at surgery as an acoustic neuroma.

Conclusions

The evaluation of patients suspected of (C)APD requires a multidisciplinary team including audiologists, otolaryngologists (and often other medical specialists including pediatric neurologists), speech-language pathologists, primary care providers, and teachers, parents, and other family members. The medical evaluation begins once audiologic testing indicates the presence of (C)APD and aims at understanding possible causes of the altered processing of the auditory signal. This chapter reviewed the four primary components of the medical evaluation, including patient history, physical examination, laboratory testing, and neuroimaging. Based on an exhaustive medical evaluation, appropriate medical or surgical treatments may be employed to complement audiologic and speech-language intervention.

References

Bamiou, D., Musiek, F., & Luxon L. (2001). Aetiology and clinical presentations of auditory processing disorders: A review. *Archives of Disease in Childhood*, *85*, 361–365.

Bellis, T. J., Brannen, S. J., Chermak, G. D., Ferre, J. M., Musiek, F. E., & Rosenberg, G. G. (2005). *(Central) auditory processing disorders*. Technical report. http://www.asha.org/members/deskref-journals/deskref/default

Chermak, G. D. (2002). Deciphering auditory processing disorders in children. *Otolaryngologic Clinics of North America*, *35*, 733–749.

Davies, R. (2004). Bedside neuro-otological examination and interpretation of commonly used investigations. *Journal of Neurology Neurosurgery and Psychiatry*, *75*, 32–44.

Demanez, L., Boniver V., Dony-Closon B., Lhonnex-Ledoux, F., & Demanez, J. P. (2003). Central auditory processing disorders: Some cohorts studies. *Acta Oto-rhino-laryngologica Belgica*, *57*(4), 291–299.

Demanez, L., & Demanez, J. (2003). Central auditory processing assessment. *Acta Oto-rhino-laryngologica Belgica*, *57*(4), 243–252.

Hone, S. W., & Smith, R. J. H. (2002). Medical evaluation of pediatric hearing loss. Laboratory, radiographic, and genetic testing. *Otolaryngologic Clinics of North America*, *35*, 751–764.

Kelsell, D. P., Dunlop, J., Stevens, H. P. O., Lench, N. J., Liang, J. N., Parry, G., Mueller, R. F., & Leigh, I. M. (1997). Connexin 26 mutations in hereditary non-syndromic sensorineural hearing deafness. *Nature*, *387*, 80–87.

Lehmann, M., Charron K., Kummer A., & Keith, R. (1979). The effects of chronic middle ear effusion on speech and language development—a descriptive study. *International Journal of Pediatric Otorhinolaryngology*, *1*(2), 137–144.

Masquelier, M. (2003). Management of auditory processing disorders. *Acta Oto-rhino-laryngologica Belgica*, *57*(4), 301–310.

Munchnik, C., Ari-Even Roth D., Othman-Jebara R., Putter-Katz, H., Shabtai, E. L., & Hildesheimer, M. (2004). Reduced medial olivocochlear bundle systems function in children with auditory processing disorder. *Audiology and Neuro-Otology*, *9*(2), 107–114.

Phillips, J. O., & Backous, D. D. (2002) Evaluation of vestibular function in young children. *Otolaryngologic Clinics of North America*, *35*, 765–790.

Rosenfeld, R. M., Culpepper L., Doyle K. J., Grundfast, K. M., Hoberman, A., Kenna, M. A., Lieberthal, A. S., Mahoney, M., Wahl, R. A., Woods, C. R., Yawn, B; American Academy of Pediatrics Subcommittee on Otitis Media with Effusion; American Academy of Family Physicians; American Academy of Otolaryngology—Head and Neck Surgery. (2004). Clinical practice guideline: Otitis media with effusion. *Otolaryngology-Head and Neck Surgery*, *130*(5 Suppl.), S95–S118.

Strauss, D., Delb, W., & Plinkert P. (2004). Objective detection of the central auditory processing disorder: A new machine learning approach. *IEEE Transactions on Biomedical Engineering*, *51*(7), 1147–1155.

SECTION V

Future Directions

CHAPTER 19

FUTURE DIRECTIONS IN THE IDENTIFICATION AND DIAGNOSIS OF (CENTRAL) AUDITORY PROCESSING DISORDER

FRANK E. MUSIEK and GAIL D. CHERMAK

The future directions to be taken in the identification and diagnosis of (central) auditory processing disorder (C)APD are difficult to predict. Without a crystal ball, the projections offered in this chapter are somewhat speculative, although they are derived from our clinical experiences and they evolve logically from the tremendous research advances in auditory neuroscience and related areas.

Early Advances in Central Auditory Assessment

Perhaps one of the best ways to predict the future is to study the past. In this regard, (C)APD has a varied and interesting history. In introducing the concept of central auditory assessment, Bocca and his colleagues (Bocca et al., 1954) affirmed several pivotal principles which are likely to continue to guide central auditory testing in the future. One key principle guiding their work was their recognition of the limited value of pure tone sensitivity measures in detecting and revealing compromise of the central auditory nervous system (CANS). This principle led Bocca and his associates to develop auditory tests placing greater challenge on the CANS and therefore more sensitive than pure tone thresholds to central auditory dysfunction. To increase the challenge, they developed low-redundancy speech tests (e.g., filtered speech). Although we now know that the utility of filtered speech tests for CANS evaluation may be compromised by the effects of peripheral hearing loss, Bocca's understanding of the need to challenge the

CANS has been confirmed over the years. (See Tests Abandoned or of Limited Value below.).

Shortly after Bocca and colleagues began developing their test strategies, another breakthrough was achieved in 1961 when Doreen Kimura published her seminal article on dichotic listening. Based on a relatively large population of patients with temporal lobe damage, Kimura (1961) reported poorer performance for the ear contralateral to the involved cerebral hemisphere, findings that were consistent with Bocca's inferences regarding the structure of the CANS. Shortly after Kimura's dichotic studies, Katz and colleagues (1963) introduced the Staggered Spondaic Word (SSW) test, also grounded in the anatomy and physiology of the CANS, which became a widely used test of central auditory function. Using a dichotic listening paradigm, Milner (1968) demonstrated the role of the corpus callosum in dichotic listening, an important principle that later was well solidified in the areas of neuroscience and audiology (Musiek et al., 1984). At about the same time, Pinheiro and Ptacek (1971) introduced the original paradigm for testing pattern perception.

In the mid-1970s, Willeford (1977) observed that children with learning disabilities may be at risk for central auditory dysfunction, an association that has been documented over the years (ASHA, 2005). Also evolving in the 1970s was the auditory brainstem response (ABR), which would become a major clinical and research tool. Sensitive to dys-synchrony of the brainstem, the ABR continues in use today to assess the integrity of this more caudal portion of the CANS (Musiek et al., 1988). Throughout the 1980s and 1990s, the sensitivity of other auditory

evoked potentials to dysfunction of the CANS was demonstrated for purposes of research (e.g., mismatched negativity [MMN]) as well as research and clinical application (e.g., middle latency response [MLR], late-latency responses, N1, P2 response, and P300). (See Musiek & Lee, 1999 for a review.)

Progress Demands Communication and Change

For research to continue to advance, it is important to take a retrospective look to examine where the field has been in order to identify unanswered questions, as well as the advances that have occurred. Based on that retrospective, decisions can be reached as to what kind of research efforts should be emphasized in the future. Unfortunately, it seems clear that in the area of (C)APD, basic science has advanced at a much faster pace than clinical research and application. Advances in auditory neuroscience have been striking, whereas clinical application of these developments has lagged. Perhaps communication shortcomings between researchers and clinicians, as well as clinical resistance to change, have contributed to the slower pace in the clinical domain.

Developments in central auditory processing are at least partially dependent on clinicians' ability to embrace change. It seems clear that many basic and clinic science advances have never been translated into clinical use (e.g., click lateralization, tests of localization, cross-channel gap detection, backward masking, interaural timing procedures). This is a curious and unfortunate phenomenon, as it slows the pace of improvements in clinical services. However, the problem is not one-sided: researchers must consider the practical needs of clinicians. Diagnostic tests must be developed that are clinically feasible, that can be incorporated within the constraints and conditions of typical clinical settings, and thus can appeal to clinicians, not just to other researchers. Failure to consider these issues leads to delays or, worse yet, rejection of promising new clinical tools. Basic researchers and clinical scientists interested in advancing new clinical tests and procedures must develop paradigms that are not only sensitive and specific, but also easy to administer and score, time efficient, and use equipment that is commonly available in most audiology clinics. Moving a procedure from the laboratory to the clinic must proceed incrementally and with generous communication between the scientist and the clinician.

Although some procedures are quickly adapted for clinical use (e.g., dichotic listening), others require extended periods of time to integrate fully into the clinical test battery. In our own experience, we have noticed that the frequency pattern test is still viewed by some as a *new procedure* even though it has existed for over 25 years and has been used clinically for almost that long (Chermak, Traynham, Seikel, & Musiek, 1998). Researchers can hasten clinicians' adoption of new tools by developing them for clinical (as opposed to laboratory) application and then explaining their use in clinical terms and forums. Clinicians must be ready to critically evaluate new tools, and, if determined to be better than what currently is available, they must accept and embrace these new tools and secure the continuing education that might be necessary to fully implement the new procedure. Failure to incorporate efficient tools will not only slow down the pace of clinical improvements for our patients, but may also discourage creative and innovative approaches in the basic and clinical science arenas. Change can be unsettling; however, as clinicians committed to quality patient care, we must be willing to put away older and perhaps more comfortable approaches in favor of better approaches and tools.

Clinicians' Knowledge and Interpretation of Test Outcomes

Test interpretation is crucial to improved diagnostic capability. Clinicians must be well versed in the strengths and limitations of the tests in their battery and the bases (e.g., anatomy, physiology, and pathophysiology) of these strengths and limitations. Passing or failing a test(s) may not be the only factor guiding diagnosis. In fact, it is clinically feasible that two different clinicians with different depths of knowledge could render two different diagnoses for the same patient presenting the same test results. This would likely mean that a misdiagnosis would occur with significant consequences to the patient. Both the efficiency of the test and the knowledge brought to bear by the clinician *interpreting* the test are essential to accurate diagnosis. To advance our diagnostic precision, our knowledge of underlying mechanisms, both normal and pathologic, must be grounded firmly.

To improve (C)APD diagnostics, clinicians must be attuned to patients' complaints, and conceptualize those complaints within a broad context, which includes test results, symptoms, history, and family, workplace, and educational and recreational issues that may bear on the situation. The current central auditory test battery does not allow us to probe every type of auditory processing problem. Indeed, the number and types of auditory processes might actually exceed those currently identified (ASHA, 2005). Fortunately, patients' symptoms are invaluable indicators of processing deficits, particularly if the symptoms are interpreted correctly.

To optimally utilize information pertaining to the patient's symptomatology, the clinician must understand and apply knowledge of anatomy, physiology, and psychoacoustics. For example, for some patients with central auditory deficits secondary to a neurologic insult, the clinician might be able to *predict* the patient's performance on certain central auditory tests based on the patient's symptoms and an accompanying magnetic resonance image (MRI). We are not suggesting that one can or should diagnose (C)APD without confirming deficits using efficient central auditory tests; rather, we are emphasizing that by properly interpreting a thorough case history combined with careful testing using efficient tests and procedures we can obtain the maximum amount of information and insight to best serve the patient. To maximize the information gleaned from the history and best interpret test results, however, clinicians must be knowledgeable. Improving diagnosis of (C)APD is not just a matter of developing better tests; improving diagnostic capability also is dependent on more insightful interpretation of efficient tests.

Auditory Psychophysics and Confounds of Behavioral Tests

Test Development: Language and Other Confounds

Behavioral tests of central auditory function have both advantages and disadvantages. Behavioral tests allow the patient (in most instances) to relate what/how they hear, which can be very enlightening for the clinician. Also, behavioral tests often approximate real listening situations which enhance their relevancy. In addition, behavioral tests usually require less time to administer relative to electrophysiologic procedures and often are easier to score and interpret. However, because successful performance on behavioral tests, even those employing simple responses, requires the coordination of many systems (e.g., attention, memory, motor control, and sometimes language), there are liabilities associated with behavioral testing of central auditory function.

Interpreting performance on behavioral central auditory tests that use speech stimuli (i.e., language) can be difficult, especially with pediatric populations, nonnative speakers, and older adults following cerebral vascular accidents or affected by other conditions that compromise language and/or cognitive function. One must consider that performance on behavioral tests that employ speech stimuli might reflect language, memory, and attention factors as well as true auditory function. In children, this potential confound is underscored by the frequency with which children suspected of having (C)APD also have language processing problems (see Sloan, 1992). Most would agree that language difficulties can manifest as auditory processing deficits and that (C)APD can manifest as a language problem. These two entities also can coexist (ASHA, 2005; Sloan, 1992).

To avoid the potential confounding effects of language, audiologists should select behavioral central auditory tests that employ nonspeech stimuli (e.g., frequency and duration patterns, gap detection) or low-level language stimuli (e.g., dichotic digits). (Electrophysiologic procedures are also useful in this regard as long as they employ nonspeech stimuli.) Expanding the variety of tests and procedures in the central auditory battery that use nonspeech stimuli (and are not highly dependent on attention and memory) and are focused on specific auditory processes (e.g., lateralization, cross-channel gap detection) will provide the audiologist with additional options to examine multiple central auditory processes and augment our ability to differentially diagnose the range of comorbidly presented disorders (e.g., [C]APD, attention deficit-hyperactivity disorder, language impairment, etc.).

One such test that may soon emerge in the clinical arena involves interaural timing. In this procedure, clicks are presented to both ears with differing time delays and intensity levels resulting in defined changes in intracranial lateralization. Under experimental conditions this procedure has been shown to be highly sensitive to lesions of the CANS (Pratt et al., 1998). Moving this procedure from the lab to the clinic will require some procedural streamlining and attention to the issues discussed above.

Developing tests that use nonspeech stimuli and do not therefore require native language proficiency will serve the needs of the growing number of countries around the world that have begun establishing programs for evaluation and management of (C)APD. By developing tests that can be used universally, insightful comparisons can be made about potential cultural differences and their influences on auditory processing outcomes.

As noted above, in selecting and interpreting tests audiologists must take into consideration the potential confounding effects of systems other than audition. The interdependencies among these systems suggest, however, that multidisciplinary assessment is essential to fully evaluate and differentially diagnose a range of *look-alike* conditions. For example, recognizing the potential confound imposed by language, as well as the frequency with which (C)APD and language problems co-occur, it is essential that a full speech and language evaluation be completed on all children referred for (C)APD testing. Having this information in hand at the time of audiologic testing should assist the audiologist in the selection and interpretation of tests. If multidisciplinary evaluations are to provide useful information, the data provided by our colleagues in other disciplines must meet the same high standards of sensitivity and specificity as audiologists require of central auditory tests.

The Role of Tests Using Speech Stimuli in the Central Auditory Test Battery

Ironically, some of our most efficient tests of central auditory function involve speech stimuli (e.g., dichotic tests) and are, therefore, linked to language processes

(Musiek, 1983). Despite the potential for confounding effects, there is no question that tests using speech stimuli should remain in the central auditory test battery, given the primacy of speech as stimulus to the CANS and the likely coevolution of the speech and auditory systems.

When properly interpreted, certain performance patterns on tests using speech stimuli can help the audiologist differentiate auditory system versus other system deficits. For example, central auditory dysfunction is commonly manifested by depressed performance in only one ear or asymmetric performance across ears, with one ear's performance much poorer than the other. When this pattern of result is observed, it is highly likely that the source is an auditory problem, as speech, language, and memory deficits would not lateralize (see Chermak & Musiek, 1997 for review). More research is needed to explore lateralization in procedures using speech stimuli, such as dichotic listening. Moreover, speech-evoked auditory potentials (see Auditory Evoked Potentials below) may soon offer additional clinical applications for differential diagnosis.

Tests of the *Missing* Central Auditory Processes

Ironically, our current central auditory test battery does not contain a test of auditory discrimination nor of localization. Despite the fact that auditory discrimination is one of the most basic hearing functions, it is seldom clinically evaluated. So basic is auditory discrimination

to auditory processing, that frequency, intensity, and duration discrimination should be assessed as part of both the peripheral and the central auditory test batteries. No doubt, auditory discrimination problems are likely to be present in many children and adults with (C)APD; therefore, our failure to assess this fundamental auditory process limits our ability to gain a full understanding of the patient's difficulties.

There has been some groundwork accomplished on the development of a frequency discrimination procedure for clinical use—but with little uptake by the clinical community (Cranford, Stream & Rye, 1982). Cranford et al. (1982) demonstrated that frequency discrimination is severely degraded, especially when there are temporal restrictions, in patients with damage of the CANS. Developing a clinically useful measure of auditory discrimination is all the more important given the considerable evidence that auditory discrimination can be improved with training (Delhommeau et al., 2005).

The psychoacoustic tuning curve is another test procedure that involves frequency analysis and could be developed for clinical use in the future. This procedure, which has been commonly used in psychoacoustics research, provides an indication of the status of the frequency selectivity of the auditory system.

A clinically feasible test of sound localization also is needed and may emerge in the future. Sound localization as a central auditory test holds great promise, given that even informal tests of sound localization appear to be highly sensitive to dysfunction of the CANS (Sanchez-Longo & Forester, 1958). Because measures of sound localization are usually obtained in heavily sound-treated rooms or anechoic chambers, the clinical feasibility of localization in the clinical setting is questionable. On the horizon, however, are virtual reality techniques that can be applied to sound localization in the clinical setting (Besing & Koehnke, 1995).

Tests Abandoned or of Limited Value

Temporal processing is fundamental to audition and involves many subprocesses and abilities, only a few of which are tested clinically (e.g., temporal sequencing, temporal resolution or discrimination). Additional measures are needed to fully explore temporal processes, including temporal masking and temporal integration. In this context, it is interesting to note the fate of a test of temporal integration, around which there was a flurry of activity in the late 1970s. The test was called brief tone audiometry (Wright, 1978). This technique, though it seemed useful to many, did not survive as a clinical procedure, despite some compelling reports on its use with central auditory disorders (Baru & Karaseva, 1972). Given this history, a test of temporal integration may not re-emerge soon as a clinical audiologic test procedure.

Monaural low-redundancy speech tests (e.g., filtered speech, compressed speech, speech in noise) are among the oldest types of central auditory tests. Unfortunately, they have been shown to be highly confounded by hearing loss and language disorders. These confounds combined with their relatively mediocre sensitivity and specificity has led to a continued decline in their use, with continuing decline projected into the future.

Multimodality Testing

Recent interest in cross-modality testing to assist in the differential diagnosis of (C)APD has stimulated much debate. Proponents assert that (C)APD must be defined as an exclusively modality-specific perceptual disorder that can only truly exist if it can be demonstrated that the auditory system is the only modality involved (Cacace & McFarland, 2005). Others, including the authors of this chapter, define (C)APD as a *primarily* modality-specific perceptual dysfunction that cannot be attributed to peripheral hearing loss or higher order, global cognitive, attention, or related disorders (ASHA, 2005).

To fully examine these competing conceptualizations of (C)APD, other modalities must be assessed with the same rigor applied to the auditory modality to ascertain fully the status of these other modalities, as well as the status of supramodal systems (i.e., attention and memory) that influence processing across modalities (Musiek, Bellis, & Chermak, 2005). Limiting cross-modality measurement and comparisons at this time are a number of theoretical, procedural, and professional scope of practice issues. For example, the equivalence of multimodal tests that differ only in sensory stimulus has not yet been demonstrated. Moreover, if audiologists are not presently qualified to test other modalities and determine possible interactions with pansensory systems, broader based training for audiologists or increased dependence on other professionals to evaluate individuals suspected of (C)APD will be required. Additional issues may emerge with more research and clinical trials. Nonetheless, it is important to work toward this more comprehensive assessment as it would augment the specificity of the (C)APD diagnosis. (See Musiek et al., 2005 for elaboration of issues related to multimodal testing.).

Auditory Evoked Potentials

Topographic Mapping as a Clinical Instrument

As we move forward, it is likely that auditory evoked potentials (AEPs) will serve an increasingly larger role in the diagnosis of (C)APD. Testing with AEPs affords the clinician the advantage of little contamination from language, cognition, or other potential confounds. Also advantageous, AEPs permit testing of various levels of the CANS.

Although AEPs provide precise temporal information about CANS activity, topographic mapping provides spatial as well as temporal detail. Topographic mapping is the process of viewing evoked potential responses from multiple electrode arrays (often 64-128 electrodes) placed on the scalp. Not only can the generator sites across the scalp be analyzed, but also the time course of these potentials can be observed. Activity across the scalp is color coded, usually with lighter, brighter colors indicating high-amplitude response and darker colors conveying lower amplitudes.

Topographic mapping will continue to serve as a valuable research tool to explore the neurophysiology underlying (C)APD. The key question, however, is whether topographic mapping or some modification can become a *clinically* useful procedure for diagnosing (C)APD. Clin-

ical trials in regard to its diagnostic test efficiency must be conducted. If proven efficient for diagnosis of (C)APD, the procedure would need to be streamlined so that it could become a clinical tool. Technologically, topographic mapping could, in all likelihood, be streamlined to make it a clinically feasible procedure; however, the issue then becomes whether the cost of a topographic procedure could be tolerated by third-party or even private payers.

Middle and Late Auditory Evoked Potentials

The MLR and the late (N1, P2) AEPs have been used successfully in the evaluation of (C)APD (see Musiek & Lee, 1999 for review); however, these evoked potentials (EPs) can likely become more diagnostically powerful with certain alterations. For example, by recording the EPs in the presence of acoustic competition and/or using some form of abbreviated speech as stimulus rather than clicks and tonal stimuli—both of which would increase the practical relevance of these EPs— MLR and N1, P2 could provide valuable indices and insights regarding CANS function, particularly through comparisons with results obtained without competition and for nonspeech stimuli. In fact, recent investigations using short speech segments with an ABR paradigm have reported impressive findings in individuals with learning problems (Russo, Nicol, Zecker, Hayes, & Kraus, 2005) (see Chapter 4). Longer speech segments could be employed with the late EPs—for which there is a good experimental track record in identifying CANS dysfunction using standard click and tonal stimuli (see Musiek & Lee, 1999 for review).

Another EP that holds promise for the future is the Auditory Steady-State Response (ASSR). The ASSR is triggered by the depth of frequency, intensity, or both frequency and intensity modulation. Comparison of the ASSR with behaviorally obtained measures of modulation (e.g., frequency difference limen [DL] defined as the smallest modulation depth discerned by the listener) might offer a powerful pair of physiologic and psychoacoustic measures to diagnose frequency discrimination problems and central auditory dysfunction. Some preliminary research already has been conducted on this technique (John et. al., 2001). Also promising, ASSR threshold and behavioral threshold comparisons may help differentiate central versus peripheral involvement. In contrast to subjects with normal hearing or cochlear hearing loss where the ASSR-behavioral threshold correlation is good (Shinn, 2005), there is some evidence that subjects with CANS involvement demonstrate poor correlation between behavioral and ASSR thresholds.

P300 and Multimodality Testing

Given the issues raised above regarding behavioral measurement of multimodal performance, perhaps the most promising means to conduct multimodal measures would be via the P300. It is well known that P300s can be obtained using auditory, visual, and tactile stimulation (Regan, 1989). Therefore, with sufficient normative data, the auditory, visual, and tactile P300s could be compared to help determine the modality specificity of a processing deficit. Although cross-modality P300s have been examined (Regan, 1989), this technique has not received clinical application.

The Role of Imaging Techniques

Functional magnetic resonance imaging (fMRI) and positron emission tomography (PET) are the two main imaging techniques commonly used in auditory research. Both techniques reflect changes in metabolic activity for various regions of the brain, generally in response to some type of stimulation. In the future, both of these techniques will play an increasing role in (C)APD diagnosis and in communication disorders in general.

In regard to (C)APD, imaging will reveal the areas of the brain that are activated during a particular central auditory test procedure. In so doing, imaging will advance our understanding of the physiologic and anatomic correlates of test procedures and subject performance. Imaging may also allow monitoring recovery or treatment progress. Combining behavioral tests with functional imaging should allow us to determine the neurophysiologic basis for changes observed in patient performance. Correlating functional imaging results with behavioral test results may also provide a basis for differentiating auditory, language, and attention deficits. Cost and equipment issues are likely to determine whether imaging emerges as a clinical tool.

Education and Training

If the area of (C)APD is to advance, a major change must occur in the education and training of audiologists. The education and clinical training for most audiology students in the area of (C)APD and its neuroscience foundations have been inadequate. In one survey, 80% of the respondents reported not to have taken even one course as a graduate student that was dedicated to (C)APD (Chermak et al., 1998). In that same survey 20% of the respondents reported that they had never taken even one graduate course in the structure and function of the CANS. Although our recently completed follow-up survey revealed some change in graduate students' education over 30% of respondents had not completed a course devoted to the assessment of the CANS or diagnosis of (C)APD, despite the replacement of master's programs with the more extensive AuD degree program. Also troubling is the lack of diversity in the populations students evaluate for (C)APD. Commonly, student clinical experience with (C)APD is restricted to children with learning problems. Even within this limited population, experiences are meager, with the vast majority of students obtaining less than 5 clock hours in this category (Chermak et al., 1998), a finding replicated in our recent follow-up survey. Patients with neurologic involvement (e.g., strokes, closed head injuries, epilepsy, and mass lesions) are seldom seen and yet it is this population that perhaps allows us to learn the most about the nature of (C)APD. It is ironic that such serious training issues are prevalent in one of the most demanding areas within audiology. Recognizing that many AuD programs include specific courses in (C)APD and its underlying anatomy and physiology, we remain hopeful that readministration of the survey in 5 to 10 years will reveal the benefits of the transition of audiology to a doctoral level profession,

It is beyond the scope of this chapter to detail the courses and training experiences needed to properly prepare students to serve patients with (C)APD, although a recent technical report offers some guidance in this regard (ASHA,

2005). At a minimum, undergraduate students aspiring to the audiology profession should focus on biological and physical sciences, as well as courses in psychology focused on the physiologic, experimental, and perceptual foundations. At the graduate level, the neurosciences should be pursued along with focused courses on anatomy and physiology of the CANS. Psychoacoustics and pediatric audiology courses also are crucial, in addition to a heavy dose of courses devoted to (C)APD, including electrophysiology.

In addition to more extensive course work and clinical experiences, it is probably as important that faculty and clinical supervisors instill in their students an appreciation of the essential role of science in professional practice. As elaborated above, a strong relationship between the scientist and clinician needs to be nurtured.

A specialty certification in the area of (C)APD (as well as strong continuing education programs) may be needed to achieve the considerable enhancements and consistency in education and training that emphasize neuroscience and pathophysiology. A specialty certification could require certain types of clinical experiences and courses prior to delivering services in the area of (C)APD. Alternatively, or in conjunction with specialty certification, one could make opportunities available to clinicians to work alongside *master* clinicians who have proven knowledge and experience in (C)APD, either during or after university training.

Underserved Clinical Populations with (C)APD

One of the most exciting facets of future diagnostic work in the area of (C)APD is the potential for expansion of the clinical population base. Currently, children with learning problems comprise the largest component of audiologic referrals for central auditory testing. Although audiologists must continue to serve this clinical population, there are other clinical populations that currently are underserved to the detriment of both the patients and the clinician.

Head Trauma

Many patients with head injury have a compromised CANS and when tested demonstrate central auditory deficits (Musiek et al., 2004). Unfortunately, most often these patients receive no audiologic evaluation of any sort. This is especially unfortunate given the emerging evidence that auditory training techniques can help these patients (Musiek et al., 2004). From an audiologic viewpoint, this population is clearly underserved and efforts should be made to expand services to this population in the future.

Surgery of the CANS

In the field of otology it is commonplace to conduct pre- and postsurgical audiologic evaluations. For example, pre- and post-hearing testing allows one to measure the effect of myringotomy and tubes for otitis media. Strikingly, however, auditory testing seldom precedes neurosurgical procedures that remove portions or all of the temporal lobe, despite risk to the CANS imposed by these major surgical procedures. Inroads must be made here to better serve the audiologic needs of these patients.

Stuttering

Renewed interest in investigating the CANS of individuals who stutter may be on the horizon. Historically, some postulated that those who stutter might experience CANS dysfunction. Implicating the possible linkage of stuttering and the CANS have been reports of differences in dichotic listening and temporal processing between those who stutter and controls (Cimorell-Strong, Gilbert, & Frick, 1983; Meyers, Hughes, & Schoney, 1989; Sommers, Brady, & Moore, 1975). More recently, delayed auditory feedback as well as frequency transposition feedback techniques have demonstrated clear effects on stuttering severity (Stuart & Kalinowski, 2004). Although most current auditory-stuttering research is directed toward auditory evoked potentials, behavioral techniques likely will continue to reveal interesting central auditory relationships in those with fluency disorders. Future studies should employ extensive testing with efficient procedures, both behavioral and electrophysiologic. In addition, those who stutter and represent various age groups should be studied.

Auditory Hallucinations

Although the primary population experiencing auditory hallucinations are those with psychiatric disorders (schizophrenia) (Johns et al., 2002), audiologists' interest in auditory hallucinations has emerged recently, especially in Europe. Recent studies demonstrate that auditory hallucinations involve the CANS and can be precipitated by hearing loss (i.e., deprivation) and or damage to the CANS (Berrios, 1990). Functional imaging studies have shown activation of auditory areas of the cortex during auditory hallucinations (Shergill et al., 2004). This intriguing area may one day involve audiologists in the evaluation and treatment of central auditory dysfunction with a fascinating and complex population.

Screening and Early Identification

Better screening tools and earlier detection of (C)APD are essential to minimize the functional consequences of (C)APD. Certainly the earlier (C)APD can be identified, the earlier intervention can be started—a key to success. Given the variability of young, normal children's performance on the currently available behavioral measures of central auditory function, it is difficult to identify those young children in need of follow-up. Contributing to much of this variation is the long maturational course of the CANS (Thompson et al., 2003). Sensitive and specific screening procedures must be developed that can be readily administered and easily completed by young children. Developing such procedures is difficult while still maintaining the level of difficulty required to challenge the CANS. This indeed will be one of our great challenges, but one that must be met.

Several studies suggest that evoked potentials, perhaps paired with traditional behavioral paradigms assessing central auditory behaviors that have a short maturational course, may hold promise as a tool for early identification. For example, infrequent stimuli with silent gaps modulated P2 and generated MMN in normal 6-month-old infants (Trainor, Samuel, Desjardins, & Sonnadara, 2001). Also illustrating the potential to identify

CANS dysfunction in younger children, Trehub, Schneider, and Henderson (1995) reported that normal 6-month-old infants detected gaps down to 12 ms using visual reinforcement audiometry.

Summary and Conclusions

The future of (C)APD is one with many challenges, but also one with many opportunities. It is necessary that we continue to develop tests that are highly sensitive and specific to central auditory dysfunction. This may mean depending more on electrophysiologic procedures, as well as behavioral tests that are resistant to confounds such as language and attention. Our clinical doctoral (AuD) programs must better educate tomorrow's clinicians. Clinicians must embrace change and become better grounded in the neurosciences. Likewise, researchers hoping to advance clinical practices must understand clinical needs and constraints. Improvements in all of these areas will yield dividends for our patients as well as our discipline and profession. The challenges ahead will be exciting and advances will come. We must be steadfast, patient, and proceed with strong science and enthusiasm.

References

American Speech-Language-Hearing Association. (2005). *(Central) auditory processing disorders.* Available at http://www.asha.org/members/deskref-journals/deskref/default

Baru, A. V., & Karaseva, T. (1972). *The brain and hearing: Hearing disturbances asso-*

ciated with local brain lesions. New York: Consultants Bureau.

Berrios, G. E. (1990). Musical hallucinations: A historical and clinical study. *British Journal of Psychiatry, 156,* 188-194.

Bocca, E., Calearo, C., & Cassinari, V. (1954). A new method for testing hearing in temporal lobe tumors: Preliminary report. *Acta Otolaryngologica, 44*(3), 219-221.

Cacace, A., & McFarland, D. (2005). The importance of modality specificity in diagnosing central auditory processing disorder. *American Journal of Audiology, 14,* 112-123.

Chermak, G. D., & Musiek, F. E. (1997). *Central auditory processing disorders: New perspectives.* San Diego, CA: Singular Publishing Group.

Chermak, G. D., Traynham, W. A., Seikel, J. A., & Musiek, F. E. (1998) Professional education and assessment practices in central auditory processing. *Journal of the American Academy of Audiology, 9*(6), 452-465.

Cimorell-Strong, J., Gilbert, H., & Frick, J. (1983). Dichotic speech perception: A comparison between stuttering and nonstuttering people. *Journal of Fluency Disorders, 8,* 77-91.

Cranford, J., Stream, R., & Rye, C. (1982). Detection versus discrimination of brief duration tones: Findings in patients with temporal lobe damage. *Archives of Otolaryngology, 108,* 350-356.

Delhommeau, K., Micheyl, C., & Jouvent, R. (2005). Generalization of frequency discrimination learning across frequencies and ears: Implications for underlying neural mechanisms in humans. *Journal of the Association for Research in Otolaryngology, 6*(2), 171-179.

John, M., Dimitrijevic, A., van Roon, P., & Picton, T. (2001). Multiple auditory steady-state responses to AM and FM stimuli. *Audiology and Neuro-Otology, 6,* 12-27.

Johns, L. C., Hemsley, D., & Kuipers, E. (2002). A comparison of auditory hallucinations in a psychiatric and non-psychiatric group. *British Journal of Clinical Psychology, 41*(Pt. 1), 81-86.

Katz, J., Basil, R. A., & Smith, J. M. (1963). A staggered spondaic word test for detecting central auditory lesions. *Annals of Otolaryngology, 72,* 908-918.

Kimura, D. (1961). Some effects of temporal lobe damage on auditory perception. *Canadian Journal of Psychology, 15,* 157-165.

Meyers, S. C., Hughes, L. F., & Schoeny, Z. G. (1989). Temporal-phonemic processing skills in adult stutterers and nonstutterers. *Journal of Speech and Hearing Research, 32,* 274-280.

Milner, B., Taylor, S., & Sperry, R. (1968). Lateralized suppression of dichotically presented digits after commissural section in man. *Science, 161,* 184-185.

Musiek, F. E. (1983). The results of three dichotic speech tests on subjects with intracranial lesions. *Ear and Hearing, 4,* 318-323.

Musiek, F. E., Baran, J. A., & Shinn, J. (2004). Assessment and remediation of an auditory processing disorder associated with head trauma. *Journal of the American Academy of Audiology, 15*(2), 117-132.

Musiek, F., Bellis, T., & Chermak, G. (2005). Nonmodularity of the CANS: Implications for central auditory processing disorder. *American Journal of Audiology, 14,* 128-138.

Musiek, F. E., Gollegly, K. M., Kibbe, K. S., & Verkest, S. B. (1988). Current concepts on the use of ABR and auditory psychophysical tests in the evaluation of brainstem lesions. *American Journal of Otology, 9,* 25-33.

Musiek, F. E., Kibbe, K., & Baran, J. (1984). Neuroaudiological results from split-brain patients. *Seminars in Hearing, 5*(3), 219-229.

Musiek, F. E., & Lee, W. W. (1999). Auditory middle and late potentials. In F. E. Musiek & W. F. Rintelmann (Eds.), *Contemporary perspectives in hearing assessment* (pp. 243-271). Boston: Allyn & Bacon.

Pinheiro, M. L., & Ptacek, P. H. (1971). Reversals in the perception of noise and tone patterns. *Journal of the Acoustical Society of America, 49,* 1778-1783.

Pratt, H., Polyakov, A., Aharonson, V., Korczyn, A. D., Tadmor, R., Fullerton, B., Levine, R. A., & Furst, M. (1998). Effects of localized pontine lesions on auditory brain-stem evoked potentials and binaural processing in humans. *Electroencephalography and Clinical Neurophysiology, 108*, 511-520.

Regan, D. (1989). *Human brain electrophysiology*. New York: Elsevier.

Russo, N., Nicol, T., Zecker, S., Hayes, E., & Kraus, N. (2005). Auditory training improves neural timing in the human brainstem. *Behavioural Brain Research, 156*, 95-103.

Sanchez-Longo, L. P., & Forster, F. M. (1958). Clinical significance of impairment of sound localization. *Neurology, 8*, 119-125.

Shergill, S. S., Brammer, M. J., Amaro, E., Williams, S. C., Murray, R. M., & McGuire, P. K. (2004). Temporal course of auditory hallucinations. *British Journal of Psychiatry, 185*, 516-527.

Shinn, J. B. (2005). *The auditory steady state response in individuals with neurological insult of the central auditory nervous system*. Ph.D dissertation, University of Connecticut, Storrs.

Sloan, C. (1992). Language, language learning, and language disorder: Implications for central auditory processing. In J. Katz, N. Stecker, & D. Henderson (Eds.), *Central auditory processing: A transdisciplinary view* (pp.179-186). St. Louis, MO: Mosby Year Book.

Sommers, R. K., Brady, W. A., & Moore, W. H. (1975). Dichotic ear preferences of stuttering children and adults. *Perceptual and Motor Skills, 41*, 931-938.

Stuart, A., & Kalinowski, J. (2004). The perception of speech naturalness of post-therapeutic and altered auditory feedback speech of adults with mild and severe stuttering. *Folia Phoniatrica et Logopaedica, 56*(6), 347-357.

Thompson, P., Narr, K., Blanton, R., & Toga, A. (2003). Mapping structural alterations of the corpus callosum during brain development and degeneration. In E. Zaidel & M. Iacoboni (Eds.), *The parallel brain: The cognitive neuroscience of the corpus callosum* (pp. 93-130). Cambridge, MA: The MIT Press.

Trainor, L. J., Samuel, S. S., Desjardins, R. N., & Sonnadara, R. R. (2001). Measuring temporal resolution in infants using mismatch negativity. *NeuroReport, 12*(11), 2443-2448.

Trehub, S. E., Schneider, B. A., & Henderson, J. L. (1995). Gap detection in infants, children, and adults. *Journal of the Acoustical Society of America, 98*, 2532-2541.

Willeford, J. (1977). Assessing central auditory behavior in children: A test battery approach. In R. W. Keith (Ed.), *Central auditory dysfunction* (pp. 43-72). New York: Grune & Stratton.

Wright, H. N. (1978). Brief tone audiometry. In J. Katz (Ed.), *Handbook of clinical audiology* (1st ed., pp. 218-232). Baltimore: Williams & Wilkins.

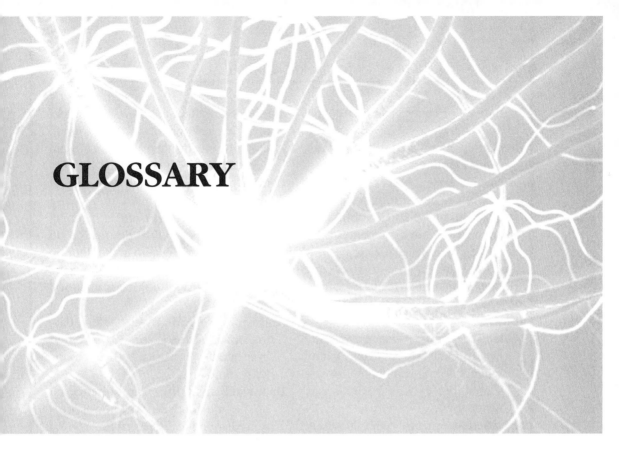

GLOSSARY

Absorption. Property of a material or an object whereby sound energy is converted into heat by propagation in a medium or when sound strikes the boundary between two media. It is determined for a specified frequency or for a stated frequency band.

Accommodation. Making facilities and programs accessible to and usable by persons with disabilities through appropriate modifications, including policy modifications, task restructuring, modified schedules, equipment acquisition or modification, training, or provision of qualified readers or interpreters, and other similar accommodations.

Acoustic access. Access through the auditory channel, either unaided or aided, to acoustic information.

Acoustic saliency. An acoustically salient phoneme (speech sound) or word is one that is obvious and prominent in an utterance. In a sentence context, acoustically nonsalient morphemes are shorter in duration and softer than louder phonemes in adjacent portions of the utterance.

Afferent. Used to refer to neurons carrying information to the brain, such as those in the ascending auditory pathways.

Amplitude modulation (AM). Variation in the envelope of a sound over time.

Analog. Refers to a signal that varies continuously over time.

Assessment. Formal and informal procedures to collect data and gather evidence; delineation of functional areas of strength or weakness and/or determination of ability or capacity in associated areas.

Assistive listening system. A device that delivers sound to individuals with peripheral or central auditory deficits to mitigate listening problems (e.g., frequency modulated [FM] systems, personal amplifiers, infrared systems).

Association area. Areas of the cerebral cortex not believed to receive direct sensory inputs or send outputs to motor neurons, but communicate with other cerebrocortical areas.

Attention. Gateway to conscious experience; maintains primacy of certain information in ongoing information processing.

> **Selective (focused) attention.** Ability to focus on relevant stimuli while ignoring simultaneously presented, but irrelevant stimuli (i.e., distractors).
>
> **Divided attention.** Ability to attend to multiple stimuli simultaneously.
>
> **Sustained attention (vigilance).** Ability to inhibit interference; requires sustained focus for a period of time while awaiting the occurrence of a target stimulus.

Attention deficit hyperactivity disorder (ADHD). Persistent pattern of inattention and/or hyperactivity-impulsivity that is more frequent and severe than is typically observed in individuals at a comparable level of development; manifested in at least two settings; interferes with developmentally appropriate social, academic, or occupational functions; and has been present before age 7 years.

> **Combined type.** Attention deficit characterized by hyperactivity-impulsivity and inattention.
>
> **Predominantly inattentive type.** Presents primary symptoms of inattention.
>
> **Predominantly hyperactive-impulsive type.** Behavioral regulation disorder.

Attenuation. Reduction in magnitude of a physical quantity such as sound, either by electronic means (e.g., by an attenuator), or by a physical barrier, including various absorptive materials. It is usually measured in decibels.

Auditory cortex. Area of the cerebral cortex that is the final destination of auditory inputs; located in the floor of the lateral sulcus in the superior temporal gyrus; *see also* Primary auditory area.

Auditory discrimination. Differentiating similar acoustic stimuli that differ in frequency, intensity, and/or temporal parameters.

Backward masking. The presence of one sound renders a previously presented sound less detectable.

Binaural interaction. Central auditory processing of intensity or time differences of acoustic stimuli presented diotically to the two ears.

Binaural masking level difference. A measure of the advantage in signal detection that can result from the use of binaural cues; the difference in signal threshold between a situation in which the masker and signal have the same interaural time difference and interaural level difference, and a situation in which the interaural time and/or level differences for the masker and the signal differ.

Bottom-up processing. Information processing that is data driven; properties of the data are primary determinants of higher level representations and constructions.

Brain imaging. Procedures used to map the structure and metabolic and electrophysiologic properties of the brain; includes computed tomography, magnetic resonance imaging, positron emission topography, regional cerebral blood flow, and brain electrical activity mapping.

Central auditory nervous system (CANS). The auditory brainstem, subcortical pathways, auditory cortex, and corpus callosum.

Central auditory processes. Auditory system mechanisms and processes that underlie the following abilities or skills: sound localization and lateralization; auditory discrimination; auditory pattern recognition; temporal aspects of audition including, temporal integration, temporal discrimination (e.g., temporal gap detection), temporal ordering, and temporal masking; auditory performance with competing acoustic signals (including dichotic listening); and auditory performance with degraded acoustic signals.

(Central) auditory processing disorder ([C]APD). Difficulties in the perceptual processing of auditory information in the central nervous system, that cannot be *attributed to* higher order language, cognitive, or related supramodal confounds, and manifest as poor performance in one or more of the central auditory processes, with associated changes in the neurobiologic activity underlying those processes that give rise to the auditory evoked potentials.

Characteristic frequency. The pure tone frequency to which a given place on the basilar membrane, or a given neuron in the auditory system, is most sensitive at low stimulation levels.

Clear speech. Speech produced by a speaker who has been instructed to speak as clearly as possible, as if trying to communicate in a noisy background.

Closure. The ability to subjectively complete and make whole an incomplete form. Listeners use language knowledge and inductive and deductive reasoning, as well as auditory and grammatic closure to derive the meaning of words and messages.

Auditory closure. The ability to recognize a whole word despite the absence of certain elements.

Grammatic closure. The ability to complete phrases or sentences despite missing words or morphemes (e.g., filling in the verb form *are* versus *is* to conjugate with the subject *they*).

Verbal auditory closure. The ability to use spoken contextual information to facilitate speech recognition.

Cognition. Activity of knowing, encompassing the acquisition, organization, and use of knowledge; automatic and unconscious processes that transform, reduce, elaborate, store, recover, and use sensory input; processes involved in knowing, including perceiving, recognizing, conceiving, judging, sensing, and reasoning; primary phase in the development of knowledge.

Cognitive style. An individual's approach to processing information, problem-solving, and cognitive tasks (e.g., bottom-up/top-down, impulsive/reflective, field dependent/field independent).

Commissure. A group of axons of neurons passing from one side of the brain, usually, to a similar structure on the opposite side of the brain.

Commissurotomy. The medical term for surgical sectioning of a brain commissure, usually the corpus callosum.

Comorbidity. Existence of two or more disorders, diseases, or pathologic processes in an individual that are not necessarily related.

Compensation. Rehabilitative approach directed toward reducing the negative impact of a disorder or disease not amenable to complete recovery through treatment.

Consonant-vowel (CV) Syllable. Nonsense syllable comprised of a consonant followed by a vowel (e.g., ba, da, ga).

Corpus callosum. Principal commissure of the cerebral hemispheres.

Critical distance. Distance from a sound source at which direct sound level and reverberant sound level are equal.

Damping. Dissipation of energy with time or distance; loss of energy in a system resulting from friction (internal or external) or other resistance.

Deductive inferencing. Reasoning from the general to the specific.

Depolarization. An increase in the electric potential of a hair cell or neuron from a negative resting potential.

Diagnosis. Identification and categorization of impairment/dysfunction; determination of presence and nature of a disorder.

Dichotic. Simultaneous presentation of two different acoustic events, one to each ear.

Difference limen (DL). Just noticeable difference or smallest detectable change in a stimulus, usually pertaining to frequency, intensity, or duration; the difference in a quantity that a listener can just detect at some criterion level of performance.

Differential diagnosis. Distinguishing between two or more conditions presenting with similar symptoms or attributes.

Diffraction. Bending of sound waves around obstacles whose dimensions are smaller than the wavelength of the sound; the spreading out of waves beyond openings that are smaller than the wavelength of the sound. Diffraction involves a change in direction of a wave as it passes through a small opening or around a barrier in its path.

Diffusion. Process of spreading or dispersing radiated energy so that it is less direct or coherent. In acoustics, diffusion is caused by sound waves reflected from an uneven surface.

Distortion. Undesired change of a waveform resulting in the presence of some frequency components in the output signal that are not present in the input signal.

Dynamic assessment. Approach to evaluation focused on the different ways by which an individual achieves a score rather than the score achieved; approach is characterized by guided learning to determine an individual's potential for change.

Effectiveness. Effects of treatment; how well a treatment works in real-world settings.

Effect size. Calculated measure used to determine the extent of practical significance for particular research results.

Efferent system. The portion of the auditory system, also called the descending system, that courses from the brain down to the cochlea following a similar pathway as the afferent system.

Efficacy. Effects of treatment; how well a treatment can work under ideal circumstances and adequate control; documenting treatment efficacy requires demonstrating that a particular treatment produces the desired outcomes or behavior change in an efficient manner (e.g., cost effective) as a result of the treatment.

Efficiency. A measure of a test's combined sensitivity and specificity; ability of a test to identify correctly those individuals who have the dysfunction and correctly identify those individuals who do not have the dysfunction.

Electroacoustic measures. Recordings of acoustic signals from within the ear canal that are generated spontaneously or in response to acoustic stimuli (e.g., otoacoustic emissions, acoustic reflexes).

Electrophysiologic measures. Recordings of electrical potentials that reflect synchronous activity generated by the central nervous system in response to a wide variety of acoustic events (e.g., auditory brainstem response, steady-state evoked potentials, auditory middle-latency response, frequency following response, cortical auditory event-related potentials [P1, N1, P2, P300]).

Endogenous. Refers to evoked potentials (e.g., P300) that are relatively invariant to changes in the eliciting physical stimulus, but are highly influenced by subject state and require an internal or mental activity (e.g., perceptual or cognitive process) to generate the potential.

Evaluation. Interpretation of assessment data, evidence, and related information.

Evidence-based practice. Explicit and judicious use of current best evidence in making decisions about the care of individual patients by integrating individual clinical expertise with the best available external clinical evidence from systematic research; a systematic method to evaluate and implement best practices for assessment and treatment in clinical fields.

Executive function. Component of metacognition; set of general control processes that coordinate knowledge (i.e., cognition) and metacognitive knowledge, transforming such knowledge into behavioral strategies, which ensure that an individual's behavior is adaptive, consistent with some goal, and beneficial to the individual; self-directed actions of an individual that are used to self-regulate so as to accomplish self-control, goal-directed behavior, and maximize future outcomes.

Exogenous. Refers to evoked potentials that are highly dependent on acoustic features of the stimulus.

Extra-axial. Lesions of the brainstem that do not arise from within the brainstem, but from near structures that encroach upon the brainstem.

Forward masking. The presence of one sound renders a subsequent sound less detectable.

Free field. A sound environment in which there are no significant effects on sound propagation from boundaries and the medium (air) is homogeneous and motionless; under free field conditions, the loss of energy with distance may be predicted by the inverse square law.

Gyrus (pl. gyri). Bulge on the surface of the cerebral cortex consisting of gray matter with an inner core of white matter.

Impedance. Quotient of a dynamic field quantity (e.g., sound pressure) by a kinematic field quantity (e.g., particle velocity), at a specified frequency; total opposition to energy flow expressed in ohms.

Individuals with Disabilities Education Act (IDEA). A federal education act that guarantees special education and related services to children with disabilities.

Induction learning. Discovery learning; a three-step process through which a learner recognizes a pattern or relationship, explains the pattern or relationship, and hypothesizes the rule governing the pattern or relationship.

Inductive inferencing. Reasoning from the particular facts to a general conclusion.

Inferencing. Reaching a conclusion on the basis of facts or evidence.

Information processing. Assigning meaning to sensory input based on the extraction of cues or constraints through various processes or stages of cognition, including encoding, organizing, storing, retrieving, comparing, and generating or reconstructing information; these stages involve the interaction between sensory (e.g., auditory processes) and central processes (e.g., cognitive and linguistic processes) through feedback and feedforward loops.

Interaural timing. Refers to a behavioral task requiring the subject to determine the order of two acoustic events presented to each ear separately at slightly different times.

Intervention. Comprehensive, therapeutic treatment and management of a disorder.

Intra-axial. Refers to lesions of the brainstem that evolve from the brainstem tissue itself, as opposed to extra-axial lesions that arise from nonbrainstem tissue. Extra-axial lesions often are in contact with the brainstem.

Inverse square law. Principle whereby under free field conditions, sound intensity varies inversely with the square of the distance from the source; sound intensity I (in W/m^2) measured at distance r (in m) from the source producing the power P (in W) is described as $I = P/(4\pi r^2)$. Thus, if distance is doubled, sound intensity decreases by a factor of four. When expressed in decibels, level decreases by 6 dB for each doubling of the distance from the source to the point of measurement.

Isolation point. A real-time word recognition processing event, which occurs at the gate when the listener initially identifies the target word.

Latency. The time between occurrence of a physiologic event, usually a spike or evoked potential, and a stimulus.

Learning disabilities. A heterogeneous group of disorders, presumed to be due to central nervous system dysfunction, manifested by significant difficulties in the acquisition and use of listening, speaking, reading, writing, reasoning, or mathematical abilities.

Learning style. An individual's characteristic cognitive, affective, modality, and physiologic behaviors and preferences employed in perceiving, interacting with, and responding to the learning environment.

Lexical access. A spoken language processing event in which a percept comes in contact with various features of stored lexical representations.

Lexical activation. Some change in status of a subset of word candidates contained in the mental lexicon.

Linguistic-contextual information. Anything that influences the a priori probability of an upcoming utterance or the post hoc, retroactive recognition of an ongoing utterance.

Management. Procedures (e.g., compensatory strategies, environmental modifications) targeted toward reducing the effects of a disorder and minimizing the impact of the deficits that are resistant to remediation.

Masking. Process by which the threshold of one sound is raised by the presence of another (masking) sound; presence of one sound renders a subsequent sound less detectable.

Memory. Capacity to encode, process, and retrieve events, knowledge, feelings, and decisions of the past.

> **Short-term memory.** Brief storage of limited capacity with minimal processing requirements.

> **Working memory.** Temporary storage of information used during reasoning and planning; involves both storage and executive processing and manipulation of information.

> **Long-term memory.** Declarative or explicit memory and procedural or implicit memory; long-term storage of unlimited capacity; involves both storage and processing of information.

>> **Declarative or explicit memory.** Conscious awareness or recollection of previously acquired information, retrieved on demand.

>> **Procedural or implicit memory.** Use of previous experience or knowledge, in the absence of conscious awareness or recollection, to support learning and guide performance.

Mesencephalic. Referring to the midbrain, just rostral to the pons.

Meta-analysis. Synthesis of treatment efficacy literature (randomized controlled trials) on a given topic using mathematical procedures to integrate results from multiple studies.

Metacognition. Awareness and appropriate use of knowledge; awareness of the task and strategy variables that affect performance and the use of that knowledge to plan, monitor, and regulate performance, including attention, learning, and the use of language; second phase (following cognition) in the development of knowledge which is active and involves conscious control over knowledge.

Metalinguistics. Aspects of language competence that extend beyond unconscious usage for comprehension and production; involves ability to think about language in its abstract form—to reflect on aspects of language apart from its content, analyze it, and make judgments about it; metalinguistic knowledge underlies performance on a number of tasks, including phonologic awareness (e.g., segmentation, rhyming), organization and storage of words (e.g., multiple meaning words), and figurative language (e.g., metaphor, idiom, humor); may be considered a subset of metacognition as using language is one of the goals of metacognitive processes.

Metamemory. Knowledge and awareness of one's own memory systems and strategies.

Minimum audible angle. The smallest detectable angular separation between two sound sources relative to the head.

Mnemonics. Artificial or contrived memory aids for organizing information (e.g., acronyms, rhymes, verbal mediators, visual imagery, drawing).

Myogenic. A response that is generated by muscle contractions.

Neural synchrony. Pattern of neural activity in which large populations of neurons fire simultaneously; this type of neural activity generates the electric activity giving rise to auditory evoked potentials.

Neurobiology. Encompasses neuroanatomy, physiology, neurochemistry, and neuropharmacology.

Neuropharmacology. Effects of drugs on neuronal tissue.

Neurotransmitter. Chemical agent released by vesicles of a nerve cell that permits synaptic transmission between neurons, between sensory cells and neurons, and between neurons and muscle cells.

No Child Left Behind Act (NCLB). A federally mandated statute enacted in 2002 designed to improve student achievement in the public schools.

Otoacoustic emissions. Subaudible sounds generated by the cochlea either spontaneously or evoked by sound stimulation.

Pansensory. Referring to higher level mechanisms that are common to and that support processing across all modalities.

Perceptual training. Regimens in which basic perceptual attributes (e.g., sound frequency or duration) are trained through repeated exposure to a task (typically discrimination or identification).

Pharmacology. Sources, chemistry, actions, and uses of drugs.

Phase. Proportion of a period through which the waveform of a sound has advanced relative to a given time.

Phase-locking. Tendency of an auditory neuron to fire at a particular time (or phase) during each cycle of vibration on the basilar membrane.

Phonemic analysis. Separating words or syllables into a sequence of phonemes.

Phonemic synthesis. Blending of discrete phonemes into the correctly sequenced, coarticulated sound patterns.

Phonologic awareness. Explicit awareness of the sound structure of language, including the recognition that words are composed of syllables and phonemes.

Plasticity. Reorganization of the cortex by experience, often reflected in behavioral change (i.e., learning); alter-ation of neurons to conform better to immediate environmental influences, often associated with a change in behavior; changes in the properties of individual neurons or neuronal assemblies following specific use, pattern of stimulation, injury or during development; neural reorganization may be possible to some extent across the life span, as well as following injury (compensatory plasticity), and in response to learning.

Precedence effect. Refers to the dominance of information from the leading sound (as opposed to delayed or reflected versions of that sound) for the purpose of sound localization; the effect occurs for stimulus time delays varying from fractions of a millisecond to the upper limit for auditory fusion, after which separate sounds are perceived.

Prevalence. Total number of cases of a specific disease or disorder existing in a given population at a certain time.

Prevention. Procedures targeted toward reducing the likelihood that impairment will develop.

Primary auditory area (or cortex). The main auditory area of the brain, typically considered to be Heschl's gyrus.

Problem-solving. Generating a variety of potentially effective responses to a situation and recognizing and implementing the most effective response.

Prosody. Suprasegmental aspects of spoken language; the dynamic melody, timing, rhythm, and amplitude fluctuations of fluent speech.

Psychoacoustics. The study of the relation between sound (i.e., physical parameters) and perception (i.e., psychological correlates) using behavioral measurement techniques.

Real-time speech. The transitory, ephemeral nature of an ongoing speech signal; when speech is presented in a real-time manner, listeners must quickly recognize phonemes, syllables, and words based on preceding linguistic-contextual cues and ongoing acoustic-phonetic information.

Reasoning. Evaluation of arguments, drawing of inferences and conclusions, and generation and testing of hypotheses.

Reciprocal teaching. Alternating roles between the client and clinician, allowing the client to assume the role of teacher as well as learner.

Reflection. Acoustical phenomenon that occurs whenever sound strikes a surface; reflected sound is the portion of the sound energy striking the surface that bounces off the surface.

Reliability. The consistency, dependability, reproducibility, or stability of a measure.

Remediation (or treatment). Procedures targeted toward resolving an impairment.

Reverberation. Persistence or prolongation of sound in an enclosed space, resulting from multiple reflections of sound waves off hard surfaces after the source of the sound has ceased. Reverberation time (RT_{60}) refers to the time required for a steady-state sound to decay 60 dB from its initial peak amplitude offset.

Schema. Structured cluster of concepts and expectations; an abstract and generic knowledge structure stored in memory that preserves the relations among constituent concepts and generalized knowledge about a text, event, message, situation, or object.

Formal schema. Linguistic form that organizes, integrates, and predicts relationships across propositions (e.g., additives [*and, furthermore*], adversative [*although, nevertheless, however*], causal [*because, therefore, accordingly*], disjunctive [*but, instead, on the contrary*], and temporal connectives [*before, after, subsequently*], as well as patterns of parallelism and correlative pairs [*not only/but also*; *neither/nor*]).

Content or contextual schema. Provides a generalized interpretation of the content of experience; organizes facts and establishes a framework that imposes certain structures on events, precepts, situations, and objects and facilitates interpretation.

Screening. Procedures used to identify individuals who are *at risk* for an impairment.

Segmentation. Parsing spoken language into its constituent and successive segments; parsing sentences, words, or syllables into their constituent phonetic units; the manner in which listeners demarcate the ongoing spoken utterance into units of lexical access.

Self-regulation. Encompasses metacognitive knowledge and skills, as well as affective/emotional, motivational, and behavioral monitoring and self-control processes.

Semantic network. Construct representing a mental system of nodes and links connecting lexical units; vocabulary building in such a network involves adding new nodes and links, as well as changing activation values of the links between nodes (e.g., building synonymy by strengthening the relationships between nodes).

Sensitivity. The ability of a test to yield positive findings when the person tested truly has the dysfunction; ability of a test to identify correctly those individuals who have the dysfunction.

Signal-to-noise ratio. Relationship between the sound levels of the signal and the noise at the listener's ear, commonly reported as the difference in decibels between the intensity of the signal and the intensity of the background noise (e.g., if the speech signal is measured at 70 dB and the noise is 64 dB, the signal-to-noise ratio is +6 dB).

Sound field. The area and/or pattern of air pressure disturbance caused by the compression and rarefaction of energy in the audio frequency range.

Specificity. Ability of a test to identify correctly those individuals who do not have the dysfunction.

Spectrum level. Level of sound contained in a 1-Hz wide band; a measure of spectral density.

Speech intelligibility. Percentage of words, sentences or phonemes correctly received out of those transmitted; an important measure of the effectiveness or adequacy of a communication system or of the ability of people to communicate in noisy environments.

Spoken language processing. An interactive system of peripheral and central functions used to recognize and understand real-world transitory utterances as meaningful speech.

Standing wave. Phenomenon resulting from the interference of sound waves of the same frequency and kind traveling in opposite directions; characterized by the absence of propagation and the existence of nodes and antinodes that are fixed in space.

Sulcus. Infoldings on the cerebral surface separating gyri.

Synapse. Junction where information is transmitted between two neurons.

Synaptic transmission. Passage of an electrical impulse across a synapse through transduction to a chemical neurotransmitter presynaptically and transduction back to an electrical signal postsynaptically.

Systems theory. Study of systems as an entity rather than a conglomeration of parts; provides a conceptual framework for understanding the organization, interaction, and dynamic nature of elements comprising systems.

Temporal integration. Refers to the relationship between stimulus duration and intensity within a time frame of less than one-half second; integration of energy sampled within a time frame of approximately 200 milliseconds; sensitivity improves as signal duration increases up to approximately 200 to 300 milliseconds, after which thresholds remain essentially constant; also known as temporal summation.

Temporal masking. Masking that occurs when the signal and the masker do not overlap in time; also known as nonsimultaneous masking.

Temporal ordering. *See* Temporal sequencing.

Temporal processing. Auditory mechanisms and processes responsible for temporal patterning (e.g., phase locking, synchronization) of neural discharges and the following behavioral phenomena: temporal resolution (i.e., detection of changes in durations of auditory stimuli and time intervals between auditory stimuli over time), temporal ordering (i.e., detection of sequence of sounds over time), temporal integration (i.e., summation of power over durations less than 200 milliseconds), and temporal masking (i.e., obscuring of probe by pre- or post-stimulatory presentation of masker).

Temporal resolution. Refers to the shortest time period over which the ear can discriminate two signals; also known as temporal discrimination.

Temporal sequencing. The ability to discern the correct order of rapid acoustic events as they occur over time.

Temporal summation. *See* Temporal integration.

Tonotopic. Organization of auditory neurons in a particular structure according to their responsiveness to specific frequencies; a system of sound frequency representation in which the frequency determines the place (for example, in a neural array) of activation.

Top-down processing. Information processing that is knowledge or concept driven such that higher level constraints guide data processing, leading to data interpretation consistent with these constraints.

TORCH+S complex. A group of perinatal medical problems often linked to hearing loss. T = toxoplasmosis; O = other (e.g., associated ophthalmologic disease); R = rubella; C = cytomegalovirus; H = herpes; S = syphilis.

Total acceptance point. A late event in the real-time word recognition process when a listener recognizes the target word with a high level of confidence.

Treatment (remediation). Procedures targeted toward resolving an impairment.

Treatment outcomes. General term to denote change on measurements from pre- to postintervention.

Tuning curve. A graph depicting the response of a neuron, plotted as a function of stimulus intensity and frequency. The lowest sound level to which the neuron responds is represented by the tip of the tuning curve (i.e., characteristic frequency).

Validity. The degree to which a test measures what it is intended to measure.

Wernicke's area. The receptive auditory-language associational area of the cortex that may include part of the planum temporale and the posterosuperior temporal gyrus.

Word predictability. Amount of *fill-in-the blank* meaningfulness in a preceding spoken context. In predictability-high (PH) sentences, preceding semantic-contextual information is presented in the form of clue words; no such clue words are available in predictability-low (PL) sentences.

Word recognition. A spoken language processing event marking the conclusion of the word selection phase; also refers to a listener's ability to perceive and correctly identify a set of words usually presented at suprathreshold hearing level.

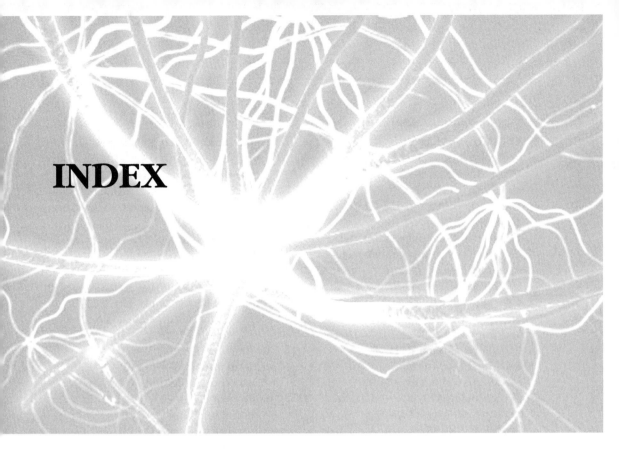

INDEX

W